SMART BUYS DRUG-WISE

Smart Buys Drug-Wise

**HOW TO SAVE A FORTUNE ON PRESCRIPTION
AND OVER-THE-COUNTER DRUGS**

▼

Lee Brian Haak, R.Ph., Rick Melcher, R.Ph.
Deborah S. Romaine

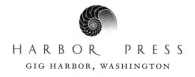

HARBOR PRESS
GIG HARBOR, WASHINGTON

LIBRARY OF CONGRESS CATALOGING-IN-PUBLICATION DATA

Haak, Lee Brian, 1966–
    Smart buys drug-wise : how to save a fortune on prescription and over-the-counter drugs/Lee Brian Haak, Rick Melcher, Deborah S. Romaine.
        p. cm.
    Includes index.
    ISBN 0-936197-46-3 (alk. paper)
    1. Drugs—Purchasing—Popular works. 2. Drugs, Nonprescription—Purchasing—Popular works. 3. Consumer education. I. Title: Smart buys drug wise. II. Melcher, Rick, 1950– III. Romaine, Deborah S., 1956– IV. Title.

RM301.15 .H315 2003
615'.1'029673—dc21   2002027263

IMPORTANT NOTICE

The authors of this book are not medical doctors, and nothing contained herein should be construed as medical advice, as a prescription, as a promise of benefits or of results to be achieved, or as a guarantee by the author or publisher of safety or efficacy. You should never attempt self-diagnosis or self-treatment of any kind without qualified medical supervision. Never take any drug that has not been prescribed for you by a medical doctor or an equally qualified physician. Despite the authors' and publisher's best efforts to make the contents of this book as accurate and error-free as possible, this book may contain unintentional errors, omissions, or misstatements of fact. Never implement any of the advice in this book without first consulting a medical doctor or an equally qualified physician. Nothing contained herein should be construed as advice to violate the laws or statutes of any municipality, state, province or nation. If you are not willing to be bound by these disclaimers, please return your copy of this book to the publisher for a full refund.

Printed in the United States of America
10 9 8 7 6 5 4 3 2 1

Harbor Press, Inc.
P.O. Box 1656
Gig Harbor, WA 98335

Visit us on the Internet at
www.smartbuysdrugwise.com
or www.harborhealth.com

Contents

Foreword   ix

Acknowledgments   xi

Introduction   xiii

PART 1   SAVE YOUR MONEY, SAVE YOUR HEALTH

Chapter 1   How Much Is Too Much?   3

Chapter 2   Protecting Yourself
from Common Prescription Mistakes   13

Chapter 3   Wired for Savings: Internet Pharmacies   27

Chapter 4   Savings on Drugs Across the Border   37

Chapter 5   When You Can't Afford to Buy
the Prescription Drugs You Need   51

PART 2   SAVING MONEY ON PRESCRIPTION DRUGS

Chapter 6   Rx SOS: Smart Options for Saving Money
on Prescription Drugs   67

Chapter 7   Prescription Drugs to Treat Infections   89

Chapter 8   Prescription Drugs to Treat Heart Conditions   119

Chapter 9   Prescription Hormones and Drugs
to Treat Hormone-Based Conditions   155

Chapter 10   Prescription Drugs to Treat Genitourinary Conditions   183

Chapter 11   Prescription Drugs to Treat Allergies, Asthma, and Coughs   193

Chapter 12 Prescription Drugs that Affect the Central
Nervous System   209

Chapter 13 Prescription Drugs to Treat Pain and Inflammation   239

Chapter 14 Prescription Drugs to Treat Gastrointestinal Conditions   257

Chapter 15 Prescription Drugs to Treat Conditions of the Eyes and Skin   269

PART 3   SAVING MONEY ON OVER-THE-COUNTER DRUGS

Chapter 16 SOS Over-the-Counter: Smart Options
for Saving Money on Over-the-Counter Drugs   297

Chapter 17 Over-the-Counter Cold, Flu, Cough,
and Allergy Preparations   315

Chapter 18 Over-the-Counter Pain Relief   341

Chapter 19 Over-the-Counter Gastrointestinal Remedies   359

Chapter 20 Over-the-Counter Treatments for Eyes,
Ears, Mouth, and Skin   383

Chapter 21 Other Over-the-Counter Products   421

Chapter 22 Over-the-Counter Drugs for Children   459

Index   489

In a country as great as ours, it is unacceptable that older Americans or families without insurance have to choose between food and medicine because drug prices are exorbitant—and they're rising. These spiraling prices are also forcing businesses to scale back their health plans or cut prescription drug coverage entirely because the premiums have become unaffordable—putting even more families at risk.

It's important to remember that the larger story of prescription drug prices is made up of millions of individual human stories – often stories of life and death. I've seen them. I remember taking a bus trip to Canada to compare drug prices with a group of seniors. One of the women on board—a breast cancer survivor named Barbara Morgan of Livonia, Michigan—was stunned to find that her vital anti-cancer drug Tamoxifen, which was priced at $136 a month in Michigan, was just $15 a month in Canada.

This is outrageous. The bulk of United States consumers do not have easy access to Canada. And for all those millions of people, drugs that are unaffordable are unavailable—and that is unacceptable.

With *Smart Buys Drug-Wise*, pharmacists Lee Haak and Rick Melcher, and medical writer Deborah S. Romaine have made an important contribution in the battle to rein in prescription drugs prices by writing a book that gives consumers detailed strategies they can use to lower their bills without sacrificing their health.

In Part 1 of the book, the authors detail how the prescription drug companies have over the past decade used their huge advertising budgets and other marketing ploys— like ski trips and expensive dinners for doctors and pharmacists—as a way of steering consumers to more expensive drugs when less expensive alternatives would be just as effective. The authors urge their readers to write their state and federal legislators and demand an end to these practices that drive up drug prices while doing nothing for a patient's health.

The voice of the consumer must be heard. As head of the U.S. Senate's Prescription Drug Task Force, I know that every time Congress has tried to stop these practices, armies of lobbyists—almost seven for every Senator—have been able to stall, dilute or kill legislation the prescription drug companies don't like.

For instance, toward the end of the 107th Congress in 2002, the Senate passed legislation that would allow pharmacists, wholesalers and consumers to import safe, FDA-approved drugs from Canada at substantial savings. The legislation also closed legal loopholes that name-brand drug companies use to keep lower-priced generic drugs off the market, and permitted states to extend Medicaid rebates and discounts to their residents who lack prescription drug coverage. But the legislation died in the House.

In Parts 2 and 3, the authors present meticulously detailed strategies that show consumers how they can lower their prescription—as well as over-the-counter—drug bills, and they discuss hundreds of specific drugs. Examples include shopping on the Internet, buying older, less expensive, but therapeutically equivalent drugs, and asking for generics instead of name-brand drugs. The book also provides detailed plans for dealing with specific conditions like asthma, diabetes, heart disease and allergies. There is even a chapter on ways that consumers can protect themselves from prescription mistakes, which can have deadly consequences.

Each chapter is accompanied by easy-to-understand charts and worksheets that will help consumers understand their options and communicate more effectively with their doctor or pharmacist.

I recommend this book to consumers as well as all my colleagues in the U.S. Senate and U.S. House of Representatives. And if you find this book helpful, I ask you to share your experiences by going to the Web site www.fairdrugprices.org and telling your story. This site is maintained by a broad coalition of public interest and consumer groups who, like the authors of *Smart Buys Drug-Wise*, believe it is critical to bring some sanity back to the prescription drug marketplace.

Informed consumers are crucial in the effort to lower prescription drugs prices, and the information contained in *Smart Buys Drug-Wise* can help us all get there.

U.S. Senator Debbie Stabenow
East Lansing, Michigan

Acknowledgments

We thank the many people whose efforts have taken this book from concept to publication. Our publisher, Harry Lynn, for his support, patience, and belief in our book's potential. Our editor, Debby Young, for her extraordinary vision and talent in shaping and developing our ideas into the form and structure that have become the book you hold in your hands. The dedicated staff at Harbor Press. Cheryl Haak for her amazing proofreading abilities that put spellcheck to shame. Dick Joss for his eye for detail. Pam Fator and Debbie Parries for covering Lee and Rick so they had time to work on this project. Louise Achey, Pharm.D., and Sota Omoigui, M.D., for their thorough technical review of the book.

We give special thanks to our families for putting up with late nights spent researching and writing: Lee his wife Beth, Rick his wife Karol, Debbie her husband Mike and children Chris and Cass. Finally, we acknowledge with deep appreciation the wonderful working relationship we have enjoyed as coauthors.

T wo hundred dollars. Five hundred dollars. A thousand dollars. Two thousand dollars—or more. How much do *you* spend on prescription and over-the-counter drugs *every month?* Millions of Americans fork out more at the pharmacy than they spend for any other living expense, including housing! And while you struggle to budget enough money to put food on the table, the big pharmaceutical companies are spending billions of dollars on efforts to get you to spend even more. Drug companies continue to roll in record profits, as they have for the past decade, earning billions of dollars and making their executives and stockholders wealthy, while you juggle your finances to buy the medications you need.

It doesn't have to be this way. We can show you how to save hundreds, even thousands, of dollars each year on the prescription and over-the-counter drugs you buy— legally, safely, and consistently. The recommendations in this book come from our many years of experience as pharmacists helping people like you. We know how this industry works from the inside out. And we want to share this inside knowledge with you so you can beat the high cost of keeping yourself healthy.

In this book, we show you:

how to counter the influence drug companies have over your doctor's drug choices to make sure you get the right medications *for you*, not just the ones that boost drug-company profits.

how to get your doctor to include cost as a factor in making prescribing decisions.

how to read between the lines of drug-company advertising that targets *you*.

how to use all the resources modern technology makes available, including the Internet, to save 50 percent or more on expensive drugs that treat a wide range of health conditions.

how to get the best prices from your local pharmacies.

how to keep up with changes in the pharmaceutical industry with "Smart Buy" recommendations on our Web site at www.smartbuysdrugwise.com for the latest information.

how to take charge of your health and control the cost of maintaining it!

To make this book easy to use, we provide simple tables listing hundreds of drugs and health conditions. And for every class of drugs we discuss, we offer a Smart Buy recommendation. As you leaf through *Smart Buys Drug-Wise,* look for the Smart Buy symbol **$**. This symbol highlights the drugs, stores, and Web sites we think offer the best value for your dollar.

This book is organized as a quick reference: You needn't read it from cover to cover to find the information you want. Refer to the table of contents or look up a health condition in the index to find what you're looking for quickly and easily.

This book's three parts make it easy for you to look up virtually any drug and any common health condition for which you must take medication.

Part 1 provides critical background information on the drug industry, demonstrating how and why drug costs have gone through the roof. We show you how to protect yourself from dangerous—even life-threatening—prescription mistakes. We list the advantages and disadvantages of purchasing drugs in Canada and Mexico, and over the Internet, including how to get the biggest discounts and avoid common problems. Part 1 also features a chapter on discount plans for those with special needs, including lists of many state-sponsored programs, with addresses, phone numbers, and eligibility requirements. If you qualify for one of these programs, signing on can save you a lot of money.

Part 2 offers information and money-saving advice on prescription drugs, organized by health condition. We describe medications commonly prescribed for hundreds of conditions. Our tables organize pertinent facts, including strength, dose, active ingredient, typical price per dose, and potential savings, for each class of drugs we discuss, so you can locate information quickly and easily. Although we point out the Smart Buys in each group of drugs, the facts we provide will prepare you to make your own informed decisions.

Part 3 covers over-the-counter drugs. Like Part 2, it's organized by health condition. You'll learn the secrets of saving money on hundreds of common over-the-counter medications and health-related products. Again, our easy-to-use tables provide all the information you need to make informed purchasing decisions about drugs for health conditions as diverse as the common cold, chronic pain, and nausea. At the end of each chapter, we sum up our Smart Buy recommendations. Look for the Smart Buy symbol in the margin to locate these summaries easily.

Americans pay more for prescription drugs than people in any other country. And because drug companies have their hands in the pockets of so many elected leaders and officials, efforts to regulate drug costs go down to defeat again and again. No other

American industry wields such political clout! It's time to end this unfairness. And it can end with you, when you become a smart and savvy consumer and make purchasing choices that benefit *you*, not drug companies. *It's time to educate yourself* before you spend your hard-earned dollars on medications, just as you do with other products you buy. You can spend less, *far* less, on prescription and over-the-counter drugs without putting your health at risk.

If you, like millions of Americans, are fed up with how much of your paycheck, your retirement fund, or your savings you spend on medications, read on! Let us show you how to make smart buys drug-wise.

PART 1

Save Your Money, Save Your Health

Chapter 1

How Much Is Too Much?

B y any measure, the pharmaceutical industry is the most wildly profitable business in the U.S. Americans now spend a staggering $125 billion dollars a year for prescription drugs—that's $430 for every man, woman, and child in the country.

The billions that drug companies rake in translate to profits so massive, other industries in the Fortune 500 can only drool with envy. Drug-industry profit margins are five times higher than those in the automotive industry. On top of that, pharmaceutical manufacturers get enormous tax breaks for research and development, and benefit from billions of dollars in taxpayer money for research. The icing on the industry's cake is that its profits are recession-proof. In good economic times or bad, drug sales remain locked into a high-speed profit-and-growth pattern.

With salaries ranging from $6 million to $40 million a year (not including stock options), you'd think drug-company executives would be satisfied. But it's not enough. Prices for the most prescribed medications for older Americans are spiraling upward at twice the rate of inflation and four times the rate of other healthcare costs.

If you find this state of affairs outrageous, you're not alone. The U.S. Congress has tried for years to pass legislation bringing drug prices under control, but has met with little success. It's no wonder: The pharmaceutical industry employs a small army of lobbyists—more than the number of U.S. senators and congressional representatives combined—at a cost of more than $200 million a year! These lobbyists, backed up by lavish drug-industry contributions to political campaigns, aggressively squelch any and all efforts on Capitol Hill to impede the industry's profitability. Even though those profits come at the expense of *your* finances—and your health. Escalating drug costs affect the price of health care services across the board, from insurance rates to Medicare. Everywhere you turn, you pay more—more for prescription drugs, more for drugstore services, more for health insurance.

The Pharmaceutical Research and Manufacturers of America (PhRMA) claims the industry's pricing is necessary to pay the average $800 million cost of bringing a new drug to market. Without huge profits, adds PhRMA, drug makers will have no incentive to develop new products. What PhRMA fails to mention is that the drug industry spends more than twice that amount on advertising, marketing, and administration. And nearly 80 percent of the their so-called "new" drugs are not appreciably different from drugs already on the market.

According to U.S. Food and Drug Administration (FDA) data, barely 20 percent of newly patented drugs offer any significant improvement over those already in use. How much more can you afford to pay for the prescription drugs you need to safeguard your health? If you're among the 70 million Americans who lack prescription drug insurance coverage, you can't afford today's high prices, let alone higher prices tomorrow.

As a smart consumer, you know you're being had. But there's nothing you or anybody else can do about it. Right?

Wrong! The truth is, you have more choice than you think! We can show you ways to save up to 75 percent on your drug expenses—in some cases, even more. But first you need to understand the inner workings of the pharmaceutical industry, from manufacturing to marketing to sales.

GUARANTEED EXCLUSIVE SALES

As compensation for bringing new drugs to market, U.S. patent law grants pharmaceutical companies exclusive rights to manufacture and sell their drugs for a certain period of time. Prescription drug patents are good for years from the date of application; during this time, no one else can produce and sell the same drug. And under certain circumstances, this period can be extended. This gives the patent holder the opportunity to price the drug to recover the costs of research and development and generate a profit. Thus, drugs under patent are quite expensive. This is true even if you have prescription insurance coverage, because most plans require you to pay a percentage of the total cost.

The drugs shown in the following table were new to the market between 1998 and 2000 and have lengthy time periods remaining on their patents.

A drug patent is virtually a license to print money. A hot new drug can catapult a drug company's revenues into the financial stratosphere. The arthritis drug Vioxx is a good example of how this works. This drug debuted in 1999. One year later, after the most aggressive marketing campaign in pharmaceutical history exposed the American public to $160 million in advertising and promotion, Vioxx sales soared to more than $1.5 billion.

Sample Costs for Patented Drugs New to the Market

Drug	Typical Quantity	Typical Retail Cost	Prescribed to Treat
Protonix 40mg	30	$96.49	Stomach ulcers
Tequin 400mg	7	$54.29	Respiratory infections
Vioxx 25mg	30	$86.49	Inflammation/Pain
Trizivir	60	$847.99	HIV (AIDS)
Enbrel (injectable liquid)1-month supply		$1,123	Rheumatoid arthritis

THE POWER OF ADVERTISING

In times past, when a patient needed a prescription drug, the doctor researched what would work best and wrote a prescription; the drugstore pharmacist took the prescription and ten or fifteen minutes later handed over a bottle of pills. Things are very different today. With billions of dollars at stake, drug companies will try almost anything to get your money. And with so many similar products on the market, their efforts have reached frightening levels.

Until the late 1990s, severe restrictions governed how and where pharmaceutical companies could advertise. When new regulations removed these limits, the pharmaceutical industry started making up for lost time. In 2000, pharmaceutical manufacturers spent nearly $2.5 billion to influence your doctor, your pharmacy, and *you*. The payoff? Sales of the most advertised drugs soared by 25 percent, compared to an increase of just over percent in sales of all other drugs combined. No wonder drug companies now spend more on advertising and promotion than they do on research and development.

HOW DRUG COMPANIES INFLUENCE DOCTORS

Once upon a time, pharmaceutical sales representatives, or drug reps, were welcome partners in the healthcare industry. They were knowledgeable not only about the products they represented, but also about competing products. The rep's role was to educate doctors about drugs so doctors could make therapeutically appropriate drug choices— in other words, to give doctors the information they needed to keep abreast of new drugs and pick the ones that were best for their patients. Most reps were honest enough to say which products were genuinely better and which were more hype than help.

But that was the "good old days," and those days are gone. The pharmaceutical industry has become a behemoth beholden primarily to stockholders and investors. The role of today's drug rep is solely and entirely to sell. To make money, pharmaceutical companies must convince doctors to prescribe their drugs.

To win doctor loyalty, thirty-five or so major pharmaceutical companies have launched a small army of 70,000 drug reps. Their mission—to visit each of the country's 756,000 doctors and change their prescribing patterns to match the company's sales objectives. That's one drug rep for every 10.5 doctors! If only the ratio of teachers to children were that high! Certainly drug reps remain sources of information. But the information they provide focuses largely on products the rep *wants* the doctor to prescribe. Although this can introduce doctors to newer, more effective products than those they're in the habit of prescribing, often the products are simply different, not better.

Today, with revenue stakes spiking well into the billions of dollars, efforts to generate new business know no limits. Drug companies commonly offer free ski trips, golf outings, dinners at expensive restaurants, and travel packages in efforts to get doctors to prescribe and pharmacists to recommend their products. These practices are legal, although many in the healthcare industry question whether they're ethical.

Not only does this strategy contribute to higher drug costs, but you could also wind up taking a medication that's not really right for you. Certainly doctors won't admit to any influence from drug-company "freebies." We know a number of doctors (and pharmacists) who've been the guests of drug companies for ski trips and golf outings—luxurious vacations with all expenses paid. We receive frequent invitations to dinners at our area's most expensive restaurants—ostensibly to learn the "benefits" of the drugs the sponsoring manufacturer wants to promote. And you can bet that the drug reps who attend have their guests' full attention when it comes time to pitch their products.

How Drug Companies Influence Pharmacies and Drugstores

Drug companies have learned that, from giving advice to requesting changes in prescribed medications, pharmacists often have the doctor's ear. Because the direct approach—encouraging pharmacists to recommend or request specific drugs—tends to be less than successful, drug companies target the drugstores and pharmacies that employ pharmacists by offering financial incentives, usually in the form of rebates, for selling certain quantities of their products. Chain pharmacies, in particular, often become willing partners in this scheme—the corporate America ideal of making a buck any way you can.

In concept, a rebate sounds like a great idea. Buy a certain product, get some money back for doing so. If you need the product anyway, what's the harm? Most of us have received manufacturer rebates for purchasing everything from automotive products to toothpaste. You buy the product, fill out the request form, attach the proof of purchase, and mail it all off. In time, your check arrives in the mail. You may appreciate the manufacturer's "generosity," but this process provides marketing information that far exceeds the rebate's value. And when it comes to drug rebates, consumers rarely see any savings: The check goes to the drugstore.

Here's how it works. The manufacturer establishes a special promotion. For a specified amount of time, it offers rebates (typically percent) based on the volume of a certain product a drugstore sells. The drugstore purchases a quantity of the product from the manufacturer (usually through a wholesaler). The drugstore then completes the rebate paperwork and mails it, along with the invoice, to the manufacturer. Finally, the drugstore receives a rebate—either a check or a credit to its account. Because the financial incentives can be great, many drugstores encourage their pharmacists to sell as much rebate-eligible product as possible. Sometimes this "encouragement" becomes outright pressure, with directives instructing pharmacists to call physicians and request permission to change prescriptions to the preferred products.

But what about the *patient?* Do you think you'll receive the drug that's best for you and your health condition when the pharmacy filling your prescription stands to make more money by switching you to another drug? We don't. Always ask for an explanation if a pharmacist asks you to substitute. There may be good reason. If there isn't, don't switch.

HOW DRUG COMPANIES USE YOUR PHARMACY TO INFLUENCE YOU

Recent years have seen the emergence of a disturbing new trend in marketing. It's now possible to use a pharmacy's prescription records to contact consumers directly. This practice is at best ethically questionable and at worst downright illegal. In fact, a number of lawsuits challenging it are underway at this writing.

What happens is this: A manufacturer offers to pay a drugstore chain a fee of as much as $3 for each "informational" letter it sends or phone call it makes to its customers. Then, using its prescription records, the store identifies and contacts everyone who has purchased drugs made by that manufacturer. This means big money: A large chain that sends 200,000 letters could receive $300,000!

The manufacturer makes out even better. Recently, *The Wall Street Journal* reported on Merck's "patient information" campaign encouraging consumers who take Fosamax for osteoporosis to switch from the daily drug, the patent for which has been challenged in the courts, to the weekly drug, which is a different formulation and clearly under patent. Over 85 percent of those contacted switched, nearly doubling the sales for weekly Fosamax (from $844 million to $1.25 billion in just over a year). Did patients benefit from switching? Some may have; the cost often balances out, and sometimes even comes out less for the weekly dose than for a daily one. And many people like the convenience of taking a pill just once a week. But weekly isn't good for people who have trouble remembering to take their medications, and in the case of some drugs, it can cost from $7 to $10 *more* per week to take the weekly pill than the daily pill—an extra expense of $520 over the course of a year.

Several big chains have come under fire for this practice—Eckerd, Longs Drugs, Wal-Mart, and Walgreens, for example—as well as smaller regional chains and even independent pharmacies that find the money too good to pass up. Privacy laws in most states prohibit healthcare providers from sharing private information without permission. This is why the letters usually come from drug*stores,* rather than drug manufacturers. But the line is a fine one, and consumer-protection groups contend that this practice walks the wrong side of it, no matter what. It's a claim the attorneys general of several states, including Florida and Massachusetts, are actively investigating.

Consumer-protection laws generally require all businesses to permit customers to opt out of contact for marketing purposes. What this means and how it works in reality is another thing. Some pharmacies insist that the signature you provide when picking up your prescription authorizes them to contact you for "patient education" and "informational" purposes. The fine print at the bottom of the form says so. Others contend that, because they contact you to provide education and information and not to market anything, they don't need your consent. We feel these are weak arguments that rationalize unethical actions on the part of both drug manufacturers and drugstores. Any communication that attempts to get you to refill a prescription or to ask your doctor to change you to a different drug is *marketing,* pure and simple, no matter what the pharmacy or manufacturer wants to call it. When better drug choices actually exist, as can happen when you've been taking the same drug for a long time to treat a chronic condition, your doctor or pharmacist usually will tell you in person—not by phone or mail.

What can you do about this? Plenty! First, remember that you can always take your business to another pharmacy. You don't have to accept intrusive mailings and telephone calls. And take the following steps:

1. Ask your doctor to explain the medical benefits of changing your prescriptions, and make sure they really apply to *you.*

2. Contact the pharmacy that fills your prescription, and ask the manager to remove you from the mailing or calling list.

3. When you fill your prescriptions, request that the pharmacy *not* contact you for patient information, patient education, or other such reasons.

4. Read carefully anything you sign at the pharmacy. Look for fine print at the bottom of the page. If you can't read it, or if it doesn't make sense to you, ask the pharmacist (not the technician or cashier) to read and explain it to you.

5. Next to your signature on any pharmacy form, write "Do not contact me for patient education, information, refill reminder, or any marketing purposes." If letters or phone calls continue, file formal complaints with your local Better Business Bureau, state pharmacy association, and state attorney general's office.

6. Write your legislators and press for laws that clearly and unmistakably protect your privacy and outlaw such contact.

Drug manufacturers and pharmacies want you to believe they contact you because they have your best interests at heart. Sadly, though, the real motivator is almost always money. Guess whose?

HOW DRUG COMPANIES
USE ADVERTISING TO INFLUENCE YOU

The pharmaceutical industry spends nearly $3 billion a year to influence you through what the marketing industry calls "direct-to-consumer" advertising. They know that the power of such advertising can be summed up in to two words: It works. Surveys show that one patient in three asks the doctor about a specific advertised drug—and in about half such instances, the doctor prescribes that drug. Think about that when you watch a TV commercial for an anti-impotence pill after having just paid $45 for an antibiotic made by the same company. Although drug companies insist that each drug's cost corresponds only to the expense of bringing that particular drug to market, the bottom line is that the more a drug company spends on advertising and marketing, the more you'll pay for *any* drug the company manufactures.

But the costs don't end there. The advertised product—often the newest and most expensive of its kind—may well be no more effective than less costly, more familiar drugs. Yet the marketers would have us believe that, if we're not taking this drug, we're not getting the best modern medicine has to offer. Yes, every advertisement includes cautions and warnings. But how many of us really listen to the rapid-fire recital of potential side effects at the commercial's end, or read the fine print in the magazine ad? Even when we do, we find our attention drawn to the healthy, robust models touting their now-wonderful lives!

The risk here is twofold. First, people request—and receive—prescriptions for drugs that aren't necessarily the most appropriate or least costly choices. Second, the money invested in such extensive advertising efforts drives the cost of prescription drugs even higher. You need to know *why* your doctor chooses to prescribe a particular drug, and to learn about alternatives that can accomplish the same therapeutic result at a lower price. But don't rely on commercials and magazine ads for information! Remember, they exist only to convince consumers to buy. Question your doctor about drug choices before you walk out with a prescription, and if, at the drugstore, you learn that a drug is very expensive, discuss possible alternatives with your pharmacist.

Contact Your Legislators

Contact your elected state and federal representatives to let them know you oppose drug-company marketing practices. These tactics are good for manufacturers but bad for consumers. They influence doctors and pharmacists to base their drug choices on factors that may be unrelated to what's best for the patient. And, in the end, you must spend even more money for the medications you need to maintain your health and well-being.

TRY IT, YOU'LL LIKE IT: SAMPLES

Here's another popular ploy: A drug rep leaves the doctor samples of new drugs to give to patients to try. On the surface, this seems like a strategy with multiple benefits. Your doctor becomes familiar with the product, and you get to try something for free. This is especially beneficial if you have no insurance coverage for prescription drugs and must pay for your medications yourself.

But the risks, too, are multiple. First, sample packages seldom contain enough doses of a drug to complete a course of treatment. If the drug works for you, you must fill a prescription for the remainder of the treatment period. You still end up buying the drug—which, as a new product, is likely to be quite expensive. Second, your doctor's prescribing patterns are subtly influenced and changed. Along with the free samples, the doctor may issue a prescription for the same drug—or at least instruct you to call the office for a prescription if the sample works for you. Even should the sample *not* work for you, the doctor is now in the habit of thinking about and writing prescriptions for the drug. And what happens when the samples run out? The drug company hopes the doctor continues writing those prescriptions!

When your doctor offers you drug samples, ask whether it's the drug he or she would prescribe if those samples weren't available. If the answer is no, then ask about cost. We'll bet that the purchase price of the sample drug is significantly higher than the drug your doctor would prescribe otherwise. Request a prescription for the drug your doctor would prefer to use, instead. Although accepting free samples can be a good way to find out whether an expensive new drug works for you, a doctor who has a bountiful supply of samples may be a getting little too cozy with drug-company sales reps—and that can cost you plenty when you pay for your prescriptions.

MAKE INFORMED CHOICES

Naturally, it's important that you trust in your doctor's medical expertise and believe he or she has your best interests at heart. But rarely does only a single option exist for treating any health condition. It's *your* health: Take charge! Be active in your care, especially when it comes to prescription drugs. After all, your bank account and your well-being are at stake. When your doctor wants to prescribe a drug for you, learn as much as you can before you accept the prescription. Ask pointed questions, such as:

1. How expensive is this drug?
2. Is there anything that might work better for me, or which would work as well but cost less?
3. What advantages or disadvantages are there to this medication compared to those of less expensive medications that do the same thing?
4. Why do you think this particular drug is right for me?
5. What side effects might I expect?
6. Have I tried anything similar before?

These questions will cause your doctor to think before writing that prescription. And don't be surprised if you wind up with a different drug. Sometimes doctors don't realize how they select the drugs they prescribe until they're forced to explain their reasoning.

THE BOTTOM LINE

There's no way around it: Right now, the drugs you need to maintain your health are expensive. But we can show you how to spend far less for the drugs you buy—whether prescription or over-the-counter—without jeopardizing your health and safety.

In reading the chapters that follow, you'll learn which factors to consider when you choose or take medications, and how to find the best deals. Our Smart Options for Savings—your "SOS" for finding the best savings options for *you*—and our Smart Buy recommendations will help you get the most for your money. We provide easy-to-use one-page worksheets, one for prescription drugs and one for over-the-counter drugs. Photocopy these forms and use them to keep track of what you spend and save.

Follow our simple guidelines, and you'll find you save a *lot*.

Chapter 2

Protecting Yourself from Common Prescription Mistakes

I n life, some mistakes are inevitable. But prescription mistakes occur more often than they should, and they can have very serious consequences: According to the National Academy of Sciences Institute of Medicine, medication errors account for tens of thousands of deaths each year. Reasons for prescription errors include:

+ Illegible physician handwriting
+ Errors in transcribing verbal orders to written orders (misunderstanding)
+ Misinterpretation of abbreviations

Other errors involve inappropriate substitutions, drug interactions, allergies, and problems due to the age of the patient.

WHAT DOES THAT SAY?

Physician handwriting is notoriously poor—so poor, in fact, that many hospitals and medical centers are moving away from handwritten records to automated or computerized systems. A doctor may key a prescription into a computer or a special hand-held device, which either prints the prescription or transmits it electronically to a pharmacy equipped to receive it. Use of such technology remains more the exception than the rule, however, and most prescriptions are still written by hand. This leaves you vulnerable to mistakes that can result from illegible writing, unclear instructions, and even confusion about which medication the doctor is prescribing.

Philip, newly diagnosed with type 2 diabetes, brought in a prescription for the commonly used medication Glucophage, which lowers blood sugar. The doctor's handwritten prescription was difficult to read, but the pharmacy technician and the pharmacist agreed that it said "500mg i bid"—that is, Glucophage in the 500mg strength, 1 tablet to be taken twice a day. The pharmacist dispensed the medication to Philip and provided cautions and warnings related to the drug. When Philip went back to his doctor for a routine blood-sugar test after two weeks on Glucophage, however, both Philip and his doctor were astonished to find that Philip's blood sugar was still dangerously high.

The doctor looked at Philip's prescription bottle, which Philip had brought with him. When he compared the label to notes in Philip's medical record, the mistake became clear: The pharmacist's dosage instructions were wrong. He had written "500mg ii bid"—2 500mg-strength pills twice a day. But the "ii"—an abbreviation commonly used to denote the number of pills—had looked to the pharmacy staff like a single "i," indicating a single tablet. Because high blood sugar can cause problems ranging from cataracts to coma, Philip could have suffered serious health consequences!

Always ask your doctor and your pharmacist what results to expect from a prescription drug, when to expect them, and what to do if you don't experience those results. Philip was lucky that his doctor scheduled a follow-up visit and caught the mistake in his prescription. All too often, such errors are discovered only after they've caused serious health problems.

Put yourself to the test! Can you figure out what these prescriptions say?

SAMPLE 1

SAMPLE 2

SAMPLE 3

How did you do? If you were able to make out the letters and numbers, give your-self a pat on the back. And if you could interpret the symbols and abbreviations, reward yourself with the treat of your choice! These aren't the worst we've seen, but, unfor-tunately, they're representative. Here are the solutions.

SAMPLE 1 SOLUTION

This prescription is for eye drops.

MEDICAL VERSION	WHAT IT MEANS
Sulfacetamide Ophth. 10% 1-2 gtts 5x/day for 5-6 days To R eye	Sulfacetamide ophthalmic (eye) 10% solution Put 1 to 2 drops into the *right* eye 5 times per day for 5 to 6 days.

SAMPLE 2 SOLUTION

This prescription is for a product that is most likely less expensive if purchased as the over-the-counter drug diphenhydramine (or Benadryl).

MEDICAL VERSION	WHAT IT MEANS
Diphenhydramine 25mg Sig: 1 q 6_ PRN itching & rash Disp: 20	Diphenhydramine, 25mg strength Instructions: Take 1 every 6 hours as needed for itching and rash. Dispense quantity of 20.

SAMPLE 3 SOLUTION

This one was a real doozy, with the doctor making every effort to get the most from a single piece of paper: This prescription is for eight different drugs! And don't feel bad if you couldn't get all of them; neither could we. Not only is the handwriting illegible, but it's also hard to tell what quantity goes with which drug. Furthermore, anyone tak-ing six or more drugs risks some type of drug interaction. Such interactions may not be serious or life-threatening, but they still may be unpleasant and are certainly unwanted. This person is taking Prozac (an antidepressant) and Xanax (an antianxiety drug related to Valium). Xanax taken long term will somewhat dampen the effective-ness of the Prozac. The Vicodin pain medication could increase the drowsiness that may be present already because of the Xanax and Prozac, if the Prozac is a new med-ication for this patient.

Needless to say, we had to call on this one—or, rather, these eight. If your doctor wants to give you more than one prescription at the same time, make sure he or she writes each one separately! Here's what the doctor ordered, line by line:

MEDICAL VERSION	WHAT IT MEANS
Lipitor 10mg 1 po, HS #30	Lipitor, 10mg strength. Take 1 by mouth at bedtime. Quantity: 30 pills
Tiazac 180mg 1 Po, BID #60	Tiazac, 180mg strength. Take 1 by mouth twice daily. Quantity: 60 pills
Albuterol 90mcg 2 puffs q as needed, taper 2 /…	Albuterol inhaler, 90 mcg/dose strength. Take 2 puffs (every) as needed. (Remainder is illegible.)
#60 Isosorbide 20mg 1 Po, BID	Isosorbide, 20mg strength. Take 1 by mouth twice daily. Quantity: 60 pills
Vicodin 5mg 1 Po, TID #90	Vicodin, 5mg strength. Take 1 by mouth 3 times daily. Quantity: 90 pills
Monopril 10mg 1 Po, BID #60	Monopril, 10mg strength. Take 1 by mouth twice daily. Quantity: 60 pills
Xanax 0.5mg 1 Po, BID #60	Xanax 1/2mg strength. Take 1 by mouth twice daily. Quantity: 60 pills
Prozac 20mg 2 Po, QD #60	Prozac, 20mg strength. Take 2 by mouth once daily. Quantity: 60 capsules

COMMONLY CONFUSED DRUGS

With more than 11,000 pharmaceutical products on the market already, it's an extreme understatement to say that it's challenging to come up with unique names for new ones. Many drugs have similar-sounding or looking names. Generic versions present their own problems, because their names often resemble that of a drug's chemical structure or family. For example, fluoxetine (generic Prozac) and fluvoxamine (generic Luvox) sound similar when you hear them spoken over the telephone, and, as you can see, their spellings are very close. Furthermore, both are antidepressants, so a smart consumer who double-checks the pharmacist by asking what a medication is used for may be less likely to catch the mistake.

Sometimes these similarities are intentional, designed to capture market share by capitalizing on popular names. Most often, however, similar names are unintentional—

potentially a very dangerous situation. The FDA, through its Center for Drug Evaluation and Research, tracks medication errors. Their findings to date include these mistakes:

+ A pharmacy dispensed Lanoxin, a heart medication, instead of levothyroxine, a thyroid supplement. The mistake was fatal.
+ Because of illegible handwriting, a prescription for Volmax 4mg, a drug used to treat bronchial spasms, was filled instead with Flomax 0.4mg, a drug prescribed to treat benign prostatic hyperplasia. According to the FDA, one patient who took Flomax instead of Volmax developed insomnia, tiredness, weakness, dizziness, a runny nose, frequent urination, and a chronic sinus infection and a vocal-cord polyp, both of which required surgery to remedy.
+ More than 100 cases of name confusion have been reported involving the drugs Celebrex (for arthritis), Cerebryx (an antiseizure drug), and Celexa (an antidepressant). If Cerebryx isn't taken when it should be, dangerous seizures may result. And if Cerebryx is taken instead of either Celebrex or Celexa, severe drowsiness, headaches, difficulty in walking or speaking, and/or a decrease in cognitive ability may result.
+ The FDA reports that prescription errors have been associated with Zantac and Zyrtec syrups. Of the seven such errors on record, most involved children from 7 days to 15 months of age. In all these cases, Zantac syrup (an H2 blocker that reduces stomach acid) was the intended drug, and Zyrtec syrup (an antihistamine for allergies) was dispensed, instead. Patients experienced effects ranging from difficulty sleeping to becoming "violently ill," with decreased appetite, diarrhea, and vomiting.

In an effort to prevent such potentially dangerous sound-alike and look-alike confusion, the FDA has established an Office of Postmarketing Drug Risk Assessment to review the names of new drugs before they come to market. Only time will tell whether this reduces medication errors.

In the meantime, be diligent. *Always*

...ask questions, and persist until you get answers that satisfy you.

...ask your doctor to print the name of the drug clearly on the prescription form and on a separate piece of paper for you, so you can double-check the prescription label at the store.

...look at the bottle to make sure that the name and strength match what's on the piece of paper. If it doesn't, ask your pharmacist why.

...ask the pharmacist what the medication is for to ensure you get the right drug type. If you expected medicine to treat an infection and the pharmacist says you're getting something to thin your blood, send up a red flag!

…ask the pharmacist if it's OK to take this new medication with the other things you're taking. Pharmacists *should* check this before filling the prescription, but prompting from the customer sometimes helps alert them to drug interactions they might have missed.

TRANSCRIBING ERRORS

To save time, doctors or their aides often relay prescription information to the pharmacy via telephone. It's easy for this communication to go awry on either end. Often the person phoning the prescription in is in a hurry. The pharmacist at the other end might not hear all that the doctor says, or might assume the doctor meant one thing when something else was said, or might make inadequate notes that cause confusion later. Transcription errors can occur for a variety of reasons.

The most effective way to reduce the incidence of phone mistakes is for the pharmacist to insist on letter-by-letter spellings. For your part, make sure you know which drug your doctor has prescribed and what condition it's supposed to treat. Ask your doctor to write out a copy of this information. Compare this with the label on your prescription container. If the two don't match, ask the pharmacist to recheck the prescription against the drug you've been given.

THAT'S NOT WHAT I MEANT

Medical shorthand is a blessing and a curse. Although common abbreviations speed and simplify the process for healthcare professionals, they can lead to potentially serious problems if they're misinterpreted. A good example is the abbreviation "QD," short for the Latin phrase *quaque die*—"once a day." Written quickly or carelessly, this can instead look like "QID," short for the Latin phrase *quater in die*—"four times a day." This is particularly challenging for non-medical folks to make sense of; few people know Latin anymore! But Latin is the language of medicine (and science in general). Taking a drug 4 times a day when you're supposed to take it once can be lethal. Although the reverse misinterpretation isn't usually as dangerous, the patient won't get enough of the prescribed drug. If it's to treat high blood pressure, diabetes, or even hypercholesterolemia (high cholesterol), for example, consequences can be serious.

Sometimes the number of tablets or capsules is misread. Handwriting Sample 3 is a perfect example of medical shorthand—and the challenge of deciphering it. Many doctors write "ii" (looking like a capital "T" with two dots above) to indicate 2 tablets. In this example, the shorthand behind the 20mg strength of Prozac is an abbreviation that tells the pharmacist to instruct the patient to take 2 capsules for each dose. This easily could be misread as *one* capsule, especially with so many medications listed on the same prescription form. Sometimes doctors write the Roman numeral "iv" for the quantity four. A pharmacist in a hurry easily might type one for the other—two for the four or four for the two. Someone who's a little lazy or in a hurry might read the doctor's scribbled "v" as "ii," and so the patient will take half the dose prescribed.

Commonly confused abbreviations include:

- **mcg** (micrograms) and **mg** (milligrams): This can lead to a serious dosage error—100mcg is equivalent to 0.1mg.
- **QD** and **QID**: Once a day or 4 times day—the difference is likely to be important.
- **QOD** (every other day) and **QID** (4 times a day) and **QD** (once daily): Again, the potential is great for a serious misdosing error.
- **SC** (subcutaneous, or under the skin) and **SL** (sublingual, or under the tongue).
- **TIW** (3 times a week) and **TID** (3 times a day).
- **HS** (hour of sleep; that is, at bedtime) and **HS** (half-strength).
- **AU** (both ears) and **OU** (both eyes).
- **AS** (left ear) and **OS** (left eye).
- **AD** (right ear) and **OD** (right eye).
- **PCN** (penicillin) and **TCN** (tetracycline): Confusion here could be disastrous if the patient is severely allergic to one or the other drug.

Ask your doctor how often you're supposed to take your medication. If this doesn't match the instruction on your prescription label, ask the pharmacist to call your doctor for clarification. You might have to wait a bit longer, but it will be worth it.

INAPPROPRIATE SUBSTITUTIONS

Substituting a generic drug for a name-brand drug or changing brands with refills can be cost-effective moves with no adverse therapeutic effects. Usually the drugs will be chemically equivalent, and they'll have the same effect no matter which company manufactures them.

For some drugs, however, this isn't true. Healthcare professionals identify these drugs as having "narrow therapeutic indexes," or NTIs. (Refer to Chapter 4, "Savings on Drugs Across the Border," for more information about NTIs.) These drugs are very sensitive and their levels in the bloodstream require close monitoring when they're taken. Usually the pharmacist will recommend against changing brands if your doctor has prescribed such a drug. But it's prudent for you to find out which NTI drugs are commonly prescribed. (You'll find a list in Chapter 6, "Rx SOS: Smart Options for

Saving Money on Prescription Drugs.") If you're taking an NTI, change brands only under close supervision from your doctor, and be aware that you might find yourself back at square one for establishing an effective dose.

Sue had been taking Synthroid 0.175 mg, a purple pill, for about years. When she got a recent refill, she noticed the pills she received were turquoise. When Sue questioned the pharmacist, she learned she'd been given Levothroid, a different brand. The pharmacist explained that the pharmacy, which was affiliated with a hospital, had a contract with the company that manufactures Levothroid and that it routinely dispensed that product unless the physician specifically ordered a different brand. Well, Sue's physician had specifically ordered Synthroid; the pharmacist had made a mistake. And because thyroid-replacement drugs aren't really generically equivalent, this was in fact a *serious* mistake. Were Sue to switch to another brand of thyroid drug intentionally, she would need regular lab tests, over a period of usually 3 to 6 months, until her blood levels stabilized. Had Sue not noticed that she'd received a different drug when she refilled her prescription, she could have ended up with either too much or too little thyroid replacement, and experienced adverse health effects.

Although a different brand of drug might cost less than the one your doctor has prescribed, the savings aren't always in your best interest. In Sue's case, the pharmacy appeared to have a greater interest in dispensing large volumes of Levothroid than in making sure Sue got the drug her doctor prescribed. Although it passed its cost savings on to consumers, the pharmacy likely had a volume purchasing contract with the manufacturer: The more of the drug the pharmacy sells, the lower the manufacturer's purchasing price. (We discuss the sometimes too-cozy relationships between drug companies and the doctors and pharmacists to whom they market their products in Chapter 1, "How Much Is Too Much?")

DRUG INTERACTIONS AND ALLERGIES

Many drugs should not be taken in combination with one another. Computer programs exist to help pharmacists screen for them, but these are only as useful as the data they contain. If you get your prescriptions at different pharmacies or switch from one drugstore to another, your records might be incomplete. When you take a new prescription drug for the first time, tell the pharmacist about all the other drugs (including those you buy over the counter) that you take.

Here are some examples of potentially dangerous combinations:

✦ Coumadin, a drug used to thin the blood to prevent heart attacks and strokes, can become deadly if taken with aspirin. Sometimes doctors will use this combination carefully if Coumadin alone can't do the job, but patients who take blood thinners should avoid treating their fevers and headaches with over-the-counter aspirin.

✦ If you're taking the cholesterol-lowering drug Lipitor and your doctor also prescribes the antibiotic Biaxin, commonly used for sinus infections or bronchitis, you could end up with a rare but serious complication in which muscle tissue breaks down and the kidneys fail. Biaxin can slow liver enzymes enough to cause blood levels of Lipitor to rise, with dangerous consequences.

✦ Tagamet, a medication commonly used to treat stomach ulcers or acid reflux, should not be taken with theophylline unless the dose of the theophylline is reduced and blood theophylline levels are monitored closely. If this is not done, theophylline blood levels can elevate quickly, causing life-threatening seizures. Tagamet slows theophylline metabolism so the drug stays in the body longer and at higher than usual levels.

Often patients attribute unpleasant—but entirely normal—reactions to drugs to allergies. The narcotic pain reliever, codeine, for example, is notorious for causing nausea. But this isn't an allergy; it's simply the nature of the drug. To be sure, this effect can be intolerable, and that's reason enough to try a different pain reliever. Certain antibiotics also are likely to cause nausea and even vomiting; again, this is not an allergic response, but a not-uncommon bodily reaction to these drugs.

When you're *allergic* to a drug, your body's immune system perceives the drug as an "invader" and attacks it; this results in symptoms of an allergy. Doctors are uncertain why this occurs. If you experience any of these signs of an allergy, stop taking the drug and contact your doctor immediately:

✦ Itching or rash, particularly on your belly and the insides of your arms and legs
✦ Hives (raised welts)
✦ Feeling of numbness, thickness, or swelling on your lips and tongue and in your mouth (This can be life-threatening. Seek medical attention immediately.)
✦ Difficulty breathing, a feeling that your throat is swelling (Again, this can be life-threatening. Seek medical attention immediately.)

Typically, an allergic reaction to a drug occurs *after* the first time you take it—on the second, third, or even tenth time. This is because it takes time for your body to develop the histamine response that will attack the drug when it enters your system. However, a severe allergic reaction can manifest as soon as the second dose. Always stop taking the drug and contact your doctor immediately if you believe you're having an allergic reaction.

SPECIAL CONSIDERATIONS IF YOU'RE OVER AGE 65

We're all getting older. Aging is just a fact of life. And although modern medical methods, especially drugs, have made longer lives possible and enjoyable, advancing age still comes with special concerns.

As we age, many of our body systems function less and less efficiently. Liver and kidney functions are especially important for metabolizing drugs, and with increased age, these systems slow down. These organs become less efficient at filtering your blood, which can extend the amount of time a drug stays in your body. This increases your risk for side effects. Doctors typically reduce standard dosages of many drugs when they prescribe them for older patients. If you're over age 65, ask your doctor or pharmacist if your age will have any effect on how your body uses a given drug. And if you're taking any of the drugs shown in the following chart, question your doctor or pharmacist about your dosage to make sure it's appropriate for your age.

Drugs That Have Increased Risk In the Elderly

DRUG	COMMON BRANDS	COMMON USES	POTENTIAL RISKS
Amitriptyline	Elavi	Depression Nerve pain relief	Anticholinergic effects* Very sedating
Belladonna alkaloids	Donnatal	Stomach cramps	Anticholinergic effects*
Carisoprodol	Soma	Muscle spasm	Anticholinergic effects* Very sedating Weakness
Chlordiazepoxide	Librium	Anxiety	Prolonged drowsiness that can lead to falls and fractures
Chlorpheniramine	Chlor-trimeton	Allergies	Anticholinergic effects*
Chlorpromazine	Thorazine	Psychosis	Anticholinergic effects Nausea Very sedating Hiccups Increased movement disorders
Chlorpropamide	Diabinese	Diabetes	Hypoglycemia Excessively low sodium levels
Chlorzoxazone	Parafon Forte	Muscle spasms	Anticholinergic effects* Very sedating Weakness

DRUG	COMMON BRANDS	COMMON USES	POTENTIAL RISKS
Cimetidine	Tagamet	Stomach ulcers	Confusion
Clidinium-chlordiazepoxide	Librax	Stomach cramps	Anticholinergic* effects
Cyclobenzaprine	Flexeril	Muscle spasms	Anticholinergic effects* Very sedating Weakness
Cyproheptadine	Periactin	Allergies	Anticholinergic effects*
Diazepam	Valium	Anxiety Insomnia	Prolonged drowsiness that can lead to falls and fractures
Dicyclomine	Bentyl	Stomach cramps	Anticholinergic effects*
Diphenhydramine	Benadryl	Allergies	Anticholinergic effects*
Dipyridamole	Persantine	Blood-clot prevention	Light-headedness
Doxepin	Sinequan	Depression Nerve-pain relief	Anticholinergic effects* Very sedating
Famotidine	Pepcid	Stomach ulcers	Confusion
Flurazepam	Dalmane	Insomnia	Prolonged drowsiness that can lead to falls and fractures
Haloperidol	Haldol	Psychosis	Anticholinergic effects* Very sedating Increased movement disorders
Hydroxyzine	Atarax	Allergies	Anticholinergic effects.*
Hyoscyamine	Levsin Levsinex	Stomach cramps	Anticholinergic effects*
Indomethacin	Indocin	Inflammation Arthritis	Confusion Dizziness
Iron supplements	Feosol Slow Fe Ferrous sulfate Ferrous gluconate	Anemia	Constipation
Meperidine	Demerol	Pain relief	Confusion
Metaxalone	Skelaxin	Muscle spasms	Anticholinergic effects* Very sedating Weakness
Methocarbamol	Robaxin	Muscle spasms	Anticholinergic effects* Very sedating Weakness
Methyldopa	Aldomet	High blood pressure	Slowed heartbeat Depression
Nizatidine	Axid	Stomach ulcers	Confusion

DRUG	COMMON BRANDS	COMMON USES	POTENTIAL RISKS
Oxybutynin	Ditropan	Bladder control	Anticholinergic effects* Very sedating Weakness
Pentazocine	Talwin	Pain relief	Confusion Hallucinations
Promethazine	Phenergan	Nausea	Anticholinergic effects*
Propantheline	Pro-Banthine	Stomach ulcers	Anticholinergic effects* Stomach cramps
Propoxyphene	Darvon Darvocet	Pain relief	Constipation Drowsiness Confusion
Ranitidine	Zantac	Stomach ulcers	Confusion
Reserpine	Hydropres Regroton Salutensin	High blood pressure	Depression Impotence Sedation Dizziness
Thioridazine	Mellaril	Psychosis	Anticholinergic effects* Very sedating Increased movement disorders
Thiothixene	Navane	Psychosis	Anticholinergic effects* Very sedating Increased movement disorders
Trimethobenzamide	Tigan	Nausea	Abnormal movements of the arms, legs, and body

* "Anticholinergic" side effects include blurred vision, constipation, dry mouth, light-headedness, difficulty with urination, and confusion.

The older you are, the more medications you're likely to take. This further increases your risk for unpleasant or even fatal drug reactions and interactions. The FDA reports that nearly half of all deaths related to drug interactions and errors occur in people over age 65. We can't stress this enough: Always tell your doctor and your pharmacist about *all* the drugs you take, including those you buy without prescriptions (over the counter). To make this easier, write them down and carry the list in your wallet. If you like, photocopy the form provided here, fill it out, and carry it with you.

SAFEGUARDING YOURSELF

The more you know about how and when mistakes happen, the better equipped you are to make sure they *don't* happen to you. Take these basic steps to protect yourself from common prescription mistakes:

Prescription Drugs I Take

Drug Name and Strength	When and How I Take This Drug	Why I Take This Drug	Name and Phone Number of Doctor Who Prescribed This Drug

Over-the-Counter Drugs I Take

Drug Name and Strength	When and How I Take This Drug	Why I Take This Drug

✦ Ask your doctor about the drug he or she is prescribing. What is its exact name? What is it used to treat? What are its possible side effects and risks? Why has your doctor selected this drug for you?

✦ Remind your doctor about other drugs you're taking— prescription and over-the-counter medications.

✦ Have your doctor *print* the name and strength of the drug on a piece of paper you can take with you. (The back of the doctor's business card works well.) When you pick up your prescription at the pharmacy, check the label against what the doctor wrote down for you. If anything is different, ask the pharmacist to explain why.

✦ When you refill a prescription for a drug you take regularly or have taken before, examine the pills or capsules before you leave the store. If they look different from what you've been taking, ask the pharmacist to recheck the prescription.

✦ Let the pharmacist tell you about the drug when you pick up your prescription. If a technician hands your prescription to you and asks whether you want to talk with the pharmacist, say *yes*. Then say to the pharmacist, "Tell me about this drug." This kind of "patient counseling" forces us to take one more look at your prescription, and it gives you a chance to question anything that's unclear or different from what your doctor has told you.

✦ Fill your prescriptions at a pharmacy near your doctor's office, if this is practical. A pharmacy familiar with your doctor's handwriting and prescribing patterns is more likely to note inconsistencies.

✦ Use the same pharmacy for all of your drug needs (prescription and over the counter). Most pharmacies and drugstores use computer records to keep track of prescriptions and drug purchases. This helps the pharmacist red-flag potential drug interactions and other problems, including allergies.

✦ Take your medications properly! Read the label instructions carefully. If you don't understand them or have questions, talk with your pharmacist. Find out what to do if you miss a dose, and make sure you know how long you should take the drug.

✦ Read the product literature information that comes with your prescriptions so you know what adverse reactions to look for and whether potential food or drug interactions exist.

It's great having one of the world's most sophisticated healthcare systems. In the end, though, your health is *your* responsibility. Learn as much as you can about the drugs you take, so you can be your own best protector.

Chapter 3

Wired for Savings: Internet Pharmacies

The practice of buying drugs from a pharmacy without going to an actual store and standing in line has been around for decades. We used to call it "mail order": A patient or doctor sent a written prescription to a warehouse-based "drugstore," which then sent the drugs to the patient through the mail. Most of these mail-order pharmacies were connected in some way to insurance plans or special membership programs. The savings could be phenomenal, but the programs were available to relatively few people.

Sample Internet Pharmacy Savings

DRUG	STRENGTH	QUANTITY	COMMON USE	TRADITIONAL RETAIL PHARMACY	INTERNET PHARMACY	SAVINGS
Aerobid Inhaler	250mcg	7 grams	Asthma	$74.39	$62.65	$11.74 16%
Allegra	60mg	60 tablets	Allergies	$78.69	$64.92	$13.77 17%
Buspar	10mg	60 tablets	Anxiety	$92.59	$84.31	$8.28 9%
Celebrex	200mg	30 capsules	Arthritis	$91.99	$71.73	$20.26 22%
Celexa	20mg	30 tablets	Depression	$74.89	$63.84	$11.05 15%
Coumadin	5mg	100 tablets	Blood thinner	$72.99	$63.40	$9.59 13%

DRUG	STRENGTH	QUANTITY	COMMON USE	TRADITIONAL RETAIL PHARMACY	INTERNET PHARMACY	SAVINGS
Covera-HS	240mg	30 tablets	High blood pressure	$63.79	$54.62	$9.17 14%
Depakote	250mg	60 tablets	Epilepsy	$67.09	$56.35	$10.74 16%
Detrol-LA	2mg	30 capsules	Bladder control	$90.49	$75.21	$15.28 17%
Effexor XR	150mg	30 capsules	Depression	$92.89	$73.89	$19 20%
Estrace	1mg	30 tablets	Estrogen replacement therapy	$22.99	$17.87	$5.12 22%
Flonase Nasal Spray	50mcg	16 grams	Sinus congestion	$58.79	$50.43	$8.36 14%
Fosamax	10mg	30 tablets	Osteoporosis	$77.99	$58.74	$19.25 25%
Glucophage	500mg	100 tablets	Diabetes	$84.69	$70.13	$14.56 17%
Hyzaar	50/12.5mg	30 tablets	High blood pressure	$49.99	$38.85	$11.14 22%
Imitrex	50mg	9 tablets	Migraine headaches	$149.99	$134.70	$15.29 10%
Lescol	20mg	30 capsules	High cholesterol	$51.69	$43.65	$8.04 16%
Norvasc	5mg	100 tablets	High blood pressure	$139.59	$118.34	$21.25 15%
Premarin	0.625mg	100 tablets	Estrogen replacement	$65.99	$59.97	$6.02 9%
Prevacid	30mg	30 capsules	Acid reflux and ulcers	$134.59	$110.31	$24.28 18%
Prilosec	20mg	30 capsules	Acid reflux and ulcers	$119.99	$108.03	$11.96 10%
Relafen	500mg	100 tablets	Arthritis	$132.79	$118.28	$14.51 11%
Viagra	100mg	5 tablets	Erectile dysfunction	$49.99	$41.85	$8.14 16%
Vioxx	25mg	100 tablets	Arthritis	$259.99	$228.80	$31.19 12%
Zocor	40mg	60 tablets	High cholesterol	$246.79	$231.06	$15.73 6%

In our electronic age, "virtual" shopping via the Internet has become a way of life. From automobiles to exotic foods, just about anything you might want is just a few keystrokes away. Studies show that you can find significant savings in cyberspace—if you know where to look and how to shop. This is as true for drugs as for any other product. Prices at online drugstores average 14 percent cheaper than prices at discount retail drugstores, as the chart shows.

Because you can't just reach through your computer and grab your drugs, mail order is the mode of delivery. Order and pay for your medicines electronically, and the Internet pharmacy has them delivered to you by mail or shipping service. Most Internet pharmacies also offer options for those who have no computer access or who prefer to handle transactions the conventional way: First telephone the pharmacy to set up an account, and then mail a check or money order to pay for your drugs. Many Internet pharmacies will also bill your insurance company or prescription plan, if you have coverage for prescription drugs.

The "store" for some Internet pharmacies, such as www.drugstore.com, is really a Web site—an electronic location on the Internet. Using a computer, you "visit" the Web-site address (URL), which usually starts with "www" (short for World Wide Web, the technical name for the Internet). Most Web sites feature several "pages" of information, usually organized like a physical store might be, with a legend or navigation key to help you find your way around. Have your doctor fax, phone, or mail your prescriptions to the Internet pharmacy. Then establish your account, choosing your delivery and payment preferences. It's most efficient to do this at the Internet pharmacy's Web site, but you can handle these details by telephone, if you prefer. A few Internet pharmacies remain phone-in models; that is, a doctor must phone or fax prescriptions, and then patients must call a toll-free number to complete the transaction. It probably won't be long, however, before all Internet pharmacies offer Website *and* telephone access.

A growing number of traditional "brick-and-mortar" pharmacies—those in buildings where you can go physically to shop—also operate Internet pharmacies, usually as Web sites. Eckerd Drug Stores, for example, operates www.Eckerd.com. Typically, you use a computer to order your drugs online, and then either have them mailed to you or made available for you to pick up at a convenient store location. If you choose the store pick-up option, though, you generally lose any savings you might have gained by shopping on the Internet.

A number of large health insurance companies own or maintain arrangements with Internet pharmacies (which they usually call "mail-order pharmacies") through which subscribers can receive prescription drugs at significant discounts. In theory, these arrangements save money for insurance companies and consumers. The Internet pharmacy is guaranteed business in exchange for offering discounted prices to the insurance plan.

Most of the time this works to your advantage—as it did for Roger, for example. He discovered that if he filled his prescription for blood-pressure medication through our local pharmacy he could get a 30-day supply for a $10 co-payment—not a bad deal. But if he ordered his prescription through the Internet drugstore his insurance company recommended, he could get a 90-day supply for the same $10 co-pay mailed right to his house—clearly, a better deal!

PLAN AHEAD

One drawback to using an Internet pharmacy is the time it usually takes for your drugs to reach you after you place your order. If your medications don't arrive before your current supply runs out, or if your doctor wants you to start taking a new drug right away, you'll have to fill a second prescription for the drug at a local pharmacy so that you'll have medicine to tide you over until your shipment arrives in the mail. This is a hassle for you, a hassle for your doctor, *and* you may end up paying the full cost yourself. Insurance companies typically won't pay for double prescriptions, which is what it looks like when they receive two bills for the same prescription from two different drugstores. So much for your mail-order savings! Yes, you can request overnight or next-day delivery. But, as the table on page 34 shows, this is an expensive option that can eat up (and even exceed) any savings you might have enjoyed from using an Internet pharmacy in the first place. To avoid this problem, plan ahead. Reorder when you still have a two-week supply left. And if taking your prescription medication right way is important, as with an antibiotic, use your local pharmacy.

> ### ▶ If It Sounds Too Good to Be True...
>
> Avoid any online pharmacy source that advertises the availability of prescription drugs without requiring a prescription. For example, numerous Web sites offer Viagra, an anti-impotence drug, without a prescription. These sales are illegal in the U.S. But because these sites typically are located in other countries, there is little U.S. regulators can do about them. Your best protection if you're going to buy your drugs online is to look for the VIPPS seal. It's great to save money, but don't do it at the risk of buying drugs of questionable potency or that could jeopardize your health. ◀

CONSUMER CAUTIONS

As with any shopping environment, the first rule of Internet shopping is *buyer beware*. Purchase only from reputable Web sites. A number of Internet pharmacies are affiliated with familiar traditional drugstores, such as Eckerds.com and CVS.com. Other Internet pharmacies, such as Drugstore.com, have built strong reputations and successful businesses exclusively on the Web. Make sure the online pharmacy you select participates in a certification program administered by the National Association of Boards of Pharmacy (NABP), which requires participating Internet pharmacies to undergo an inspection that evaluates 17 criteria to determine the quality and consistency of their procedures. You can double-check an Internet pharmacy's VIPPS status at the NABP Web site, http://www.NABP.net/. Among the criteria NABP inspectors consider is how the pharmacy protects customer confidentiality. Online pharmacies that have no procedures in place to protect customer information won't gain VIPPS certification. Once the online pharmacy passes inspection, it may advertise itself as a Verified Internet Pharmacy Practice Site and may display the VIPPS seal.

▶ Illegal Drug Sales via the Internet

The Internet has become a favorite venue for unscrupulous business ventures that take advantage of people looking for low prescription-drug prices. Even though certain drugs might be available legally over the counter in the country where the Web site is based, if they're considered prescription-only drugs in the U.S., then it's illegal to market them here.

The FDA has taken an aggressive enforcement position with such marketing. Each year it sends out hundreds of warnings to the operators of Web sites located in countries around the world. For the latest FDA warnings, alerts, and other information related to buying medical products over the Internet, go to the FDA Web site at http://www.fda.gov/.

No matter where you shop, find out about the company's customer-service procedures before you spend your money. Know the answers to these questions *before* you place your order:

+ What happens if you have a question about or a problem with a medication? Will you be able to talk with a "live person" who can resolve your problem quickly?

+ What happens if you get the wrong pills in the mail, your package doesn't arrive, or it's stolen? How quickly will the pharmacy get the right drugs out to you?

+ How much information do you need about the drugs you're taking? If you want to talk with a pharmacist, is one available? Is there a charge for this service?

+ What are the shipping charges? Many Internet pharmacies offer free shipping for standard mail deliveries, but if you need your medicine quickly, you'll pay a hefty fee for rapid delivery. In fact, you could end up paying more than it would have cost you to fill your prescriptions at the local drugstore.

+ Will the pharmacy bill your insurance company? If not, will your insurance company reimburse you? Many insurance companies require that you obtain your prescriptions from network pharmacies. Know what your insurance covers and what it doesn't, no matter where you buy your drugs!

SAFE CREDIT CARD SHOPPING

Many people worry that online credit card transactions, which make Internet shopping so easy and convenient, are risky. So far, no evidence exists to support this concern. Studies show that online credit card purchases are typically *safer*, in fact, than traditional in-store credit card purchases. Thieves can acquire credit card information from the records traditional stores throw away in the trash. Because electronic transactions leave no such paper trails, acquiring this information is much harder. Of course, the potential exists for security breaches, and certainly there have been some high-profile reports of stolen credit card data. But the precautions you should take when you shop on the Internet are no different than those for in-store credit card purchases.

+ Go over your credit card statement each month.

+ Immediately report inconsistencies to the issuing credit card company. Most will suspend billing for questionable charges until the situation is resolved.

+ Use a low-limit card for online purchases. This limits the amount a thief could charge against it should the data be stolen.

If using a credit card online makes you nervous, or if you don't have a credit card, ask whether you can send a check or money order by mail to pay for your prescriptions. Most Internet pharmacies offer this option, although your order might take longer to process as a result. Most commercial venues at a distance (from mail-order merchandisers to book clubs) will wait for your check to clear before shipping your purchases. Once you become a regular customer, however, the Internet pharmacy may relax its procedures and ship your drugs when it receives your order, trusting that you'll send payment promptly. Ask about its policies in this regard.

WATCH FOR HIDDEN COSTS

Most Internet pharmacies charge extra for shipping, and fees for rapid delivery can add up fast. Some provide free shipping for standard ground delivery via the U.S. Postal Service or a carrier such as United Parcel Service (UPS). This typically takes two weeks. If you can plan well in advance, this won't be a problem; look for Internet pharmacies that offer free shipping to enjoy the greatest savings. If you must pay for shipping, though, either because you need your order quickly or because the Internet pharmacy you like charges for it, factor in this extra expense when you compare its prices to other pharmacies "virtual" and traditional.

Some Internet pharmacies offer membership plans or fee-based programs. You might have to pay an annual fee (as with Merck Medco's "Your Plan," for example), or a co-payment for each prescription, or a combination of fee and co-pay. Most insurance plans that use Internet pharmacies require co-payments for drugs. Some offer a lower co-pay if you use the Internet pharmacy to encourage you to use the venue that's less expensive for the insurance company.

If you take a lot of prescription drugs over the course of a year, especially if they're "maintenance" medications—that is, drugs you'll take for a long time or even for the rest of your life (for heart disease, high blood pressure, thyroid disease, or diabetes, for example)—then the average 14 percent you'll save when you purchase your drugs through an Internet pharmacy instead of a brick-and-mortar store probably will offset any membership fee. If you use prescription drugs only occasionally, however, such savings may be insufficient to offset the fee.

$ SMART BUY
Internet Pharmacies

Your Smart Buy over the Internet is Express Pharmacy Services (www.eckerd.com). The Web site is user-friendly, offers free shipping (offsetting any price differences when compared to other Internet pharmacies), has a pharmacist available to answer questions, and bills insurance companies. The AARP (American Association of Retired Persons) pharmacy seems to be a Smart Buy as well, although at this writing, its Web site operation hasn't received VIPPS certification. AARP is one of the nation's largest consumer

Internet Pharmacies

NAME	HOW TO CONTACT	VIPPS	MEMBERSHIP OR SERVICE FEES	SHIPPING & HANDLING FEES	COMMENTS
AARP	http://www.aarppharmacy.com/ (800) 456-2277 (800) 530-5014 Fax	No	$15/year	Standard (2 weeks) $2.25 2nd-day not available Overnight $13.99	Bills numerous insurance plans. Provides information from pharmacists. Must be at least 50 years old. Spouse joins free.
Cigna Tel-Drug	http://www.cigna.com/ consumer/services/ pharmacy/tel_drug.html (800) 835-3784	Yes	Available for people who have Cigna insurance or no insurance.	Standard (2 weeks) free. 2nd-day $3.75 Overnight $18	90-day supply available per co-pay. Web site provides a link with drugstore.com for discounts on over-the-counter products. Bills only Cigna insurance plans. Prescriptions may only be mailed or faxed (no telephone orders). Mailed-in prescriptions are preferred. Difficult to reach on the telephone.
Costco	http://www.costco.com/ (800) 607-6861 (800) 633-0334	No	The $45 fee for a standard annual Costco membership is not required.	Standard (6 to 11 days) free 2 to 6 day $6.95 Overnight $8.95	Online prescriptions may be picked up at any warehouse. Membership isn't required if prescriptions are shipped to your home.
CVS Washington	http://www.cvs.com/ (888) 607-4287 (401) 233-7059 Fax	Yes	None	Standard (5 to 10 days) $3.95 if prescription is less than $40. Over $40, shipping is free. 2nd-day $9.95 Overnight $14.95	Good info provided on the Web site. Customers may ask pharmacist questions. Bills most insurance plans. Records maintained for receipts needed for tax purposes and insurance billing.
Drugstore.com and Rite-Aid	http://www.drugstore.com/ (800) 378-4786 (800) 373-6013 Fax	Yes	None	Standard (10-12 days) free 3-day $5.95 2-day $8.95 Overnight $16.95	Questions answered by a pharmacist. Bills most insurance companies. Records maintained for receipts for taxes. Prescriptions may be sent through the mail or picked up at any Rite-Aid. If you pick up at Rite-Aid, you will pay the Rite-Aid price.
Express Pharmacy Services/Eckerd .com	http://www.eckerd.com/ (800) 325-3737 (800) 323-0161 Fax	Yes	None	Free via UPS ground (14 days) 2nd-day delivery $7.95 Overnight $10.95	Good information provided on the Web site. Customers may ask pharmacists questions. Bills most insurance plans. You may either pick up your prescription at one of their stores or have it sent through the mail. Site warns that the online price will not be what you pay if you pick up at the store, but it's safe to assume that the store price will be higher.

Name	How to Contact	VIPPS	Membership or Service Fees	Shipping & Handling Fees	Comments
Familymeds.com	http://www.familymeds.com/ (888) 787-2800 (888) 787-2822 Fax	Yes	None	Standard (10 to 14 days) free 2nd-day $8.95 Overnight $12.95	Good information provided on Web site. Able to ask pharmacist questions. Takes a long time to get through on the telephone.
GLD Pharmaceuticals	http://www.gldpharmacy.com/ (888) 692-6928 (888) 692-6925 Fax	No	None	Standard (7 to 10 days) free 3rd-day $3.50 2nd-day $15.99 Overnight $29.95	No insurance billing provided. Pharmacists are available to answer questions. Claims savings of up to 70%.
Longs Drugs	http://www.longs.com/ (800) 865-6647 no fax is available	No	None	Standard (3 to 5 business days) $1.95 2nd-day $7.95 Overnight $14.95	Pharmacists are available to answer questions. Bills most insurance plans. Prescriptions must be called or mailed in. Faxed prescriptions are not allowed. Prescriptions may be picked up at a Longs store for a higher price.
Postal Prescription Services	http://www.ppsrx.com (800) 552-6694 (800) 723-9023 Fax	No	Available only through membership or through medical insurance drug benefit. There is a one time $10 membership fee	Standard (2 weeks) free 2nd-day $8.50 Overnight $23.50	No price quotes appeared to be available online. Pharmacists are available to answer questions. Services uninsured customers and those with insurance. Bills most insurance plans.
PrecisionRX	http://www.precisionrx.com/ (800) 905-9818 (800) 905-9815 Fax	No	None	Standard (14 days) via U.S. mail or UPS 3rd-day $8 2nd-day $10 Overnight $15	Bills some insurance plans. Pharmacists are available to answer questions. Prefers that the customer arrange for the doctor to contact the pharmacy.
Prescriptions By Mail	http://www.prescriptionsbymail.com/ (888) 726-4496 (877) 906-7005 Fax	No	None	Standard (14 days) free 2nd-day $12.50 Overnight $25	Good information provided on Web site. Pharmacist is available to answer questions. Pet supplies are available.
RXMPSS	http://www.rxmpss.com/ (800) 438-2014 (402) 342-4425 Fax	No	None	Standard (5 days) free 2nd-day $3.75 Overnight $12.45	Provides a 24-hour help desk. Pharmacist is available to answer questions. Very user-friendly Web site.
Walgreens	http://www.walgreens.com/ (877) 345-1985 (800) 332-9581 Fax	Yes	None	Standard (2 weeks) $1.95 2nd-day $5.95 Overnight $12.95	Good info provided on the Web site. Pharmacists are available to answer questions. Bills most insurance plans.
"Your Plan" by Merck Medco	http://www.yourplan.com/ (877) 733-6765 (888) 327-9791 Fax	Yes	Available only through membership or medical-insurance drug benefit. Fees for membership in Your Plan are $25 per year for one person, $40 for a family.	Standard (11 business days) free 3rd-day $9 2nd-day and overnight not available.	Very cumbersome and difficult to get through to a real person if you have a problem. Prices for prescription drugs are said to be 12% to 20% less than traditional pharmacy prices.

organizations, however, and it's known for its strong consumer advocacy positions and actions. And AARP's low annual fee covers access to a range of other discounts and services, as well.

VIRTUAL PHARMACIES: WHAT YOU NEED TO KNOW

Technology makes life easier in many ways, and it can make life less expensive, too. Be sure to evaluate carefully the integrity of the source you choose. Remember the adage, "If it sounds too good to be true, then it usually is."

Keep the following tips in mind when you shop for medications on the Internet:

+ When buying drugs online, make sure the Web site carries the VIPPS seal of approval. If it doesn't, confirm the pharmacy's credibility or shop elsewhere.
+ When your drugs will be shipped to you via street mail or parcel delivery service (such as FedEx or UPS), make sure you know the shipping charges, times, and conditions.
+ Know where the Internet pharmacy is based. Sites not located in the U.S. are not bound by U.S. regulatory oversight. Although at present Internet pharmacies located in Canada often offer the biggest savings, there are risks to consider. (See Chapter 4, "Savings on Drugs Across the Border.")
+ Check our Web site for updates on prescription and over-the-counter drugs at http://www.smartbuysdrugwise.com.

Savings on Drugs Across the Border

Prescription drugs are dramatically cheaper in Canada and Mexico. For many years, Americans have traveled across both borders to take advantage of these savings. Now they can even order Canadian drugs via Internet mail-order pharmacies.

This chapter provides you with all you need to know to take advantage of these low drug prices while avoiding problems and pitfalls.

NORTH OF THE BORDER: BUYING DRUGS IN CANADA

Drugs are significantly cheaper in Canada than name-brand counterparts sold in America. In fact, though, most of them come from American manufacturers. Canadian price controls and increase limits allow Canadian pharmacies to buy and sell American name-brand drugs far more cheaply than their U.S. counterparts. Although savings average about 50 percent across the spectrum of prescription drugs, it's possible to save as much as 60 to 80 percent on many drugs you buy there.

Americans can take advantage of these savings in two ways. They can cross the Canadian border and purchase drugs in person at a Canadian pharmacy, or they can buy drugs via the Internet from mail-order pharmacies located in Canada.

TRAVELING NORTH

Every month, we hear stories in the news about senior citizens groups who travel to Canada to find big savings on prescription drugs. Savings range from hundreds of dollars for drugs such as Zocor, which lowers blood cholesterol levels, to a thousand dollars or more for drugs such as the breast-cancer medication Tamoxifen. Sixty tablets of Tamoxifen 10mg that costs $156 at a drugstore in the U.S. are only $13 in Canada! If you take multiple prescription drugs, as many older Americans must, your savings can add up to hundreds or even thousands of dollars.

On average, Canadian drugs are only half the price of their American equivalents. Even more surprising is the number of generic versions of name-brand drugs available in Canada that aren't sold in the U.S. Among the 50 commonly prescribed drugs we surveyed, seven were available as generics in the U.S., while were available in generic forms in Canada—at significant savings, of course.

Commonly Prescribed Name-Brand Drugs Available in U.S. and Canada

DRUG	STRENGTH	QUANTITY	COMMON USE	TYPICAL U.S.PRICE	TYPICAL CANADIAN PRICE (IN U.S.DOLLARS)	YOU SAVE
Accupril (quinapril)	20mg	30	High blood pressure	$34.69	$25.24	27%
Actos (pioglitazone)	15mg	30	Diabetes	$104.99	$63.61	39%
Allegra (fexofenadine)	60mg	60	Allergies	$82.24	$33.06	60%
Altace (ramipril)	5mg	30	High blood pressure	$45.39	$28.25	38%
Amaryl (glimepiride)	4mg	30	Diabetes	$29.99	$26.64	11%
Augmentin (amoxicillin with clavulanic acid)	500mg	20	Bacterial infections	$96.99	$30.06	69%
Avandia (rosiglitazone)	4mg	30	Diabetes	$89.49	$60.69	33%
Celebrex (celecoxib)	200mg	60	Arthritis	$172.34	$72.07	58%
Celexa (citalopram)	20mg	30	Depression	$73.17	$39.85	46%
Cipro (ciprofloxacin)	500mg	20	Bacterial infections	$96.79	$44.95	54%
Claritin (loratadine)	10mg	30	Allergies	$83.49	$29.77	64%
Coumadin (warfarin)	5mg	30	Blood thinner	$30.19	$15.72	48%
Cozaar (losartan)	50mg	30	High blood pressure	$49.29	$36.77	25%
Effexor XR (venlafaxine)	150mg	30	Depression	$84.79	$50.16	41%
Evista (raloxifene)	60mg	30	Osteoporosis	$76.99	$48.50	37%
Flonase Nasal Spray (fluticasone)	50mcg	1 bottle	Sinus congestion	$57.99	$28.94	50%

DRUG	STRENGTH	QUANTITY	COMMON USE	TYPICAL U.S. PRICE	TYPICAL CANADIAN PRICE (IN U.S. DOLLARS)	YOU SAVE
Flovent oral inhaler (fluticasone)	220mcg	1 inhaler	Asthma	$104.19	$68.42	34%
Fosamax (alendronate)	10mg	30	Osteoporosis	$69.99	$57.59	18%
Glucophage (metformin)	500mg	60	Diabetes	$50.99	$20.01	61%
Lanoxin (digoxin)	0.25mg	30	Congestive heart failure	$14.99	$12.99	13%
Levaquin (levofloxacin)	500mg	10	Infections	$96.99	$51.20	47%
Lipitor (atorvastatin)	20mg	30	High cholesterol	$97.24	$58.57	40%
Lotensin (benazepril)	10mg	30	High blood pressure	$39.99	$26.78	33%
Monopril (fosinopril)	10mg	30	High blood pressure	$44.79	$26.23	41%
Neurontin (gabapentin)	300mg	60	Epilepsy and neuropathy	$84.99	$57.36	33%
Norvasc (amlodipine)	5mg	30	High blood pressure	$47.94	$34.35	28%
Ortho Tri-Cyclen (norgestimate with ethinyl estradiol)	N/A	1 pack	Oral contraceptive	$33.54	$26.54	21%
Paxil (paroxetine)	20mg	30	Depression	$89.79	$48.38	46%
Plavix (clopidogrel)	75mg	30	Blocks platelet aggregation	$125.49	$70.99	43%
Pravachol (pravastatin)	20mg	30	High cholesterol	$79.99	$58.26	27%
Premarin (conjugated estrogens)	0.625mg	30	Estrogen replacement therapy	$26.80	$11.08	59%
Prempro (conjugated estrogen with medroxy progesterone)	0.625/2.5mg	1 pack	Estrogen and progestin replacement therapy	$42.22	$22.55	47%
Prevacid (lansoprazole)	30mg	30	Stomach acid	$135.99	$57.02	58%
Prilosec (omeprazole) called Losec in Canada	20mg	30	Stomach acid	$128.59	$66.17	49%
Prinivil (lisinopril)	10mg	30	High blood pressure	$39.99	$29.69	26%

DRUG	STRENGTH	QUANTITY	COMMON USE	TYPICAL U.S. PRICE	TYPICAL CANADIAN PRICE (IN U.S. DOLLARS)	YOU SAVE
Protonix (pantoprazole)	40mg	30	Stomach acid	$89.79	$56.25	37%
Prozac (fluoxetine)	20mg	30	Depression	$98.19	$48.62	50%
Risperdal (risperidone)	2mg	60	Psychosis	$139.99	$113.20	19%
Serevent oral inhaler(salmeterol)	25mcg	1 inhaler	Asthma	$78.99	$50.40	36%
Singulair (montelukast)	10mg	30	Asthma	$89.49	$60.13	33%
Synthroid (levothyroxine)	0.1mg	100	Thyroid supplement	$35.69	$15.36	57%
Viagra (sildenafil)	100mg	10	Erectile dysfunction	$102.49	$89.99	12%
Vioxx (rofecoxib)	25mg	30	Arthritis	$93.14	$39.47	58%
Wellbutrin SR (bupropion)	150mg	60	Depression	$104.19	$49.87	52%
Zestril (lisinopril)	10mg	30	High blood pressure	$40.69	$29.73	27%
Zithromax (azithromycin)	250mg	6	Bacterial infections	$53.04	$32.69	38%
Zocor (simvastatin)	20mg	30	High cholesterol	$148.59	$63.50	57%
Zoloft (sertraline)	100mg	30	Depression	$74.99	$49.00	35%
Zyprexa (olanzapine)	5mg	30	Psychosis	$179.99	$93.27	48%
Zyrtec (cetirizine) called Reactine in Canada	10mg	30	Allergies	$70.64	$30.90	56%

What's going on? Why are the generic companies allowed to put products on the market in Canada but not in the U.S.? Don't patent laws apply everywhere?

Surprisingly, they don't.

In order to have its patent honored in Canada—or in any other country—a drug company must apply to the government of that country for a "unique patent." Although treaties currently in place speed and simplify this process, most countries also require that a patented product be manufactured in its own country within at least three years of receiving the patent; otherwise, the patent may become void. Hence, most drug companies opt to forgo their patent rights outside the U.S. The cost of locating a factory in every country to maintain a patent is just too great.

This means most of the name-brand drugs you pay big money for in the U.S. are available in Canada in cheaper generic versions. It also means that, because many of the drugs you buy in Canada are manufactured here, they're exactly the same drugs you'd get if you bought them from an American pharmacy. Often even the labeling is the same!

> ### Check the Currency Exchange

The currency exchange rate affects the actual cost of drugs you buy in Canada. Since the late 1990s, the exchange rate has been very favorable for Americans spending American currency in Canada, running from 35 percent to as high as nearly 60 percent at times. A 35 percent exchange rate means that $1 American is worth $1.35 Canadian. The rate changes daily; any commercial bank can give you the current rate. Often credit card purchases receive the most favorable exchange rates. Check with your card's issuing financial institution to be sure. And remember to convert Canadian prices to American dollars before you compare them to those for products available in the U.S. The Canadian dollar amount may look much higher until you factor in the exchange rate.

THE LEGALITIES OF IMPORTING DRUGS INTO THE U.S.

Every country has laws regulating the purchase and use of drugs and controlled substances, such as narcotics. In the U.S., the Food and Drug Administration (FDA) is responsible for regulating the drugs we can import from foreign countries. Foreign-made drugs that haven't received FDA approval can't be imported into the U.S. legally.

However, according to the FDA document *Coverage of Personal Importations,* "FDA personnel may use their own discretion to allow entry of shipments of violative FDA regulated products when the quantity and purpose are clearly for personal use, and the product does not present an unreasonable risk to the user."

For years, efforts have been made on Capitol Hill to make it legal for Americans to purchase drugs from Canada for their own use. In 2000, Congress passed a bill not only allowing individuals to re-import U.S.-made drugs from Canada, but also allowing pharmacies to re-import such drugs and sell them in the U.S. at reduced prices. Although President Clinton signed the bill, his Secretary of Health and Human Services, citing "serious flaws and loopholes," refused to enforce the measure. Congressional efforts to pass another, enforceable, measure continue.

So, strictly speaking, it's not legal at this time for you to go to Canada, get your prescriptions filled, and bring them back home, or to order drugs from a Canadian pharmacy and have them shipped to your home. And, although the FDA does have authority to exercise discretion and allow you to purchase drugs from Canada for your own use, it has issued no formal policy statement giving you a go-ahead.

In actual practice, the FDA seems sympathetic to the plight of elderly Americans who shoulder most of the burden of high drug prices. At the time of this writing, the FDA doesn't interfere as Americans routinely cross the border with small quantities of American-made drugs purchased in Canada, and even order and receive prescriptions from Canadian pharmacies by mail-order or via the Internet. A recent NBC newscast quoted an unnamed FDA official as saying the FDA "looks the other way," because "we don't want to punish seniors."

American pharmacies and drug manufacturers complain loudly and often about the revenues they lose because so many people buy their drugs from foreign countries. So be forewarned. Before you decide to purchase prescriptions from Canada, you should understand and accept the possibility that the FDA, under pressure from the pharmaceutical industry, could crack down at any time with tough enforcement measures. If that happens, your drug purchase could be confiscated at the border, and you could lose the money you paid.

If you feel, as many American do, that U.S. pharmaceutical companies are guilty of price gouging, and that you should have the legal right to purchase prescription drugs from Canada, make your opinion heard by writing to your elected representatives in Washington.

Perhaps Congress will enact a law in the not-too-distant future that allows you to share in the drug price advantages Canadians enjoy. In the meantime, though, as long as vast cost disparities and inequities exist, Americans in large numbers are likely to continue crossing borders in search of the lower prices.

TRADITIONAL PHARMACIES IN CANADA

If you live near the Canadian border, the best way to cash in on Canada's low drug prices is to travel to a Canadian pharmacy in person. Until recently, all you needed to buy your drugs in Canada was a prescription from your American doctor. Now Canada has tightened its rules. If you, as an American, want to purchase drugs in Canada, you'll need to have a prescription written by a Canadian doctor, and most Canadian doctors won't write prescriptions for you unless they examine you. To play by the rules, you'll need to find a Canadian doctor who'll see you and rewrite the prescriptions that your U.S. doctor wants you to take.

Here are some ways to find a Canadian doctor.

1. If you live near the Canadian border, ask your U.S. doctor if he or she knows any Canadian physicians to refer you to.
2. Check the "courtesy services" listings in Canadian hotels and motels. Many include telephone numbers for local physicians who will provide medical care for foreign visitors.
3. Look in the telephone directory. (A number of directories are available via the Internet.)
4. If you can visit a Canadian pharmacy, ask the pharmacist to recommend a physician.
5. Contact a Canadian provincial or local medical association for a list of Canadian doctors who provide services for non-Canadians.

It may seem like overkill to see doctors in both the U.S. and Canada, but doing so can make for considerable savings. For example, suppose you're taking Glucophage 500mg for diabetes. Because you take 2 tablets a day, you need 60 tablets to last you one month. A typical price for this amount in the U.S. is around $49. In Canada, it's just under $11. Your annual cost for this prescription through a U.S. drugstore will be $588, but in Canada it's just $132! The cost of having a Canadian doctor examine you is a small price to pay for such huge savings.

An alternative to traveling to Canada is to find a physician practicing in the U.S. who is licensed in Canada, as well. Unfortunately, no directory exists for this, and there's no easy way to identify one; most people locate them by word-of-mouth. These physicians will review your medications and rewrite your prescriptions under their Canadian licensure and fax the prescriptions to a Canadian pharmacy, which will set up an account for you, bill you (usually requiring credit card payment), and mail you your prescriptions.

MAIL-ORDER AND INTERNET PHARMACIES IN CANADA

Opportunities are multiplying for savings using mail-order and Internet pharmacies based in Canada. These sources fill prescriptions from U.S. doctors and ship the drugs directly to you. Some of these pharmacies are Web-site extensions of traditional stores,

Canadian Mail-Order and Internet Pharmacies

WEB SITE	PHONE NUMBER	MEDICAL RECORDS REVIEW CHARGE	SHIPPING AND HANDLING FEES (IN U.S. DOLLARS)	COMMENTS
canadameds.com	(877) 542-3330	None	$13	Good links available. Online shipment tracking available.
canadianmedsusa.com	(877) 933-0505	None	$10 per package	Transactions conducted through U.S. location. Charges 1% service fee for personal checks.
canadarx.com	(866) 262-2174	None	$13	Online shipment tracking available.
crossborderpharmacy.com	(888) 626-0696	None	$10	Online tracking available. Offers many of the best prices.
doctorsolve.com (Web site provides information only; you must order by mail or phone)	(866) 732-0305	$39	$20	Advertises savings of up to 90%. Very limited price quotes available online. Request prices by phone.
healthmeds.com	(866) 444-6337	None	$10	Provides excellent information about healthcare and related matters.
realfastdrugstore.com	(866) 412-6262	None	$10 for the first prescription, $3 for each additional prescription.	Price quotes are available only through e-mail.
thecanadiandrugstore.com	(888) 372-2252	None	$12 for the first 2 prescriptions, $6 for each additional prescription.	Long list of drugs that aren't available. Very limited number of drug prices available online.

others are Internet-based operations, and at least one is mail-order only. All allow you to transact business by phone, mail, fax, or online. Typically, they'll ask you to sign forms that constitute authorization (a limited power of attorney) that gives the pharmacy the right to act on your behalf—to have a Canadian physician review your medical history and your prescriptions, and to fill and mail you your prescriptions. Some Canadian online pharmacies charge for this review, but most don't. If this option interests you, telephone the pharmacy for more information. That's what we did, and we were surprised to discover huge differences among mail-order and Internet pharmacies—from prices to levels of service. To help you narrow the field, we provide you with a list of what we feel are the cream of the crop. You may recognize the names of some of these Web sites, such as Doctorsolve.com. Doctorsolve.com is good, but there may be better choices.

We made our selections based on which and how many services were offered, how user-friendly the site is, the amount and quality of its information, how many and how valuable the links are, and how easy it is to reach a real person on the phone. Then we considered fees and prices to make our Smart Buy recommendations. To explore the possibility of purchasing your drugs from Canada over the Internet, or by mail or phone, look over the pharmacy's Web site carefully, or call and request printed information. Prices for individual drugs can vary substantially from one pharmacy to another, so compare.

One interesting difference between U.S.-based mail-order and Internet pharmacies and those based in Canada is that Canadian mail-order and Internet prices tend to be higher than those in Canadian brick-and-mortar pharmacies. If you live near the border, it might be worth your while to make the trip to a Canadian pharmacy, at least to compare prices.

$ SMART BUY
Canadian Mail-Order and Internet Pharmacies

Crossborderpharmacy.com is the Smart Buy among Canadian-based mail-order and Internet pharmacies. It offers most of the best prices, the shipping fee is low, there's no doctor fee, you can transact business at its Web site or via mail or telephone, and the Web site offers online tracking, so you can check the status of your order.

Savings can be phenomenal. Doctorsolve.com, for example, advertises 90 tablets of the cholesterol-lowering drug Lipitor 20mg for $134, compared to $250 in the U.S.

Be aware of these key points:

1. Factor in the cost of a medical records/history exam when you compare prices. Say you can buy your Lipitor for $134 (U.S. dollars). Even if you must pay $39 U.S. for an "exam" and another $20 for shipping and handling, you're still ahead of the U.S. price.

2. If your health insurance covers prescription drugs, it won't pay for drugs you receive through Canadian sources.

3. Canadian pharmacies may not ship prescriptions for controlled substances, such as narcotics, to the U.S.

4. Not all drugs available in the U.S. are available in Canada, so check the Web sites for current drug listings.

5. It takes one to two weeks for Canadian online pharmacies to process prescriptions. If you have a prescription for a drug you must start taking right away, get one prescription from your doctor to fill at a local pharmacy and another you can send to the Canadian pharmacy.

There has been much discussion on both sides of the border about the appropriateness of buying prescription drugs in this way. Health organizations in both countries have expressed concern about the ethics of doctors in Canada writing prescriptions without physically examining patients, citing the risks of incomplete medical records. Because Canadian authorities are moving toward tightening regulations and guidelines, it's uncertain at this time how much longer Internet purchases from Canadian drugstores will continue to be an option for Americans.

Prescription Drugs Need a Prescription!

As in the U.S., a drug that requires a prescription from a doctor requires a prescription from a doctor—period. Any mail-order or Internet pharmacy based in Canada that offers to sell prescription drugs without a prescription is operating in violation of Canadian law.

$ SMART BUY
Buying Drugs in Canada

It's hard to beat the prices you can find in Canada, if you can accommodate the inconveniences of getting them. In general, the Smart Options for Savings that apply for drug purchases in the U.S. also apply to drug purchases in Canada. Finding a doctor in the U.S. who's also licensed in Canada gives you the best of both worlds: You keep your regular doctor who oversees and manages your medical care, you don't have to travel out of the country, and you can have your prescriptions sent right to your home—all in absolute compliance with current regulations in both countries.

Price Savings from Mail-Order and Internet Pharmacies in Canada

DRUG	STRENGTH	QUANTITY	COMMON USE	TYPICAL U.S. PHARMACY PRICE	TYPICAL U.S. GENERIC PRICE (IF AVAILABLE)	TYPICAL CANADIAN MAIL-ORDER /INTERNET PRICE (IN U.S.DOLLARS)	TYPICAL CANADIAN GENERIC PRICE (IN U.S. DOLLARS)
Accupril (quinapril)	20mg	30	High blood pressure	$34.69	N/A	$25.24	N/A
Actos (pioglitazone)	15mg	30	Diabetes	$104.99	N/A	$63.61	N/A
Allegra (fexofenadine)	60mg	60	Allergies	$82.24	N/A	$33.06	N/A
Altace (ramipril)	5mg	30	High blood pressure	$45.39	N/A	$28.25	N/A
Amaryl (glimepiride)	4mg	30	Diabetes	$29.99	N/A	$26.64	N/A
Augmentin (amoxicillin with clavulanic acid)	500mg	20	Bacterial infections	$96.99	N/A	$30.06	$22.27
Avandia (rosiglitazone)	4mg	30	Diabetes	$89.49	N/A	$60.69	N/A
Celebrex (celecoxib)	200mg	60	Arthritis	$172.34	N/A	$72.07	N/A
Celexa (citalopram)	20mg	30	Depression	$73.17	N/A	$39.85	N/A
Cipro (ciprofloxacin)	500mg	20	Bacterial infections	$96.79	N/A	$44.95	N/A
Claritin (loratadine)	10mg	30	Allergies	$83.49	N/A	$29.77	$24.52
Coumadin (warfarin)	5mg	30	Blood thinner	$30.19	$20.49	$15.72	$13.77
Cozaar (losartan)	50mg	30	High blood pressure	$49.29	N/A	$36.77	N/A
Effexor XR (venlafaxine)	150mg	30	Depression	$84.79	N/A	$50.16	N/A
Evista (raloxifene)	60mg	30	Osteoporosis	$76.99	N/A	$48.50	N/A
Flonase Nasal Spray(fluticasone)	50mcg	1 bottle	Sinus congestion	$57.99	N/A	$28.94	N/A
Flovent oral inhaler (fluticasone)	220mcg	1 inhaler	Asthma	$104.19	N/A	$68.42	N/A
Fosamax (alendronate)	10mg	30	Osteoporosis	$69.99	N/A	$57.59	N/A
Glucophage (metformin)	500mg	60	Diabetes	$50.99	$32.99	$20.01	$11.30
Lanoxin (digoxin)	0.25mg	30	Congestive heart failure	$14.99	$9.99	$12.99	$7.99

DRUG	STRENGTH	QUANTITY	COMMON USE	TYPICAL U.S. PHARMACY PRICE	TYPICAL U.S. GENERIC PRICE (IF AVAILABLE)	TYPICAL CANADIAN MAIL-ORDER /INTERNET PRICE (IN U.S.DOLLARS)	TYPICAL CANADIAN GENERIC PRICE (IN U.S. DOLLARS)
Levaquin (levofloxacin)	500mg	10	Infections	$96.99	N/A	$51.20	N/A
Lipitor (atorvastatin)	20mg	30	High cholesterol	$97.24	N/A	$58.57	N/A
Lotensin (benazepril)	10mg	30	High blood pressure	$39.99	N/A	$26.78	N/A
Monopril (fosinopril)	10mg	30	High blood pressure	$44.79	N/A	$26.23	N/A
Neurontin (gabapentin)	300mg	60	Epilepsy and neuropathy	$84.99	N/A	$57.36	46.88
Norvasc (amlodipine)	5mg	30	High blood pressure	$47.94	N/A	$34.35	N/A
Ortho Tri-Cyclen (norgestimate with ethinyl estradiol)	N/A	1 pack	Oral contraceptive	$33.54	N/A	$26.54	N/A
Paxil (paroxetine)	20mg	30	Depression	$89.79	N/A	$48.38	N/A
Plavix (clopidogrel)	75mg	30	Blocks platelet aggregation	$125.49	N/A	$70.99	N/A
Pravachol (pravastatin)	20mg	30	High cholesterol	$79.99	N/A	$58.26	$39.29
Premarin) (conjugated estrogens)	0.625mg	30	Estrogen replacement therapy	$26.80	N/A	$11.08	N/A
Prempro (conjugated estrogen with medroxypro-gesterone)	0.625 /2.5mg	1 pack	Estrogen and progestin replacement therapy	$42.22	N/A	$22.55	N/A
Prevacid) (lansoprazole	30mg	30	Stomach acid	$135.99	N/A	$57.02	N/A
Prilosec (omeprazole) called Losec in Canada	20mg	30	Stomach acid	$128.59	N/A	$66.17	N/A
Prinivil (lisinopril)	10mg	30	High blood pressure	$39.99	$29.99	$29.69	$27.05
Protonix (pantoprazole)	40mg	30	Stomach acid	$89.79	N/A	$56.25	N/A
Prozac (fluoxetine)	20mg	30	Depression	$98.19	$47.99	$48.62	$32.90
Risperdal (risperidone)	2mg	60	Psychosis	$139.99	N/A	$113.20	N/A

DRUG	STRENGTH	QUANTITY	COMMON USE	TYPICAL U.S. PHARMACY PRICE	TYPICAL U.S. GENERIC PRICE (IF AVAILABLE)	TYPICAL CANADIAN MAIL-ORDER /INTERNET PRICE (IN U.S.DOLLARS)	TYPICAL CANADIAN GENERIC PRICE (IN U.S. DOLLARS)
Serevent oral inhaler (salmeterol)	25mcg	1 inhaler	Asthma	$78.99	N/A	$50.40	N/A
Singulair (montelukast)	10mg	30	Asthma	$89.49	N/A	$60.13	N/A
Synthroid (levothyroxine)	0.1mg	100	Thyroid supplement	$35.69	$24.99	$15.36	$12.48
Viagra (sildenafil)	100mg	10	Erectile dysfunction	$102.49	N/A	$89.99	N/A
Vioxx (rofecoxib)	25mg	30	Arthritis	$93.14	N/A	$39.47	N/A
Wellbutrin SR (bupropion)	150mg	60	Depression	$104.19	N/A	$49.87	N/A
Zestril (lisinopril)	10mg	30	High blood pressure	$40.69	$29.99	$29.73	$24.29

$ SMART OPTIONS FOR SAVINGS
Buying Prescription Drugs in Canada

Buying drugs in Canada can cut your prescription costs to a fraction of what you'd pay in the U.S. Here are some tips for making sure you get all the benefits available:

1 Carefully evaluate the integrity of the source you choose—whether it's a physical pharmacy, a mail-order or Internet pharmacy, or a third-party facilitator.
2 Don't take any drug your doctor hasn't prescribed for you.
3 You're on more solid ground legally in Canada if you obtain an examination and written prescription from a Canadian physician.
4 Stay within the limits on the quantities of drugs you can bring back into the U.S.

SOUTH OF THE BORDER: GETTING DRUGS FROM MEXICO

Because it borders the southwestern U.S., Mexico offers an enticing opportunity for Americans to find bargains of all kinds, and drugs are no exception. The very low prices in Mexico can be an irresistible draw. We want to make it clear from the start: We recommend that you do not buy drugs in Mexico. We consider Mexico here only because we know many Americans already buy drugs there to save money. If they get what they think they're getting, then they do save money. But if not, as is often the case, then they might as well just throw their money—and their health—away.

One reason Mexican drugs are so inexpensive is that Mexico is considered a developing country. American drug manufacturers sell at deep discounts because that's what the Mexican economy will support. But because controls and manufacturing standards are lax in Mexico, drugs made within that country are often of questionable quality and may not be what you think they are. Many drugs available in Mexico contain ingredients not found in American versions with the same names, and some drugs are produced in combinations that don't exist elsewhere. And the sale of counterfeit drugs—drugs made to look like the real deal but which might contain none of the genuine drug's active ingredients—is a huge problem. They might be cheap by American standards, but counterfeit drugs make a lot of money for unethical sellers in Mexico.

Language can be a barrier, as well. Spanish drug names can be tricky, and many times the person selling the product doesn't speak English, so you're on your own. If you don't read the label carefully, or if you can't read the Spanish names, serious problems can result. Many drugs that require prescriptions in the U.S. are available without a prescription or without even seeing a doctor in Mexico. Although at first this might seem like a blessing, it can easily be a health risk. Understanding potential side effects and drug interactions is essential. (Later chapters in this book cover these issues in detail.) If you live near the Mexican border, speak fluent Spanish, and are convinced you're knowledgeable enough to separate the opportunity from the opportunist, be sure that you

> ...check the active ingredients, which should resemble or match the drug name or generic name of its U.S. counterpart.
> ...confirm that the product was made in the U.S. (and don't buy it if you can't or it wasn't).
> ...look for an expiration date (and don't buy the drug if there isn't one or if it has passed).
> ...take *nothing* your doctor hasn't prescribed for you.

Most people find ways to save money safely without heading to Mexico to buy their prescription drugs. You can, too.

We offer no Smart Buy recommendation here because we believe buying drugs in Mexico is an unacceptable option.

Chapter 5

When You Can't Afford to Buy the Prescription Drugs You Need

E very week, thousands of Americans must choose between buying their medications and putting food on the table. It's an unfair, no-win situation. Fortunately, a number of avenues exist for those who are genuinely in need to get the medications they need at low (or even no) cost.

DRUG COMPANY PATIENT ASSISTANCE PROGRAMS

Believe it or not, the very drug companies that want to take your money—so *much* of your money—have a compassionate side. More than 100 pharmaceutical manufacturers offer free medications for those who can't afford to buy them. So why, you might ask, do so many people go without the drugs they need? Mostly because they don't know this help is available.

Drug companies don't hide these programs, but they don't exactly promote them, either. Each company's program is different, sometimes because of its product line. Some provide maintenance medications for as long as you need them and continue to meet the qualification criteria. Others provide a time-limited supply, typically 90 days. Each drug company's qualifying criteria are different, but most require that you

...have no insurance coverage for prescription drugs.
...meet income guidelines (usually tied to federal poverty guidelines).
...have your doctor contact the drug company.

Drug Company Patient Assistance Programs

MANUFACTURER	TELEPHONE NUMBER	GUIDELINES	COMMENTS
Abbott	(800) 222-6855	1. Physician calls to request an enrollment form. 2. Doctor completes and signs the form. 3. Patient must sign the form and provide financial and insurance information. 4. Form is mailed to the address shown (no prescription needed). 5. Medicine is sent to the doctor's office. 6. Patient picks up medicine from the doctor.	This program is only for low-income patients who have no prescription insurance coverage. If the patient doesn't meet these guidelines, rejection letter from Medicaid is required.
Bayer Corporation Pharmaceutical Division	(800) 998-9180	Anyone may call to enroll. 1. Over the telephone, provide physician's name, address, and DEA number. 2. Also, provide patient's name, address, phone number, Social Security number, and date of birth. 3. Provide household size, annual income, and monthly out-of-pocket expenses. 4. Operator will inform caller of approval or denial. 5. Application is sent to the physician with a pharmacy card. 6. Patient may take the card to any pharmacy to obtain the medication.	Applicant must be a U.S. citizen, have no insurance coverage for prescription drugs, and must be taking the drug for FDA approved indication. Further, applicant annual income must be at or below the Federal Poverty Level.
Boehringer-Ingelheim Pharmaceuticals	(800) 556-8317	1. Anyone may call for an application. 2. Physician must submit a prescription with the application. 3. Patients must provide documentation of income. 4. Mail application to address on the form. 5. Medication is sent to the physician's office. 6. Patient picks up medication from doctor.	Applicant must be a U.S. citizen ineligible for prescription insurance coverage. Product must meet approved label indications and recommended dosage. Maximum 3-month supply may be provided for each request. Patient must reapply every year.
Bristol-Myers Squibb	(800) 736-0003 (800) 344-8792 Fax	1. Physician's office may call to obtain a form. 2. Physician and patient complete the form. Doctor must provide a DEA number and sign the form. 3. Patient must provide financial information. 4. Form may be mailed or faxed. 5. The doctor and the patient are notified by mail of application status. 6. Medication is sent to the doctor's office.	Applicant must be a U.S. citizen or a legal resident. For quicker service, the manufacturer recommends faxing forms instead of mailing. Patient may receive 90 days of medication at one time. A new application form must be submitted every 180 days of assistance.
Eli Lilly and Company	(800) 545-6962	1. Physician calls to obtain a form. 2. Physician must fill out a prescription and provide information. A DEA number is required. 3. Patient must provide information and sign the form. 4. Medication is sent to the doctor's office. 5. Patient picks up medication from the doctor.	Applicant must be a U.S. resident unable to afford medication and without prescription insurance and must be an outpatient (not in a hospital or nursing facility). Call to see whether the needed drug is available. Quantity is determined by the type of product prescribed.

MANUFACTURER	TELEPHONE NUMBER	GUIDELINES	COMMENTS
Glaxo Wellcome	(800) 722-9294 (800) 750-9832 Fax	1. Patient calls to receive enrollment form. 2. Patient and doctor must fill out the form and mail into Glaxo. 3. Patient must designate a doctor, nurse, pharmacist or social worker as an advocate. 4. Advocate calls to supply information, obtain eligibility, and to receive initial authorization (usually within a few minutes). 5. Once approved, advocate is instructed by Glaxo to present the patient with a prescription benefit card (attached to the application). This card may be used at any local pharmacy to obtain the medication for a $5 or $10 co-payment.	Applicant must be a U.S. resident who is ineligible for private or government prescription assistance. Applicant must meet financial eligibility criteria. Enrollment form must be received within 30 days of the advocate's phone call. Initially only a 30-day supply of medication is authorized; 90-day increments are available with additional documentation.
Merck & Company	(800) 994-2111	1. Physician calls the company to obtain an application and must enter a DEA number to obtain a form. 2. Physician and patient complete and sign the form. 3. The physician must write a prescription to include with the form, which is then mailed to the program. 4. Medication is sent to the physician within weeks. 5. Patient picks up medication from physician.	This program is for low-income patients who have no prescription insurance coverage only. Refills are allowed, but a new application must be completed. Vaccines and injectable drugs aren't included.
Parke-Davis	(908) 725-1247	1. Physician must enroll the patient using enrollment form. 2. Physician must include a signature, DEA number, and a prescription with original signature. 3. Patient must fill out and sign the form, and mail to the address shown on the form. 4. Medication will be sent to the physician's office. 5. Patient picks up medication from doctor.	Program limited to those who can't qualify for local, state, or federal drug programs, and who aren't covered by any prescription insurance. Annual income for a single household must be less than $16,000, or $25,000 for a family. Patient must reapply four times a year. Benefit includes a three-month supply of medication. Allow six weeks for delivery.
Roche Pharmaceuticals	(800) 285-4484	1. Physician must call to obtain an application form. 2. Physician and patient must sign the form and the doctor's DEA number must be included. 3. Medication is sent to physician's office by FedEx within 48 hours. 4. Patient picks up medication from doctor.	Patient must be an outpatient to qualify. Cannot be eligible for any federal assistance for prescription drugs. Repeat requests require additional applications.
Schering Laboratories/Key Pharmaceuticals	(800) 656-9485	Anyone may call for an application form. 1. Physician must attach a prescription for three months of medication and sign the form. 2. Patient must fill out and sign the form. 3. Attach proof of income (zero income must be verified in writing by physician or social worker). 4. A maximum of three months of medication will be sent to the physician's office. 5. Patient picks up medication from the doctor.	Patient must not be eligible for insurance reimbursement and unable to afford treatment. Call for availability of drugs. Repeat requests require a new application, a new prescription, and current income documentation.

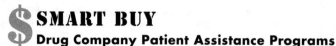

$ SMART BUY
Drug Company Patient Assistance Programs

The most important factor here is knowing that these programs exist. The Smart Buy is the program for which you qualify. Always ask your doctor how much a prescription will cost. If you can't afford the drug, ask your doctor whether less expensive options are available. If none exist, or if you can't afford even those, then ask your doctor to submit an application to the manufacturer's patient-assistance program. Remember, though, that these programs are for those who truly lack the resources to pay for prescription drugs.

IDENTIFYING PROGRAMS FOR WHICH YOU QUALIFY

Doctors don't always know which drug-company patient-assistance programs are available or what their criteria are. Several Internet-based services keep track of all these programs and can help you identify those for which you might qualify. They'll gather the forms that you and your doctor need to fill out and facilitate your application process. Some services charge a fee to cover administrative costs. Here are three that don't.

ASSISTANCE SERVICES

PROGRAM	SERVICES	FEE	COMMENTS
RxAssist http://www.rxassist.org	Comprehensive, up-to-date listing of manufacturer programs and their requirements.	None	Sponsored by the Robert Wood Johnson Foundation, a reputable agency that funds many health programs.
http://www.needymeds.com	Extensive listing of manufacturer programs and their requirements.	None	Maintains a very user-friendly Web site.
http://www.phrma.org/patients	Thorough listing of manufacturer programs and their requirements.	None	Sponsored by a national association of drug manufacturers; not as user-friendly as other sites.

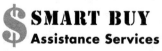

$ SMART BUY
Assistance Services

RxAssist is the Smart Buy among services that can help you identify drug-manufacturer assistance programs you may qualify for. It's user-friendly, doesn't charge for its assistance, and keeps a comprehensive and current list of assistance programs and their requirements. RxAssist will even help you complete the necessary paperwork. Check the Web site at http://www.rxassist.org/ for the latest information, qualifying criteria, and application procedures. If you don't have a computer, visit your local public library and ask a librarian for help in connecting with the Web site on a library computer.

Assistance for Veterans

Veterans honorably discharged from military service may receive prescription drugs at no charge through any Veteran's Administration (VA) hospital. The catch here is one of convenience: VA hospitals are located regionally. Unless you live nearby, your travel expenses could outweigh any savings you gain by using this service. You'll need to get an annual physical exam from a VA doctor, and a VA doctor must write your prescriptions. Several hundred VA hospitals and medical centers are located throughout the U.S.; every state has at least one. Call 877-222-8387 to find the VA medical center nearest you. The VA will send your drugs through the mail, or veterans who live near a VA hospital can pick up their prescriptions directly. Although any retail pharmacy can fill a prescription written by a VA doctor, it can't bill the VA for the drug's cost. The veteran must pay out-of-pocket and in full for the drug. Nonveterans can't fill prescriptions at VA hospital pharmacies.

Programs for Seniors

Despite all the political debate, Medicare still doesn't cover the cost of prescription drugs. About the only break seniors can get right now are the discounts, typically 10 percent, that many drugstores and pharmacies offer. A 2001 study conducted by the U.S. Government Accounting Office found that prescription drug plans that target seniors offer few, if any, tangible benefits. Most of the time, the plan saves only a few dollars at best—significant, perhaps, on prescriptions that cost under $10, but not especially helpful when the prescription runs $100 or more, as is often the case. And all too often the drugstore's purchase price is less than the plan's price or co-payment amount.

These plans attempt to offer seniors buying power. When a plan has a sufficient number of members, it can approach pharmacies and say, "If you agree to charge our customers our contract prices, we'll put you on our list of participating pharmacies, and you'll get our business." Small independent drugstores tend not to agree to this; they simply can't meet contract prices that often end up below their own cost for the drugs. Chain stores can afford to sign on, though, and they make money as a result. In fact, it's not uncommon for a chain drugstore's regular prices to be cheaper than the contract prices it agrees to charge plan members!

Anne brought in one of these plans to see whether it would save her money on Pravachol 40mg. She was surprised—and disappointed—to learn that her membership price was $11 *more* than the regular retail price—$117 through the plan and $106 without it.

The American Association of Retired Persons (AARP), the best-known assistance plan for seniors, has a membership large enough to lend it substantial bargaining power. The plan can obtain lower prices for its members on a vast number of items and services. Just $15 a year guarantees discounts on items ranging from airline tickets to life insurance, including contract pharmacy prices. Like any other plan, this seems like a good deal, and it probably is. Just don't be surprised if you don't save 50 percent on your prescription bills. Instead, expect $2 or $3 savings here and there. You may purchase your prescription drugs through AARP's Internet pharmacy (by telephone or on the Web site) or through your local pharmacy. In general, you'll save more when you use the online pharmacy.

Most other membership plans require you to pay a small monthly fee, usually less than $10, to take advantage of their contract pricing. The more prescriptions you buy, the more likely it is that such a plan will result in savings for you; three or more prescriptions a month seems to be the point at which you at least recoup any fees you've had to pay. If you fill few prescriptions, though, these plans are unlikely to save you money.

STATE PHARMACEUTICAL ASSISTANCE PROGRAMS

Some states sponsor pharmaceutical assistance programs of their own to help people who can't afford to buy the prescription drugs they need. These plans are separate from state welfare programs. Most are intended to aid seniors who meet the low-income criteria but who don't qualify for public assistance (welfare or Medicaid). Typically they charge some sort of co-payment or fee, so the drugs aren't free. And most state pharmaceutical programs cover only the drugs on their formularies, which can be quite restrictive.

State Pharmaceutical Assistance Programs

STATE	NAME OF PROGRAM	CONTACT NUMBER	ELIGIBILITY REQUIREMENTS	BENEFITS	FEES OR PREMIUMS	COMMENTS
California	Discount Prescription Medication Program	(800) 434-0222*	Applicant must qualify for Medicare.	Most prescription drugs are covered at a discounted price.	There is no fee to join this program.	Prices are guaranteed to be only 15 cents above what the state welfare program pays to pharmacies.
Connecticut	Connecticut Pharmaceutical Assistance Contract to the Elderly and Disabled (ConnPACE)	800) 423-5026*	Applicant: • must have resided in Connecticut in the preceding six months • must be 65 years of age or older, or over 18 and disabled • must earn an annual gross income of less than $20,000 (single), $27,100 (married) • must have no other prescription insurance coverage. Medicaid recipients are ineligible.	Covers most prescription drugs, as well as insulin and insulin syringes.	Annual registration fee of $25 per person. Co-payment of $12 each time a prescription is filled (new and refill).	Applications may be obtained at most pharmacies and senior centers. Drugs not covered include: antihistamines, contraceptives, cough-suppressants, diet pills, multiple vitamins, drugs for cosmetic purposes, and smoking cessation gum.
Delaware	Delaware Prescription Drug Assistance Program	(800) 996-9969* ext. 17	Applicant: • must be age 65 or older, or disabled • annual income must be less than 200% of federal poverty level, unless prescription expense is greater than 40% of annual income.	Program pays 75% of prescription cost, to a maximum of $2,500 per year.	There is no fee to join the program. Patient co-pays $5 each time a prescription is filled	State residents who buy drugs through Nemours clinics in Wilmington and Mitford call (800) 292–9538 or (new and refill) (800) 763-9326.
Florida	Prescription Assistance Program for Seniors	(800) 963-5337*	Applicant: • must be 65 or older and eligible for Medicare Savings Programs • income must be between 90 to 120% of the federal poverty level.	Pays for $80 worth of prescription drugs every month.	There is no fee to join this program. A co-payment of 10% is required for each prescription (new and refill).	Ask about the Medicare Prescription Discount Program for discounts for Medicare beneficiaries.
Illinois	Pharmaceutical Assistance Program	(800) 624-2459*	Applicant: • must be a resident of Illinois • must be age 65 or older, or disabled • annual income must be less than $21,218 if single or $28,480 if married.	Up to $2,000 worth of prescription drugs for a minimum co-pay if single and income is less than $8,950 or married and income is less than $11,610.	Charges a one-time $5 fee for low-income individuals and $25 fee for middle-income individuals; $5 minimum co-pay for each prescription (new and refill).	Program covers drugs for heart and blood pressure problems, arthritis, cancer, glaucoma, Alzheimer's disease, diabetes, Parkinson's disease, osteoporosis, and lung disease.

STATE	NAME OF PROGRAM	CONTACT NUMBER	ELIGIBILITY REQUIREMENTS	BENEFITS	FEES OR PREMIUMS	COMMENTS
Illinois (continued)					$25 co-pay if annual income is greater than $8,590 (singles) or $11,610 (couples). Once the $2,000 benefit is met, co-payments increase to 20%.	
Indiana	HoosieRx	(866) 267-4679*	Applicant: • must be age 65 or older and have no prescription drug insurance coverage • annual income must be below $11,604 (single) or $15,684 (couples) Welfare recipients are ineligible.	Participants receive quarterly refunds for purchases up to $1,000.	There is no fee to join this program.	On-the-spot discounts will soon be available using discount cards that will replace the current refund program.
Iowa	The Iowa Priority Prescription Savings Program	(866) 282-5817*	Applicant must qualify for Medicare.	Participants receive a discount card to use at participating pharmacies to receive varying discount prices.	Participants pay an annual fee of $20 to join this program.	There are no income restrictions.
Kansas	Kansas Senior Pharmacy Assistance Program	(800) 432-3535*	Applicant: • must reside in the state and be 67 years of age or older • must be eligible for Medicare Beneficiary Programs • annual income must be less than 150% of the federal poverty level.	Participants receive refunds for 70% of out-of-pocket expenses, up to $1,200 a year.	There is no fee to join this program.	Participants must reapply three times a year.
Maine	Low Cost Drugs for the Elderly Program	(888) 600-2466*	Applicant: • must reside in Maine • must be 62 years of age or older or disabled • annual income must be less than $15,989 (single) or $21,541 (couples).	Participants receive discount of 80% on all generic drugs and selected name-brand drugs at participating pharmacies.	There is no fee to join this program.	Ask about the "Healthy Maine Prescriptions" program to receive discounts of up to 25%.
Maryland	Maryland Pharmacy Assistance Program	(800) 492-1974*	Applicant: • must reside in Maryland and be ineligible for welfare • annual income must be less than $10,300 (single) or $11,150 (couples).	After the co-payment, this program covers 100% of prescription drug cost for chronic conditions, anti-infective drugs, including AZT, and insulin.	There is no fee to join this program. Participants are charged a $5 co-pay for each prescription (new and refill).	Ask about the "Senior-Short-Term Prescription Drug Plan," a privately run insurance program.

STATE	NAME OF PROGRAM	CONTACT NUMBER	ELIGIBILITY REQUIREMENTS	BENEFITS	FEES OR PREMIUMS	COMMENTS
Massachusetts	Prescription Advantage Plan	(800) 243-4636*	Applicant: • must reside in Massachusetts • must be 65 years of age or older, or disabled.	After paying $2,000 (single) or $3,000 (couple) in a year, or 10% of annual gross income, participants receive all remaining prescriptions for the year free of charge.	There is no fee to join this program.	There is no income limit, but income levels affect fees.
Michigan	Elder Prescription Insurance Coverage (EPIC)	(517) 373-8230	Applicant: • must be 65 years of age or older • must have resided in Michigan in the last three months • must have a maximum household income level not greater than 200% of the federal poverty level • can have no other prescription insurance coverage, except Medicare. Medicaid recipients are ineligible.	Covers most prescription drugs, insulin, and insulin syringes. Doesn't cover non-essential or "lifestyle" drugs such as for hair loss or wrinkles.	Program charges an annual non-refundable $25 administrative fee. Monthly co-payments range from 1/12th of 1% of annual income, for those with incomes at or below 100% of the federal poverty level, to 1/12th of 5%, for those between 175 and and 200% of the poverty level.	For more information, including a list of the types of drugs not covered, go to the website: http//www.miepic.com/.
Minnesota	Senior Citizen Drug Program	(800) 333-2433*	Applicant: • must be 65 years of age or older • must have resided in Minnesota for at least six months • must be ineligible for Medigap or other prescription insurance • must currently receive or apply for either Qualified Medicare Beneficiary or Service Limited Medicare Beneficiary • income must be less than 120% of the federal poverty guidelines.	Program covers all drugs included in the contract between the state and drug companies.	There is no fee to join this program. Participants pay a monthly deductible of $35.	Assets that don't count toward limits include: • homestead property • mobile home, if used as the primary residence • prepaid burial fund up to $1,500 • one motor vehicle, under certain conditions This program is for senior citizens only.
Missouri	Missouri SenioRx Program	(866) 556-9316*	Applicant: • must reside in Missouri • must be 65 years of age or older • annual income must	After member meets the annual deductible, program pays 60% of prescription costs, up to $5000.	Participants pay a fee of $25 to $35 to join, depending on income level. Depending on	Apply April 1 through May 30, or January 1 through February 28.

STATE	NAME OF PROGRAM	CONTACT NUMBER	ELIGIBILITY REQUIREMENTS	BENEFITS	FEES OR PREMIUMS	COMMENTS
Missouri (continued)			be less than $17,000 (single) or $23,000 (couples).		income level, program charges an annual deductible of $250 to $500 and a co-pay of 40%.	
Nevada	Senior Citizen Subsidy for Drugs	(775) 688-2964	Applicant: • must reside in Nevada and be 62 years of age or older • annual household income must be less than $21,500. Welfare recipients are ineligible.	Program provides prescription insurance coverage with varying benefits for free and pays the $100 deductible.	There is no fee to join this program.	For more information, see the web site at http://www.nevada seniorrx.com/.
New Hampshire	New Hampshire Prescription Drug Discount Program	(888) 580-8902*	Applicant must reside in New Hampshire and be 65 years of age or older.	Participants receive discounts of up to 15% on name-brand drugs and 40% on generic drugs at participating pharmacies.	There is no fee to join this program.	There are no income limits to join this program.
New Jersey	Pharmaceutical Assistance for the Aged and Disabled (PAAD)	(800) 792-9745*	Applicant • must reside in New Jersey • must be 65 years of age or older, or disabled • annual income must be less than $19,739 (single) or $24,203 (couples).	Members pay discounted prices at participating pharmacies.	There is no fee to join this program. Members pay a $5 co-payment for each prescription (new and refill).	Members must present discount cards at the pharmacy to receive the discounted prices.
New York	Elderly Pharmaceutical Insurance Coverage (EPIC)	(800) 332-3742*	Applicant: • must be at least 65 years of age • must have an annual income of less than $20,000 (single), $26,000 (married) to qualify for the Fee Plan (see "Fees or Premiums" column) • must have annual income of less than $35,000 (single), $50,000 (married) to qualify for the Deductible Plan (see "Fees or Premiums" column) • may have no other prescription insurance coverage.	Plan covers most prescription drugs, as well as insulin and insulin syringes. Participants may obtain up to 100 tablets or a 30-day supply at a time.	Seniors with moderate incomes pay an annual fee. This is called the "Fee Plan." Seniors with higher incomes pay an annual deductible and a co-payment for each prescription. This is called the "Deductible Plan."	This plan is for senior citizens only. Co-payments range from $3 for prescription cost of $15 or less to $20 for prescriptions that cost more than $55. Annual fees range from $8/person for annual incomes of less than $6,000 to $300 for incomes as high as $26,000. Deductibles range from $530 to $1,230 for singles, and $650 to $1,715/person if married. For more information, refer to the web site at http://www.health.state.ny.us/nysdos/epic/faq.htm.

STATE	NAME OF PROGRAM	CONTACT NUMBER	ELIGIBILITY REQUIREMENTS	BENEFITS	FEES OR PREMIUMS	COMMENTS
North Carolina	Prescription Drug Assistance Program	(919) 715-3338	Applicant: • must reside in North Carolina, and be 65 or older • annual income must be less than $17,180 (single) or $23,220 (couples)	Members receive a 60% discount on on prescription drugs, up to an annual maximum of $1,000.	There is no cost to join this program	Applicant must have heart disease, chronic obstructive pulmonary disease, or diabetes to be eligible. A new program called Carolina Cares is planned for the near future.
Pennsylvania	Pharma-ceutical Assistance Elderly (PACE)	(800) 255-7223*	Applicant: • must reside in Pennsylvania and be 65 years of age or older. • annual income must be less than $14,000 (single) or $17,200 (couples) Welfare recipients are ineligible.	Programs cover prescription drugs, insulin, and syringes	There is no fee to join this program. Members pay a $6 co-payment for each pre-scription (new and refill).	Also available: the PACENET pro-gram, which has more stringent eligibility criteria and higher fees.
Rhode Island	Rhode Island Pharma-ceutical Assistance for the Elderly (RIPAE)	(800) 322-2880*	Applicant: • must reside in Rhode Island and be 65 or older • annual income must be between $16,490 and $36,225 (single) or $20,613 and $41,400 (couples).	Participants receive discount cards that provide 15 to 60% discounts on pre-scription drugs at participating phar-macies.	There is no fee to join this program.	This program is intended to cover drugs to treat most chronic conditions and some select conditions. Call for details.
South Carolina	SilveRxCard South Carolina Senior Prescription Drug Program	(877) 239-5277*	Applicant: • must reside in South Carolina • must be 65 years of age or older • must have no other prescription drug coverage • must have an annual income between $8,861 and $15,505 if (single) and $11,941 and $20,895 (couples).	Program covers most name-brand and generic drugs at participating pharmacies.	There is no fee to join this program. Members pay an annual de-ductible of $500 and a $10 co-payment for each prescription for generic drugs, $21 for name-brand drugs (new and refill).	For more information, refer to the program's Web site at http://www.silverxcard.com.
Vermont	Vermont Health Access Program (VHAP)	(800) 529-4060*	Applicant: • must reside in Vermont and be 65 years of age or older, or disabled • annual income must be less than $13,368 (single) or $17,988 (couples).	Participants receive discount cards to be honored at parti-cipating pharmacies.	There is no cost to join this program. Participants pay a co-payment of $1 to $3 per prescription (new and refill), de-pending on the drug.	Also available: the VSCRIPT program, which has more stringent eligibility criteria and higer fees.

STATE	NAME OF PROGRAM	CONTACT NUMBER	ELIGIBILITY REQUIREMENTS	BENEFITS	FEES OR PREMIUMS	COMMENTS
West Virginia	Golden Mountaineer Discount Card	(877) 987-3646*	Applicant must reside in West Virginia and be 60 years of age or older.	Participants receive a discount card they may use at participating pharmacies to receive varying discounts on prescription drugs.	There is no fee to join this program.	There are no income restrictions to be eligible for this program.
Wyoming	Minimum Medical Program	(800) 442-2766*	Applicant: • must be a U.S. citizen or eligible immigrant • reside in Wyoming • may not be in a public institution • may have received no prescription insurance coverage in the last month • income must be linked to federal poverty guidelines.	Participants are limited to three prescriptions per month. Program covers the same prescription drugs covered by the state Medicaid program.	There is no fee to join this program. Participants are charged a co-payment of $25 per prescription.	Assets that don't count toward income limits include one house and car.

SMART BUY
State Pharmaceutical Assistance Programs

State residency is a requirement for all of these programs. Because they're publicly funded, their criteria (and even their existence) are subject to change. Many of these programs are set up to be resources of last resort—that is, for use only when you can get no assistance from any other source, and you don't qualify for public assistance (welfare or Medicaid). The kinds of medications covered or provided typically are severely restricted, and the program is likely to have some sort of co-payment structure. Always investigate other options before turning to these programs.

SMART BUY
When You Can't Afford to Buy the Prescription Drugs You Need

Often you can save a lot of money by purchasing your prescription drugs from non-traditional or "alternative" sources. Be sure to evaluate carefully the integrity of the source you choose.

Keep these important tips in mind:

+ Programs offered through drug manufacturers generally base their requirements on federal poverty guidelines. Your first step in qualifying for assistance is to make sure you meet the annual income restrictions.

✦ If you believe you might qualify for an assistance program, ask your doctor about it before he or she writes your prescriptions. This way you can start out using medications made by the manufacturer that offers the program, and avoid the inconvenience and possible expense of switching drugs later.

✦ If you must wait for approval, ask your doctor for samples of the prescribed drug to tide you over. If no samples are available in the office, your doctor might be able to contact the company's representative to obtain samples for you.

✦ New programs are set up and existing programs discontinued on a regular basis. It pays to persist, especially if you *just* missed the qualification mark.

✦ If you couldn't qualify for one manufacturer's assistance program, but you have a fixed income, ask your doctor to find out whether comparable drugs are available from manufacturers with assistance programs you might qualify for. Do this each time your doctor renews your prescriptions.

PART 2 ▼

Saving Money
on Prescription Drugs

Chapter 6

Rx SOS: Smart Options for Saving Money on Prescription Drugs

When you pay for your prescription medications, do you wonder, *Are these prices for real, or am I being ripped off?* Well, drug prices certainly are for real: Pharmacies are charging them and people are paying them. And if you have chronic health conditions, you could be paying hundreds or even thousands of dollars for drugs every year.

It's true that finding the best buy isn't always easy. And when it comes to your health, you should take no risks. But neither should you pay unnecessary costs.

Our Rx SOS approach can help you make the best choices and find the biggest savings. In this chapter, we explain how you can save money without jeopardizing your health. We provide a simple worksheet at the end that you can photocopy and take with you to the pharmacy. Using it can help you identify specific savings that are best for *you*.

Rx SOS #1: Buy Generic

As long as a drug remains under patent, only the manufacturer that holds the patent can produce it. The manufacturer can charge what it wants for the drug, according to what the market will bear: With no competition, the sky's the limit. But after a drug's patent expires, other manufacturers can make and sell the same drug under different names. These are *generic* drugs; they contain the same active ingredients as their name-brand counterparts, but they typically cost about half as much, or even less than that. Sometimes generic forms of drugs have their own trade names (store brands, for example), and sometimes they go by the drug's generic name. The following table shows representative examples of the cost differences between name-brand and generic drugs.

Name-Brand and Generic Drug Comparisons

NAME-BRAND DRUG	PRESCRIBED TO TREAT	TYPICAL QUANTITY	TYPICAL NAME-BRAND RETAIL COST	GENERIC FORM	TYPICAL GENERIC RETAIL COST	TYPICAL SAVINGS USING GENERICS
Ativan 1mg	Anxiety	30	$41.55	Lorazepam	$25.99	$15.56—37%
Bactrim DS	Infections	20	$38.19	SMZ/TMP DS	$11.41	$26.78—70%
Cardizem CD 180mg	High blood pressure	30	$54.99	Diltiazem ER	$35.99	$19—35%
Diabeta 5mg	Diabetes	30	$29.49	Glyburide	$14.49	$15—51%
Elavil 25mg	Depression	30	$20.19	Amitriptyline	$7.49	$12.70—63%
Feldene 20mg	Arthritis	30	$101.09	Piroxicam	$19.99	$81.10—80%
Glucotrol 5mg	Diabetes	30	$17.59	Glipizide	$13.99	$3.60—20%
Halcion 0.25mg	Insomnia	30	$46.71	Triazolam	$26.99	$19.72—42%
Lasix 40mg	High blood pressure	30	$14.39	Furosemide	$7.49	$6.90—48%
Ortho-Novum 1/35	Contraception	28	$31.67	Necon 1/35	$21.99	$9.68—31%
Pamelor 25mg	Depression	30	$63.99	Nortriptyline	$14.89	$49.10—77%
Pepcid 20mg	Stomach acid	60	$132.19	Famotidine	$45.99	$86.20—65%
Procardia XL 30mg	High blood pressure	30	$45.99	Nifedipine XL	$36.99	$9—20%
Relafen 500mg	Arthritis	30	$51.69	Nabumetone	$35.79	$15.90—31%
Sinemet 25/100	Parkinson's disease	60	$69.99	Carbidopa with levodopa	$44.79	$25.20—36%
Tegretol 200mg	Epilepsy	60	$36.89	Carbamazepine	$23.49	$13.40—36%
Tenormin	High blood pressure	30	$41.79	Atenolol	$10.89	$30.90—74%
Vasotec 5mg	High blood pressure	30	$34.99	Enalapril	$25.69	$9.30—27%
Wellbutrin 75mg	Depression	60	$60.99	Bupropion	$49.99	$11—18%
Xanax 0.5mg	Anxiety	30	$44.39	Alprazolam	$14.79	$29.60—67%

You won't find every generic prescription alternative automatically, and sometimes doing so can be a real challenge. You might have to ask your doctor to write a prescription specifically for the generic product you want, or explicitly ask the pharmacist to use a generic drug. Laws regulating generic drugs are different from state to state. Most require physicians to state on the prescription form whether a pharmacist may substitute a generic equivalent. Some allow doctors to check a box on the form; others require them to write the prescription for the drug by its generic name. And some states *require* pharmacies to pass generic cost savings on to their customers. Pharmacies tend to do this anyway; it's good business to be able to offer lower prices.

What Is a Generic Drug and Is It as Good as the "Real Thing"?

Generic drugs are drugs the FDA has determined to be equivalent to their name-brand counterparts. This means that, when compared to a name-brand product, the generic product has the same amounts of the same active ingredients and should produce the same results. Notice we say "should." Although the vast majority of generic drugs produce precisely the same results as their name-brand counterparts, a few may not—and you need to know which ones they are.

Physicians and pharmacists measure a drug's relative safety according to its *therapeutic index*. This is the dosage range, measured as a ratio, for which the drug provides the desired results without producing undesired (and often dangerous) side effects. For most drugs, the therapeutic index is wide enough to accommodate the unavoidable differences among manufacturers in the production process, and the generic and name-brand forms of the drug will be essentially the same. (No two products of any kind can be *exactly* the same. Think of it in terms of ice cream: Two manufacturers might make vanilla ice cream from essentially the same recipe, but the results will taste a little different.)

Most of the time, variations between name-brand and generic drugs are subtle and irrelevant. Certain drugs, however, have a *narrow therapeutic index* (NTI); that is, there's a fine line between the dose that achieves the desired effect and one that causes problems. (Medical professionals say these drugs "have NTIs.") Although several factors determine whether a drug has an NTI, the FDA regulation defines a narrow therapeutic ratio as less than a twofold difference between the median lethal dose and the median effective dose. This isn't something you should worry about; your doctor and your pharmacist keep very close track of your treatment and progress if you take an NTI drug.

When your doctor prescribes a drug with a narrow therapeutic index, often he or she will monitor the level of the drug in your body by measuring how much of it is in your blood. You have your blood drawn at a lab, and your doctor will adjust your dosage to reach the desired therapeutic level. This process may take several weeks to months, but once your blood levels stabilize, your doctor will ask to have your blood tested only every few months to once a year, depending on the drug and your health.

Not all NTIs require monitoring this closely; your doctor or pharmacist will know whether blood tests are necessary. (Ask, if you're concerned or uncertain.) If you're taking an NTI drug, neither your doctor nor your pharmacist should change the brand of drug you take without repeating this assessment process. No two drugs are exactly alike, even when they have the same ingredients, and with NTIs, even the subtlest differences can matter. Once you start taking an NTI drug, don't change brands.

Some Commonly Prescribed NTI Drugs

DRUG	GENERIC NAME	COMMON USE
Alupent	Metaproterenol	Asthma
Cardioquin	Quinidine	Irregular heartbeats
Catapress	Clonidine	High blood pressure
Choledyl	Oxtriphylline	Asthma
Cleocin	Clindamycin	Bacterial infections
Cordarone	Amiodarone	Irregular heartbeats
Coumadin	Warfarin	Blood thinner
Depakene	Valproic acid	Epilepsy
Depakote	Divalproex sodium	Epilepsy
Dilantin	Phenytoin	Epilepsy
Elixophyllin	Theophylline	Asthma
Eskalith	Lithium	Bipolar disorder
Ismelin	Guanethidine	High blood pressure
Lanoxin	Digoxin	Congestive heart failure
Levothroid	Levothyroxine	Thyroid disease
Lithobid	Lithium	Bipolar disorder
Lithonate	Lithium	Bipolar disorder
Loniten	Minoxidil	High blood pressure
Minipress	Prazosin	High blood pressure
Mysoline	Primidone	Epilepsy

DRUG	GENERIC NAME	COMMON USE
Neoral	Cyclosporine	Organ transplant rejection prevention
Norpace	Disopyramide	Irregular heartbeats
Pacerone	Amiodarone	Irregular heartbeats
Procan	Procainamide	Irregular heartbeats
Pronestyl	Procainamide	Irregular heartbeats
Quibron	Theophylline	Asthma
Quinaglute	Quinidine	Irregular heartbeats
Quinidex	Quinidine	Irregular heartbeats
Sandimmune	Cyclosporine	Organ transplant rejection prevention
Slo-bid	Theophylline	Asthma
Slo-phyllin	Theophylline	Asthma
Synthroid	Levothyroxine	Thyroid disease
T-phyl	Theophylline	Asthma
Tegretol	Carbamazepine	Epilepsy
Theo-24	Theophylline	Asthma
Theobid	Theophylline	Asthma
Theochron	Theophylline	Asthma
Theo-Dur	Theophylline	Asthma
Theolair	Theophylline	Asthma
Uniphyl	Theophylline	Asthma

BUYING GENERIC CAN MEAN BIG SAVINGS

For most generic drugs, the real difference is in the price. Again, on average, generic drugs cost half of what their name-brand counterparts do. For example, Rhonda was taking the blood-pressure medication Vasotec 10mg, for which she paid $75.99 for 60 tablets. When a generic form of this drug came out, Rhonda's doctor authorized its use—and Rhonda saved 72 percent ($55) on her next prescription! Sometimes the price of a name-brand drug drops when other manufacturers begin to market generic forms. Even when this is the case, however, the generic usually is cheaper.

> ## ▶ A New "Gold Standard"?
>
> Zofran is an extremely expensive drug used for nausea other drugs can't control, such as that
> which accompanies chemo and radiation therapies. In fact, Zofran is so expensive that customers
> often say, "Wow! What's in it, gold?" Not quite. Ounce for ounce, the cost of Zofran tablets is almost 10
> times more than gold! While an ounce of gold might cost around $270, an ounce of Zofran
> (109 tablets) is $2,677!
>
> Good thing Zofran works for nausea. Its cost makes it a hard pill to swallow. ◀

Not all drugs are available in generic versions. Some drugs are so difficult to manufacture or have such a specialized use that it doesn't make sense to create competing products. And, of course, as we mentioned in Chapter 1, generic forms of drug products may be manufactured and sold only after the patents expire for the name brands. Fortunately, the numbers of drugs available in generic form continues to increase as patents expire. It can be daunting for the average consumer to try to keep up with this lengthening lists of generics, but pharmacists always know which drugs are available as generic products. If your doctor prescribes a name-brand drug, ask your pharmacist whether a generic form is available. Often he or she will phone your doctor for approval to switch to the less expensive generic (again, except for drugs with narrow therapeutic indexes).

Rx SOS #2: Buy the Right Amount

One measure of prescription drug expense is the *per-unit* cost. This is the price you pay divided by the number of tablets, capsules, or doses you get. Most of the time, the larger the quantity you buy, the less the drug will cost per unit. If you must take a drug for a long time—for hypertension or a thyroid condition, for example—it makes good sense to buy it in larger quantities.

Whether this is a good option for you depends on how much you can afford to spend at one time on prescription drugs. Although you spend more to buy the greater amount when you fill your prescription, you're paying less per dose, and so you get more for your money. The examples in the following table demonstrate how this works.

Because the savings for buying in quantity can be substantial, you'll find it worth your while to ask your pharmacist about it before you get your prescription filled.

Sample Savings When Buying Larger Quantities

DRUG	RETAIL COST FOR QUANTITY 30	RETAIL COST FOR QUANTITY 100	SAVINGS
Dilantin 100mg	$12.99 (43¢ each)	$29.99 (30¢ each)	30%
Famotidine 20mg	$21.99 (73¢ each)	$69.79 (70¢ each)	4%
Furosemide 40mg	$7.49 (25¢ each)	$15.99 (16¢ each)	36%
Gemfibrozil 600mg	$17.99 (60¢ each)	$54.99 (55¢ each)	8%
Glucotrol XL 5mg	$15.99 (53¢ each)	$41.49 (41¢ each)	13%
Hydrochlorothiazide 25mg	$5.49 (18¢ each)	$8.99 (9¢ each)	50%
Imipramine 25mg	$14.99 (50¢ each)	$34.79 (35¢ each)	30%
Lanoxin 0.25mg	$10.99 (37¢ each)	$23.99 (24¢ each)	35%
Levoxyl 0.1mg	$8.49 (28¢ each)	$15.79 (16¢ each)	43%
Lipitor 10mg	$63.99 ($2.13 each)	$199.09 ($1.99 each)	7%
Monopril 20mg	$39.99 ($1.33 each)	$123.99 ($1.24 each)	7%
Pamelor 25mg	$63.89 ($2.13 each)	$123.99 ($2.02 each)	5%
Potassium chloride tablets 10 mEq	$8.99 (30¢ each)	$19.99 (20¢ each)	33%
Procardia XL 30mg	$45.99 ($1.53 each)	$144.99 ($1.45 each)	6%
Relafen 500mg	$51.59 ($1.72 each)	$161.49 ($1.61 each)	6%
Tegretol 200mg	$20.99 (70¢ each)	$58.09 (58¢ each)	17%
Trazodone 50mg	$10.99 (37¢ each)	$19.99 (20¢ each)	46%
Vasotec 5mg	$35.99 ($1.20 each)	$104.29 ($1.04 each)	14%
Xanax 0.5mg	$44.39 ($1.48 each)	$132.47 ($1.32 each)	11%
Zocor 40mg	$117.49 ($3.92 each)	$365.89 ($3.65 each)	7%

It isn't always practical to buy in larger quantities, however. Buying in bulk isn't a good option under the following circumstances:

+ Some drugs, such as antibiotics, are prescribed for a limited time, so buying more than you need to take to complete the course of treatment won't benefit you.
+ If you're taking a drug for the first time, buy no more than a 30-day supply, in case it doesn't do what your doctor expects, or you have an adverse reaction. (To protect consumers from tampering and contamination, in most states, pharmacies may not take back drugs once they've left the premises.)
+ Many insurance plans restrict coverage to a certain supply, such as 30, 60, or 90 days' worth.
+ Controlled substances, such as narcotic pain medications, usually must be filled in limited quantities because they can be addictive.

Rx SOS #3: LESS EXPENSIVE ALTERNATIVES

Everybody wants the latest and greatest when it comes to personal health. And technology offers us wonderful ways both to extend our life and to improve its quality. Drugs are key to most medical treatments, and have, in fact, made it possible for thousands of people to live relatively normal lives in the wake of medical conditions that would have meant severe disability or early death just decades ago. Health conditions such as diabetes, heart disease, and cancer once sentenced their victims to misery and early death. For much of the last half of the twentieth century, each decade—and sometimes each year—brought exciting and life-changing discoveries in drugs, from new and powerful antibiotics to medications that can prevent transplant organ rejection. If you're older than forty, roughly 90 percent of the drugs you accept as commonplace today didn't even exist when you were born! Drugs have transformed the practice of medicine, and our lives are much the better for them.

But *newer* isn't necessarily *better*, and this is true of more and more drugs that come on the market today. Dozens, even hundreds, of new drugs go on sale each year, many intended to replace drugs already in use. Often the new drugs offer improvements over the old ones: They might have fewer side effects, require fewer or less frequent doses, or have different actions that make them more effective.

But sometimes these replacements offer benefits merely of convenience. And sometimes they're created to compete with existing similar products just to make money! The drug's packaging might be fancier or it might come in five fruit flavors, but the new product does exactly what the old standby did. It just costs more.

Millions of allergy sufferers embraced the new generations of "nondrowsy" antihistamines, for example. But these drugs can cost up to 10 times as much as conventional antihistamines already in use, while offering no therapeutic improvement. Yes, it's nice to feel alert, but it has nothing to do with how well the product suppresses your body's allergic responses. And many health insurance companies don't feel the convenience is worth the steep cost; often your doctor must write a letter explaining why you need the expensive antihistamine before your health insurance will pay for it.

Ask your doctor whether a new drug offers any therapeutic advantage over the older one. If the answer is no, then don't waste your money.

Those who work in the medical community often joke that new drug discoveries lead to new health conditions to treat. There's a grain of truth in this: Once treatments become available, we want to use them to make us feel better. The nondrowsy antihistamines we just mentioned provide a case in point. Thousands of people with seasonal allergies refused to take antihistamines because they made them sleepy. These people got through each allergy season without medication, uncomfortable but alert. But when the new antihistamines hit the market, suddenly everyone wanted to take them. The drug companies created a need, and consumers responded.

▶ Do Drug Companies Create Markets for New Drugs?

Some consumer advocates accuse drug companies of creating markets for new drugs through intense marketing to physicians and direct advertising to consumers. This increases the demand for the drugs, and results in thousands or even millions of prescriptions that would not have been written otherwise. The pharmaceutical industry spends billions of dollars a year in advertising. Some studies suggest this spending accounts for as much as 30 percent of the increased costs of drugs.

In response to ever-greater leaps in cost, many insurance companies refuse to pay for many new drugs when less expensive alternatives exist, unless your doctor can provide a clinically sound reason for prescribing them. Many HMOs and health insurance plans attempt to counter the effects of pharmaceutical advertising by covering only the drugs they include in their formularies (lists of drugs and the conditions for which they may be prescribed).

New drugs that offer little therapeutic advantage over drugs already on the market, especially those available in generic form, seldom make it onto such formularies. Many formularies exclude the new, very expensive, nondrowsy antihistamines, for example. The doctor must write a letter to the HMO or insurance company to justify prescribing a drug that isn't in their formulary. This restriction often draws the ire of physicians who feel it interferes with their ability to select the most appropriate drug for a patient's condition. However, the approach has proven effective in controlling drug costs—for the insurer, at least, although consumers who pay a predetermined co-payment or fee won't see much savings.

As a consumer, you may find there's little you can do about formulary restrictions beyond paying the full cost of the excluded drug. The restriction isn't on what your doctor can prescribe, but on what your health plan will pay for. You and your doctor might feel strongly that a nonformulary drug is the best therapeutic choice for you; if your insurance plan disagrees, you can still pay for the drug yourself.

Rx SOS #4: Compare to Over-the-Counter Drugs

Over the years, the FDA has moved about 200 drugs from prescription-only status to over-the-counter availability, and more make the transition each year. This means that you can now walk into a drugstore or even a grocery store and buy products to treat cold and flu symptoms, headaches, digestive upset, and other common ailments without first visiting a doctor. Yet the fact that certain drugs are available over the counter doesn't always deter doctors from writing prescriptions for them.

For instance, Lorna's doctor wrote her a prescription for 60 tablets of Pepcid 20mg for her gastric reflux problems. As a prescription, this would cost $102.89. However, Lorna could buy 120 tablets of Pepcid 10mg—the over-the-counter strength—for just $33.98, and save herself 67 percent! Because the over-the-counter strength is half what the doctor ordered, Lorna must take two such pills to get the correct dose. But the slight inconvenience of taking two pills instead of one makes for quite a savings!

The prescription drugs in the following list are currently under consideration for over-the-counter status:

✦ Carafate	✦ Feldene	✦ Prilosec	✦ Voltaren
✦ Claritin	✦ Flexeril	✦ Proventil	✦ Zithromax
✦ Clinoril	✦ Lodine	✦ Questran	✦ Zyrtec
✦ Diflucan	✦ Naprosyn	✦ Soma	
✦ Dolobid	✦ Prevacid	✦ Ventolin	

Once Prescription-Only Drugs Now Available Over the Counter

PRESCRIPTION VERSION	TYPICAL COST FOR 30-DAY SUPPLY	OVER-THE-COUNTER VERSION	TYPICAL COST FOR 30-DAY SUPPLY	USED TO TREAT
Anusol HC ointment	$9.49 for 20 grams	Anusol HC	$5.79 for 21 grams	Hemorrhoids
Axid 150mg	$72.79 for 25 capsules	Axid AR (75mg)	$15.99 for 50 tablets	Stomach acid
Benadryl 25mg	$9.09 for 24 capsules	Benadryl 25mg	$4.29 for 24	Allergy symptoms
Gyne-Lotrimin vaginal cream	$12.69 for 1 box	Gyne-Lotrimin vaginal cream	$10.99 for 1 box	Yeast infections
Hydrocortisone cream	$8.49 for 30 grams	Cortaid	$4.29 for 30 grams	Rashes and itching
Lamisil cream	$38.99 for 15 grams	Lamisil AT	$14.99 for 12 grams	Topical fungal infections
Lotrimin cream	$21.89 for 15 grams	Lotrimin AF cream	$11.99 for 24 grams	Topical fungal infections
Monistat vaginal cream	$18.29 for 1 box	Monistat-7 vaginal cream	$11.99 for 1 box	Yeast infections
Motrin 600mg	$34.99 for 83 tablets	Advil, Motrin-IB, Nuprin all 200mg tablets	$15.99 for 250 count	Arthritis, pain, inflammation, fever
Naphcon A eye drops	$13.99 for 15ml	Naphcon A	$8.99 for 15ml	Red, itchy eyes
Naprosyn 500mg	$91.79 for 50 tablets	Aleve 275mg tablets	$8.49 for 100	Arthritis, pain, inflammation, fever
Nasalcrom nasal spray	$28.49 for 1 box	Nasalcrom	$9.99 for 1 box	Allergy symptoms
Nicoderm patches 21mg	$54.79 for 1 box of 14	Nicoderm CQ	$49.99 for 1 box of 14	Nicotine addiction
Nicorette gum 2mg	$54.79 for 1 box of 96	Nicorette	$49.99 for 1 box of 108	Nicotine addiction
Nizoral shampoo 2%	$29.99 for 120ml	Nizoral shampoo (1%)	$14.99 for 200ml	Topical fungal infections of the scalp
Orudis 75mg	$16.79 for 8 capsules	Orudis KT (12.5mg)	$6.99 for 50	Arthritis, pain, inflammation, fever
Pepcid 20mg	$36.69 for 15 tablets	Pepcid AC (10mg)	$9.29 for 30	Stomach acid
Rogaine shampoo	$41.29 for 1 box	Rogaine	$29.99 for 1 box	Baldness
Tagamet 300mg	$12.79 for 10 tablets	Tagamet HB (100mg)	$9.99 for 30	Stomach acid
Tavist 2.68mg	$19.79 for 12 tablets	Tavist allergy (1.34mg)	$4.99 for 24 tablets	Allergy symptoms
Zantac 150mg	$34.79 for 15 tablets	Zantac 75	$8.99 for 30	Stomach acid

Even certain oral contraceptives soon may be available over the counter!

Often, the over-the-counter medication comes in a lower strength than the prescription version, as with Lorna's Pepcid. This is true, as well, for the popular anti-inflammatory pain reliever ibuprofen. The over-the-counter strength of this drug is 200mg, although prescription-only versions are available in 400mg, 600mg, and 800mg. If your doctor writes you a prescription for a drug that's available over-the-counter in a different strength, ask whether the over-the-counter form will work as well, if you take the same dose. The difference between taking 2 or 3 tablets per dose and taking a single, stronger tablet per dose can mean savings well worth the minor inconvenience.

Many insurance companies won't pay for prescriptions if the drugs are also available over-the-counter. It pays to find out your company's policy—and be sure to read the section "Rx SOS #6: Make the Most of Your Insurance Benefits" later in this chapter.

▶ Check Expiration Dates

Don't try to save money by taking drugs that have lasted beyond their expiration dates. Expired drugs may deteriorate, which can affect their potency (making them stronger or weaker than the indicated dose) or the rate at which your body absorbs them.

You'll find the drug's expiration date on your prescription container label. If you want to know whether a drug is still good, take it to your pharmacy and ask the pharmacist.

Rx SOS #5: Cut Tablets to Cut Costs

You can save hundreds of dollars a year by purchasing some drugs as tablets in a strength that's twice what your doctor prescribes, and then cutting them in half. This doubles the quantity you get, usually for not much more money than you'd have paid for pills in the originally prescribed strength. Many drugs come in a variety of strengths that, oddly enough, manufacturers price at close to the same cost per tablet. The popular antidepressant Paxil is one example. A typical dose is one 20mg tablet daily—between $80 and $100 for a 30-day supply. But the manufacturer also makes a 40mg tablet that can be cut in half. Buying 15 of the 40mg tablets costs $40 to $50, saving about $50 a month, or $600 a year! This is a savings of 50 percent.

Your savings can be even more dramatic, depending on what and how many kinds of prescription drugs you take. We stress, however, that cutting tablets won't work for everybody or with all medications. Consider these crucial caveats:

✦ Work with your pharmacist to be sure you can get the proper dose and absorption if you split tablets. It's also a good idea for your pharmacist to check with your doctor (and some states require this).

✦ Use a tablet cutter to split tablets evenly for medications. If your pharmacist doesn't normally sell them, he or she can easily order one for you. Unevenly cut tablets give you uneven, and unknown, amounts of the drug. Many tablets are scored—they have a line across the center along which the tablet will break evenly.

✦ Don't split capsules. Even if you manage to pull a capsule apart, it's nearly impossible to divide its powdered contents into even doses.

✦ Don't split most time-release products. For some, doing so destroys the coating, which is what delays the drug's absorption into your bloodstream: You'll risk getting a dangerously high dose of the drug immediately instead of a therapeutic dose released into your body at a safe rate.

Passing the Savings on to You

You might think that pharmacies would discourage their customers from buying a stronger drug and cutting it in half, but in fact they rarely do. The drugstore's gross profit margin will be the same regardless of the strength you purchase. Most pharmacists sincerely want to help people save money on their medications. Customers appreciate these efforts and will come back, and that's good for business. (It also cuts down on complaints about high prices!)

The common medications shown in the following table come in strengths that should be safe for splitting. Products change from time to time, however, so check with your pharmacist each time you refill your prescription just to be sure this money-saving approach isn't harming your health. Again, this is an option *you first must discuss with your doctor.* It's not appropriate for every drug or every person.

Potential Savings of Splitting Drugs

DRUG	PRESCRIBED STRENGTH	NUMBER OF TABLETS	BUY THIS STRENGTH TO SPLIT	ARE TABLETS SCORED?	NUMBER OF TABLETS	POTENTIAL SAVINGS FOR 30-DAY SUPPLY
Accolate	10mg	60	20mg	No	30	$33.90—50%
Accupril	5mg	30	10mg	No	15	$12.29—50%
	10mg	30	20mg	No	15	$12.29—50%
	20mg	30	40mg	No	15	$12.29—50%
Aceon	2mg	30	4mg	Yes	15	$15.75—50%
	4mg	30	8mg	Yes	15	$10.50—26%
Actos	15mg	30	30mg	No	15	$17.70—17%
Aldactone	25mg	30	50mg	No	15	$2.04—7%
	50mg	30	100mg	No	15	$4.80—13%
Amaryl	1mg	30	2mg	Yes	15	$1.15—8%
	2mg	30	4mg	Yes	15	75¢—5%
Ambien	5mg	30	10mg	No	15	$22.05—31%
Aricept	5mg	30	10mg	No	15	$51.02—50%
Atacand	4mg	30	8mg	No	15	$20.10—50%
	8mg	30	16mg	No	15	$20.01—50%
	16mg	30	32mg	No	15	$27.01—57%
Avandia	2mg	30	4mg	No	15	$13.70—21%
	4mg	30	8mg	No	15	$6.75—8%
Avapro	75mg	30	150mg	No	15	$18.45—38%
	150mg	30	300mg	No	15	$16.50—34%
Baycol	0.2mg	30	0.4mg	No	15	$22.20—50%
	0.4mg	30	0.8mg	No	15	$12.45—22%
Bumex	0.5mg	30	1mg	No	15	$3.45—29%
	1mg	30	2mg	No	15	$2.25—13%
Buspar	5mg	60	10mg	Yes	30	$6.60—13%
Calan	40mg	90	80mg	Yes	45	$10.80—24%
Calan SR	120mg	30	240mg	Yes	15	$33.60—83%
Capoten	12.5mg	90	25mg	Yes	45	$41.85—43%
	25mg	90	50mg	Yes	45	$13.50—13%
	50mg	90	100mg	Yes	45	$56.38—31%
Cardura	1mg	30	2mg	Yes	15	$15.90—50%
	2mg	30	4mg	Yes	15	$15.15—53%
	4mg	30	8mg	Yes	15	$15.75—52%
Celexa	20mg	30	40mg	Yes	15	$31.05—52%

DRUG	PRESCRIBED STRENGTH	NUMBER OF TABLETS	BUY THIS STRENGTH TO SPLIT	ARE TABLETS SCORED?	NUMBER OF TABLETS	POTENTIAL SAVINGS FOR 30-DAY SUPPLY
Coreg	3.125mg	60	6.25mg	No	30	$48.60—50%
	6.25mg	60	12.5mg	No	30	$48.60—50%
	12.5mg	60	25mg	No	30	$48.60—50%
Cozaar	25mg	30	50mg	No	15	$20.40—50%
	50mg	30	100mg	No	15	$11.55—50%
Cylert	18.75mg	30	37.5mg	Yes	15	$7.05—25%
	37.5mg	30	75mg	Yes	15	$7.20—16%
Cytotec	100 mcg.	120	200 mcg.	Yes	60	$25.80—33%
Detrol	1mg	60	2mg	No	30	$39.60—53%
Diabeta	1.25mg	30	2.5mg	Yes	15	5¢—0.2%
	2.5mg	30	5mg	Yes	15	$1.20—9%
Effexor	25mg	60	50mg	Yes	30	$39—45%
	37.5mg	60	75mg	Yes	30	$38.20—44%
	50mg	60	100mg	Yes	30	$38.40—41%
Estrace	0.5mg	30	1mg	Yes	15	$4.35—33%
	1mg	30	2mg	Yes	15	$4.50—26%
Fosamax	5mg	30	10mg	No	15	$33.65—50%
Glucophage	500mg	60	1000mg	Yes	30	$1.50—3%
Glucotrol	5mg	30	10mg	Yes	15	30¢—2%
Glynase	1.5mg	30	3mg	Yes	15	$2.28—15%
	3mg	30	6mg	Yes	15	$5.25—20%
Halcion	0.125mg	30	0.25mg	Yes	15	$15.30—42%
Hyzaar	50/12.5mg	30	100/25mg	No	15	$11.55—27%
Imdur	30mg	30	60mg	Yes	15	$22.05—42%
	60mg	30	120mg	No	15	$14.85—27%
Inderal	10mg	60	20mg	Yes	30	$7.50—30%
	20mg	60	40mg	Yes	30	$12.90—34%
	40mg	60	80mg	Yes	30	$11—22%
Kerlone	10mg	30	20mg	No	15	$7.37—21%
Lamictal	100mg	60	200mg	Yes	30	$61.50—37%
Lasix	20mg	30	40mg	Yes	15	$1.80—29%
	40mg	30	80mg	No	15	$1.80—20%
Lipitor	10mg	30	20mg	No	15	$13.80—20%
	20mg	30	40mg	No	15	$41.70—42%
	40mg	30	80mg	No	15	$52.50—49%
Lopressor	50mg	60	100mg	Yes	30	$11.70—25%

DRUG	PRESCRIBED STRENGTH	NUMBER OF TABLETS	BUY THIS STRENGTH TO SPLIT	ARE TABLETS SCORED?	NUMBER OF TABLETS	POTENTIAL SAVINGS FOR 30-DAY SUPPLY
Lotensin	5mg	30	10mg	No	15	$13.50—50%
	10mg	30	20mg	No	15	$13.50—50%
	20mg	30	40mg	No	15	$13.50—50%
Lotensin HCT	5/6.25mg	30	10/12.5mg	Yes	15	$13.50—50%
	10/12.5mg	30	20/25mg	Yes	15	$13.50—50%
Lozol	1.25mg	30	2.5mg	No	15	$11.25—37%
Luvox	25mg	30	50mg	Yes	15	$38.85—44%
	50mg	30	100mg	Yes	15	$48—48%
Mavik	1mg	30	2mg	No	15	$12.75—50%
	2mg	30	4mg	No	15	$12.75—50%
Mevacor	10mg	30	20mg	No	15	$5.40—11%
	20mg	30	40mg	No	15	$7.95—10%
Micronase	1.25mg	30	2.5mg	Yes	15	$1.95—20%
	2.5mg	30	5mg	Yes	15	$2.55—18%
Monoket	10mg	60	20mg	Yes	30	$26.10—50%
Monopril	10mg	30	20mg	No	15	$14.70—50%
	20mg	30	40mg	No	15	$14.70—50%
Normodyne	100mg	60	200mg	Yes	30	$10.20—27%
Norvasc	2.5mg	30	5mg	No	15	$21.15—148%
	5mg	30	10mg	No	15	$9.75—21%
Ogen	0.625mg	30	1.25mg	Yes	15	$7.35—29%
	1.25mg	30	2.5mg	Yes	15	$4.35—12%
Ortho-Est	0.75mg	30	1.5mg	Yes	15	$4.65—23%
Paxil	10mg	30	20mg	No	15	$37.20—46%
	20mg	30	40mg	No	15	$37.35—44%
Pepcid	20mg	60	40mg	No	30	$3.60—3%
Pletal	50mg	60	100mg	No	30	$49.20—48%
Prandin	0.5mg	90	1mg	No	45	$37.35—50%
	1mg	90	2mg		45	$37.35—50%
Precose	25mg	90	50mg	No	45	$26.10—45%
	50mg	90	100mg	No	45	$18.90—32%
Prinivil	2.5mg	30	5mg	No	15	$4.80—23%
	5mg	30	10mg	No	15	$14.25—44%
	10mg	30	20mg	No	15	$14.10—41%
	20mg	30	40mg	No	15	$8.70—25%
Prinzide	10/12.5mg	30	20/25mg	No	15	$15.30—42%

DRUG	PRESCRIBED STRENGTH	NUMBER OF TABLETS	BUY THIS STRENGTH TO SPLIT	ARE TABLETS SCORED?	NUMBER OF TABLETS	POTENTIAL SAVINGS FOR 30-DAY SUPPLY
Provera	2.5mg	30	5mg	Yes	15	$4.50—28%
	5mg	30	10mg	Yes	15	$10.50—39%
Provigil	100mg	30	200mg	Yes	15	$53.45—44%
Remeron	15mg	30	30mg	Yes	15	$38.55—47%
Risperdal	1mg	30	2mg	No	15	$30.90—21%
	2mg	30	4mg	No	15	$14.10—15%
Rythmol	150mg	90	300mg	Yes	45	$15.30—9%
Serzone	50mg	60	100mg	Yes	30	$38.70—44%
	100mg	60	200mg	No	60	$38.40—42%
Singulair	5mg	30	10mg	No	15	$41.25—50%
Tenormin	25mg	30	50mg	No	15	$17.05—49%
	50mg	30	100mg	No	15	$8.70—26%
Toprol-XL	25mg	30	50mg	Yes	15	$9.42—50%
	50mg	30	100mg	Yes	15	$9.45—45%
	100mg	30	200mg	Yes	15	15¢—0.5%
Univasc	7.5mg	30	15mg	Yes	15	$11.70—50%
Valium	5mg	90	10mg	Yes	45	$13.05—14%
Vasotec	2.5mg	30	5mg	No	15	$9.75—35%
	5mg	30	10mg	No	15	$16.05—44%
	10mg	30	20mg	No	15	$10.35—26%
Viagra	25mg	30	50mg	No	15	$130.34—50%
	50mg	30	100mg	No	15	$130.34—50%
Vioxx	12.5mg	30	25mg	No	15	$39.30—50%
	25mg	30	50mg	No	15	$24.98—30%
Xanax	0.25mg	90	0.5mg	Yes	45	$33.30—38%
	0.5mg	90	1mg	Yes	45	$36.45—33%
	1mg	90	2mg	Yes	45	$22.05—15%
Zaroxolyn	2.5mg	30	5mg	No	15	$10.12—36%
	5mg	30	10mg	No	15	$9.81—31%
Zestoretic	10/12.5mg	30	20/25mg	No	15	$15.30—41%
Zestril	5mg	30	10mg	Yes	15	$14.25—44%
	10mg	30	20mg	No	15	$14.10—42%
	20mg	30	40mg	No	15	$8.70—26%
Ziac	2.5mg	30	5mg	No	15	$19.65—50%
	5mg	30	10mg	No	15	$19.65—50%
Zocor	5mg	30	10mg	No	15	$10.65—20%
	10mg	30	20mg	No	15	$5.40—7%

DRUG	PRESCRIBED STRENGTH	NUMBER OF TABLETS	BUY THIS STRENGTH TO SPLIT	ARE TABLETS SCORED?	NUMBER OF TABLETS	POTENTIAL SAVINGS FOR 30-DAY SUPPLY
	20mg	30	40mg	No	15	$37.50—29%
	40mg	30	80mg	No	15	$37.50—50%
Zoloft	25mg	30	50mg	Yes	15	$104.40—50%
	50mg	30	100mg	Yes	15	$35.25—48%
Zyrtec	5mg	30	10mg	No	15	$29.70—49%

Rx SOS #6: Make the Most of Your Insurance Benefits

Insurance plans seldom pick up the full tab for prescriptions, leaving you to pay either a flat fee or a percentage of the cost, known as your co-payment (or "co-pay"). Although at first glance it seems silly to bypass your insurance when getting prescriptions, under some circumstances this makes sense—and saves you money.

The co-pay structure that can cost you big bucks is the *flat fee*. It applies to each prescription you fill or refill, regardless of whether the drug costs $10 or a hundred. At first glance, a fixed-fee co-payment of $5 or $10 doesn't seem so bad. But if you're filling 3 or 4 or 5 prescriptions at a time, your co-pays instantly can exceed the cost of dinner out and a movie! And most insurance companies limit the supply of medication you can receive at one time—usually to 30, 60, or 90 days, depending on which plan you have. You must fork out an additional co-pay if you purchase more than the limit. Your insurance company essentially forces you along a path that isn't necessarily the most economical for you—or even for the insurance company.

Robert, for example, takes a common diuretic, a generic form of hydrochlorothiazide. His doctor prescribes a hundred tablets of the 25mg strength with directions to take one-half tablet daily. Robert's insurance plan has a $5 co-pay and limits prescriptions to a 30-day supply, which for Robert is 15 tablets. Although the noninsurance cost for 100 tablets is only $9.49, Robert's cost for the same quantity, billed through his insurance company with a $5 co-pay for every 15 tablets, is $30—three times as much! Robert can save more than $40 a year by buying the full 100 tablets, which for him is a 6-month supply.

Whether your insurance plan charges you a flat fee or a percentage of cost, it's almost always less expensive to buy your prescriptions in larger, rather than smaller, quantities. Not only will you save on drug costs, but you'll also make fewer trips to the pharmacy. Many insurance plans limit you to a certain quantity, however, such as a 30- or 60-day supply. Some allow larger quantities for drugs that you take on a regular basis, such as medications for high blood pressure or hypothyroidism.

> ### ▶ Insurance Savings on Generic Drugs
>
> Many insurance plans now offer tiered co-payments, where you pay a lesser flat co-pay for generic
>
> products than for name-brand items. A typical tiered co-payment structure is $10 for brand items and
>
> $5 for generics. You save on your co-pays and your insurance company saves because generics cost
>
> less than name-brand equivalents—a rare instance where everybody wins.

PRESCRIPTION MEMBERSHIP PROGRAMS

A number of prescription card and membership programs have emerged in recent years to help consumers save money on their medications. You can sign on for prescription coverage tied to your medical insurance, or get separate prescription insurance (or join a plan) to cover drugs alone. Either way you'll have a co-pay or receive special contract prices.

Unfortunately, studies show that the savings are seldom what the program's advertising implies or what people expect. When Paul brought in a prescription for Enalapril 20mg 100 tablets for his high blood pressure, he wanted to use his prescription plan. So we ran it through the computer, and the plan showed Paul would owe a co-payment of $110. Yet just by buying the prescription as a direct purchase, Paul would pay only $32! This happens all too often with such plans, which often charge enrollment, membership, or service fees in addition to co-pays for drug purchases. Always have the pharmacist calculate your costs with and without your prescription card or membership plan, if you have one.

RX SOS #7: COMPARE PRICES

Do you know, right now, which grocery store in your area has milk or bread or soft drinks on sale? Odds are, you do! Do you know which pharmacy offers the best price for the prescription drugs you take, or even how much your own pharmacy charges you? Odds are, you don't.

Most people fail to comparison-shop when they fill their prescriptions. One reason for this is that, when you're sick, you need your prescriptions *now*. You don't feel like calling around to see who has the best price, or you might not be able to. In such circumstances, shopping around probably isn't worth the effort, because you'll probably take the prescription drugs you need for only a limited time.

When it comes to drugs you take regularly, however, comparing prices can save you a lot of money.

▶ IRS Deduction for Prescription Drugs

The IRS considers prescription drugs tax deductible if they (along with all other medical expenses) exceed 7.5 percent of your annual gross income. Medical expenses below 7.5 percent aren't deductible. Many senior citizens benefit from this deduction. If you're unsure whether your medical expenses qualify, contact a tax consultant or accountant before filing your federal income tax return. And be sure to save all of your drug receipts, so you have accurate records of your prescription expenses.

$ PUTTING YOUR KNOWLEDGE TO USE: Your Rx SOS Savings Worksheet

Your own Rx SOS worksheet is on page 88. Using it can help you save money on your prescription drug purchases. Photocopy the form and carry it with you when you go to the pharmacy. Use a separate worksheet for each prescription drug you buy. Planning your savings is as easy as 1–2–3:

1. Use this book. For each drug, refer to the book to determine whether the drug is available in a generic form, has a narrow therapeutic index (NTI), can be cut, or is available in a less expensive or over-the-counter form. Then pick the Smart Buy for that category of drug.
2. Check your insurance coverage and note any limits it imposes.
3. Call three pharmacies to get price quotes. Also, check the tables in this book for reasonable prices. If you aren't finding those prices, keep shopping. (Our Web

site, www.smartbuysdrugwise.com, will always provide up-to-date information about prescription and over-the-counter drugs.)

Write all this information on your "SOS Worksheet for Smart Buys on Prescription Drugs" to find the greatest savings when you buy your prescription drugs.

SOS WORKSHEET FOR SMART BUYS ON PRESCRIPTION DRUGS
Use a separate worksheet for each drug.

Prescribed Drug	Name, strength, quantity, and directions for use of the drug your doctor has prescribed.
	_____

SOS #1

Buy Generic

1. Is this drug available in generic form? ❏ YES ❏NO
2. Does this drug have a narrow therapeutic index (NTI)? ❏ YES ❏NO
3. Did (or will) your doctor authorize a generic substitution? ❏ YES ❏NO

If you answer yes to items 1 and 3, and no to item 2, generic is an option for you.

SOS #2

Quantity

What is the largest quantity of this drug your insurance company will cover? _____

What is the largest quantity of this drug your pharmacy will let you buy? _____

SOS #3

ARE LESS EXPENSIVE ALTERNATIVES AVAILABLE? IF SO, LIST THEM HERE.

Less Expensive Alternatives

_____

_____

SOS #4

Over-the-Counter

Is this drug available without a prescription? ❏ YES ❏NO

If so, in what strengths? _____

What quantity of the over-the-counter drug would you need to buy

to take the prescribed dose? _____

What would it cost to buy this quantity? _____

SOS #5

Cutting Tablets

Can you buy a higher strength of this drug and cut the tablets in half? ❏ YES ❏NO

SOS #6

DO YOU HAVE INSURANCE COVERAGE FOR PRESCRIPTION DRUGS? ❏ YES ❏NO

Get the Most from Your Insurance

What is your co-payment? _____

What is the limit for the quantity of the drug your insurance will cover? _____

SOS #7

Compare Prices (include alternative sources)	PHARMACY 1	PHARMACY 2	PHARMACY 3
	_____	_____	_____
	_____	_____	_____
	_____	_____	_____

Smart Buy

LIST SMART BUYS FOR THE CATEGORIES OF PRODUCTS YOU NEED.

[$]

_____

_____

Your Best Choices	PRODUCT	QUANTITY	PRICE	STORE
	_____	_____	_____	_____
	_____	_____	_____	_____

Chapter 7

Prescription Drugs to Treat Infections

Barely 50 years ago, infection was the leading cause of death in most of the world. Health problems—from sore throats to cuts and cavities—that for us today mean little more than a trip to the doctor or dentist were once the kiss of death. Common infections such as tonsillitis and strep throat killed thousands of children and adults each year. More soldiers died from infections than from gunshot wounds in all the nation's wars through World War II. It wasn't until 1943 that the first antibiotic debuted—sulfa. Despite its myriad unpleasant side effects, this miraculous drug saved thousands of lives. Penicillin followed a few years later. Today there are dozens of different antibiotics on the market, each targeting one or more of the 75 strains of bacteria known to cause infections in people.

TOO MUCH OF A GOOD THING CAN BE VERY, VERY BAD

We've become accustomed to popping a few pills and having whatever ails us disappear. So we want doctors to prescribe the pills that will make us feel better. But sometimes too much of a good thing ends up doing harm, instead. Bacteria, the targets of antibiotics, can develop *resistance*. That is, over the course of numerous generations (measured in days or even hours, not decades like us slow-growing humans), bacteria can change their chemical and physical structures so that a particular kind of antibiotic is no longer effective in killing them. Scientists call this a survival mutation. Although they're primitive life forms, bacteria can adapt to changes in their environment (mutate) to improve their ability to survive. When they've been exposed continually to a particular hazard, such as an antibiotic, bacteria can develop mechanisms to protect themselves from that hazard.

The number of antibiotics available today is perhaps the most alarming evidence of how serious this problem is. Each time a strain of bacteria develops resistance to one antibiotic, researchers must develop another. Healthcare professionals refer to these as "generations" of antibiotics. Typically, each generation is more powerful than the one before. With some antibiotics, this power is a double-edged sword; stronger activity can bring with it the potential for more significant side effects. On the other hand, many new antibiotics actually have far fewer side effects than their predecessors. (We cover this in greater detail later in this chapter.)

The issue of resistance is of particular concern with children. Cassie started taking amoxicillin for ear infections when she was 6 months old. She's 2 years old now, and amoxicillin no longer works on her infections. Instead, her doctor has to prescribe the more powerful, and more expensive, antibiotic Augmentin. Although Cassie is scheduled to have drain tubes placed in her ears to help prevent future infections, we have no way of knowing whether infections she might develop later in her life will be resistant to the first or even second line of antibiotics typically used to counter them.

THE CAUSE OF YOUR INFECTION: BACTERIA OR VIRUS?

Although we worry most about the bacteria that cause infections, such as Streptococcus or Staphylococcus, other agents can cause infections, too. The most common of these are viruses. Viruses cause the most unpleasant and common of these infections, colds and influenza (the "flu"). Antibiotics have no effect on viruses. This fact is so important, we want to say it again: Antibiotics have no effect against viruses.

The problem is that sometimes it's difficult, if not downright impossible, for you or your doctor to distinguish between a viral infection and a bacterial infection. The symptoms can be very much alike; only a laboratory test called a culture can tell conclusively. Bacteria will grow in the lab but viruses won't. This is why doctors often want to do a throat culture before prescribing an antibiotic to treat a sore throat. If bacteria such as strep or staph are causing your symptoms, you need an antibiotic. If a virus is the culprit, antibiotics won't help. Most bacterial infections respond immediately to treatment with antibiotics—within hours to a day or two. But here's the rub: Most viral infections only last a week or so. By the time you feel sick enough to go to the doctor, if your infection is viral, you actually may be on the mend.

Say you've had a killer sore throat for five days. You go to the doctor. The doctor prescribes an antibiotic, which you start taking right away. A day or two later, you're feeling fine. Proof your sore throat was bacterial, right? Not necessarily. Because most viruses run their course in 7 to 10 days, by the time you started taking the antibiotic, a viral sore throat could be nearing the end of its natural existence. Its demise may well be a coincidence.

Although only a lab test can tell for sure, these charts show the typical symptoms of, and differences between, viral and bacterial infections.

Upper Respiratory Infection: Common (Viral) Cold or Bacterial Infection?

Symptom	Viral Cold	Bacterial Infection
Cough	Sometimes; may bring up clear or white sputum	Often persistent; may bring up yellow or green sputum
Duration	5-10 days	7 days
Fatigue	Mild	Strong
Fever	Seldom or slight	Sudden onset, with temperature over 102 degrees
Headache	Mild	Strong
Muscle or joint pain	Mild	Strong
Runny nose	Often	Not usually
Sneezing	Often	Not usually
Sore throat	Often	Often
Stuffy nose	Often	Not usually

Viral Versus Bacterial Sore Throat

Symptom	Viral Sore Throat	Bacterial Sore Throat
Duration	5-10 days	7 days
Lymph-node involvement	Slightly enlarged, not tender	Large and tender
Onset	Slow (takes several days to develop)	Fast
Other cold symptoms	Often	Not usually
Pain	Mild to moderate	Intense

Doctors commonly prescribe antibiotics for sore throats and upper respiratory infections that have produced symptoms for a week or longer, presuming that such infections are likely bacterial. They're usually right; viruses tend to go away on their own within a week or so. Sometimes a viral infection sets the stage for a bacterial infection, so what started as a virus ends up as a bacterial infection that needs antibiotic treatment. Some doctors use quick, in-office tests for strep throat, the most common bacterial throat infection. Because these tests are less accurate than laboratory cultures, though, other doctors consider them a waste of time and money.

> ## Watch for Pneumonia After the Flu
>
> If you recently had the flu and recovered, but now you have a high fever, call your doctor immediately.
>
> People who have had the flu tend to be more susceptible to bacterial pneumonias, which can become
>
> dangerous quite quickly.

DO YOU NEED AN ANTIBIOTIC?

How can you tell whether you need an antibiotic? The short answer is that *you* can't, really. But you *can* look at the same clues your doctor would evaluate. (See the tables of symptoms on page 91.) Give your body time to heal itself. If you have a cold or a viral upper-respiratory infection, expect to be sick for at least five days. Rest and drink lots of fluids, and perhaps try an over-the-counter cold preparation to relieve your symptoms. (Refer to Chapter 17, "Over-the-Counter Cold, Flu, Cough, and Allergy Preparations.") If you still feel sick after five days, or if you suddenly develop a high fever, or if your symptoms get significantly worse, *then* see a doctor.

If your doctor wants to put you on an antibiotic without doing a culture first, ask how he or she concluded that your infection is bacterial. If the reasons make sense, an antibiotic is probably a good choice. If your doctor can't give you a good reason or says something like, "There's a lot of this going around and this is what I've been giving people," consider waiting a few more days before you fill that prescription. Taking an antibiotic when you don't need it isn't likely to cause much trouble down the road if you only do it occasionally, but doing it often can be a prescription for disaster.

Ask your doctor how soon you can expect your symptoms to start going away once you start taking the antibiotic. If your infection hasn't begun to clear up within that time frame, your doctor may need to prescribe a different antibiotic. (And if this turns out to be the case, ask the doctor to do a culture.) Do your part to reduce bacterial resistance. This benefits everyone, because ultimately we all wade in the same germ pools.

Don't insist on an antibiotic if your doctor doesn't seem inclined to prescribe one. At the very least, be grateful that your doctor is saving you some money.

> ## Let Your Doctor Know About Drug Allergies
>
> Be sure to tell your doctor about *any* drug allergies you have, whether you react to antibiotics or to other drugs. You may have cross-sensitivities, which means that your allergy to one drug can rear its ugly head when you take certain other drugs.

When your doctor prescribes an antibiotic for you, ask these five vital questions:

1. Why are you choosing this particular antibiotic?
3. Does this antibiotic have any potentially serious side effects?
4. About how much will this antibiotic cost?
5. Is this drug available in generic form? If it is, will you authorize the pharmacy to dispense it?
6. Is there a less expensive but equally effective antibiotic I could take instead?

Don't be surprised if your doctor can't answer these questions. Not many people ask them. Doctors should know the costs, forms, and potential side effects of the drugs they prescribe, but often they rely on pharmacists to handle these details. As we noted in earlier chapters, many factors influence physicians' prescribing practices, from insurance-company formularies that restrict drug choices to pharmaceutical representatives who work hard to promote the newest drugs. If your doctor says, "Here, try these," and offers you samples, then you know the drug rep was a recent visitor. Go back to the five vital questions. If you don't get answers from your doctor, ask your pharmacist.

Sometimes doctors prescribe antibiotics *prophylactically*—that is, to *prevent* infection. This is done most commonly before and following surgery (including certain dental surgeries and when you get your teeth cleaned). Always take a prescribed antibiotic according to the directions on the label and until you have taken all of the prescription, unless your doctor instructs you otherwise. Some antibiotics must be taken on an empty stomach; with others, it doesn't matter what you've eaten. Some antibiotics are particularly irritating to the stomach, so generally they're taken with food to reduce discomfort.

> ### Take Antibiotics Until They're Gone
>
> Take your antibiotic until it's completely used up! This is crucial when fighting infections.
>
> If you start to feel better after the first couple of days, *don't* stop taking the medication.
>
> Even though most of the bacteria have been killed, enough may be left to come back with
>
> a vengeance if you stop taking the antibiotic.

STICKER SHOCK!

Your doctor has chosen your antibiotic, and you go to the pharmacy to purchase the prescription—only to learn that the 10-day supply you need will cost you *over $100*. Is that really *necessary?* Or will a less expensive drug do the same job? Often doctors are unaware that certain drugs are as expensive as they are. Or your pharmacist may discover that your insurance company will pay more of the cost for a different antibiotic than for the one your doctor prescribed. Does the insurance company know something you don't? Probably.

Often less expensive antibiotics exist that will do the same job. This was the case for Jerry, who came in with a prescription for Augmentin 500mg. The cost of a 10-day supply of 30 tablets came to $118. This was too expensive for Jerry, so he asked us to call the doctor and request a less expensive drug. The doctor was somewhat reluctant at first, but agreed to give cephalexin a try. This prescription for 40 capsules (also a 10-day supply) came to only $25, saving Jerry 79 percent. When Jerry came into the pharmacy a month later, we asked him how the cephalexin worked. He said, "Great!"

How could cephalexin work as well (in this instance) as Augmentin at a fraction of the price? Well, as a generic drug, cephalexin simply costs less than the name-brand Augmentin. But it also costs less because *it kills far fewer types of bacteria* than Augmentin. Jerry's doctor probably prescribed Augmentin because he didn't know exactly what strain of bacteria was causing Jerry's infection. Rather than spend the money on and wait the extra time for the results of a culture, the doctor chose a broad-brush antibiotic instead. This approach is certainly valid from a clinical perspective, but it overlooks other factors that should contribute to the antibiotic choice. Even though cephalexin has a narrower range of effectiveness in terms of the number of bacteria strains it can kill, it's just as potent as Augmentin against those strains for which it is effective.

Of course, if the strain of bacteria causing Jerry's infection had not been susceptible to cephalexin, using cephalexin would have been a waste of time and money. This is one reason we believe that doing a culture before prescribing an antibiotic for most infections is the best way to go, both in terms of your health and your pocketbook. We also believe that by reserving powerful antibiotics, such as Augmentin, for second-round therapy (for use when a less powerful antibiotic doesn't work), you and your doctor will help slow the inevitable development of bacterial resistance to the stronger antibiotics. If you have an infection that hasn't been a problem for you before, ask your doctor about starting you on one of the less potent and less expensive antibiotics first. The following table can help you and your doctor consider alternatives.

Antibiotics and Potential Savings

TYPE OF INFECTION	PRODUCTS COMMONLY USED	STRENGTH PER DOSE	ACTIVE INGREDIENT	USUAL DOSAGE	TYPICAL QUANTITY	TYPICAL PRICE	PRICE PER DOSE
Bladder							
	Cephalexin (generic Keflex)	500mg	Cephalexin	Take 1 capsule every 6 hrs.	40	$25	63¢
	Cipro	500mg	Ciprofloxacin	Take 1 tablet twice a day.	20	$102	$5.10
	Doxycycline	100mg	Doxycycline	Take 1 tablet twice a day.	20	$12	60¢
	Floxin	400mg	Ofloxacin	Take 1 tablet twice a day.	20	$119	$5.95
	Levaquin	500mg	Levofloxacin	Take 1 tablet daily.	10	$97	$9.70
	SMZ/TMP DS (generic Septra)	160/800mg	Sulfamethoxazole and trimethoprim	Take 1. tablet twice a day.	20	$11	55¢

TYPE OF INFECTION	PRODUCTS COMMONLY USED	STRENGTH PER DOSE	ACTIVE INGREDIENT	USUAL DOSAGE	TYPICAL QUANTITY	TYPICAL PRICE	PRICE PER DOSE
Breast							
	Augmentin	875mg	Amoxicillin with clavulanic acid	Take 1 tablet twice a day.	20	$123	$6.15
	Ceftin	500mg	Cefuroxime	Take 1 tablet twice a day.	20	$178	$8.90
	Clindamycin	150mg	Clindamycin	Take 2 capsules every 6 hrs.	80	$82	$2.05
	Dicloxacillin	500mg	Dicloxacillin	Take 1 capsule every 6 hrs.	40	$37	93¢
Bronchitis							
	Amoxicillin	500mg	Amoxicillin	Take 1 capsule 3 times daily.	30	$16	53¢
	Augmentin	875mg	Amoxicillin with clavulanic acid	Take 1 tablet twice a day.	20	$123	$6.15
	Biaxin	500mg	Clarithromycin	Take 1 tablet twice a day.	20	$90	$4.50
	Cefaclor (generic Ceclor)	500mg	Cefaclor	Take 1 capsule 3 times daily.	30	$40	$1.333
	Doxycycline	100mg	Doxycycline	Take 1 tablet twice a day.	20	$15	75¢
	SMZ/TMP DS (generic Septra)	160/800mg	Sulfamethoxazole and trimethoprim	Take 1 tablet twice a day.	20	$11	55¢
External Ear Canal							
	Cipro HC ear drops	0.2% and 1%	Ciprofloxacin and hydrocortisone	Place 4 drops in affected ear(s) 4 times a day.	10ml	$75	$3
	Floxin ear drops	3mg/ml	Ofloxacin	Place 4 drops in affected ear(s) 4 times a day.	5ml	$45	$3.60

TYPE OF INFECTION	PRODUCTS COMMONLY USED	STRENGTH PER DOSE	ACTIVE INGREDIENT	USUAL DOSAGE	TYPICAL QUANTITY	TYPICAL PRICE	PRICE PER DOSE
	Hydrocortisone, Neomycin, Polymyxin B (generic Cortisporin) ear drops	N/A	Hydrocortisone, Neomycin, Polymyxin B	Place 4 ear drops in affected ear(s) 4 times a day.	10ml	$20	80¢
Eye (contact lens wearers)							
	Ciloxan eye drops	0.3%	Ciprofloxacin	Place 2 drops in affected eye(s) every 4 hrs.	5ml	$41	$1.64
	Gentamicin eye drops (generic Garamycin)	0.3%	Gentamicin	Place 2 drops in affected eye(s) every 4 hrs.	5ml	$10	40¢
	Ocuflox eye drops	0.3%	Ofloxacin	Place 2 drops in affected eye(s) every 4 hrs.	5ml	$41	$1.64
	Sulfacetamide eye drops (generic Sulamyd)	10%	Sulfacetamide	Place 2 drops in affected eye(s) every 4 hrs.	15ml	$9	12¢
	Tobramycin eye drops (generic Tobrex)	0.3%	Tobramycin	Place 2 drops in affected eye(s) every 4 hrs.	5ml	$14	56¢
Foot (diabetics)							
	Augmentin	875mg	Amoxicillin with clavulanic acid	Take 1 tablet twice a day.	20	$123	$6.15
	Ceftin	500mg	Cefuroxime	Take 1 tablet twice a day.	20	$178	$8.90
	Cephalexin (generic Keflex)	500mg	Cephalexin	Take 1 capsule every 6 hrs.	80	$60	75¢
	Clindamycin	150mg	Clindamycin	Take 2 capsules every 6 hrs.	80	$82	$2.05

TYPE OF INFECTION	PRODUCTS COMMONLY USED	STRENGTH PER DOSE	ACTIVE INGREDIENT	USUAL DOSAGE	TYPICAL QUANTITY	TYPICAL PRICE	PRICE PER DOSE
Kidney							
	Augmentin	875mg	Amoxicillin with clavulanic acid	Take 1 tablet twice a day.	28	$169	$6.04
	Cephalexin (generic Keflex)	500mg	Cephalexin	Take 1 capsule every 6 hrs.	42	$31	74¢
	Cipro	500mg	Ciprofloxacin	Take 1 tablet twice a day.	20	$102	$5.10
	SMZ/TMP DS (generic Septra)	160/800mg	Sulfamethoxazole and trimethoprim	Take 1 tablet twice a day.	28	$14	50¢
	Tequin	400mg	Gatifloxacin	Take 1 tablet daily.	7	$62	$8.86
Middle Ear Canal							
	Amoxicillin	250mg/5ml	Amoxicillin	Take 1 dose 3 times a day.	150ml	$10	33¢
	Augmentin	250mg/5ml	Amoxicillin with clavulanic acid	Take 1. dose 3 times a day.	150ml	$85	$2.83
	Ceftin	250mg/5ml	Cefuroxime	Take 1 dose twice a day.	100ml	$73	$3.65
	Omnicef	125mg/5ml	Cefdinir	Take 1 dose twice a day.	100ml	$76	$3.80
	SMZ/TMP (generic Septra)	40/200mg per 5ml	Sulfamethoxazole and trimethoprim	Take 1 dose twice a day.	100ml	$20	$1
	Vantin	100mg/5ml	Cefpodoxime	Take 1 dose twice a day.	100ml	$91	$4.55
Mouth							
	Augmentin	875mg	Amoxicillin with clavulanic acid	Take 1 tablet twice a day.	20	$123	$6.15
	Ceftin	500mg	Cefuroxime	Take 1 tablet twice a day.	20	$178	$8.90

TYPE OF INFECTION	PRODUCTS COMMONLY USED	STRENGTH PER DOSE	ACTIVE INGREDIENT	USUAL DOSAGE	TYPICAL QUANTITY	TYPICAL PRICE	PRICE PER DOSE
	Clindamycin	150mg	Clindamycin	Take 2 capsules every 6 hrs.	80	$82	$2.05
$	Penicillin V	500mg	Penicillin	Take 1 tablet every 6 hrs.	40	$10	40¢
Pneumonia							
	Augmentin	875mg	Amoxicillin with clavulanic acid	Take 1 tablet twice a day.	20	$123	$6.15
	Biaxin	500mg	Clarithromycin	Take 1 tablet twice a day.	20	$90	$4.50
$	Doxycycline	100mg	Doxycycline	Take 1 tablet twice a day.	28	$17	61¢
	Zithromax	250mg	Azithromycin	Take 2 tablets on day 1 and then 1 tablet daily.	6	$50	$8.33
Prostate							
	Cipro	500mg	Ciprofloxacin	Take 1 tablet twice a day.	28	$142	$5.07
$	SMZ/TMP DS (generic Septra)	160/800mg	Sulfamethoxazole and trimethoprim	Take 1 tablet twice a day.	28	$14	50¢
Sinusitis							
$	Amoxicillin	500mg	Amoxicillin	Take 1 capsule 3 times daily.	30	$16	53¢
	Augmentin	875mg	Amoxicillin with clavulanic acid	Take 1 tablet twice a day.	20	$123	$6.15
	Biaxin	500mg	Clarithromycin	Take 1 tablet twice a day.	20	$90	$4.50
	Ceftin	250mg	Cefuroxime	Take 1 tablet twice a day.	20	$100	$5.00

TYPE OF INFECTION	PRODUCTS COMMONLY USED	STRENGTH PER DOSE	ACTIVE INGREDIENT	USUAL DOSAGE	TYPICAL QUANTITY	TYPICAL PRICE	PRICE PER DOSE
	Omnicef	300mg	Cefdinir	Take 1 capsule twice daily.	20	$96	$4.80
	Vantin	200mg	Cefpodoxime	Take 1 tablet twice a day.	20	$110	$5.50
Skin—bites from bats, raccoons, and skunks							
	Augmentin	875mg	Amoxicillin with clavulanic acid	Take 1 tablet twice a day.	20	$123	$6.15
	Doxycycline	100mg	Doxycycline	Take 1 tablet twice a day.	20	$15	75¢
Skin —cat bites							
	Augmentin	875mg	Amoxicillin with clavulanic acid	Take 1 tablet twice a day.	20	$123	$6.15
	Ceftin	500mg	Cefuroxime	Take 1 tablet twice a day.	20	$178	$8.90
	Doxycycline	100mg	Doxycycline	Take 1 tablet twice a day.	20	$15	75¢
Skin —dog bites							
	Augmentin	875mg	Amoxicillin with clavulanic acid	Take 1 tablet twice a day.	20	$123	$6.15
	Clindamycin	150mg	Clindamycin	Take 2 capsules every 6 hrs.	80	$82	$2.05
Skin —infected wounds							
	Augmentin	875mg	Amoxicillin with clavulanic acid	Take 1 tablet twice a day.	20	$123	$6.15
	Biaxin	500mg	Clarithromycin	Take 1 tablet twice a day.	20	$90	$4.50
	Clindamycin	150mg	Clindamycin	Take 2 capsules every 6 hrs.	80	$82	$2.05
	Erythromycin	500mg	Erythromycin	Take 1 tablet 4 times a day.	40	$18	45¢

TYPE OF INFECTION	PRODUCTS COMMONLY USED	STRENGTH PER DOSE	ACTIVE INGREDIENT	USUAL DOSAGE	TYPICAL QUANTITY	TYPICAL PRICE	PRICE PER DOSE
	Levaquin	500mg	Levofloxacin	Take 1 tablet daily.	10	$97	$9.70
	Zithromax	250mg	Azithromycin	Take 2 tablets on day 1 and then 1 tablet daily.	6	$50	$8.33
Skin—rat bites							
	Augmentin	875mg	Amoxicillin with clavulanic acid	Take 1 tablet twice a day.	20	$123	$6.15
	Doxycycline	100mg	Doxycycline	Take 1 tablet twice a day.	20	$15	75¢
Throat							
	Biaxin	500mg	Clarithromycin	Take 1 tablet twice a day.	20	$90	$4.50
	Erythromycin	500mg	Erythromycin	Take 1 tablet 4 times a day.	40	$18	45¢
	Penicillin V	500mg	Penicillin	Take 1 tablet every 6 hrs.	40	$10	40¢
	Zithromax	250mg	Azithromycin	Take 2 tablets on day 1 and then 1 tablet daily.	6	$50	$8.33

*Outpatient infections in adults, except children for ear infections

When **all other factors are equal**, it almost always makes sense to go with the least expensive antibiotic option. This is an important qualifier! When it comes to choosing antibiotics, cost isn't always the most appropriate factor to consider. If the doctor prescribes an expensive antibiotic, it's worth asking for an explanation. Most doctors are willing to consider other options if there are no clinical reasons for you to take the more costly antibiotic.

Here is a summary of our Smart Buy recommendations for antibiotics, based just on cost when there is no clinical justification for a high-powered, expensive drug:

✦ For bladder infections, the best choice for your money is the familiar standard SMZ/TMP DS, the generic form of Septra, which can save you $108, or a whopping 91 percent over the high-priced Floxin.

✦ For breast infections, another familiar standard is the Smart Buy: dicloxacillin. At just $37 for a 10-day course of treatment, this choice saves you $141, or 79 percent over the cost of Ceftin.

✦ For bronchitis, SMZ/TMP DS again gets the Smart Buy award, saving you $112 (91 percent) compared to popular but costly Augmentin.

✦ For infections of the external ear canal, our Smart Buy recommendation is the generic formula Hydrocortisone, Neomycin, Polymyxin B ear drops, a savings of $55 or 73 percent over Cipro HC ear drops.

✦ For eye infections if you wear contact lenses, we recommend sulfacetamide eye drops. This generic form of the brand-name product Sulamyd is a $32-savings (78 percent) over Ciloxan eye drops.

✦ For foot infections related to diabetes, your Smart Buy is cephalexin, the generic form of the brand-name drug Keflex. At $60 for a typical 10-day course of treatment this drug is still pricey, but a 66-percent savings, or $118 compared to Ceftin.

✦ For kidney infections, we once again recommend SMZ/TMP DS, a savings of $155 (92 percent) over Augmentin.

✦ For infections of the middle ear canal, amoxicillin gets our vote for Smart Buy, giving you a savings of $81 or 89 percent compared to Vantin.

✦ For mouth infections, the standard penicillin VK will save you $168, or 94 percent, compared to Ceftin.

✦ For pneumonia, doxycycline will save you $106, or 86 percent, over Augmentin.

✦ For infections of the prostate, SMZ/TMP DS can save you 90 percent ($127) compared to Cipro.

✦ For sinusitis, simple amoxicillin features savings of up to $107 or 87 percent over its supercharged but superpriced cousin Augmentin.

✦ For infections caused by bites from bats, raccoons, rats, or skunks, choosing doxycycline can save you $108 or 88 percent over Augmentin. For infected cat bites, the same choice saves you $163 (92 percent) over the very expensive Ceftin.

✦ For infected dog bites, save 33 percent, or $41, by choosing clindamycin over Augmentin.

✦ For other skin infections, erythromycin is the Smart Buy, featuring savings of up to $105 or 85 percent compared to Augmentin.

✦ For bacterial infections of the throat, your Smart Buy is penicillin VK, a choice that can save you $80 or 89 percent compared to Biaxin.

WEIGHING THE RISKS: COMMON SIDE EFFECTS

All drugs carry a risk of potential side effects, and antibiotics are no exception. In fact, antibiotics lead the list when it comes to drug allergies. Antibiotic side effects can be merely annoying (stomach upset), or they can manifest as serious problems. It's important to understand these potential risks.

HYPERSENSITIVITY (ALLERGIC REACTION)

Hypersensitivity, or an allergic reaction, is probably the most frequent and potentially the most severe problem related to any antibiotic. Common hypersensitivity reactions include rash, photosensitivity (increased sensitivity to sunlight that results in a rash), and anaphylaxis (difficulty in breathing, sometimes severe enough to be life-threatening). If you believe you're having an allergic reaction to an antibiotic, stop taking it and call your doctor. Take no more of the antibiotic until your doctor evaluates your reaction.

A potential complicating factor when it comes to drug allergies is that of *cross-sensitivity*. This means that your allergy to one antibiotic increases the likelihood that you're also allergic to certain other antibiotics. A percentage of people who are allergic to penicillin, for example, are also allergic to later-generation antibiotics such as cephalosporins. It's important to discuss any adverse reactions you've had with any antibiotic (or any drug) with any doctor who prescribes an antibiotic for you, as well as with your regular doctor. He or she might not remember, or the information might not be noted prominently in your medical record. Pharmacies always ask about and document in your file (now computerized in most stores) any allergies or reactions you may have to certain drugs. This is why filling your prescriptions regularly at the same pharmacy or drugstore gives you another layer of protection. When Maria developed a bacterial infection, her doctor prescribed the commonly used antibiotic penicillin. When we typed Maria's name into the computer to prepare the label for her prescription, her records displayed a warning that she was allergic to penicillin. We called Maria's doctor, who confirmed the allergy and changed the prescription to sulfa.

GASTRIC AND INTESTINAL UPSET

Many antibiotics cause nausea, vomiting, and diarrhea. This can be due to simple irritation of the gastrointestinal tract or from the antibiotic killing the bacterial flora naturally present in the intestines. We all have "good" or beneficial bacteria in our intestines to help with the processing of waste products. If you kill these bacteria, severe diarrhea can result. Quite often, any strong antibiotics you take to fight an infection also will kill the beneficial bacteria.

To counteract this problem, doctors and pharmacists often tell patients who are starting a course of strong antibiotics to take *Lactobacillus acidophilus* as well. This will replenish the normal bacteria in the intestines and prevent diarrhea. Various forms of *Lactobacillus acidophilus* are available, including some fairly expensive tablet forms in health food stores. But here you can safely save yourself some money. Just go to your regular grocery store and stock up on yogurt that contains live cultures (this is on the label) and eat a cup a day during the time you take the antibiotic. Most *flavored* yogurts don't contain these cultures; purchase plain unflavored yogurt.

YEAST AND FUNGAL INFECTIONS

For some women, an antibiotic prescription becomes an invitation for a vaginal yeast infection. This is another good bacteria-bad bacteria story. Antibiotics can upset the natural balance of bacterial flora that exist in the vagina, and this allows yeast and fungal infections to flourish. Antibiotics most likely to do this include:

+ Augmentin
+ Avelox
+ Cedax
+ Cipro

+ Floxin
+ Levaquin
+ Maxaquin
+ Omnicef

+ Suprax
+ Tequin
+ Trovan
+ Vantin

Fortunately, products are now available over the counter that will cure yeast infections. For more information on these remedies, see Chapter 21, "Other Over-the-Counter Products."

Antibiotics Can Cause Yeast Infections

Have you developed a yeast infection as a result of taking your antibiotic? Watch for these symptoms:

+ Moderate to intense itching in the vaginal area

+ White vaginal discharge—thick, like paste, or lumpy, like cottage cheese

+ Swollen, cracked, or reddened skin around the vagina

+ Soreness or a burning sensation inside the vagina

PHOTOSENSITIVITY

Another side effect common to many antibiotics is an increase in sensitivity to sunlight. This is different from a hypersensitivity (allergic) photosensitive reaction. Rather than develop a rash, you'll simply experience an increased tendency to sunburn. If you're taking any of the following antibiotics, apply a good sunscreen before you go outside (even when it's cloudy), and limit your exposure to the sun. (Chapter 20, "Over-the-Counter Treatments for Eyes, Ears, Mouth, and Skin," provides details on over-the-counter sunscreens.)

+ Cipro
+ Clindamycin
+ Doxycycline
+ Floxin
+ Levaquin
+ Maxaquin
+ Sulfa drugs
  (Bactrim, Septra,
  SMZ/TMP)
+ Tequin
+ Tetracycline
+ Trovan

INTERFERENCE WITH BIRTH CONTROL PILLS

Some antibiotics can decrease the effectiveness of birth control pills—so much so that pregnancy can occur. The list that follows includes some common culprits:

+ Amoxicillin
+ Ampicillin
+ Cloxacillin
+ Dicloxacillin
+ Dynabac
+ Doxycycline
+ Minocycline
+ Penicillin
+ Tetracycline

If you're taking one of these antibiotics, you may want to take extra precautions to prevent a pregnancy. Assume the antibiotic will interfere with the contraceptive properties of your birth control pills for 2 to 4 weeks, depending on how long you take it, and supplement your birth control pills with another method during that time.

ANTIBIOTIC FAMILIES

The six families of antibiotics commonly used in outpatient settings today are:

+ Cephalosporins
+ Fluoroquinolones
+ Macrolides
+ Penicillins
+ Sulfas
+ Tetracyclines

Each antibiotic family is most effective against certain kinds of bacteria. Doctors first will determine which family of antibiotic is appropriate for use against an infection, and then will select a drug within that family that they feel will provide the desired results with minimal side effects.

PENICILLINS

Penicillins generally are used for mild to moderately severe infections of the ears, sinuses, teeth, lungs, and throat. Often penicillins also are used to prevent infections of the heart valves when dental work is done, (people who have had rheumatic fever or other infections of the heart valves are at risk), and to treat sexually transmitted diseases. Members of the penicillin family include penicillin V, dicloxacillin, amoxicillin, ampicillin, and Augmentin.

Over time, penicillins have progressed from penicillin G to penicillin V, and on to ampicillin and dicloxacillin, and then into amoxicillins and augmentins and the semi-synthetics, such as cephalosporins (such as Keflex, known generically as cephalexin). Penicillin V is acid stable, but penicillin G is not and must be taken on an empty stomach. As bacteria mutated and became resistant to each new penicillin, they learned to produce an enzyme called *penicillinase*, which "deactivates" penicillin. This forced scientists to develop new penicillinase-resistant penicillins. Such penicillins include methicillin, nafcillin, oxacillin, cloxacillin, and dicloxacillin. Some of these still must be taken on empty stomach.

Augmentin is a combination of amoxicillin and clavulanic acid. Clavulanic acid makes the amoxicillin more potent, allowing it to kill bacteria that have developed a resistance to normal penicillins. This increased potency comes at a price, though: A prescription for 30 capsules of amoxicillin 500mg usually sells for around $15, while the same quantity of Augmentin 500mg costs a hefty $120. Another drawback to Augmentin is that it can cause some pretty bad diarrhea, not seen with amoxicillin. Take it with food to limit this problem. And, if you're giving this to an infant, make sure he or she drinks plenty of water (to avoid dehydration), and watch for diaper rash.

Dicloxacillin is a penicillin used mostly for staph infections of the skin. It's resistant to an enzyme made by staph bacteria that breaks down regular penicillins. Finally, of all the penicillins (except Augmentin), ampicillin covers the greatest number of a specific type of bacteria called gram-negative, which includes the type of bacteria that causes urinary tract infections. Because of this, ampicillin is generally a better choice among the antibiotics in this family for treating urinary tract infections.

Common side effects when taking any drug in the penicillin family include a sore mouth and tongue, "furry" tongue, abnormal taste sensations, abdominal pain, nausea, vomiting, and diarrhea. Take penicillins (other than Augmentin, which should be taken with food) on an empty stomach (one hour before eating) to increase absorption. Take heed: Penicillins can decrease the effectiveness of oral contraceptives. Finally, allergic reactions to penicillins are extremely common. Watch for signs of a rash, hives, itching, or any difficulty in breathing.

Antibiotics in the Penicillin Family

PRODUCT	STRENGTH PER DOSE	ACTIVE INGREDIENT	USUAL DOSAGE	TYPICAL QUANTITY	TYPICAL PRICE	PRICE PER DOSE
Amoxicillin	250mg	Amoxicillin	Take 1 capsule 3 times a day.	30	$10	33¢
Amoxicillin	500mg	Amoxicillin	Take 1 capsule 3 times a day.	30	$16	50¢
Ampicillin	250mg	Ampicillin	Take 1 capsule 3 times a day.	30	$10	33¢
Ampicillin	500mg	Ampicillin	Take 1 capsule 3 times a day.	30	$10	33¢
Augmentin (amoxicillin with clavulanic acid)	250mg	Amoxicillin with clavulanic acid	Take 1 tablet 3 times a day.	30	$100	$3.33
Augmentin (amoxicillin with clavulanic acid)	400mg	Amoxicillin with clavulanic acid	Take 1 tablet twice a day.	20	$90	$4.50
Augmentin (amoxicillin with clavulanic acid)	500mg	Amoxicillin with clavulanic acid	Take 1 tablet 3 times a day.	30	$120	$4
Augmentin (amoxicillin with clavulanic acid)	875mg	Amoxicillin with clavulanic acid	Take 1 tablet twice a day.	20	$123	$6.15
Dicloxacillin	250mg	Dicloxacillin	Take 1 capsule every 6 hrs.	40	$35	88¢
Dicloxacillin	500mg	Dicloxacillin	Take 1 capsule every 6 hrs.	40	$37	93¢
$ Penicillin VK	250mg	Penicillin	Take 1 tablet every 6 hrs.	40	$10	25¢
$ Penicillin VK	500mg	Penicillin	Take 1 tablet every 6 hrs.	40	$10	25¢

$ SMART BUY
Among the Penicillins

Unless a culture has been taken to identify the specific bacteria, or symptoms provide clues to which bacteria type is the probable culprit (for example, skin infections usually are due to *Staphylococcus*, which calls for dicloxacillin), we suggest starting with either penicillin or amoxicillin as your Smart Buy. These are by far the least expensive penicillins and usually will do the job. Switch to Augmentin if the infection doesn't clear.

CEPHALOSPORINS

The cephalosporin family is closely related to the penicillin family—so much so, in fact, that many cephalosporins cover the same bacteria as penicillins. Cephalosporins are different enough, however, that people who are allergic to penicillin generally can take them, although there's a risk of cross-sensitivity. About 2 in 25 people who are allergic to penicillin drugs are also allergic to cephalosporin drugs. There are three categories of cephalosporins.

First generation cephalosporins commonly prescribed include Keflex (generic name cephalexin), Velosef (generic name cephradine), and Duricef (generic name cefadroxil). These are the first cephalosporins that came onto the market, and all are now available in less expensive generic forms. They're used to treat bronchitis and infections of the skin, ears, bladder, throat, and sinuses.

Second generation cephalosporins commonly prescribed include Ceclor (generic name cefaclor), Lorabid (generic name loracarbef), Cefzil (generic name cefprozil), and Ceftin (generic name cefuroxime). These antibiotics came on the market in the 1990s and cover a broader range of infections. Most are available in lower cost generic versions. They cover the same types of infections as first-generation cephalosporins, but usually are not prescribed until one of the first-generation members has failed to cure the problem (resistant bacteria).

Third generation cephalosporins commonly prescribed include Omnicef (generic name cefdinir), Suprax (generic name cefixime), Vantin (generic name cefpodoxime), and Cedax (generic name ceftibuten). These are the newest antibiotics in the cephalosporin family, and the most expensive. These drugs treat the same types of infections as first- and second-generation cephalosporins but are reserved for infections not cured by them. They also work well for pneumonia, bites, and infections of the mouth, feet (diabetics), breast, prostate, and kidneys.

With the increase in gram-negative coverage comes a substantial increase in cost: A 10-day course of treatment of first-generation cephalexin 500mg (40 capsules) sells for around $25, and of third-generation Suprax 400mg (10 tablets) for about $90.

Cephalosporins are similar in structure to penicillins and cover a greater number of different bacteria than penicillins. Because cephalosporins are biosynthesized penicillins, their structure is similar but still different. Because of this, allergic responses, if any, differ, too. Allergic reactions to cephalosporins may occur if you're allergic to penicillins, but they're far less likely.

Common uses for cephalosporins include infections of the ears, urinary tract, sinuses, lungs, throat, and skin. Side effects resemble those of the penicillin family. For most cephalosporins, it doesn't matter whether doses are taken with food. Exceptions are Vantin and Ceftin; in both cases, food increases the amount absorbed into the bloodstream, so take them with meals. Allergic reactions to cephalosporins tend to be less frequent than with penicillins, but they still can occur. Watch for symptoms such as those listed in the earlier section on penicillin.

Antibiotics in the Cephalosporin Family

PRODUCT	GENERATION	STRENGTH PER DOSE	ACTIVE INGREDIENT	USUAL DOSAGE	TYPICAL QUANTITY	TYPICAL PRICE	PRICE PER DOSE
Ceclor (cefaclor)	Second	250mg	Cefaclor	Take 1 capsule 3 times a day.	30	$80	$2.67
Ceclor (cefaclor)	Second	500mg	Cefaclor	Take 1 capsule 3 times a day.	30	$86	$2.87
Cedax (ceftibuten)	Third	400mg	Ceftibuten	Take 1 capsule daily.	10	$95	$9.50
Cefaclor	Second	250mg	Cefaclor	Take 1 capsule 3 times a day.	30	$40	$1.33
Cefaclor	Second	500mg	Cefaclor	Take 1 capsule 3 times a day.	30	$40	$1.33
Cefadroxil	First	500mg	Cefadroxil	Take 1 capsule twice daily.	20	$40	$2
Ceftin (cefuroxime)	Second	250mg	Cefuroxime	Take 1 tablet twice a day.	20	$100	$5
Ceftin (cefuroxime)	Second	500mg	Cefuroxime	Take 1 tablet twice a day.	20	$178	$8.90
Cefzil (cefprozil)	Second	250mg	Cefprozil	Take 1 tablet twice a day.	20	$85	$4.25
Cefzil (cefprozil)	Second	500mg	Cefprozil	Take 1 tablet twice a day.	20	$160	$8
Cephalexin	First	250mg	Cephalexin	Take 1 capsule every 6 hrs.	40	$20	50¢
Cephalexin	First	500mg	Cephalexin	Take 1 capsule every 6 hrs.	40	$30	75¢
Cephradine	First	250mg	Cephradine	Take 1 capsule every 6 hrs.	40	$30	75¢
Cephradine	First	500mg	Cephradine	Take 1 capsule every 6 hrs.	40	$30	75¢
Duricef (cefadroxil)	First	500mg	Cefadroxil	Take 1 capsule twice daily.	20	$95	$4.75
Duricef (cefadroxil)	First	1 gram	Cefadroxil	Take 1 tablet daily.	10	$105	$10.50
Keflex (cephalexin)	First	250mg	Cephalexin	Take 1 capsule every 6 hrs.	40	$75	$1.88

PRODUCT	GENERATION	STRENGTH PER DOSE	ACTIVE INGREDIENT	USUAL DOSAGE	TYPICAL QUANTITY	TYPICAL PRICE	PRICE PER DOSE
Keflex (cephalexin)	First	500mg	Cephalexin	Take 1 capsule every 6 hrs.	40	$140	$3.50
Lorabid (loracarbef)	Second	200mg	Loracarbef	Take 1 capsule twice a day.	20	$95	$4.75
Lorabid (loracarbef)	Second	400mg	Loracarbef	Take 1 capsule twice a day.	20	$130	$6.50
Omnicef (cefdinir)	Third	300mg	Cefdinir	Take 1 capsule twice a day.	20	$96	$4.80
Suprax (cefixime)	Third	200mg	Cefixime	Take 1 tablet twice a day.	20	$90	$4.50
Suprax (cefixime)	Third	400mg	Cefixime	Take 1 tablet daily.	10	$90	$9
Vantin (cefpodoxime)	Third	100mg	Cefpodoxime	Take 1 tablet twice a day.	20	$80	$4

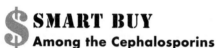

$ SMART BUY
Among the Cephalosporins

Your Smart Buy among these antibiotics is to start with a generic version of cephalexin. Don't take a second- or third-generation cephalosporin unless less powerful antibiotics have failed or a culture indicates a specific sensitivity. Because treating infections is time sensitive, alternative sources typically are not useful options.

FLUOROQUINOLONES

The fluoroquinolones comprise a fairly new family of antibiotics that have been a true blessing. Far more effective than most other antibiotics against gram-negative, anaerobic, and resistant bacteria, they've saved many lives. These are the "big guns" doctors use when other types of antibiotics prove ineffective. Fluoroquinolones are used mostly for infections of the urinary tract, lungs, sinuses, skin, bones, intestines, and for sexually transmitted diseases. Another use that came to light recently is Cipro's effectiveness at treating anthrax. Commonly used members of the fluoroquinolone family include:

- ✦ Avelox (generic name moxifloxacin)
- ✦ Cipro (generic name ciprofloxacin)
- ✦ Floxin (generic name ofloxacin)
- ✦ Levaquin (generic name levofloxacin)
- ✦ Tequin (generic name gatifloxacin)
- ✦ Trovan (generic name trovafloxacin)

Common side effects in this family include nausea, diarrhea, headaches, and dizziness. You may become more vulnerable to sunburn, as well, so wear a good sunscreen. (See Chapter 20, "Over-the-Counter Treatments for Eyes, Ears, Mouth, and Skin.")

The potential exists for liver damage (watch for signs of jaundice) and irregular heart-beats (mostly with Tequin and Avelox. Convulsions (use caution if you have epilepsy), and tendon rupture (ruptures of the shoulder, hand, and Achilles tendons) also can occur. Children should take fluoroquinolones *only* in emergency situations: These drugs can cause lesions in weight-bearing joints of adolescents that may cause lameness.

Take fluoroquinolones with lots of water and with little or no food in the stomach. Don't take antacids or iron products (including multiple vitamins) within 2 hours of taking any fluoroquinolone. Caffeine may accumulate in the blood when products containing caffeine are ingested with fluoroquinolones, so avoid coffee, black tea, cola drinks, and other such stimulants. Allergic reactions to fluoroquinolones are possible, but infrequent.

Antibiotics in the Fluoroquinolone Family

PRODUCT	STRENGTH PER DOSE	ACTIVE INGREDIENT	USUAL DOSAGE	TYPICAL QUANTITY	TYPICAL PRICE	PRICE PER DOSE
Avelox (moxifloxacin)	400mg	Moxifloxacin	Take 1 tablet a day.	10	$100	$10
Cipro (ciprofloxacin)	250mg	Ciprofloxacin	Take 1 tablet twice a day.	20	$85	$4.25
Cipro (ciprofloxacin)	500mg	Ciprofloxacin	Take 1 tablet twice a day.	20	$102	$5.10
Floxin (ofloxacin)	200mg	Ofloxacin	Take 1 tablet twice a day.	20	$95	$4.75
Floxin (ofloxacin)	300mg	Ofloxacin	Take 1 tablet twice a day.	20	$115	$5.75
Floxin (ofloxacin)	400mg	Ofloxacin	Take 1 tablet twice a day.	20	$119	$5.95
Levaquin (levofloxacin)	250mg	Levofloxacin	Take 1 tablet a day.	10	$80	$8
Levaquin (levofloxacin)	500mg	Levofloxacin	Take 1 tablet a day.	10	$97	$9.70
Tequin (gatifloxacin)	400mg	Gatifloxacin	Take 1 tablet a day.	7	$62	$8.86
Trovan (trovafloxacin)	100mg	Trovafloxacin	Take 1 tablet a day.	10	$70	$7
Trovan (trovafloxacin)	200mg	Trovafloxacin	Take 1 tablet a day.	10	$85	$8.50

$ SMART BUY
Among the Fluoroquinolones

The "quinolone" that's been around the longest and is most likely to become generic soon is Cipro. It's also the most likely to cover your infection if your doctor considers antibiotics from this family. We consider it the Smart Buy.

TETRACYCLINES

The tetracycline family contains a group of antibiotics used mostly against gram-negative bacteria and several unusual bacteria (including *Rickettsia*, which causes Rocky Mountain spotted fever and typhus, and *Mycoplasma pneumonia*, which causes a dangerous form of pneumonia). Tetracyclines are most commonly used to treat sexually transmitted diseases, intestinal infections, meningitis, acne, pneumonia, and to prevent "traveler's diarrhea." Commonly prescribed members of this family include tetracycline, doxycycline, and minocycline.

Common side effects of tetracyclines include skin rashes, nausea and vomiting, and ulcers of the esophagus. Because of this last potential problem, remain upright for at least 90 seconds after taking a tetracycline antibiotic to be sure it completely clears the esophagus. Tetracyclines can make you more apt to get a sunburn, so, again, wear a good sunscreen. (See Chapter 20, "Over-the-Counter Treatments for Eyes, Ears, Mouth, and Skin.") In children, tetracycline can cause permanent discoloration of the teeth (yellow gray-brown), so these drugs usually aren't prescribed for children 8 years old or younger.

Take tetracyclines on an empty stomach (one hour before or 2 hours after eating) to increase the amount of the drug you absorb into your system. Dairy products (milk and cheese), antacids such as Maalox or Mylanta, and iron-containing products interfere with absorption, so allow the recommended time to elapse between taking tetracyclines and ingesting any of these products. These restrictions aren't as crucial for doxycycline and minocycline as for regular tetracycline. Like penicillins, tetracyclines can reduce the effectiveness of oral contraceptives, so use extra protection. As with fluoroquinolones, allergic reactions to tetracyclines are possible but not common.

$ SMART BUY
Among the Tetracyclines

Even though many tetracyclines are still produced in name-brand forms (such as Achromycin), they're produced in such vast quantities that they're often used as the generic because pricing to wholesalers is so low. Ask your doctor to authorize a generic version; this should get you the least expensive product and save you money. Buying tetracycline in bulk will save you money, as well. Purchasing this way is your Smart Buy. Finally, buying doxycycline and minocycline in generic forms will save huge amounts of money. And, because minocycline is used mostly for acne, a chronic condition, buy this drug in bulk to save even more.

Antibiotics in the Tetracycline Family

PRODUCT	STRENGTH PER DOSE	ACTIVE INGREDIENT	USUAL DOSAGE	TYPICAL QUANTITY	TYPICAL PRICE	PRICE PER DOSE
$ Achromycin (tetracycline)	250mg	Tetracycline	Take 1 capsule twice a day.	100	$10	10¢
$ Achromycin (tetracycline)	500mg	Tetracycline	Take 1 capsule twice a day.	100	$10	10¢
Doxycycline	100mg	Doxycycline	Take 1 tablet twice a day.	20	$15	75¢
Minocin (minocycline)	50mg	Minocycline	Take 1 capsule a day.	100	$200	$2
Minocin (minocycline)	100mg	Minocycline	Take 1 capsule a day.	100	$320	$3.20
Minocycline	50mg	Minocycline	Take 1 capsule a day.	100	$55	55¢
Minocycline	100mg	Minocycline	Take 1 capsule a day.	100	$70	70¢
Sumycin (tetracycline)	250mg	Tetracycline	Take 1 capsule twice a day.	100	$15	15¢
Sumycin (tetracycline)	500mg	Tetracycline	Take 1 capsule twice a day.	100	$15	15¢

MACROLIDES

For many years, erythromycin was the only macrolide antibiotic available. Commonly used for infections in patients that couldn't tolerate penicillin, this antibiotic quickly became known for its strong tendency to cause intestinal irritations (nausea, diarrhea, cramping). Newer macrolides are much easier on the stomach. These include Biaxin (generic name clarithromycin) and Zithromax (generic name azithromycin). This improvement in stomach problems comes at an increased price, though. A 10-day course of treatment with erythromycin 500mg (40 tablets) runs around $20, while 10 days of treatment with Biaxin 500mg (20 tablets) will set you back around $90.

Macrolide antibiotics usually are used for infections in people who can't tolerate penicillins or cephalosporins. They're used to treat *Helicobacter pylori*, the bacteria that causes certain types of stomach ulcers, and have shown effectiveness in treating anthrax. Side effects mostly include diarrhea, nausea, and abdominal cramping. Although such reactions are a lot less common with Biaxin and Zithromax, they still can occur. To limit this problem, take any macrolide antibiotic with food. Rarely, Biaxin causes an unusual "metallic" taste in the mouth; this annoying problem will go away once you've finished taking the medication.

Erythromycin is notorious for causing drug interactions. Because it slows liver enzymes responsible for clearing many drugs out of the body, taking erythromycin when you're taking certain other drugs can cause an overdose of other medications. Drugs to watch out for include these:

- ✦ Baycol
- ✦ Buspar
- ✦ Cyclosporine
- ✦ Digoxin
- ✦ Disopyramide
- ✦ Halcion

- ✦ Lescol
- ✦ Lipitor
- ✦ Mevacor
- ✦ Oral contraceptives
- ✦ Pravachol
- ✦ Prilosec

- ✦ Tegretol
- ✦ Theophylline products
- ✦ Valium
- ✦ Warfarin
- ✦ Xanax
- ✦ Zocor

Erythromycin is the macrolide most likely to cause problems, although Biaxin can be the culprit if you're taking a cholesterol-reducing drug. Allergic reactions to macrolide antibiotics are possible but not common.

Antibiotics in the Macrolide Family

PRODUCT	STRENGTH PER DOSE	ACTIVE INGREDIENT	USUAL DOSAGE	TYPICAL QUANTITY	TYPICAL PRICE	PRICE PER DOSE
Biaxin (clarithromycin)	250mg	Clarithromycin	Take 1 tablet twice a day.	20	$90	$4.50
Biaxin (clarithromycin)	500mg	Clarithromycin	Take 1 tablet twice a day.	20	$92	$4.60
Erythromycin	250mg	Erythromycin	Take 1 tablet 4 times a day.	40	$10	25¢
Erythromycin	333mg	Erythromycin	Take 1 tablet 4 times a day.	40	$15	38¢
Erythromycin	500mg	Erythromycin	Take 1 tablet 4 times a day.	40	$18	45¢
Zithromax Z pack (azithromycin)	250mg	Azithromycin	Take 2 tablets on day 1, then 1 tablet a day.	6	$50	$8.33

Many pharmacies stock erythromycin in name-brand forms because they're priced low and some are coated to protect against stomach irritation. One common brand is Ery-Tab, manufactured by Abbott Labs. Its reduced price and special coating make it our Smart Buy among the macrolide antibiotics.

SULFAS

Sulfa antibiotics have been around for a very long time. Since 1943, these miraculous drugs have saved millions of lives. Even though far stronger antibiotics are on the market today, sulfa drugs remain in common use. These products include Bactrim DS (generic name sulfamethoxazole/trimethoprim DS) and Septra DS (generic name sulfamethoxazole/trimethoprim DS).

Bactrim and Septra are the same sulfa manufactured by different companies. Infections treated with sulfa drugs include urinary tract infections, sinus infections, meningitis, ear infections, and sexually transmitted diseases. Unfortunately, many bacteria have become resistant to sulfa antibiotics, and this limits their effectiveness. Nonetheless, sulfas are good antibiotics to choose when you want to save money. Twenty tablets of sulfamethoxazole/trimethoprim DS usually costs around $11, while 20 Cipro 500mg tablets, a common alternative prescription, will set you back about $100. Although there's a chance that a sulfa antibiotic would be less effective than Cipro at treating a urinary tract infection, the huge cost difference certainly makes it worth a try.

Common side effects with sulfa drugs include nausea, abdominal pain, an increase in sensitivity to sunlight (wear a good sunscreen; see Chapter 20, "Over-the-Counter Treatments for Eyes, Ears, Mouth, and Skin"), and serious blood disorders, including a fatal anemia (watch for signs such as sore throat, fever, pallor, and jaundice). Allergic reactions are extremely common; watch for rash, itching, hives, or difficulty breathing. Pregnant women near the end of their pregnancies and women breastfeeding infants younger than 2 months shouldn't take sulfa drugs because of the risk of the infant's developing a severe blood disorder. Potential drug interactions include warfarin (hemorrhaging can occur), cyclosporine (decreased blood levels possibly resulting in an organ-transplant rejection), phenytoin (increased drowsiness and confusion), and methotrexate (increased risk of bone marrow suppression).

Unless you have an allergy to sulfa or a culture indicates the bacteria causing your infection are resistant to it, a sulfa antibiotic is worth trying: The cost savings can be enormous. Buy the generic! Twenty tablets of Septra DS will cost you $45; the same number of SMZ/TMP DS tablets costs $11. Compared to Bactrim and Septra, SMZ/TMP is clearly the Smart Buy.

Antibiotics in the Sulfa Family

PRODUCT	STRENGTH PER DOSE	ACTIVE INGREDIENT	USUAL DOSAGE	TYPICAL QUANTITY	TYPICAL PRICE	PRICE PER DOSE
Bactrim (sulfamethoxazole with trimethoprim)	400/80mg	Sulfamethoxazole with trimethoprim	Take 1 tablet twice a day.	20	$30	$1.50
Bactrim DS (sulfamethoxazole with trimethoprim)	800/160mg	Sulfamethoxazole with trimethoprim	Take 1 tablet twice a day.	20	$45	$2.25

PRODUCT	STRENGTH PER DOSE	ACTIVE INGREDIENT	USUAL DOSAGE	TYPICAL QUANTITY	TYPICAL PRICE	PRICE PER DOSE
Septra (sulfamethoxazole with trimethoprim)	400/80mg	Sulfamethoxazole with trimethoprim	Take 1 tablet twice a day.	20	$30	$1.50
Septra DS (sulfamethoxazole with trimethoprim)	800/160mg	Sulfamethoxazole with trimethoprim	Take 1 tablet twice a day.	20	$45	$2.25
SMZ/TMP (sulfamethoxazole with trimethoprim)	400/80mg	Sulfamethoxazole with trimethoprim	Take 1 tablet twice a day.	20	$8	40¢
SMZ/TMP DS (sulfamethoxazole with trimethoprim)	800/160mg	Sulfamethoxazole with trimethoprim	Take 1 tablet twice a day.	20	$11	55¢

CHOOSING THE RIGHT ANTIBIOTIC

No antibiotic kills all types of bacteria. Most doctors prescribe the antibiotics they feel will work most effectively against the bacteria causing your infection, based on your symptoms. If your doctor does a culture (by collecting a sample of tissue or fluid and sending it to the lab), the results will include findings of sensitivity—which antibiotics will kill the bacteria. In this case, your doctor will prescribe an antibiotic to which your bacteria are sensitive. It takes several days for culture results to be known, and that's one reason doctors often skip this test. If your doctor doesn't do a culture, he or she is making an educated guess about which antibiotics are most likely to be effective.

$ SMART OPTIONS FOR SAVINGS
Antibiotics

When choosing an antibiotic, the key, of course, is to pick one that will kill the bacteria causing *your* infection (saving the "big guns" for when you really need them), while saving as much money as possible. For most routine infections, this means starting with the weakest and least expensive drug in the appropriate antibiotic family. Most of the time this will do the job and save you money.

Remember these key points:

◆ Make sure you really need to take an antibiotic. Antibiotics have no effect against illnesses and infections caused by viruses. Taking them when you don't need them is like throwing your money out the window (and can cause other health problems).

+ Ask your doctor whether the drug he or she prescribes is the least expensive antibiotic effective against your condition. Drug allergies, possible interference with other drugs you're taking, and other aspects of your health history will influence your doctor's choice.

+ If the antibiotic you're taking doesn't work, ask your doctor to do a culture before prescribing a different one. This will identify the specific bacteria causing the infection and indicate which antibiotics will be most effective against them. Trial and error might be more convenient for your doctor, but it can be expensive for you!

+ Alternative drug sources, such as mail-order and Canadian pharmacies, usually aren't good options when you need an antibiotic, because you can't afford to wait.

+ Check our Web site at www.smartbuysdrugwise.com for the latest information and more ways to save money on these drugs.

Chapter 8

Prescription Drugs to Treat Heart Conditions

Heart disease is the leading killer of adults in America, both male and female, although many people tend to think of heart disease as a man's problem. In fact, heart disease kills more men *and* women each year than all forms of cancer combined. So it's not surprising that drugs to treat heart conditions lead the list of prescriptions that American doctors write each year—176 million prescriptions annually, costing consumers millions of dollars. Many kinds of heart disease exist, so it's not surprising that many kinds of drugs exist to treat heart problems. And because it's not uncommon to have more than one heart problem at the same time, many people must take multiple prescription drugs.

DRUGS THAT MODIFY THE BLOOD

These drugs are mostly used to thin the blood to prevent heart attacks and strokes. Some also are used to help improve blood flow to certain areas of the body. Each of the several members of this drug family differs from the others according to the part of the blood it's designed to affect. Some drugs affect the platelets, some influence clotting, and others affect the viscosity and flexibility of the actual blood cells (how "sticky" the cells are, which influences how well they flow through the blood vessels). When taking a drug to reduce your blood's clotting ability, be sure to have your blood tested routinely to make sure it clots quickly enough to prevent excessive or internal bleeding. The test that measures this is called a *prothrombin time* (or "pro-time"). Signs of internal bleeding include blood in the stool or urine, nosebleeds, or an increase in bruising. If you experience any of these, contact your doctor right away.

Many of these drugs have narrow therapeutic indexes (NTIs), which means your doctor will supervise your treatment closely and probably call for frequent blood tests. Because these drugs affect how quickly your blood clots, ask your doctor if you should stop taking them before any scheduled surgery. Tell your surgeon and the anesthesiologist what drugs you're taking.

Sometimes it takes a little creative intervention to find the savings when it comes to these expensive drugs. After a visit to his doctor, John came to the pharmacy with a prescription for Pletal, a heavy-hitter in this drug group (with a price tag to match). John was stunned when he learned the cost—$108. He just didn't have the money to buy this drug. So we offered to call John's doctor to see whether a slightly different drug, pentoxifylline, could be prescribed instead. Because John had never taken any drugs from this group, his doctor had just picked one she knew was likely to work. But the generic form of Trental we suggested would likely achieve the same therapeutic effect to help improve the flow of blood to John's legs, and it would cost John half as much—$56. That's still a hefty amount, but at least it was something John could afford. We made the switch. John did well on the pentoxifylline and was much happier about the cost.

Drugs that Modify the Blood

PRODUCT	STRENGTH PER DOSE	ACTIVE INGREDIENT	USUAL DOSAGE	TYPICAL QUANTITY	TYPICAL PRICE	PRICE PER DOSE
Coumadin (warfarin)	1mg	Warfarin	Take 1 tablet daily.	30	$25	83¢
Coumadin (warfarin)	2mg	Warfarin	Take 1 tablet daily.	30	$25	83¢
Coumadin (warfarin)	2.5mg	Warfarin	Take 1 tablet daily.	30	$28	93¢
Coumadin (warfarin)	4mg	Warfarin	Take 1 tablet daily.	30	$28	93¢
Coumadin (warfarin)	5mg	Warfarin	Take 1 tablet daily.	30	$30	$1
Coumadin (warfarin)	7.5mg	Warfarin	Take 1 tablet daily.	30	$35	$1.17
Coumadin (warfarin)	10mg	Warfarin	Take 1 tablet daily.	30	$38	$1.27
Dipyridamole	25mg	Dipyridamole	Take 1 tablet 3 times a day.	90	$15	17¢
Dipyridamole	50mg	Dipyridamole	Take 1 tablet 3 times a day.	90	$15	17¢
Dipyridamole	75mg	Dipyridamole	Take 1 tablet 3 times a day.	90	$20	22¢
Pentoxifylline	400mg	Pentoxifylline	Take 1 tablet 3 times a day.	90	$50	56¢
Persantine (dipyridamole)	25mg	Dipyridamole	Take 1 tablet 3 times a day.	90	$60	67¢
Persantine (dipyridamole)	50mg	Dipyridamole	Take 1 tablet 3 times a day.	90	$80	89¢
Persantine (dipyridamole)	75mg	Dipyridamole	Take 1 tablet 3 times a day.	90	$105	$1.17
Plavix (clopidogrel)	75mg	Clopidogrel	Take 1 tablet daily.	30	$125	$4.17

PRODUCT	STRENGTH PER DOSE	ACTIVE INGREDIENT	USUAL DOSAGE	TYPICAL QUANTITY	TYPICAL PRICE	PRICE PER DOSE
Pletal (cilostazol)	50mg	Cilostazol	Take 1 tablet twice a day.	60	$110	$1.83
Pletal (cilostazol)	100mg	Cilostazol	Take 1 tablet twice a day.	60	$110	$1.83
Ticlid (ticlopidine)	250mg	Ticlopidine	Take 1 tablet twice a day.	60	$150	$2.50
Ticlopidine	250mg	Ticlopidine	Take 1 tablet twice a day.	60	$65	$1.08
Trental (pentoxifylline)	400mg	Pentoxifylline	Take 1 tablet 3 times a day.	90	$85	94¢
Warfarin	1mg	Warfarin	Take 1 tablet daily.	30	$20	67¢
Warfarin	2mg	Warfarin	Take 1 tablet daily.	30	$20	67¢
Warfarin	2.5mg	Warfarin	Take 1 tablet daily.	30	$20	67¢
Warfarin	4mg	Warfarin	Take 1 tablet daily.	30	$22	73¢
Warfarin	5mg	Warfarin	Take 1 tablet daily.	30	$20	67¢
Warfarin	7.5mg	Warfarin	Take 1 tablet daily.	30	$28	93¢
Warfarin	10mg	Warfarin	Take 1 tablet daily.	30	$30	$1

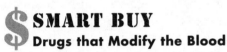

$ SMART BUY
Drugs that Modify the Blood

For drugs that work on the platelets to prevent strokes and heart attacks, we like Persantine (generic name dipyridamole) and aspirin. These two drugs are much cheaper than Ticlid (generic name ticlopidine) and Plavix (generic name clopidogrel). One month of a generic version of Persantine 50mg costs around $15 and aspirin can be bought for less than a penny a pill. By comparison, a one-month supply of a generic version of Ticlid is around $65, and Plavix will run you about $130. To save the most money, purchase the generic version of Persantine and buy it in bulk at a cost of about 17 cents a pill. Although a 100-count bottle of aspirin looks pretty cheap at $5, for just twice the cost you can get 10 times the quantity; expect to pay around $10 for a 1,000-count bottle.

For intermittent claudication, we prefer Trental (pentoxifylline). Buy a generic version in a 100-count bottle and save about 39 cents a dose, or $35 for a 30-day supply. One caution, however—some people find pentoxifylline slightly less effective than the more expensive Pletal.

> ## No Aspirin or NSAIDs with Blood Thinners
>
> Unless you're specifically told by your doctor to do so, don't take any products that contain aspirin or NSAIDs (ibuprofen, naproxen, ketoprofen) while you're taking a blood thinner. If you have a headache or are running a fever, take Tylenol (acetaminophen) instead.

CARDIOVASCULAR DRUGS

Cardiovascular drugs work on the heart and blood vessels to treat various forms of heart disease. They're extremely important, and frequently prescribed, because heart disease remains the leading cause of death in the United States. Not surprisingly, this category boasts a dozen or so *kinds* of drugs, as well as many *different* drugs.

Many cardiovascular medications are quite expensive. A 30-day supply of Cordarone (for irregular heartbeats) runs around $120, Covera (reduces blood pressure) around $60, and Diovan (reduces blood pressure) around $50. (Check our Web site at www.smartbuysdrugwise.com for updated information.) Other drugs that have been in use for decades and are available in generic versions are surprisingly inexpensive. Of course, your medical condition will determine which drugs are appropriate for you. When alternatives exist, we'll tell you how to make the choices that best meet your needs.

DIGOXIN: STRENGTHENING THE HEART'S PUMPING ABILITY

Digoxin, or digitalis, is one of the oldest cardiovascular drugs. The most common brand name is Lanoxin. This drug is obtained from a poisonous plant called foxglove, and it has been in use in some form since the time of the ancient Greek physician Hippocrates. Although proper doses of digoxin can strengthen the heart muscle and improve its pumping efficiency, excessive amounts can cause the heart to stop. Doctors usually prescribe digoxin to treat congestive heart failure (CHF), a condition in which the heart becomes inefficient and fluid builds up around the heart and lungs. Digoxin is also very good for stabilizing irregular heartbeats of the atria (upper chambers of the heart). In generic versions, this is one of the least expensive cardiovascular drugs.

Like many drugs that have therapeutic uses, digoxin is also a poison. Taking too much can slow your heart to the point of stopping, causing death. Digoxin accumulates in the body and can reach toxic levels, even when it appears to be working as intended. For this reason, doctors often use blood tests to measure the actual levels of the drug in your system. The older you are, the more sensitive your body is to the effects of digoxin. If you're taking digoxin, it's especially important that you know the signs of poisoning so you can avoid overdosing. Signs that you're taking too much digoxin include nausea, diarrhea, loss of appetite, vomiting, a slow pulse, and visual disturbances. Many people describe such visual effects as seeing a halo when looking at a light. If you're taking digoxin and experience any of these symptoms, contact your doctor immediately.

Maintaining a sufficient blood level of potassium is important when you take digoxin. Low potassium levels sensitize the heart muscle to this drug. Toxicity may develop, even though digoxin blood levels are normal. Rapid reduction of potassium (from taking a strong diuretic or due to severe vomiting and diarrhea), then, can be quite dangerous. If you're taking a diuretic (and you probably are if you have CHF), or if you experience dramatic fluid losses from vomiting or diarrhea, check with your doctor about potassium replenishment. This might be as simple and cheap as eating a banana a day (bananas are especially high in potassium) or taking a potassium supplement. We talk more about potassium supplements in the section "Diuretics ('Water Pills'): Another Approach to Treating Hypertension," later in this chapter.

Digoxin Products

PRODUCT	STRENGTH PER DOSE	USUAL DOSAGE	TYPICAL QUANTITY	TYPICAL PRICE	PRICE PER DOSE
Digitek (digoxin)	0.125mg	Take 1 tablet daily.	30	$12	40¢
Digitek (digoxin)	0.25mg	Take 1 tablet daily.	30	$12	40¢
Digoxin	0.125mg	Take 1 tablet daily.	30	$10	33¢
Digoxin	0.25mg	Take 1 tablet daily.	30	$10	33¢
Lanoxin (digoxin)	0.125mg	Take 1 tablet daily.	30	$15	50¢
Lanoxin (digoxin)	0.25mg	Take 1 tablet daily.	30	$15	50¢

$ SMART BUY
Digoxin Products

Buying generic versions of these mediations will save you money and are your Smart Buy. (Thirty tablets of name-brand Lanoxin 0.25 mg sell for about $15; generic versions cost around $10.) But remember that digoxin is an NTI drug. Because of this, don't switch brands if you're already stable on the name brand. Five dollars a month isn't worth the potential problems and blood tests that become necessary to make sure the new brand's levels are therapeutic. If you're just starting out on digoxin, though, go with the generic. You can save money by purchasing larger quantities. Expect to pay about 14 cents a dose, or $14 for a 100-count bottle (more than a 3-month supply).

DRUGS TO TREAT ARRHYTHMIAS

The group of drugs used to treat arrhythmias, or irregular heartbeats, is long and contains several families. Some of these drugs treat only irregular heartbeats; others correct irregular heartbeat and other heart problems. And some of these drugs are available in extended-release formulas, reducing the number of times a day you need to take them. As you might expect, the more the drug does, the more it costs. Older antiarrhythmia drugs are available in generic versions that are less expensive than their name-brand counterparts; newer drugs that are still under patent come in only the high-priced name-brand versions. Because your doctor might choose from any of a variety of antiarrhythmia drugs, we'll discuss the drugs first and then make our Smart Buy suggestions.

DRUGS TO TREAT IRREGULAR HEARTBEATS ONLY

First, let's look at the drugs used just for irregular heartbeats. Again, some of the older drugs—that is, drugs that have been in use for a long time—are still some of the stronger, and least expensive, agents available. All the drugs in this category are considered to have narrow therapeutic indexes (NTIs), so the dose that's correct for you must be very precise. Ask your pharmacist to avoid switching around among brands.

Clearly these drugs have saved and lengthened many lives. They're true miracle drugs. But they come with their share of problems. For example, Procan (generic name procainamide) and Tonocard (generic name tocainide) have been known to cause some deadly problems with the blood. Because of this, you should have your blood tested every week for the first 3 months you take one of these drugs and periodically thereafter. If you experience any problems, such as fever, chills, sore throat, bruising, or bleeding, report them to your doctor. Procan can also promote the development of lupus, a serious autoimmune disease.

Drugs to Treat Irregular Heartbeats Only

PRODUCT	STRENGTH PER DOSE	ACTIVE INGREDIENT	USUAL DOSAGE	TYPICAL QUANTITY	TYPICAL PRICE	PRICE PER DOSE
Amiodarone	200mg	Amiodarone	Take 1 tablet daily.	30	$56	$1.87
Cordarone (amiodarone)	200mg	Amiodarone	Take 1 tablet daily.	30	$125	$4.17
Disopyramide	100mg	Disopyramide	Take 1 capsule twice a day.	60	$14	23¢
Disopyramide	150mg	Disopyramide	Take 1 capsule twice a day.	60	$53	88¢
Mexiletine	150mg	Mexiletine	Take 1 capsule every 8 hrs.	90	$50	56¢
Mexiletine	200mg	Mexiletine	Take 1 capsule every 8 hrs.	90	$59	66¢
Mexitil (mexiletine)	150mg	Mexiletine	Take 1 capsule every 8 hrs.	90	$109	$1.21
Mexitil (mexiletine)	200mg	Mexiletine	Take 1 capsule every 8 hrs.	90	$140	$1.56
Norpace CR (disopyramide)	100mg	Disopyramide	Take 1 capsule twice a day.	60	$64	$1.07
Norpace CR (disopyramide)	150mg	Disopyramide	Take 1 capsule twice a day.	60	$75	$1.25
Procainamide	250mg	Procainamide	Take 1 tablet twice a day.	60	$23	38¢
Procainamide	500mg	Procainamide	Take 1 tablet twice a day.	60	$45	75¢
Procainamide	750mg	Procainamide	Take 1 tablet twice a day.	60	$32	53¢
Procan SR (procainamide)	250mg	Procainamide	Take 1 tablet twice a day.	60	$36	60¢
Procan SR (procainamide)	500mg	Procainamide	Take 1 tablet twice a day.	60	$58	97¢
Procan SR (procainamide)	750mg	Procainamide	Take 1 tablet twice a day.	60	$74	$1.23
Propafenone	150mg	Propafenone	Take 1 tablet every 8 hrs.	90	$140	$1.56
Propafenone	225mg	Propafenone	Take 1 tablet every 8 hrs.	90	$175	$1.94
Quinaglute (quinidine gluconate)	324mg	Quinidine gluconate	Take 1 tablet every 12 hrs.	60	$50	83¢
Quinidex (quinidine sulfate)	300mg	Quinidine sulfate	Take 1 tablet every 12 hrs.	60	$78	$1.30
Quinidine gluconate	324mg	Quinidine gluconate	Take 1 tablet every 12 hrs.	60	$31	52¢
Quinidine sulfate	300mg	Quinidine sulfate	Take 1 tablet every 12 hrs.	60	$38	63¢
Rythmol (propafenone)	150mg	Propafenone	Take 1 tablet every 8 hrs.	90	$186	$2.07
Rythmol (propafenone)	225mg	Propafenone	Take 1 tablet every 8 hrs.	90	$244	$2.71

PRODUCT	STRENGTH PER DOSE	ACTIVE INGREDIENT	USUAL DOSAGE	TYPICAL QUANTITY	TYPICAL PRICE	PRICE PER DOSE
Rythmol (propafenone)	150mg	Propafenone	Take 1 tablet every 8 hrs.	90	$186	$2.07
Rythmol (propafenone)	225mg	Propafenone	Take 1 tablet every 8 hrs.	90	$244	$2.71

$ SMART BUY
Drugs to Treat Irregular Heartbeats Only

These drugs are probably the most dangerous to substitute for. They have extremely narrow therapeutic indexes. Thus, if you're already taking one of these medications, we don't recommend changing brands or finding a generic substitute to save money. Stick with what your doctor has ordered. Likewise, we don't recommend cutting tablets to cut costs here. About the only commonsense way to save money with these drugs is to buy them in bulk, which will lower your costs somewhat. For example, 30 tablets of Rythmol 150mg typically sell for around $65 ($2.17 per dose). If you buy 90 at a time, your price should be around $180 (an even $2 per dose). (Refer to our Web site at www.smartbuysdrugwise.com for up-to-date information.) Finally, because missing doses of these drugs could be life-threatening, we don't recommend seeking alternative sources. If your package doesn't arrive in the mail on time, the consequences can be serious. And the close monitoring your doctor must do when you're taking any of these drugs makes the trip to Canada far less economical.

If your doctor is considering putting you on one of these medications, we suggest you ask about using Norpace CR. It has a generic form that will save you money, doesn't require as many blood tests as are recommended for procainamide, and you need only take it twice a day. At less than 50 cents a day for the lower dosage, it's a Smart Buy for you to ask your doctor about.

DRUGS USED TO PREVENT AND STOP ANGINA

Angina is a condition in which a limited flow of blood through the coronary arteries (arteries that supply the muscles of the heart with blood) causes a decrease in oxygen in those muscles. The patient who has angina typically complains of sharp pains in the chest. Angina is a sign of a very serious condition, because limited blood flow to the heart eventually can lead to heart attacks. To treat this condition, vasodilators often are prescribed. Vasodilators help to improve this problem simply by dilating the arteries and increasing the amount of blood and oxygen that reaches the heart muscles. To date, the only drugs used to treat angina are isosorbide (a form of nitroglycerin) and nitroglycerin. Commonly prescribed products include:

- ✦ Imdur (generic name isosorbide mononitrate)
- ✦ Ismo (generic name isosorbide mononitrate)
- ✦ Minitran patches (generic name nitroglycerin)
- ✦ Monoket (generic name isosorbide mononitrate)
- ✦ Nitro-Dur patches (generic name nitroglycerin)
- ✦ Nitrolingual spray (generic name nitroglycerin)
- ✦ Nitrostat (generic name nitroglycerin)

Products that contain isosorbide (such as Imdur and Ismo) and nitroglycerin in a patch form are prescribed to prevent angina. Nitroglycerin tablets and spray are used under the tongue in order to stop an active bout of angina and hopefully prevent a heart attack. It's important to remember that with the nitroglycerin tablets and spray you can give yourself a dose every 5 minutes, if you need to. If the third dose doesn't stop the attack, however, go to the emergency room right away.

> ### Store Nitroglycerin Carefully
>
> Nitroglycerin tablets lose potency fast. If you don't open the bottle from your pharmacy, they'll remain potent until the expiration date shown on the label. But once you've broken the seal, moisture gets in and the tablets disintegrate over time. We strongly recommend that you buy a new supply within 6 months of opening a new bottle.

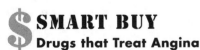

$ SMART BUY
Drugs that Treat Angina

We recommend you buy a generic product that contains isosorbide. This can cut your cost in half. And buy in bulk and ask whether the tablets can be cut. You'll probably see your cost go from $2 to 90 cents a day.

The Smart Buy to look for is the generic version of Imdur. This once-a-day tablet is more convenient and will save you money. For nitroglycerin patches, we recommend you buy the generic versions. They're equivalent to the name-brand items and cost

Drugs Used to Prevent and Stop Angina

PRODUCT	STRENGTH PER DOSE	ACTIVE INGREDIENT	USE	USUAL DOSAGE	TYPICAL QUANTITY	TYPICAL PRICE	PRICE PER DOSE
Imdur (isosorbide mononitrate)	30mg	Isosorbide mononitrate	Prevention	Take 1 tablet daily.	30	$55	$1.83
Imdur (isosorbide mononitrate)	60mg	Isosorbide mononitrate	Prevention	Take 1 tablet daily.	30	$55	$1.83
Imdur (isosorbide mononitrate)	120mg	Isosorbide mononitrate	Prevention	Take 1 tablet daily.	30	$75	$2.50
Ismo (isosorbide mononitrate)	20mg	Isosorbide mononitrate	Prevention	Take 1 tablet twice a day.	60	$65	$1.08
Isosorbide mononitrate	10mg	Isosorbide mononitrate	Prevention	Take 1 tablet twice a day.	60	$30	50¢
Isosorbide mononitrate	20mg	Isosorbide mononitrate	Prevention	Take 1 tablet twice a day.	60	$30	50¢
$ Isosorbide mononitrate	30mg	Isosorbide mononitrate	Prevention	Take 1 tablet daily.	30	$20	67¢
$ Isosorbide mononitrate	60mg	Isosorbide mononitrate	Prevention	Take 1 tablet daily.	30	$25	83¢
$ Isosorbide mononitrate	120mg	Isosorbide mononitrate	Prevention	Take 1 tablet daily.	30	$45	$1.50
Minitran (nitroglycerin) patches	0.1mg	Nitroglycerin	Prevention	Apply 1 patch daily.	30	$55	$1.83
Minitran (nitroglycerin) patches	0.2mg	Nitroglycerin	Prevention	Apply 1 patch daily.	30	$55	$1.83
Minitran (nitroglycerin) patches	0.4mg	Nitroglycerin	Prevention	Apply 1 patch daily.	30	$60	$2
Minitran (nitroglycerin) patches	0.6mg	Nitroglycerin	Prevention	Apply 1 patch daily.	30	$65	$2.17
Monoket (isosorbide mononitrate)	10mg	Isosorbide mononitrate	Prevention	Take 1 tablet twice a day.	60	$60	$1
Monoket (isosorbide mononitrate)	20mg	Isosorbide mononitrate	Prevention	Take 1 tablet twice a day.	60	$60	$1
Nitoquick (nitroglycerin)	0.4mg	Nitroglycerin	Stopping active problem	Dissolve 1 tablet under the tongue as needed.	25	$7	28¢
$ Nitoquick (nitroglycerin)	0.4mg	Nitroglycerin	Stopping active problem	Dissolve 1 tablet under the tongue as needed.	100	$10	10¢
Nitro-Dur patches (nitroglycerin)	0.1mg	Nitroglycerin	Prevention	Apply 1 patch daily.	30	$60	$2

PRODUCT	STRENGTH PER DOSE	ACTIVE INGREDIENT	USE	USUAL DOSAGE	TYPICAL QUANTITY	TYPICAL PRICE	PRICE PER DOSE
Nitro-Dur patches (nitroglycerin)	0.2mg	Nitroglycerin	Prevention	Apply 1 patch daily.	30	$60	$2
Nitro-Dur patches (nitroglycerin)	0.3mg	Nitroglycerin	Prevention	Apply 1 patch daily.	30	$65	$2.17
Nitro-Dur patches) (nitroglycerin)	0.4mg	Nitroglycerin	Prevention	Apply 1 patch daily.	30	$65	$2.17
Nitro-Dur patches) (nitroglycerin	0.6mg	Nitroglycerin	Prevention	Apply 1 patch daily.	30	$70	$2.33
Nitro-Dur patches (nitroglycerin)	0.8mg	Nitroglycerin	Prevention	Apply 1 patch daily.	30	$70	$2.33
Nitroglycerin patches	0.1mg	Nitroglycerin	Prevention	Apply 1 patch daily.	30	$25	83¢
Nitroglycerin patches	0.2mg	Nitroglycerin	Prevention	Apply 1 patch daily.	30	$27	90¢
Nitroglycerin patches	0.3mg	Nitroglycerin	Prevention	Apply 1 patch daily.	30	$27	90¢
Nitroglycerin patches	0.4mg	Nitroglycerin	Prevention	Apply 1 patch daily.	30	$30	$1.00
Nitroglycerin patches	0.6mg	Nitroglycerin	Prevention	Apply 1 patch daily.	30	$40	$1.33
Nitroglycerin patches	0.8mg	Nitroglycerin	Prevention	Apply 1 patch daily.	30	$40	$1.33
Nitrolingual spray	0.4mg	Nitroglycerin	Stopping active problem	1 spray under the tongue as needed.	1 bottle	$35	18¢
Nitrostat (nitroglycerin)	0.3mg	Nitroglycerin	Stopping active problem	Dissolve 1 tablet under the tongue as needed.	100	$15	15¢
Nitrostat (nitroglycerin)	0.4mg	Nitroglycerin	Stopping active problem	Dissolve 1 tablet under the tongue as needed.	25	$10	40¢
Nitrostat (nitroglycerin)	0.4mg	Nitroglycerin	Stopping active problem	Dissolve 1 tablet under the tongue as needed.	100	$15	15¢

about half as much. Look for generic Minitran or Nitro-Dur for your Smart Buy. To save even more money with these, buy multiple boxes at a time. For example, one box of nitroglycerin 0.1mg patches typically sells for around $25. If you buy three boxes at a time, you can expect to pay around $60—a $60 (three boxes free!) over the course of a year. Likewise, we recommend buying nitroglycerin tablets in a generic form, getting the 100-count bottle (unless you won't use them within 6 months), and buying multiple bottles. That's a truly Smart Buy.

DRUGS TO TREAT IRREGULAR HEARTBEAT AND OTHER HEART PROBLEMS

Other drugs commonly used to treat certain arrhythmias (as well as other heart conditions) include drugs called *calcium channel blockers* and *beta-blockers*. These tend to have fewer serious side effects than the other antiarrhythmia drugs, but they're also not quite as strong at regulating the heartbeat.

CALCIUM CHANNEL BLOCKERS

Calcium channel blockers are drugs that can cause the muscles of blood vessels to relax. This produces a very strong reduction in blood pressure that, in turn, decreases the work the heart must do, allowing it to function more effectively. Calcium channel blockers are an excellent choice for people who have both arrhythmias and high blood pressure, or high blood pressure alone. The market for these drugs is enormous, so of course, many manufacturers want a piece of the action.

Products available in extended-release formulas for 24-hour coverage are generally the most effective and economical. And when they become available in generic versions, the savings can really add up! When Cardizem CD became available in a generic form, people began to realize some significant savings. Jim, a customer who had been taking Cardizem, made the switch to generic and was delighted to find that his monthly bill for this drug plummeted from $55 to $36—a savings of 35 percent!

> ### ► Hold the Grapefruit!
>
> Recently it was discovered that grapefruit juice can affect enzymes in the lining of the stomach so much that dangerously high blood levels of many calcium channel blockers can occur. Oddly enough, separating the two by several hours doesn't help. Research has shown that the juice's effect can last as long as 24 hours.
>
> If you want a citrus juice with your breakfast, stick with orange.

Calcium Channel Blockers to Treat Irregular Heartbeat and Other Heart Problems

PRODUCT	STRENGTH PER DOSE	ACTIVE INGREDIENT	USUAL DOSAGE	TYPICAL QUANTITY	TYPICAL PRICE	PRICE PER DOSE
Adalat (nifedipine)	10mg	Nifedipine	Take 1 capsule 3 times a day.	90	$55	61¢
Adalat CC (nifedipine ER)	30mg	Nifedipine	Take 1 tablet daily.	30	$50	$1.67
Adalat CC (nifedipine ER)	60mg	Nifedipine	Take 1 tablet daily.	30	$80	$2.67
Adalat CC (nifedipine ER)	90mg	Nifedipine	Take 1 tablet daily.	30	$90	$3.00
Calan (verapamil)	40mg	Verapamil	Take 1 tablet 3 times a day.	90	$55	61¢
Calan (verapamil)	80mg	Verapamil	Take 1 tablet 3 times a day.	90	$70	78¢
Calan (verapamil)	120mg	Verapamil	Take 1 tablet 3 times a day.	90	$95	$1.06
Calan SR (verapamil SR)	120mg	Verapamil	Take 1 tablet daily.	30	$45	$1.50
Calan SR (verapamil SR)	180mg	Verapamil	Take 1 tablet daily.	30	$55	$1.83
Calan SR (verapamil SR)	240mg	Verapamil	Take 1 tablet daily.	30	$65	$2.17
Cardene (nicardipine)	20mg	Nicardipine	Take 1 capsule 3 times a day.	90	$65	72¢
Cardene (nicardipine)	30mg	Nicardipine	Take 1 capsule 3 times a day.	90	$90	$1.00
Cardene SR (nicardipine)	30mg	Nicardipine	Take 1 capsule twice a day.	60	$65	$1.08
Cardene SR (nicardipine)	45mg	Nicardipine	Take 1 capsule twice a day.	60	$90	$1.50
Cardizem (diltiazem)	30mg	Diltiazem	Take 1 tablet 4 times a day.	120	$70	58¢
Cardizem (diltiazem)	60mg	Diltiazem	Take 1 tablet 4 times a day.	120	$125	$1.04
Cardizem CD (diltiazem)	120mg	Diltiazem	Take 1 capsule a day.	30	$50	$1.67
Cardizem CD (diltiazem)	180mg	Diltiazem	Take 1 capsule a day.	30	$55	$1.83
Cardizem CD (diltiazem)	240mg	Diltiazem	Take 1 capsule a day.	30	$75	$2.50
Cardizem CD (diltiazem)	300mg	Diltiazem	Take 1 capsule a day.	30	$105	$3.50
Cardizem SR (diltiazem)	60mg	Diltiazem	Take 1 capsule twice a day.	60	$70	$1.17
Cardizem SR (diltiazem)	90mg	Diltiazem	Take 1 capsule twice a day.	60	$80	$1.33
Covera-HS (verapamil)	180mg	Verapamil	Take 1 tablet daily.	30	$50	$1.67
Covera-HS (verapamil)	240mg	Verapamil	Take 1 tablet daily.	30	$65	$2.17
Diltiazem	30mg	Diltiazem	Take 1 tablet 4 times a day.	120	$20	17¢
Diltiazem	60mg	Diltiazem	Take 1 tablet 4 times a day.	120	$40	33¢
Diltiazem ER	120mg	Diltiazem	Take 1 capsule a day.	30	$40	$1.33
Diltiazem ER	180mg	Diltiazem	Take 1 capsule a day.	30	$38	$1.27
Diltiazem ER	240mg	Diltiazem	Take 1 capsule a day.	30	$55	$1.83

PRODUCT	STRENGTH PER DOSE	ACTIVE INGREDIENT	USUAL DOSAGE	TYPICAL QUANTITY	TYPICAL PRICE	PRICE PER DOSE
Diltiazem ER	300mg	Diltiazem	Take 1 capsule a day.	30	$85	$2.83
Diltiazem SR	60mg	Diltiazem	Take 1 capsule twice a day.	60	$40	67¢
Diltiazem SR	90mg	Diltiazem	Take 1 capsule twice a day.	60	$45	75¢
DynaCirc (isradipine)	2.5mg	Isradipine	Take 1 capsule twice a day.	60	$70	$1.17
DynaCirc (isradipine)	5mg	Isradipine	Take 1 capsule twice a day.	60	$105	$1.75
DynaCirc SR (isradipine)	5mg	Isradipine	Take 1 capsule daily.	30	$45	$1.50
DynaCirc SR (isradipine)	10mg	Isradipine	Take 1 capsule daily.	30	$75	$2.50
Isoptin SR (verapamil SR)	120mg	Verapamil	Take 1 tablet daily.	30	$50	$1.67
Isoptin SR (verapamil SR)	180mg	Verapamil	Take 1 tablet daily.	30	$60	$2.00
Isoptin SR (verapamil SR)	240mg	Verapamil	Take 1 tablet daily.	30	$65	$2.17
Nicardipine	20mg	Nicardipine	Take 1 capsule 3 times a day.	90	$35	39¢
Nicardipine	30mg	Nicardipine	Take 1 capsule 3 times a day.	90	$55	61¢
Nifedipine	10mg	Nifedipine	Take 1 capsule 3 times a day.	90	$30	33¢
Nifedipine	20mg	Nifedipine	Take 1 capsule 3 times a day.	90	$30	33¢
Nifedipine	10mg	Nifedipine	Take 1 capsule 3 times a day.	90	$30	33¢
Nifedipine ER	30mg	Nifedipine	Take 1 tablet daily.	30	$37	$1.23
Nifedipine ER	60mg	Nifedipine	Take 1 tablet daily.	30	$60	$2.00
Nifedipine ER	90mg	Nifedipine	Take 1 tablet daily.	30	$80	$2.67
Nifedipine ER	30mg	Nifedipine	Take 1 tablet daily.	30	$40	$1.33
Nifedipine ER	60mg	Nifedipine	Take 1 tablet daily.	30	$60	$2.00
Nifedipine ER	90mg	Nifedipine	Take 1 tablet daily.	30	$80	$2.67
Norvasc (amlodipine)	2.5mg	amlodipine	Take 1 tablet daily.	30	$45	$1.50
Norvasc (amlodipine)	5mg	amlodipine	Take 1 tablet daily.	30	$45	$1.50
Norvasc (amlodipine)	10mg	amlodipine	Take 1 tablet daily.	30	$75	$2.50
Plendil (felodipine)	2.5mg	Felodipine	Take 1 tablet daily.	30	$45	$1.50
Plendil (felodipine)	5mg	Felodipine	Take 1 tablet daily.	30	$45	$1.50
Plendil (felodipine)	10mg	Felodipine	Take 1 tablet daily.	30	$70	$2.33
Procardia (nifedipine)	10mg	Nifedipine	Take 1 capsule 3 times a day.	90	$85	94¢
Procardia (nifedipine)	20mg	Nifedipine	Take 1 capsule 3 times a day.	90	$120	$1.33
Procardia XL (nifedipine ER)	30mg	Nifedipine	Take 1 tablet daily.	30	$46	$1.53

PRODUCT	STRENGTH PER DOSE	ACTIVE INGREDIENT	USUAL DOSAGE	TYPICAL QUANTITY	TYPICAL PRICE	PRICE PER DOSE
Procardia XL (nifedipine ER)	60mg	Nifedipine	Take 1 tablet daily.	30	$85	$2.83
Procardia XL (nifedipine ER)	90mg	Nifedipine	Take 1 tablet daily.	30	$95	$3.17
Sular (nisoldipine)	10mg	Nisoldipine	Take 1 tablet daily.	30	$40	$1.33
Sular (nisoldipine)	20mg	Nisoldipine	Take 1 tablet daily.	30	$40	$1.33
Sular (nisoldipine)	30mg	Nisoldipine	Take 1 tablet daily.	30	$40	$1.33
Sular (nisoldipine)	40mg	Nisoldipine	Take 1 tablet daily.	30	$40	$1.33
Vascor (bepridil)	200mg	Bepridil	Take 1 tablet daily.	30	$111	$3.70
Vascor (bepridil)	300mg	Bepridil	Take 1 tablet daily.	30	$130	$4.33
Verapamil	40mg	Verapamil	Take 1 tablet 3 times a day.	90	$35	39¢
Verapamil	80mg	Verapamil	Take 1 tablet 3 times a day.	90	$30	33¢
$ Verapamil	120mg	Verapamil	Take 1 tablet 3 times a day.	90	$50	56¢
$ Verapamil SR	120mg	Verapamil	Take 1 tablet daily.	30	$25	83¢
$ Verapamil SR	180mg	Verapamil	Take 1 tablet daily.	30	$25	83¢
$ Verapamil SR	240mg	Verapamil	Take 1 tablet daily.	30	$25	83¢

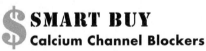

$ SMART BUY
Calcium Channel Blockers

For the money, we like the longer-acting versions of calcium channel blockers. You'll spend less (120 Cardizem 30mg, to be taken 4 times a day, is around $70 at this writing; Cardizem CD 120mg to be taken just once a day is around $50), and you'll get better results. Your blood pressure won't seesaw the way it can when you take a drug that doesn't cover you for 24 hours, and you only have to remember to take the pill once a day. When you factor in the generic forms, the short-acting products may cost you less ($20 versus $40), but because of the better coverage, we still recommend the long-acting versions as your Smart Buy. Buy in bulk to save more money when buying Cardizem in the long-acting form. That $40 for a 30-day supply ($1.33 per day) will drop to around $30 ($1 a day) if you buy at least 90 capsules at a time.

One drug *not* to jump to right away is Vascor. It can cost $4 a pill, while most of the others run about $1 a pill. Your doctor eventually may want you on Vascor, but to save money, be sure to ask why other calcium channel blockers aren't good choices.

BETA-BLOCKERS

Beta-blockers are drugs that block *beta-receptors*—points in cells of the heart muscle and blood vessels that, when triggered by epinephrine and other chemicals normally present in the body, cause the heart and blood vessels to contract. Too many contractions can result in arrhythmias and high blood pressure. Blocking these receptors slows the contractions. This stabilizes the heart's rhythm and, by relaxing the blood vessels, reduces the effort the heart must exert with each beat. Doctors also often prescribe beta-blockers to treat hypertension. (We discuss this in the next section.)

The downside to many beta-blockers is that they tend to make you feel tired. Pharmacists call this "couch potato syndrome." It can be annoying. If you experience this, ask your doctor about changing to a different type of medication.

Beta Blockers to Treat Irregular Heartbeat and Other Heart Problems

PRODUCT	STRENGTH PER DOSE	ACTIVE INGREDIENT	USUAL DOSAGE	TYPICAL QUANTITY	TYPICAL PRICE	PRICE PER DOSE
Acebutolol	200mg	Acebutolol	Take 1 capsule daily.	30	$20	67¢
Acebutolol	400mg	Acebutolol	Take 1 capsule daily.	30	$25	83¢
$ Atenolol	25mg	Atenolol	Take 1 tablet daily.	30	$10	33¢
$ Atenolol	50mg	Atenolol	Take 1 tablet daily.	30	$15	50¢
$ Atenolol	100mg	Atenolol	Take 1 tablet daily.	30	$15	50¢
Betapace (sotalol)	80mg	Sotalol	Take 1 tablet twice a day.	60	$205	$3.42
Betapace (sotalol)	120mg	Sotalol	Take 1 tablet twice a day.	60	$250	$4.17
Betapace (sotalol)	160mg	Sotalol	Take 1 tablet twice a day.	60	$270	$4.50
Betapace (sotalol)	240mg	Sotalol	Take 1 tablet twice a day.	60	$375	$6.25
Blocadren (timolol)	5mg	Timolol	Take 1 tablet twice a day.	60	$40	67¢
Blocadren (timolol)	10mg	Timolol	Take 1 tablet twice a day.	60	$50	83¢
Blocadren (timolol)	20mg	Timolol	Take 1 tablet twice a day.	60	$75	$1.25
Corgard (nadolol)	20mg	Nadolol	Take 1 tablet daily.	30	$55	$1.83
Corgard (nadolol)	40mg	Nadolol	Take 1 tablet daily.	30	$65	$2.17
Corgard (nadolol)	80mg	Nadolol	Take 1 tablet daily.	30	$90	$3
Corgard (nadolol)	120mg	Nadolol	Take 1 tablet daily.	30	$100	$3.33
Corgard (nadolol)	160mg	Nadolol	Take 1 tablet daily.	30	$115	$3.83
Inderal (propranolol)	10mg	Propranolol	Take 1 tablet 3 times a day.	90	$50	56¢
Inderal (propranolol)	20mg	Propranolol	Take 1 tablet 3 times a day.	90	$65	72¢

PRODUCT	STRENGTH PER DOSE	ACTIVE INGREDIENT	USUAL DOSAGE	TYPICAL QUANTITY	TYPICAL PRICE	PRICE PER DOSE
Inderal (propranolol)	40mg	Propranolol	Take 1 tablet daily.	30	$80	$2.67
Inderal (propranolol)	60mg	Propranolol	Take 1 tablet daily.	30	$115	$3.83
Inderal (propranolol)	80mg	Propranolol	Take 1 tablet daily.	30	$130	$4.33
Inderal LA (propranolol LA)	60mg	Propranolol	Take 1 capsule daily.	30	$40	$1.33
Inderal LA (propranolol LA)	80mg	Propranolol	Take 1 capsule daily.	30	$55	$1.83
Inderal LA (propranolol LA)	120mg	Propranolol	Take 1 capsule daily.	30	$60	$2
Inderal LA (propranolol LA)	160mg	Propranolol	Take 1 capsule daily.	30	$80	$2.67
Kerlone (betaxolol)	10mg	Betaxolol	Take 1 tablet daily.	30	$40	$1.33
Kerlone (betaxolol)	20mg	Betaxolol	Take 1 tablet daily.	30	$60	$2
Lopressor (metoprolol)	50mg	Metoprolol	Take 1 tablet twice a day.	60	$60	$1
Lopressor (metoprolol)	100mg	Metoprolol	Take 1 tablet twice a day.	60	$80	$1.33
$ Metoprolol	50mg	Metoprolol	Take 1 tablet twice a day.	60	$15	25¢
$ Metoprolol	100mg	Metoprolol	Take 1 tablet twice a day.	60	$20	33¢
Nadolol	20mg	Nadolol	Take 1 tablet daily.	30	$25	83¢
Nadolol	40mg	Nadolol	Take 1 tablet daily.	30	$30	$1
Nadolol	80mg	Nadolol	Take 1 tablet daily.	30	$35	$1.17
Nadolol	120mg	Nadolol	Take 1 tablet daily.	30	$35	$1.17
Nadolol	160mg	Nadolol	Take 1 tablet daily.	30	$35	$1.17
Propranolol	10mg	Propranolol	Take 1 tablet 3 times a day.	90	$20	22¢
Propranolol	20mg	Propranolol	Take 1 tablet 3 times a day.	90	$20	22¢
Propranolol	40mg	Propranolol	Take 1 tablet daily.	30	$20	67¢
Propranolol	60mg	Propranolol	Take 1 tablet daily.	30	$20	67¢
Propranolol	80mg	Propranolol	Take 1 tablet daily.	30	$20	67¢
Propranolol LA	60mg	Propranolol	Take 1 capsule daily.	30	$30	$1
Propranolol LA	80mg	Propranolol	Take 1 capsule daily.	30	$35	$1.17
Propranolol LA	120mg	Propranolol	Take 1 capsule daily.	30	$45	$1.50
Propranolol LA	160mg	Propranolol	Take 1 capsule daily.	30	$50	$1.67
Sectral (acebutolol)	200mg	Acebutolol	Take 1 capsule daily.	30	$50	$1.67
Sectral (acebutolol)	400mg	Acebutolol	Take 1 capsule daily.	30	$60	$2

PRODUCT	STRENGTH PER DOSE	ACTIVE INGREDIENT	USUAL DOSAGE	TYPICAL QUANTITY	TYPICAL PRICE	PRICE PER DOSE
Sotalol	80mg	Sotalol	Take 1 tablet twice a day.	60	$130	$2.17
Sotalol	120mg	Sotalol	Take 1 tablet twice a day.	60	$170	$2.83
Sotalol	160mg	Sotalol	Take 1 tablet twice a day.	60	$250	$4.17
Sotalol	240mg	Sotalol	Take 1 tablet twice a day.	60	$270	$4.50
Tenormin (atenolol)	25mg	Atenolol	Take 1 tablet daily.	30	$45	$1.50
Tenormin (atenolol)	50mg	Atenolol	Take 1 tablet daily.	30	$45	$1.50
Tenormin (atenolol)	100mg	Atenolol	Take 1 tablet daily.	30	$65	$2.17
Timolol	5mg	Timolol	Take 1 tablet twice a day.	60	$20	33¢
Timolol	10mg	Timolol	Take 1 tablet twice a day.	60	$25	42¢
Timolol	20mg	Timolol	Take 1 tablet twice a day.	60	$35	58¢
Toprol XL (metoprolol)	25mg	Metoprolol	Take 1 tablet daily.	30	$30	$1
Toprol XL (metoprolol)	50mg	Metoprolol	Take 1 tablet daily.	30	$30	$1
Toprol XL (metoprolol)	100mg	Metoprolol	Take 1 tablet daily.	30	$40	$1.33
Toprol XL (metoprolol)	200mg	Metoprolol	Take 1 tablet daily.	30	$65	$2.17

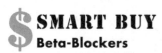

$ SMART BUY
Beta-Blockers

To save money, consider generic versions of Lopressor (generic name metoprolol) and Tenormin (generic name atenolol) for your Smart Buy. Generic versions are inexpensive, come in greater strengths, and are available in tablets that can be broken. Buying in bulk here affords you big savings, as well. Thirty tablets of the name-brand product Tenormin 50mg sells for around $45 ($1.50 a day), and 100 tablets of a generic version of atenolol 100mg sells for around $25 (just 13 cents a day if your dose is 50mg). Likewise, 60 tablets of Lopressor 50mg sells for around $60 ($1 a day), compared to 100 tablets of a generic version of metoprolol 100mg that sells for $25 (also just 13 cents a day for a 50mg dose).

DRUGS TO TREAT HYPERTENSION (HIGH BLOOD PRESSURE)

Six groups of drugs affect the circulatory system. Because the primary effect of four of these groups is to lower blood pressure, these drugs generally are not prescribed for people who also have arrhythmias. These four are:

+ Alpha-blockers
+ ACE inhibitors
+ Angiotensin II receptor antagonists
+ Vasodilators

Blood Pressure Readings

DESCRIPTION	SYSTOLIC (BOTTOM NUMBER)	DIASTOLIC (TOP NUMBER)
Normal	less than 130	less than 85
High normal	130-139	85-89
Mild hypertension	140-159	90-99
Moderate hypertension	160-179	100-109
Severe hypertension	180-209	110-119
Very severe hypertension	greater than 209	greater than 119

Calcium channel blockers and beta-blockers, discussed in the preceding section, also work to lower blood pressure, and often are used for this. Angiotensin II receptor antagonists tend to cost more than most blood-pressure drugs. (A 30-day supply of Cozaar 100mg runs around $60 at this writing; visit www.smartbuysdrugwise.com for current information.) Even though this group is probably "best," because it seems to cause the fewest side effects, we prefer the regular ACE inhibitors. You'll get close to the same side-effect profile, and you can buy generic forms. To save even more money, buy these in larger quantities and greater strengths and in tablet form. (A 30-day supply of 10mg enalapril, generic for Vasotec, will run you about $9 if you buy 100 of the 20mg tablets and cut them in half.)

You can realize big savings on beta-blockers and calcium channel blockers using the same methods. Likewise, similar savings can be had when buying alpha-blockers and vasodilators. We prefer to use the other categories of drugs first, though, because of their better side-effect profiles. Another good and inexpensive way to lower your blood pressure is to take a diuretic, or "water pill." (We discuss these in detail in the next section.) A 30-day supply of hydrochlorothiazide 25mg typically will cost about $10. This is a great price, but if you buy 100 tablets of the 50mg strength and cut them in half, your cost every month drops to just $2! Diuretics may not be sufficient for some people, but they're worth a try. You might just save yourself $60 a month!

Drugs to Treat High Blood Pressure

PRODUCT	STRENGTH PER DOSE	ACTIVE INGREDIENT	TYPE	USUAL DOSAGE	TYPICAL QUANTITY	TYPICAL PRICE	PRICE PER DOSE
Accupril (quinapril)	5mg	Quinapril	ACE inhibitor	Take 1 tablet daily.	30	$40	$1.33
Accupril (quinapril)	10mg	Quinapril	ACE inhibitor	Take 1 tablet daily.	30	$40	$1.33
Accupril (quinapril)	20mg	Quinapril	ACE inhibitor	Take 1 tablet daily.	30	$40	$1.33
Accupril (quinapril)	40mg	Quinapril	ACE inhibitor	Take 1 tablet daily.	30	$40	$1.33
Aldomet (methyldopa)	250mg	Methyldopa	Alpha 2 blocker	Take 1 tablet 3 times a day.	90	$40	44¢
Altace (ramipril)	1.25mg	Ramipril	ACE inhibitor	Take 1 capsule daily.	30	$35	$1.17
Altace (ramipril)	2.5mg	Ramipril	ACE inhibitor	Take 1 capsule daily.	30	$40	$1.33
Altace (ramipril)	5mg	Ramipril	ACE inhibitor	Take 1 capsule daily.	30	$45	$1.50
Altace (ramipril)	10mg	Ramipril	ACE inhibitor	Take 1 capsule daily.	30	$50	$1.67
Apresoline (hydralazine)	25mg	Hydralazine	Vasodilator	Take 1 tablet 4 times a day.	120	$60	50¢
Apresoline (hydralazine)	50mg	Hydralazine	Vasodilator	Take 1 tablet 4 times a day.	120	$80	67¢
Atacand (candesartan)	4mg	Candesartan	Angiotensin II receptor antagonist	Take 1 tablet daily.	30	$45	$1.50
Atacand (candesartan)	8mg	Candesartan	Angiotensin II receptor antagonist	Take 1 tablet daily.	30	$45	$1.50
Atacand (candesartan)	16mg	Candesartan	Angiotensin II receptor antagonist	Take 1 tablet daily.	30	$45	$1.50
Atacand (candesartan)	32mg	Candesartan	Angiotensin II receptor antagonist	Take 1 tablet daily.	30	$60	$2
Avapro (irbesartan)	75mg	Irbesartan	Angiotensin II receptor antagonist	Take 1 tablet daily.	30	$45	$1.50
Avapro (irbesartan)	150mg	Irbesartan	Angiotensin II receptor antagonist	Take 1 tablet daily.	30	$50	$1.67
Avapro (irbesartan)	300mg	Irbesartan	Angiotensin II receptor antagonist	Take 1 tablet daily.	30	$60	$2
Capoten (captopril)	12.5mg	Captopril	ACE inhibitor	Take 1 tablet 3 times a day.	90	$100	$1.11
Capoten (captopril)	25mg	Captopril	ACE inhibitor	Take 1 tablet 3 times a day.	90	$110	$1.22

PRODUCT	STRENGTH PER DOSE	ACTIVE INGREDIENT	TYPE	USUAL DOSAGE	TYPICAL QUANTITY	TYPICAL PRICE	PRICE PER DOSE
Capoten (captopril)	50mg	Captopril	ACE inhibitor	Take 1 tablet 3 times a day.	90	$175	$1.94
Capoten (captopril)	100mg	Captopril	ACE inhibitor	Take 1 tablet 3 times a day.	90	$225	$2.50
Captopril	12.5mg	Captopril	ACE inhibitor	Take 1 tablet 3 times a day.	90	$25	28¢
Captopril	25mg	Captopril	ACE inhibitor	Take 1 tablet 3 times a day.	90	$25	28¢
Captopril	50mg	Captopril	ACE inhibitor	Take 1 tablet 3 times a day.	90	$30	33¢
Captopril	100mg	Captopril	ACE inhibitor	Take 1 tablet 3 times a day.	90	$50	56¢
Cardura (doxazosin)	1mg	Doxazosin	Alpha-1 blocker	Take 1 tablet daily.	30	$40	$1.33
Cardura (doxazosin)	2mg	Doxazosin	Alpha-1 blocker	Take 1 tablet daily.	30	$40	$1.33
Cardura (doxazosin)	4mg	Doxazosin	Alpha-1 blocker	Take 1 tablet daily.	30	$40	$1.33
Cardura (doxazosin)	8mg	Doxazosin	Alpha-1 blocker	Take 1 tablet daily.	30	$45	$1.50
Catapress (clonidine)	0.1mg	Clonidine	Alpha-2 blocker	Take 1 tablet twice a day.	60	$55	92¢
Catapress (clonidine)	0.2mg	Clonidine	Alpha-2 blocker	Take 1 tablet twice a day.	60	$95	$1.58
Catapress (clonidine)	0.3mg	Clonidine	Alpha-2 blocker	Take 1 tablet twice a day.	60	$100	$1.67
Clonidine	0.1mg	Clonidine	Alpha-2 blocker	Take 1 tablet twice a day.	60	$15	25¢
Clonidine	0.2mg	Clonidine	Alpha-2 blocker	Take 1 tablet twice a day.	60	$15	25¢
Clonidine	0.3mg	Clonidine	Alpha-2 blocker	Take 1 tablet twice a day.	60	$25	42¢
Coreg (carvedilol)	3.125mg	Carvedilol	Alpha- and beta blocker	Take 1 tablet twice a day.	60	$115	$1.92
Coreg (carvedilol)	6.25mg	Carvedilol	Alpha- and beta blocker	Take 1 tablet twice a day.	60	$115	$1.92
Coreg (carvedilol)	12.5mg	Carvedilol	Alpha- and beta blocker	Take 1 tablet twice a day.	60	$115	$1.92

PRODUCT	STRENGTH PER DOSE	ACTIVE INGREDIENT	TYPE	USUAL DOSAGE	TYPICAL QUANTITY	TYPICAL PRICE	PRICE PER DOSE
Coreg (carvedilol)	25mg	Carvedilol	Alpha- and beta blocker	Take 1 tablet twice a day.	60	$115	$1.92
Cozaar (losartan)	25mg	Losartan	Angiotensin II receptor antagonist	Take 1 tablet daily.	30	$50	$1.67
Cozaar (losartan)	50mg	Losartan	Angiotensin II receptor antagonist	Take 1 tablet daily.	30	$50	$1.67
Cozaar (losartan)	100mg	Losartan	Angiotensin II receptor antagonist	Take 1 tablet daily.	30	$65	$2.17
Diovan (valsartan)	80mg	Valsartan	Angiotensin II receptor antagonist	Take 1 capsule daily.	30	$50	$1.67
Diovan (valsartan)	160mg	Valsartan	Angiotensin II receptor antagonist	Take 1 tablet daily.	30	$55	$1.83
Diovan (valsartan)	320mg	Valsartan	Angiotensin II receptor antagonist	Take 1 tablet daily.	30	$65	$2.17
Doxazosin	1mg	Doxazosin	Alpha-1 blocker	Take 1 tablet daily.	30	$20	67¢
Doxazosin	2mg	Doxazosin	Alpha-1 blocker	Take 1 tablet daily.	30	$20	67¢
Doxazosin	4mg	Doxazosin	Alpha-1 blocker	Take 1 tablet daily.	30	$25	83¢
Doxazosin	8mg	Doxazosin	Alpha-1 blocker	Take 1 tablet daily.	30	$25	83¢
Enalapril	2.5mg	Enalapril	ACE inhibitor	Take 1 tablet daily.	30	$20	67¢
Enalapril	5mg	Enalapril	ACE inhibitor	Take 1 tablet daily.	30	$20	67¢
Enalapril	10mg	Enalapril	ACE inhibitor	Take 1 tablet daily.	30	$25	83¢
Enalapril	20mg	Enalapril	ACE inhibitor	Take 1 tablet daily.	30	$30	$1
Guanfacine	1mg	Guanfacine	Alpha-2 blocker	Take 1 tablet daily.	30	$20	67¢
Guanfacine	2mg	Guanfacine	Alpha-2 blocker	Take 1 tablet daily.	30	$30	$1
Hydralazine	25mg	Hydralazine	Vasodilator	Take 1 tablet 4 times a day.	120	$15	13¢

PRODUCT	STRENGTH PER DOSE	ACTIVE INGREDIENT	TYPE	USUAL DOSAGE	TYPICAL QUANTITY	TYPICAL PRICE	PRICE PER DOSE
Hydralazine	50mg	Hydralazine	Vasodilator	Take 1 tablet 4 times a day.	120	$20	17¢
Hytrin (terazosin)	1mg	Terazosin	Alpha-1 blocker	Take 1 capsule daily.	30	$65	$2.17
Hytrin (terazosin)	2mg	Terazosin	Alpha-1 blocker	Take 1 capsule daily.	30	$70	$2.33
Hytrin (terazosin)	5mg	Terazosin	Alpha-1 blocker	Take 1 capsule daily.	30	$70	$2.33
Hytrin (terazosin)	10mg	Terazosin	Alpha-1 blocker	Take 1 capsule daily.	30	$70	$2.33
Labetalol	100mg	Labetalol	Alpha- and beta-blocker	Take 1 tablet twice a day.	60	$20	33¢
Labetalol	200mg	Labetalol	Alpha- and beta-blocker	Take 1 tablet twice a day.	60	$30	50¢
Labetalol	300mg	Labetalol	Alpha- and beta-blocker	Take 1 tablet twice a day.	60	$40	67¢
Lisinopril	2.5mg	Lisinopril	ACE Inhibitor	Take 1 tablet daily.	30	$17	57¢
Lisinopril	5mg	Lisinopril	ACE Inhibitor	Take 1 tablet daily.	30	$20	67¢
Lisinopril	10mg	Lisinopril	ACE Inhibitor	Take 1 tablet daily.	30	$30	$1.00
Lisinopril	20mg	Lisinopril	ACE Inhibitor	Take 1 tablet daily.	30	$39	$1.30
Lisinopril	30mg	Lisinopril	ACE Inhibitor	Take 1 tablet daily.	30	$47	$1.57
Lisinopril	40mg	Lisinopril	ACE Inhibitor	Take 1 tablet daily.	30	$50	$1.67
Loniten (minoxidil)	2.5mg	Minoxidil	Vasodilator	Take 1 tablet daily.	30	$35	$1.17
Loniten (minoxidil)	10mg	Minoxidil	Vasodilator	Take 1 tablet daily.	30	$60	$2
Lotensin (benazepril)	5mg	Benazepril	ACE inhibitor	Take 1 tablet daily.	30	$40	$1.33
Lotensin (benazepril)	10mg	Benazepril	ACE inhibitor	Take 1 tablet daily.	30	$40	$1.33
Lotensin (benazepril)	20mg	Benazepril	ACE inhibitor	Take 1 tablet daily.	30	$40	$1.33
Lotensin (benazepril)	40mg	Benazepril	ACE inhibitor	Take 1 tablet daily.	30	$40	$1.33
Mavik (trandolapril)	1mg	Trandolapril	ACE inhibitor	Take 1 tablet daily.	30	$35	$1.17
Mavik (trandolapril)	2mg	Trandolapril	ACE inhibitor	Take 1 tablet daily.	30	$35	$1.17
Mavik (trandolapril)	4mg	Trandolapril	ACE inhibitor	Take 1 tablet daily.	30	$35	$1.17
Methyldopa	250mg	Methyldopa	Alpha-2 blocker	1 tablet 3 times a day.	90	$15	17¢
Micardis (telmisartan)	40mg	Telmisartan	Angiotensin II receptor antagonist	Take 1 tablet daily.	28	$45	$1.61

PRODUCT	STRENGTH PER DOSE	ACTIVE INGREDIENT	TYPE	USUAL DOSAGE	TYPICAL QUANTITY	TYPICAL PRICE	PRICE PER DOSE
Micardis (telmisartan)	80mg	Telmisartan	Angiotensin II receptor antagonist	Take 1 tablet daily.	28	$50	$1.79
Minipress (prazosin)	1mg	Prazosin	Alpha-1 blocker	Take 1 capsule 3 times a day.	90	$50	56¢
Minipress (prazosin)	2mg	Prazosin	Alpha-1 blocker	Take 1 capsule 3 times a day.	90	$75	83¢
Minipress (prazosin)	5mg	Prazosin	Alpha-1 blocker	Take 1 capsule 3 times a day.	90	$120	$1.33
Minoxidil	2.5mg	Minoxidil	Vasodilator	Take 1 tablet daily.	30	$15	50¢
Minoxidil	10mg	Minoxidil	Vasodilator	Take 1 tablet daily.	30	$25	83¢
Monopril (fosinopril)	10mg	Fosinopril	ACE inhibitor	Take 1 tablet daily.	30	$45	$1.50
Monopril (fosinopril)	20mg	Fosinopril	ACE inhibitor	Take 1 tablet daily.	30	$45	$1.50
Monopril (fosinopril)	40mg	Fosinopril	ACE inhibitor	Take 1 tablet daily.	30	$45	$1.50
Normodyne (labetalol)	100mg	Labetalol	Alpha- and beta-blocker	Take 1 tablet twice a day.	60	$50	83¢
Normodyne (labetalol)	200mg	Labetalol	Alpha- and beta-blocker	Take 1 tablet twice a day.	60	$60	$1
Normodyne (labetalol)	300mg	Labetalol	Alpha- and beta-blocker	Take 1 tablet twice a day.	60	$75	$1.25
Prazosin	1mg	Prazosin	Alpha-1 blocker	Take 1 capsule 3 times a day.	90	$25	28¢
Prazosin	2mg	Prazosin	Alpha-1 blocker	Take 1 capsule 3 times a day.	90	$30	33¢
Prazosin	5mg	Prazosin	Alpha-1 blocker	Take 1 capsule 3 times a day.	90	$45	50¢
Prinivil (lisinopril)	2.5mg	Lisinopril	ACE inhibitor	Take 1 tablet daily.	30	$30	$1
Prinivil (lisinopril)	5mg	Lisinopril	ACE inhibitor	Take 1 tablet daily.	30	$40	$1.33
Prinivil (lisinopril)	10mg	Lisinopril	ACE inhibitor	Take 1 tablet daily.	30	$40	$1.33
Prinivil (lisinopril)	20mg	Lisinopril	ACE inhibitor	Take 1 tablet daily.	30	$40	$1.33
Prinivil (lisinopril)	40mg	Lisinopril	ACE inhibitor	Take 1 tablet daily.	30	$55	$1.83
Tenex (guanfacine)	1mg	Guanfacine	Alpha-2 blocker	Take 1 tablet daily.	30	$40	$1.33
Tenex (guanfacine)	2mg	Guanfacine	Alpha-2 blocker	Take 1 tablet daily.	30	$60	$2
Terazosin	1mg	Terazosin	Alpha-1 blocker	Take 1 capsule daily.	30	$25	83¢

PRODUCT	STRENGTH PER DOSE	ACTIVE INGREDIENT	TYPE	USUAL DOSAGE	TYPICAL QUANTITY	TYPICAL PRICE	PRICE PER DOSE
Terazosin	2mg	Terazosin	Alpha-1 blocker	Take 1 capsule daily.	30	$30	$1
Terazosin	5mg	Terazosin	Alpha-1 blocker	Take 1 capsule daily.	30	$30	$1
Terazosin	10mg	Terazosin	Alpha-1 blocker	Take 1 capsule daily.	30	$35	$1.17
Vasotec (enalapril)	2.5mg	Enalapril	ACE inhibitor	Take 1 tablet daily.	30	$35	$1.17
Vasotec (enalapril)	5mg	Enalapril	ACE inhibitor	Take 1 tablet daily.	30	$35	$1.17
Vasotec (enalapril)	10mg	Enalapril	ACE inhibitor	Take 1 tablet daily.	30	$35	$1.17
Vasotec (enalapril)	20mg	Enalapril	ACE inhibitor	Take 1 tablet daily.	30	$60	$2
Zestril (lisinopril)	2.5mg	Lisinopril	ACE inhibitor	Take 1 tablet daily.	30	$30	$1
Zestril (lisinopril)	5mg	Lisinopril	ACE inhibitor	Take 1 tablet daily.	30	$36	$1.20
Zestril (lisinopril)	10mg	Lisinopril	ACE inhibitor	Take 1 tablet daily.	30	$36	$1.20
Zestril (lisinopril)	20mg	Lisinopril	ACE inhibitor	Take 1 tablet daily.	30	$40	$1.33
Zestril (lisinopril)	40mg	Lisinopril	ACE inhibitor	Take 1 tablet daily.	30	$60	$2

$ SMART BUY
Drugs to Treat High Blood Pressure

For high blood pressure that needs more than a diuretic, we like atenolol and long-acting forms of diltiazem, verapamil, or nifedipine. See the charts on beta-blockers and calcium channel blockers for these Smart Buys. Atenolol is less likely to trigger an asthma problem, need only be taken once a day, and is available in a cheap generic version. Try to buy the generic in bulk and cut the tablets in half. Diltiazem, verapamil, and nifedipine come in generic long-acting versions that give better 24-hour coverage. Again, buy in bulk.

Among the ACE inhibitors available to treat high blood pressure, we lean toward Vasotec for the Smart Buy. Its generic form, enalapril, is much cheaper than the newer angiotensin II receptor antagonists on the market. If you develop a cough (a potential side effect), however, you'll need to switch to one of the newer products. Again, buy generic in bulk, and try cutting the tablets in half. Doing this can lower your per-dose cost to about 30 cents, or about $9 a month.

Among alpha-blockers, we like Cardura (generic name doxazosin) and Hytrin (generic name terazosin). The generic form of either will cut your costs in half, and you'll risk fewer side effects than with most of the other alpha-blockers, making them a strong Smart Buy. Buying generic Cardura in bulk and cutting tablets lowers your cost per dose to around 35 cents.

Minoxidil for Hair Growth

One side effect of minoxidil is that about 80 percent of people who take it experience enhanced growth of facial and body hair. In fact, results are so good that pharmacists used to grind up the tablets, mix the powder into a solution, and sell it as a cure for baldness. This is no longer necessary now that Rogaine (minoxidil) has arrived on the market.

DIURETICS ("WATER PILLS"): ANOTHER APPROACH TO TREATING HYPERTENSION

One commonly prescribed group of drugs for treating hypertension functions entirely differently from those that act on the circulatory system. Diuretics, also known as "water pills," work by removing fluid from your body. This helps lower the volume of blood in your blood vessels, which, in turn, lowers your blood pressure and eases your heart's workload. Your kidneys filter your blood continually to extract toxins, chemicals, and other products your body doesn't need or want and sends them to your bladder in the form of urine. Diuretics act on parts of the kidney to increase the amount of fluid they remove (and the amount of urine you produce). Doctors often prescribe diuretics with digoxin to treat congestive heart failure, and also to treat mild to moderate hypertension (high blood pressure). Diuretics come in three forms.

Thiazide diuretics, the most commonly prescribed for high blood pressure, can remove some potassium from your body. The amount is usually so small, though, that to replenish it, doctors and pharmacists often recommend that you eat foods fairly high in potassium, such as orange juice and bananas. The average banana contains about 12mEq of potassium; most potassium supplements contain 8mEq to 20mEq of potassium. So one banana a day can give you the same amount of potassium as a dose of supplement. Talk to your doctor about whether adding bananas and other high-potassium foods to your daily diet will give you a sufficient potassium boost. This is a tastier, and usually less expensive, method than taking potassium supplements (which can be hard on the stomach).

Loop diuretics are stronger than the thiazides. They're usually prescribed for people who have both congestive heart failure and severe high blood pressure. Loop diuretics, too, deplete your body's potassium levels—enough that a couple of bananas a day won't meet your body's potassium needs. Doctors almost always prescribe a potassium supplement along with a loop diuretic. Make sure your doctor monitors your potassium levels regularly through blood tests. If you experience signs of potassium depletion, such as muscle cramping, let your doctor know.

Potassium-sparing diuretics, the weakest of the three types, actually can increase potassium blood levels, so they're usually used along with a thiazide diuretic.

If you use any kind of diuretic, try to take it in the morning so you won't find yourself getting up repeatedly at night to go to the bathroom. Diuretics may trigger attacks of gout, increase blood sugar levels in people with diabetes, and increase your vulnerability to sunburn.

Diuretics ("Water Pills") to Treat High Blood Pressure

PRODUCT	STRENGTH PER DOSE	ACTIVE INGREDIENT	TYPE	USUAL DOSAGE	TYPICAL QUANTITY	TYPICAL PRICE	PRICE PER DOSE
Amiloride with HCTZ	5/50	Amiloride with HCTZ	Potassium-sparing	Take 1 tablet daily.	30	$25	83¢
Bumetanide	0.5mg	Bumetanide	Loop	Take 1 tablet daily.	30	$10	33¢
Bumetanide	1mg	Bumetanide	Loop	Take 1 tablet daily.	30	$15	50¢
Bumetanide	2mg	Bumetanide	Loop	Take 1 tablet daily.	30	$20	67¢
Bumex (bumetanide)	0.5mg	Bumetanide	Loop	Take 1 tablet daily.	30	$15	50¢
Bumex (bumetanide)	1mg	Bumetanide	Loop	Take 1 tablet daily.	30	$25	83¢
Bumex (bumetanide)	2mg	Bumetanide	Loop	Take 1 tablet daily.	30	$30	$1
Chlorothiazide	250mg	Chlorothiazide	Thiazide	Take 1 tablet daily.	30	$5	17¢
Chlorothiazide	500mg	Chlorothiazide	Thiazide	Take 1 tablet daily.	30	$10	33¢
Demadex (torsemide)	5mg	Torsemide	Loop	Take 1 tablet daily.	30	$30	$1
Demadex (torsemide)	10mg	Torsemide	Loop	Take 1 tablet daily.	30	$30	$1
Demadex (torsemide)	20mg	Torsemide	Loop	Take 1 tablet daily.	30	$30	$1
Diuril (chlorothiazide)	250mg	Chlorothiazide	Thiazide	Take 1 tablet daily.	30	$15	50¢
Diuril (chlorothiazide)	500mg	Chlorothiazide	Thiazide	Take 1 tablet daily.	30	$15	50¢

PRODUCT	STRENGTH PER DOSE	ACTIVE INGREDIENT	TYPE	USUAL DOSAGE	TYPICAL QUANTITY	TYPICAL PRICE	PRICE PER DOSE
Dyazide (triamterene with HCTZ)	37.5/25	Triamterene with HCTZ	Potassium-sparing	Take 1 capsule daily.	30	$20	67¢
Dyazide (triamterene with HCTZ)	50/25	Triamterene with HCTZ	Potassium-sparing	Take 1 capsule daily.	30	$20	67¢
Furosemide	20mg	Furosemide	Loop	Take 1 tablet daily.	30	$10	33¢
Furosemide	40mg	Furosemide	Loop	Take 1 tablet daily.	30	$10	33¢
Furosemide	80mg	Furosemide	Loop	Take 1 tablet daily.	30	$10	33¢
HCTZ	25mg	HCTZ	Thiazide	Take 1 tablet daily.	30	$10	33¢
HCTZ	50mg	HCTZ	Thiazide	Take 1 tablet daily.	30	$10	33¢
HCTZ	100mg	HCTZ	Thiazide	Take 1 tablet daily.	30	$15	50¢
HydroDIURIL (hydrochlorothiazide or HCTZ)	25mg	HCTZ	Thiazide	Take 1 tablet daily.	30	$15	50¢
HydroDIURIL (hydrochlorothiazide or HCTZ)	50mg	HCTZ	Thiazide	Take 1 tablet daily.	30	$15	50¢
HydroDIURIL (hydrochlorothiazide or HCTZ)	100mg	HCTZ	Thiazide	Take 1 tablet daily.	30	$20	67¢
Indapamide	1.25mg	Indapamide	Thiazide	Take 1 tablet daily.	30	$15	50¢
Indapamide	2.5mg	Indapamide	Thiazide	Take 1 tablet daily.	30	$15	50¢
Lasix (furosemide)	20mg	Furosemide	Loop	Take 1 tablet daily.	30	$15	50¢
Lasix (furosemide)	40mg	Furosemide	Loop	Take 1 tablet daily.	30	$15	50¢
Lasix (furosemide)	80mg	Furosemide	Loop	Take 1 tablet daily.	30	$20	67¢
Lozol (indapamide)	1.25mg	Indapamide	Thiazide	Take 1 tablet daily.	30	$40	$1.33
Lozol (indapamide)	2.5mg	Indapamide	Thiazide	Take 1 tablet daily.	30	$45	$1.50
Maxzide (triamterene with HCTZ)	37.5/25	Triamterene with HCTZ	Potassium-sparing	Take 1 tablet daily.	30	$30	$1
Maxzide (triamterene with HCTZ)	75/50 with HCTZ	Triamterene with HCTZ	Potassium-HCTZ sparing	Take 1 tablet daily.	30	$40	$1.33
Moduretic (amiloride with HCTZ)	5/50 with HCTZ	Amiloride with HCTZ	Potassium-sparing	Take 1 tablet daily.	30	$40	$1.33
Triamterene with HCTZ	37.5/25	Triamterene with HCTZ	Potassium-sparing	Take 1 tablet daily.	30	$15	50¢
Triamterene with HCTZ	75/50	Triamterene with HCTZ	Potassium-sparing	Take 1 tablet daily.	30	$10	33¢
Triamterene with HCTZ	37.5/25	Triamterene with HCTZ	Potassium-sparing	Take 1 capsule daily.	30	$15	50¢

PRODUCT	STRENGTH PER DOSE	ACTIVE INGREDIENT	TYPE	USUAL DOSAGE	TYPICAL QUANTITY	TYPICAL PRICE	PRICE PER DOSE
Triamterene with HCTZ	50/25	Triamterene with HCTZ	Potassium-sparing	Take 1 capsule daily.	30	$15	50¢
Zaroxolyn (metolazone)	2.5mg	Metolazone	Thiazide	Take 1 tablet daily.	30	$35	$1.17
Zaroxolyn (metolazone)	5mg	Metolazone	Thiazide	Take 1 tablet daily.	30	$40	$1.33
Zaroxolyn (metolazone)	10mg	Metolazone	Thiazide	Take 1 tablet daily.	30	$50	$1.67

$ SMART BUY
Diuretics ("Water Pills") to Treat High Blood Pressure

Generic hydrochlorothiazide (HCTZ) is the Smart Buy if you're taking a diuretic to treat high blood pressure. This mild diuretic effectively reduces mild to moderate high blood pressure, and it's both inexpensive and relatively side effect–free. For the best buy, purchase the generic form in bulk and ask whether you can cut the tablets. Buying HCTZ 50mg in a 100-count bottle and cutting the tablets for a 25mg dose can get the cost per dose down to about 6 cents (compared to 33 cents a dose for 30 HCTZ 25mg tablets).

> ### Stepped Approach to Drugs for High Blood Pressure
>
> Many types of drugs are used to treat high blood pressure, and doctors often prescribe from two to several in combination. Using drugs with different mechanisms of action can be more effective than using one drug alone. For high blood pressure, the American Medical Association recommends using a stepped approach: You start with one type of drug. If it doesn't work, add a second drug, and then a third, if necessary, until your blood pressure is under control.

DRUGS USED TO LOWER BLOOD CHOLESTEROL AND TRIGLYCERIDES

Elevated blood cholesterol or triglyceride levels can lead to heart disease. Health experts estimate that each 10 percent reduction in cholesterol levels corresponds to a 20 to 30 percent reduction in your risk for coronary heart disease. When a high level of cholesterol is present in the blood, hard plaques of it begin to line the blood vessel walls. This reduces vessel size and elasticity—a serious problem, because then the heart must pump harder and faster to push blood through. This increases blood pressure, which, over time, can result in strokes and even heart attacks. The following table shows commonly accepted classifications for blood cholesterol levels.

Blood Cholesterol Levels

TOTAL CHOLESTEROL	CLASSIFICATION
Less than 200	Desirable
200–239	Borderline
Greater than 240	High
HDL	
Less than 35	Low
LDL	
Less than 130	Desirable
130–159	Borderline
Greater than 160	High

The first steps to treating high cholesterol or triglyceride levels are to exercise more and reduce your intake of dietary fat. Many people can significantly improve blood levels through these lifestyle changes alone and won't have to take medications. Should diet and exercise fail, though, you'll find some very effective drugs now on the market.

Cholesterol-lowering drugs can be grouped into three categories:

+ Bile acid sequestrants
+ Statins
+ Drugs that lower blood triglyceride levels

When you look for savings when buying these drugs, first consider what you're treating. Some of these drugs lower one specific component (Tricor, for example, lowers only triglycerides); others knock down triglycerides and bad cholesterol and *raise* the good cholesterol. If you want more bang for your buck, look to the statin group of drugs. These can be far more expensive than the others, however. For an inexpensive alternative to try first, consider Lopid. It does all the aforementioned (maybe not as effectively as the statins), and a generic version usually is priced quite low. For example, a 30-day supply of Zocor 5mg (a popular statin drug) typically will cost around $65. A month's supply of gemfibrozil (generic of Lopid) will cost only around $15 if you buy it in bulk.

If your doctor wants you to take a bile acid sequestrant product, you can save a ton of money if you buy the generic in bulk cans (instead of individual packets). Buy more than one can at a time. Questran comes in bulk cans of powder that provide 4g per scoop. Each can contains 378g or about 95 doses. Questran also comes in individual 4g packets packaged in boxes of 60. That's 60 doses per box. If you buy one box of name-brand Questran, you can expect to pay about $125. Buy three cans of the generic, though, and you can expect to pay around $85. This is a real value: You'll pay about $40 less, and get 285 doses instead of 60!

BILE ACID SEQUESTRANTS

The first category of drugs used to lower cholesterol levels includes products known as bile acid sequestrants. Questran, the first of these drugs, was released in 1967. These drugs physically bind to bile acids in the intestines and force the body to eliminate them through the feces. This keeps them from reaching the liver to produce cholesterol. When taking these drugs, especially the powder forms, be sure to drink plenty of water. Failing to do so can result in severe constipation and even intestinal blockage. Commonly prescribed bile acid sequestrants include Colestid (generic name colestipol), Questran (generic name cholestyramine), and Questran Lite (generic name cholestyramine).

STATIN

Probably the strongest cholesterol-lowering drugs are the HMG-CoA reductase inhibitors, or statins. They're also the most expensive. These drugs work by blocking a key enzyme involved in the body's production of cholesterol. Mevacor, the first statin drug, was released in 1987. What's especially good about these drugs is that they do two things—lower "bad" cholesterol (LDL) *and* raise "good" cholesterol (HDL). Studies have shown that the ratio of good to bad cholesterol is more significant than the levels themselves when it comes to reducing your risk for heart disease. Because bile acid sequestrants lower only LDL, statins tend to produce better results.

Commonly prescribed statins include:

+ Lescol (generic name fluvastatin)
+ Lipitor (generic name atorvastatin)
+ Mevacor (generic name lovastatin)
+ Pravachol (generic name pravastatin)
+ Zocor (generic name simvastatin)

As with nearly all drugs, taking statins involves some risks. Because they work directly on the liver, people with liver disease should avoid these drugs. And we recommend that liver function tests be done at least yearly (or every 30 to 60 days when changing dosages). Some people have experienced severe problems with muscle tissue breaking down. Byproducts from these breakdowns can result in overloaded kidneys that can fail, a potentially fatal condition called rhabdomyolysis. One statin drug, Baycol, was removed from the market after a number of deaths due to this condition. To protect yourself, report to your doctor any muscle pain or weakness you experience while taking a statin drug.

> ## Possible Muscle Damage with Statin Drugs
>
> Drugs that slow the body's removal rate for statins can cause them to accumulate and potentially break down muscle tissue. Erythromycin, a commonly prescribed antibiotic, is one such medication. If you're taking a statin drug and your doctor feels you need an antibiotic, mention the statin you're taking. If erythromycin is the only antibiotic your doctor feels will work, then you might stop taking the statin drug until you complete the course of erythromycin.

DRUGS THAT LOWER BLOOD TRIGLYCERIDE LEVELS

The last group of drugs that help lower cholesterol also help to reduce triglycerides. This is important, because high triglyceride levels in the blood have been associated with heart attacks. One of the most commonly prescribed drugs in this group is Lopid (generic name gemfibrozil). This drug does several things: It can lower LDL levels.

Remember, LDL is the bad cholesterol, so lowering it is good. And gemfibrozil can increase HDL; that's the good cholesterol, so raising it is good. And the drug works to reduce triglyceride levels—another benefit. The downside to this drug is that it can cause some muscle problems. Like the statin drugs, gemfibrozil can cause rhabdomyolysis (muscle protein breakdown that can overload the kidneys). Nor is it as effective as the statins at lowering LDL. Because of this, doctors usually prescribe this drug when both blood cholesterol and triglyceride levels are too high.

Recent Studies into Statins

Results of studies released in August 2002 indicate that statin drugs have a rare but painful potential side effect—"polyneuropathy," nerve damage that can cause pain, tingling, loss of feeling, and weakness that may be long-lasting or even permanent. But you shouldn't stop taking your statins. These drugs can prevent heart attacks and strokes in people with high cholesterol, and that far outweighs any risk for this rare side effect.

Tricor (generic name fenofibrate) is excellent at lowering triglyceride levels, but it's rarely used to treat high cholesterol. Elevated triglyceride levels alone (without elevated blood cholesterol levels) is fairly uncommon, so this drug's usefulness is limited. Although relatively few side effects are associated with taking it, it can cause pancreatitis (inflammation of the pancreas), which can be very uncomfortable.

$ SMART BUY
Drugs to Lower Blood Cholesterol Levels

For treating high cholesterol levels, the Smart Buy is gemfibrozil. This generic form of Lopid increases HDL, lowers LDL, and lowers triglyceride levels for about half the cost of a product such as Zocor. It may not be quite as effective at reducing LDL levels as the statin drugs, but it's a good place to begin. Buy in bulk to get a per-dose cost of about 50 cents.

Drugs to Lower Blood Cholesterol and Triglyceride Levels

PRODUCT	STRENGTH PER DOSE	ACTIVE INGREDIENT	TYPE	USUAL DOSAGE	TYPICAL QUANTITY	TYPICAL PRICE	PRICE PER DOSE
Cholestyramine bulk powder	4g	Cholestyramine	Bile acid sequestrant	Take 1 scoopful daily.	1 can	$30	71¢
Cholestyramine Lite bulk powder	4g	Cholestyramine	Bile acid sequestrant	Take 1 scoopful daily.	1 can	$35	83¢
Cholestyramine Lite	4g packets	Cholestyramine	Bile acid sequestrant	Take 1 packet daily.	1 box of 60	$70	$1.17
Cholestyramine packets	4g	Cholestyramine	Bile acid sequestrant	Take 1 packet daily.	1 box of 60	$60	$1
Colestid (colestipol)	1 gram	Colestipol	Bile acid sequestrant	Take 1 tablet twice a day.	60	$35	58¢
Colestid (colestipol)	5g	Colestipol	Bile acid sequestrant	Take 1 scoopful daily.	1 bottle of 450g	$90	$1
Colestid (colestipol)	5g	Colestipol	Bile acid sequestrant	Take 1 scoopful daily.	1 bottle of 500g	$120	$1.20
Gemfibrozil	600mg	Gemfibrozil	Fibric acid derivative	Take 1 tablet twice a day.	60	$30	50¢
Lescol (fluvastatin)	20mg	Fluvastatin	Statin	Take 1 capsule daily.	30	$50	$1.67
Lescol (fluvastatin)	40mg	Fluvastatin	Statin	Take 1 capsule daily.	30	$50	$1.67
Lescol XL (fluvastatin)	80mg	Fluvastatin	Statin	Take 1 tablet daily.	30	$65	$2.17
Lipitor (atorvastatin)	10mg	Atorvastatin	Statin	Take 1 tablet daily.	30	$65	$2.17
Lipitor (atorvastatin)	20mg	Atorvastatin	Statin	Take 1 tablet daily.	30	$95	$3.17
Lipitor (atorvastatin)	40mg	Atorvastatin	Statin	Take 1 tablet daily.	30	$105	$3.50
Lipitor (atorvastatin)	80mg	Atorvastatin	Statin	Take 1 tablet daily.	30	$105	$3.50
Lopid (gemfibrozil)	600mg	Gemfibrozil	Fibric acid derivative	Take 1 tablet twice a day.	60	$100	$1.67
Lovastatin	10mg	Lovastatin	Statin	Take 1 tablet daily.	30	$40	$1.33
Lovastatin	20mg	Lovastatin	Statin	Take 1 tablet daily.	30	$50	$1.67
Lovastatin	40mg	Lovastatin	Statin	Take 1 tablet daily.	30	$70	$2.33
Mevacor (lovastatin)	10mg	Lovastatin	Statin	Take 1 tablet daily.	30	$50	$1.67
Mevacor (lovastatin)	20mg	Lovastatin	Statin	Take 1 tablet daily.	30	$80	$2.67
Mevacor (lovastatin)	40mg	Lovastatin	Statin	Take 1 tablet daily.	30	$130	$4.33
Pravachol (pravastatin)	10mg	Pravastatin	Statin	Take 1 tablet daily.	30	$70	$2.33

PRODUCT	STRENGTH PER DOSE	ACTIVE INGREDIENT	TYPE	USUAL DOSAGE	TYPICAL QUANTITY	TYPICAL PRICE	PRICE PER DOSE
Pravachol (pravastatin)	20mg	Pravastatin	Statin	Take 1 tablet daily.	30	$80	$2.67
Pravachol (pravastatin)	40mg	Pravastatin	Statin	Take 1 tablet daily.	30	$130	$4.33
Questran (cholestyramine) bulk powder	4g	Cholestyramine	Bile acid sequestrant	Take 1 scoopful daily.	1 can	$60	$1.48
Questran (cholestyramine) packets	4g	Cholestyramine	Bile acid sequestrant	Take 1 packet daily.	1 box of 60	$120	$2
Questran Lite (cholestyramine) packets	4g	Cholestyramine	Bile acid sequestrant	Take 1 packet daily.	1 box of 60	$120	$2
Questran Lite (cholestyramine) bulk powder	4g	Cholestyramine	Bile acid sequestrant	Take 1 scoopful daily.	1 can	$60	$1.48
Tricor (fenofibrate)	54mg	Fenofibrate	Fibric acid derivative	Take 1 capsule daily.	30	$35	$1.17
Tricor (fenofibrate)	67mg	Fenofibrate	Fibric acid derivative	Take 1 capsule daily.	30	$35	$1.17
Tricor (fenofibrate)	134mg	Fenofibrate	Fibric acid derivative	Take 1 capsule daily.	30	$60	$2
Tricor (fenofibrate)	160mg	Fenofibrate	Fibric acid derivative	Take 1 capsule daily.	30	$155	$5.17
Tricor (fenofibrate)	200mg	Fenofibrate	Fibric acid derivative	Take 1 capsule daily.	30	$155	$5.17
Zocor (simvastatin)	5mg	Simvastatin	Statin	Take 1 tablet daily.	30	$60	$2
Zocor (simvastatin)	10mg	Simvastatin	Statin	Take 1 tablet daily.	30	$75	$2.50
Zocor (simvastatin)	20mg	Simvastatin	Statin	Take 1 tablet daily.	30	$125	$4.17
Zocor (simvastatin)	40mg	Simvastatin	Statin	Take 1 tablet daily.	30	$125	$4.17
Zocor (simvastatin)	80mg	Simvastatin	Statin	Take 1 tablet daily.	30	$130	$4.33

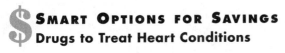

SMART OPTIONS FOR SAVINGS
Drugs to Treat Heart Conditions

These drugs can be very expensive. They also have very narrow therapeutic indexes (NTIs) and blood levels require close monitoring by your physician. If you're just starting out on them, consider buying smaller quantities through a local drugstore or pharmacy until your dosage stabilizes. This way, if your doctor changes your dose and you need a new prescription, you won't have far to go or long to wait. Once you stabilize at a certain dosage, turn to your Smart Options for Saving:

✦ Buy in bulk (at least a 90-day supply).
✦ Purchase generic versions (when available and if you're just starting to take the drug).
✦ Shop around for the lowest prices.
✦ Consider alternative sources such as virtual and Canadian pharmacies.

So many of these drugs have NTIs, we can't recommend cutting tablets (unless our Smart Buy recommendations for a particular group of drugs includes this as an option). Although ordering via mail-order or Internet drugstore (or, if you live close to the Canadian border, buying your drugs in Canada) might give you the lowest prices, make sure you order far enough in advance that you don't run out before your supply arrives. Check our Web site at www.smartbuysdrugwise.com for the latest information on ways to save money on these drugs.

Chapter 9

Prescription Hormones and Drugs to Treat Hormone-Based Conditions

Most of the drugs in this group are designed to replace substances that the body has stopped making, such as estrogen in postmenopausal women or insulin in people with diabetes. Some of these drugs come from natural sources; others are engineered in the laboratory. Regardless of how they're made, using them is crucial to the health and well-being of millions of people.

Of course, these hormone-related products come with a price tag. A year's supply of insulin costs about $675 (assuming you buy vials instead of prefilled syringes and use two types of insulin—long-lasting and short-acting). Do you take a thyroid supplement to treat hypothyroidism (underactive thyroid)? You probably pay in the neighborhood of $250 a year. And if you're a woman taking estrogen or estrogen/progesterone for menopause-related concerns, you could be spending as much as $900 each year. A year's supply of birth control pills, also hormones, adds up to about $300.

As with most prescription drugs, Smart Options for Savings can cut your costs for products that are hormone-based or treat hormone-based conditions. However, hormones vary more from product to product than many other drugs. A brand that's perfect for one person can be less effective or even cause problems for another. (We cover this in greater detail in later sections of this chapter.) When it comes to hormone products, most of the time you should stay with the brand that works best for you.

ORAL CONTRACEPTIVES (BIRTH CONTROL PILLS)

Since the "the pill" debuted in 1960, an estimated 60 million women worldwide have taken oral contraceptives. These drugs to prevent pregnancy are among the most commonly prescribed hormone products in the U.S. While research continues to search for an effective form of contraceptive drug that men can take, at present, it is women who take or use these products. Oral contraceptives today are available as either progestin-estrogen combinations or progestin-only products. Progestin-estrogen combinations are the more widely prescribed, because they're more effective. Progestin-only products (also known as the "mini-pill") are safe for breastfeeding mothers to take.

Combination products are available in three forms:

+ *Monophasic* products provide fixed amounts of progestin and estrogen throughout a woman's monthly cycle.
+ *Biphasic* products provide a fixed amount of estrogen and an amount of progestin that changes halfway through the cycle.
+ *Triphasic* products' estrogen and progestin levels vary three times during the cycle.

Biphasic pills are the more expensive. Monophasic and triphasic products price out about the same. For example, a typical price for Ortho-Novum 1/35 (monophasic) runs around $34 a month. Likewise, Ortho-Novum 777 (triphasic) typically will cost $34. But Ortho-Novum 10/11 (biphasic), made by the same company as the other two, sells for around $38 a month. This is probably the result of market factors that drive down the prices of monophasics and triphasics—supply and demand. Of all the drug types sold in the U.S., oral contraceptives are the most price-sensitive. Because pharmacists don't see many prescriptions for Ortho-Novum 10/11, the low volume probably allows the price to rise.

As you look over the following tables, you'll notice that, after progestin-only products, the biphasic group offers the fewest choices. Not many women take these products. Likewise, you'll notice few progestin-only products. And again, their prices are higher. Micronor typically sells for around $39 a pack. Regardless of the type or strength of birth control pills you take, looking for a generic version can save you big money. Necon 1/35 (generic for Ortho-Novum 1/35) sells for just $18, Necon 10/11 (generic for Ortho-Novum 10/11) sells for around $19, and Trivora (generic for Tri-Levlen) sells for around $24 a pack.

Using oral contraceptives isn't without risks. They've been associated with increased incidences of vascular disease and blood clots, especially in women who smoke. Because of this, we (and other healthcare professionals) recommend that you start on the lowest strength birth control pills available, preferably those with less than 35mcg of estrogen. If breakthrough bleeding (bleeding mid-cycle) occurs, consider switching to a product with a higher amount of estrogen or a triphasic product that more closely follows a normal menstrual cycle.

Other side effects to be aware of when taking oral contraceptives include breast tenderness and enlargement; nausea and vomiting; skin rashes; contact lens intolerance due to changes in corneal curvature; migraine headaches; and depression (taking 50mg of vitamin B_6 every day has been shown to help reduce this problem). Equivalent generic forms of many oral contraceptives are available now and we recommend using them to save money. Why pay more when you can get the same results? When it comes to oral contraceptives and generics, you get the same amounts of the same drugs for far less money. We've seen no documentation showing that generic versions of oral contraceptives are any less effective. But we *have* seen the price reduction. For example, Trivora, a generic version of Tri-Levlen, costs only $24 a month. Why pay $32 for the name-brand product Tri-Levlen?

▶ "Morning-After" Pills

Most oral contraceptives (birth control pills) combine estrogen and progestin. "Morning-after" pills, taken to prevent pregnancy after unprotected sex has taken place, are either high-dose combinations of an estrogen and progestin or a high dose of a progestin. Taking them within 24 hours of intercourse reduces the chance of pregnancy by 95 percent, or by 58 percent if taken within 72 hours. They run about $30 for the pills and the service, which includes counseling by the pharmacist (how to take the pills, what to do if side effects occur, and other relevant information). The pills are available only if the service is provided. This allows the customer to receive the pills without having to go to the doctor. The intent is to improve access to the pills, but few pharmacists provide this service. Prescribing these products requires training and a special arrangement with a local doctor, and many pharmacists find this cumbersome.

Oral Contraceptives: Monophasic

PRODUCT	STRENGTH PER DOSE (MCG/MG)	ACTIVE INGREDIENT ESTROGEN/PROGESTIN	USUAL DOSAGE	TYPICAL QUANTITY	TYPICAL PRICE	PRICE PER DOSE
Alesse	20/0.1	Ethinyl estradiol/Levonorgestrel	Take 1 tablet daily.	28	$31–$33	$1.11–$1.18
Apri	30/0.15	Ethinyl estradiol/Desogestrel	Take 1 tablet daily.	28	$22–$25	79¢–89¢
Aviane	20/0.1	Ethinyl estradiol/Levonorgestrel	Take 1 tablet daily.	28	$22–$24	79¢–86¢
Brevicon	35/0.5	Ethinyl estradiol/Norethindrone	Take 1 tablet daily.	28	$34–$38	$1.21–$1.36

PRODUCT	STRENGTH PER DOSE (MCG/MG)	ACTIVE INGREDIENT ESTROGEN/PROGESTIN	USUAL DOSAGE	TYPICAL QUANTITY	TYPICAL PRICE	PRICE PER DOSE
Demulen 1/35	35/1	Ethinyl estradiol/Norgestimate	Take 1 tablet daily.	28	$30–$38	$1.07–$1.36
Demulen 1/50	50/1	Ethinyl estradiol/Ethynodiol diacetate	Take 1 tablet daily.	28	$36–$38	$1.29–$1.36
Desogen	30/0.15	Ethinyl estradiol/Desogestrel	Take 1 tablet daily.	28	$29–$31	$1.04–$1.11
Levlen	30/0.15	Ethinyl estradiol/Levonorgestrel	Take 1 tablet daily.	28	$32–$35	$1.14–$1.25
Levlite	20/0.1	Ethinyl estradiol /Levonorgestrel	Take 1 tablet daily.	28	$31–$33	$1.11–$1.18
Levora	30/0.15	Ethinyl estradiol /Levonorgestrel	Take 1 tablet daily.	28	$25–$27	89¢–96¢
Lo/Ovral	30/0.3	Ethinyl estradiol/Norgestrel	Take 1 tablet daily.	21	$32–$34	$1.14–$1.21
Loestrin Fe 1.5/30	30/1.5	Ethinyl estradiol/Norethindrone acetate	Take 1 tablet daily.	28	$33–$35	$1.18–$1.25
Loestrin Fe 1/20	20/1	Ethinyl estradiol/Norethindrone acetate	Take 1 tablet daily.	28	$32–$34	$1.14–$1.21
Low-Ogestrel	30/0.3	Ethinyl estradiol/Norgestrel	Take 1 tablet daily.	28	$25–$28	89¢–$1
Microgestin Fe 1.5/30	30/1.5	Ethinyl estradiol/Norethindrone acetate	Take 1 tablet daily.	28	$26–$30	93¢–$1.07
Microgestin Fe 1/20	20/1	Ethinyl estradiol/Norethindrone acetate	Take 1 tablet daily.	28	$27–$30	96¢–$1.07
Modicon	35/0.5	Ethinyl estradiol/Norethindrone	Take 1 tablet daily.	28	$34–$37	$1.21–$1.32
Necon 0.5/35	35/0.5	Ethinyl estradiol/Norethindrone	Take 1 tablet daily.	28	$16–$18	57¢–64¢
Necon 1/35	35/1	Ethinyl estradiol/Norethindrone	Take 1 tablet daily.	28	$16–$18	57¢–64¢
Necon 1/50	50/1	Mestranol/Norethindrone	Take 1 tablet daily.	28	$16–$18	57¢–64¢
Nordette	30/0.15	Ethinyl estradiol/Levonorgestrel	Take 1 tablet daily.	28	$33–$35	$1.18–$1.25
Norinyl 1 + 35	35/1	Ethinyl estradiol/Norethindrone	Take 1 tablet daily.	28	$28–$32	$1–$1.14
Norinyl 1 + 50	50/1	Mestranol/Norethindrone	Take 1 tablet daily.	28	$29–$31	$1.04–$1.11
Ogestrel	50/0.5	Ethinyl estradiol/Norgestrel	Take 1 tablet daily.	28	$38–$40	$1.36–$1.43
Ortho –Novum 1/35	35/1	Ethinyl estradiol/Norethindrone	Take 1 tablet daily.	28	$32–$34	$1.14–$1.21
Ortho-Cept	30/0.15	Ethinyl estradiol/Desogestrel	Take 1 tablet daily.	28	$31–$34	$1.11–$1.21
Ortho-Cyclen	35/0.25	Ethinyl estradiol/Norethindrone	Take 1 tablet daily.	28	$30–$34	$1.07–$1.21
Ortho–Novum 1/50	50/1	Mestranol/Norethindrone	Take 1 tablet daily.	28	$32–$34	$1.14–$1.21
Ovcon-35	35/0.4	Ethinyl estradiol/Norethindrone	Take 1 tablet daily.	28	$31–$34	$1.11–$1.21
Ovcon-50	50/1	Ethinyl estradiol/Norethindrone	Take 1 tablet daily.	28	$34–$36	$1.21–$1.29
Ovral	50/0.5	Ethinyl estradiol/Norgestrel	Take 1 tablet daily.	28	$47–$49	$1.68–$1.75

PRODUCT	STRENGTH PER DOSE (MCG/MG)	ACTIVE INGREDIENT ESTROGEN/PROGESTIN	USUAL DOSAGE	TYPICAL QUANTITY	TYPICAL PRICE	PRICE PER DOSE
Yasmin	30/3	Ethinyl estradiol/Drospirenon	Take 1 tablet daily.	28	$28–$31	$1–$1.11
Zovia 1/35	35/1	Ethinyl estradiol/Ethynodiol diacetate	Take 1 tablet daily.	28	$18–$19	64¢–68¢
Zovia 1/50	50/1	Ethinyl estradiol /Ethynodiol diacetate	Take 1 tablet daily.	28	$17–$19	61¢–68¢

Oral Contraceptives: Biphasic

PRODUCT	STRENGTH PER DOSE PHASE 1 PHASE 2	ACTIVE INGREDIENT ESTROGEN (MCG)/ PROGESTIN (MG)	USUAL DOSAGE	TYPICAL QUANTITY	TYPICAL PRICE	PRICE PER DOSE
Jenest	0.5/35 1/35	Norethindrone & Ethinyl estradiol	Take 1 tablet daily.	28	$23–$27	82¢–96¢
Mircette estradiol	0.15/20 10mcg ethinyl	Desogestrel & Ethinyl estradiol	Take 1 tablet daily.	28	$30–$33	$1.07–$1.18
Necon 10/11	0.5/35 1/35	Norethindrone & Ethinyl estradiol	Take 1 tablet daily.	28	$17–$19	61¢–68¢
Ortho-Novum 10/11	0.5/35 1/35	Norethindrone & Ethinyl estradiol	Take 1 tablet daily.	28	$35–$38	$1.25–$1.36

Oral Contraceptives: Triphasic

PRODUCT	STRENGTH PER DOSE PHASE 1 PHASE 2 PHASE 3 (MCG/MG)	ACTIVE INGREDIENT ESTROGEN/PROGESTIN	USUAL DOSAGE	TYPICAL QUANTITY	TYPICAL PRICE	PRICE PER DOSE
Estrostep Fe	1/20 1/30 1/35	Norethindrone acetate & Ethinyl estradiol	Take 1 tablet daily.	28	$32–$34	$1.14–$1.21
Ortho-Novum 7/7/7	0.5/35 0.75/35 1/35	Norethindrone & Ethinyl estradiol	Take 1 tablet daily.	28	$31–$34	$1.11–$1.21
Ortho-Tri-Cyclen	0.18/20 0.75/35 1/35	Norethindrone & Ethinyl estradiol	Take 1 tablet daily.	28	$30–$34	$1.07–$1.21

PRODUCT	STRENGTH PER DOSE PHASE 1 PHASE 2 PHASE 3 (MCG/MG)	ACTIVE INGREDIENT ESTROGEN/PROGESTIN	USUAL DOSAGE	TYPICAL QUANTITY	TYPICAL PRICE	PRICE PER DOSE
Tri-Levlen	0.05/30 0.075/40 0.125/30	Levonorgestrel & Ethinyl estradiol	Take 1 tablet daily.	28	$30–$32	$1.07–$1.14
Tri-Norinyl	0.5/0.35 1/35 0.5/35	Norethindrone & Ethinyl estradiol	Take 1 tablet daily.	28	$27–$30	96¢–$1.07
Triphasil	0.05/30 0.075/40 0.125/30	Levonorgestrel & Ethinyl estradiol	Take 1 tablet daily.	28	$29–$31	$1.04–$1.11
Trivora	0.05/30 0.075/40 0.125/30	Levonorgestrel & Ethinyl estradiol	Take 1 tablet daily.	28	$21–$24	75¢–86¢

Oral Contraceptives: Progestin Only

PRODUCT	STRENGTH PER DOSE	ACTIVE INGREDIENT PROGESTIN (MG)	USUAL DOSAGE	TYPICAL QUANTITY	TYPICAL PRICE	PRICE PER DOSE
Micronor	0.35	Norethindrone	Take 1 tablet daily.	28	$37–$39	$1.32–$1.39
Nor-QD	0.35	Norethindrone	Take 1 tablet daily.	28	$35–$37	$1.25–$1.32
Ovrette	0.075	Norgestrel	Take 1 tablet daily.	28	$31–$35	$1.11–$1.25

$ SMART BUY
Oral Contraceptives (Birth Control Pills)

The Smart Buy for most women is to start with the generic version of Ortho-Novum 1/35. It has a low level of estrogen (fewer side effects) and the generic version will save you about $16 a month (a tidy $192 a year!). If breakthrough bleeding occurs, try a generic form of Triphasil. The slightly modified amounts of hormones should regulate the bleeding.

Among the oral contraceptives, generic versions often have their own "brand" names. One generic version of Ortho-Novum is Necon, and a common generic version of Triphasil is Trivora. If you're taking an oral contraceptive already, it makes sense to switch to a generic version to save money only if one is available that's nearly identical to what you're taking now.

HORMONE REPLACEMENT THERAPY

At menopause, women's bodies dramatically reduce the amounts of the hormones estrogen and progesterone they produce. During a woman's fertile years, these are the hormones that establish and regulate her menstrual cycle and make pregnancy possible. When the levels of these hormones decrease after menopause, there are a number of obvious and not so obvious results. Hormone replacement therapy uses one or the other or a combination of both of these hormones to restore some of the body's functions to their premenopausal levels.

ESTROGEN PRODUCTS

For many years, the most commonly prescribed drug in the U.S. has been the hormone replacement therapy (HRT) product Premarin. Recently, so many questions have arisen about the possible risks of taking estrogen it would take an entire book to explore the issue fully. Here we discuss only the different estrogen (and other sex-hormone) products available in the current market and provide you with what we believe are the best options in terms of cost and effectiveness.

Estrogen and Bone Loss

Estrogen does slow the process of bone loss and helps minimize osteoporosis. However, unlike a drug called Fosamax, which actually reverses bone loss, estrogen can't restore what bone has been lost already.

The most compelling reason for a woman to take estrogen after menopause is the overwhelming evidence that doing so significantly reduces the risk of osteoporosis, a potentially debilitating disease that affects up to 90 percent of postmenopausal women. In osteoporosis, bone mass and bone density decline, weakening the bones. As many as 50,000 osteoporosis-related deaths occur every year in the U.S.. Men can get osteoporosis, too, but they're less vulnerable than women because they have a larger bone mass to begin with; when *they* lose bone mass it rarely leads to fractures, because they have mass to spare. Estrogen slows the breakdown of bone cells. When a woman's estrogen levels drop, as occurs with menopause, the rate at which bone breaks down accelerates. In most women this is a slow and gradual process, but some women lose 1 percent of their bone density a year. At that rate, it doesn't take long for the situation to become critical. Studies have shown that women who take estrogen after menopause—even as long as six years after menopause—are far less likely to suffer the most common injuries related to osteoporosis, hip and wrist fractures.

For many years, health experts endorsed the long-term use of hormone replacement therapy as a hedge against heart disease. For most of their lives, women are at significantly lower risk for heart disease than men. This begins to change at menopause, and by about 10 years after menopause, the risk for heart disease becomes equal across gender. Many studies point to estrogen as the decisive factor, suggesting that estrogen plays some role in the body's manufacture of HDL (good cholesterol) and LDL (bad cholesterol). Recent studies employing newer technology were unable to substantiate this connection, however, or to provide any evidence that estrogen affects blood cholesterol levels. Thus, the medical community no longer endorses hormone replacement therapy to reduce a woman's risk of heart disease.

By far the most common reason women take estrogen is for relief from the discomforts of menopause—hot flashes, sleep disturbances, problems with concentration and memory, and decreased libido (loss of interest in sex). Although we speak of estrogen as though it were a single substance, in reality, it has several forms. Estrogen replacement therapy in humans typically involves combining these forms.

Premarin, the most commonly prescribed estrogen product, comes from an unusual natural source—pregnant mare's urine (hence the name, *pre-mar-in*) The urine is highly refined and purified, putting a vast distance between the source and the end product. Premarin contains *conjugated estrogens*—a blend of many forms of estrogen. In fact, Premarin contains at least 10 estrogenic and more than 200 individual steroidal components.

Despite its longevity and popularity, Premarin is one of the most controversial drugs on the American market today. One reason is its source. Many people feel that using pregnant horses to provide estrogen is unfair to the horses. While the manufacturer of Premarin insists that the horses receive the finest care and treatment, critics contend that using them in such a way is in itself inhumane. It's a debate unlikely to end as long as the manufacturing process remains unchanged, and if you're a woman contemplating hormone replacement therapy, you must decide for yourself whether this is an issue. Many women prefer to take products that come from other natural sources or that are synthesized in a laboratory. Like most healthcare professionals, we feel that estrogen is estrogen, whether it comes from a horse, a plant, or a lab.

Premarin's many components are another source of controversy. Because the source is natural, no one, not even Premarin's manufacturer, knows *exactly* what the product contains. But don't let this alarm you; modern technology can seem near-miraculous, but it still can't give us *all* the answers. Just as we still can't identify all the micronutrients in an apple, we can't identify all the constituents in pregnant mare's urine. So many exist, in fact, that it's proved impossible for researchers to replicate the formula to produce a generic equivalent. A number of generic products that received initial FDA approval were pulled from the market later because they produced inconsistent blood hormone levels among women who took them.

Premarin isn't the only oral form of estrogen, of course. Other products include Estrace (estradiol), Estratab (esterified estrogens), Ogen (estropipate), and Estinyl (ethinyl estradiol). These drugs come from synthetic sources—that is, they're manufactured in the laboratory to match, as closely as is possible, the chemical structure of human estrogen. Other estrogen supplements are made from plant-based estrogens similar, although not identical, to human estrogen.

Estrogen products are also available as vaginal creams and topical patches. There's no big therapeutic advantage to using one form over another; it really comes down to what you prefer and want to pay. Some women prefer patches they only need to change once a week, such as Climara. But if you have trouble with the patch sticking or if you get a rash from it, the convenience may not be worthwhile. Patches are more expensive than pills, especially generic versions. Climara patches typically cost around $40 a month, for example, while estradiol tablets cost around $15.

If the dosage form doesn't matter, you can enjoy a huge savings by using the generic form of the synthetic oral product Estrace (generic name estradiol). Especially when purchased in large quantities, oral tablets can be much less expensive than patch forms. When Bev brought in a prescription for Premarin, she mentioned that she was unhappy about its source. We phoned her doctor, who authorized a switch to a synthetic alternative. We changed her prescription to the generic form of Estrace, which made Bev especially happy, because she also saved quite a bit of money.

What about estrogen's side effects and risks? Well, certainly estrogen products have their share of both. Estrogen supplementation can promote blood clots and some forms of cancer. Studies have shown that postmenopausal women who take estrogen supplements are 4.5 to 13.9 times more likely to develop endometrial (uterine) cancer. Some studies also indicate that prolonged use (over nine years) of estrogen replacements may increase a woman's chance of developing breast cancer. Unfortunately, no study has provided *conclusive* results, and often results conflict. Because of this, many women refuse hormone replacement therapy. Other side effects of estrogen replacement products include a two- to four-fold increase in the risk of gallbladder disease that requires surgery. Estrogen supplements also have been linked to migraine headaches, depression, breast tenderness, abnormal or breakthrough vaginal bleeding, and nausea.

Estrogen Replacement Products: Transdermal (Skin Patches)

PRODUCT	RELEASE RATE (MG/24HRS)	FORM	ACTIVE INGREDIENT	USUAL DOSAGE	TYPICAL QUANTITY	TYPICAL PRICE	PRICE PER DOSE
Alora	0.05	Patch	Estradiol	Apply 1 twice weekly.	8	$36.99	$1.32
Alora	0.075	Patch	Estradiol	Apply 1 twice weekly.	8	$39.39	$1.41
Alora	0.1	Patch	Estradiol	Apply 1 twice weekly.	8	$39.49	$1.41
Climara	0.05	Patch	Estradiol	Apply 1 once weekly.	4	$35.79	$1.28
Climara	0.075	Patch	Estradiol	Apply 1 once weekly.	4	$38.99	$1.39
Climara	0.1	Patch	Estradiol	Apply 1 once weekly.	4	$38.99	$1.39
Estraderm	0.05	Patch	Estradiol	Apply 1 twice weekly.	8	$29.99	$1.07
Estraderm	0.1	Patch	Estradiol	Apply 1 twice weekly.	8	$31.99	$1.14
Estradiol	0.05	Patch	Estradiol	Apply 1 once weekly.	4	$32.39	$1.16
Estradiol	0.075	Patch	Estradiol	Apply 1 once weekly.	4	$30.99	$1.11
Estradiol	0.1	Patch	Estradiol	Apply 1 once weekly.	4	$31.99	$1.14
Vivelle	0.0375	Patch	Estradiol	Apply 1 twice weekly.	8	$39.99	$1.43
Vivelle	0.05	Patch	Estradiol	Apply 1 twice weekly.	8	$39.99	$1.43
Vivelle	0.075	Patch	Estradiol	Apply 1 twice weekly.	8	$36.39	$1.30
Vivelle	0.1	Patch	Estradiol	Apply 1 twice weekly.	8	$36.99	$1.32
Vivelle-Dot	0.0375	Patch	Estradiol	Apply 1 twice weekly.	8	$39.99	$1.43
Vivelle-Dot	0.05	Patch	Estradiol	Apply 1 twice weekly.	8	$39.99	$1.43
Vivelle-Dot	0.075	Patch	Estradiol	Apply 1 twice weekly.	8	$39.99	$1.43
Vivelle-Dot	0.1	Patch	Estradiol	Apply 1 twice weekly.	8	$40.99	$1.46

Estrogen Replacement Products: Oral

PRODUCT	STRENGTH	FORM	ACTIVE INGREDIENT	USUAL DOSAGE	TYPICAL QUANTITY	TYPICAL PRICE	PRICE PER DOSE
Cenestin	0.625mg	Tablets	Synthetic conjugated estrogens	Take 1 tablet daily.	30	$30.99	$1.03
Cenestin	0.9mg	Tablets	Synthetic conjugated estrogens	1 tab daily	30	$34.69	$1.16

PRODUCT	STRENGTH	FORM	ACTIVE INGREDIENT	USUAL DOSAGE	TYPICAL QUANTITY	TYPICAL PRICE	PRICE PER DOSE
Cenestin	1.25mg	Tablets	Synthetic conjugated estrogens	1 tab daily	30	$37.89	$1.26
Estinyl	0.02mg	Tablets	Ethinyl estradiol	1 tab daily	30	$22.99	77¢
Estinyl	0.05mg	Tablets	Ethinyl estradiol	1 tab daily	30	$33.99	$1.13
Estrace	0.5mg	Tablets	Micronized estradiol	Take 1 tablet daily.	30	$22.99	77¢
Estrace	1mg	Tablets	Micronized estradiol	Take 1 tablet daily.	30	$27.99	93¢
Estrace	2mg	Tablets	Micronized estradiol	Take 1 tablet daily.	30	$35.99	$1.20
$ Estradiol	0.5mg	Tablets	Micronized estradiol	Take 1 tablet daily.	30	$10.99	37¢
$ Estradiol	1mg	Tablets	Micronized estradiol	Take 1 tablet daily.	30	$16.99	57¢
$ Estradiol	2mg	Tablets	Micronized estradiol	Take 1 tablet daily.	30	$20.99	70¢
Estratab	0.3mg	Tablets	Esterified estrogens	Take 1 tablet daily.	30	$23.99	80¢
Estratab	0.625mg	Tablets	Esterified estrogens	Take 1 tablet daily.	30	$28.99	97¢
Estratab	2.5mg	Tablets	Esterified estrogens	Take 1 tablet daily.	30	$55.99	$1.87
Estropipate	0.75mg	Tablets	Micronized estradiol	Take 1 tablet daily.	30	$17.49	58¢
Estropipate	1.5mg	Tablets	Micronized estradiol	Take 1 tablet daily.	30	$20.99	70¢
Estropipate	2.5mg	Tablets	Micronized estradiol	Take 1 tablet daily.	30	$38.99	$1.30
Menest	0.3mg	Tablets	Esterified estrogens	Take 1 tablet daily.	30	$20.99	70¢
Menest	0.625mg	Tablets	Esterified estrogens	Take 1 tablet daily.	30	$23.99	80¢
Menest	1.25mg	Tablets	Esterified estrogens	Take 1 tablet daily.	30	$32.99	$1.10
Menest	2.5mg	Tablets	Esterified estrogens	Take 1 tablet daily.	30	$42.99	$1.43
Ogen	0.75mg	Tablets	Micronized estradiol	Take 1 tablet daily.	30	$33.99	$1.13
Ogen	1.5mg	Tablets	Micronized estradiol	Take 1 tablet daily.	30	$42.99	$1.43
Ogen	2.5mg	Tablets	Micronized estradiol	Take 1 tablet daily.	30	$71.99	$2.40
Ortho-Est	0.75mg	Tablets	Micronized estradiol	Take 1 tablet daily.	30	$26.99	90¢
Ortho-Est	1.5mg	Tablets	Micronized estradiol	Take 1 tablet daily.	30	$32.99	$1.10
Premarin	0.3mg	Tablets	Conjugated estrogens	Take 1 tablet daily.	30	$23.99	80¢
Premarin	0.625mg	Tablets	Conjugated estrogens	Take 1 tablet daily.	30	$24.99	83¢
Premarin	0.9mg	Tablets	Conjugated estrogens	Take 1 tablet daily.	30	$34.99	$1.17
Premarin	1.25mg	Tablets	Conjugated estrogens	Take 1 tablet daily.	30	$36.99	$1.23
Premarin	2.5mg	Tablets	Conjugated estrogens	Take 1 tablet daily.	30	$55.99	$1.87

$ SMART BUY
Estrogen Products

The Smart Buy when it comes to estrogen for hormone replacement is the generic form of Estrace (estradiol), which is significantly cheaper than Premarin ($15 compared to $30). This is true whether you take estrogen alone or with progesterone. Taking the two hormones separately allows you the greatest flexibility in adjusting your doses. (Also read our Smart Buys in the following sections, "Progesterone Products" and "Drugs to Treat Osteoporosis.") Likewise, oral versions of estrogen are smarter buys than the topical patch. Avoid the patches and save yourself some money (and the hassle of a possible skin rash). Buy oral forms in quantities of 100, which most pharmacies consider a three-month supply. Also, consider getting a strength that's twice the dose your doctor prescribes and cutting the tablets in half.

PROGESTERONE PRODUCTS

To help reduce the chances of estrogen causing some types of cancer, some HRT products add a second hormone, progestin, to their formulas. Progestin is also available separately. Progestin allows the lining of the uterus to build up and then shed, just as it did during menstruation. In fact, the most common complaint women have about taking progestin is that their periods start again. For most women, however, this is a temporary effect that subsides within six months or so. The premise of progestin therapy is that allowing the uterus to function as it did during your fertile years keeps endometrial cancer at bay. Most women who have their uteruses after menopause should take a progesterone supplement to offset the increased cancer risk of taking estrogen. Doctors also prescribe progestins alone (without estrogen) to regulate menstruation, treat endometriosis, and improve infertility.

$ SMART BUY
Progesterone Products

As the charts show, taking the separate components of Premarin and generic Provera will cost you about $37 for 28 days of therapy, compared to taking the Prempro at about $40 a pack. That's a savings of around $3 for every four-week cycle, $36 a year, or about 8 percent. Combination estrogen-progestin products cost more, and have the added disadvantage of limiting your ability to adjust the doses of each hormone. The trial-and-error period commonly involved in adjusting hormone levels can make combination products even more expensive. We recommend you take progestin as a separate product, even if you also take estrogen. Taking separate progestin and estrogen products affords you maximum

Progesterone Replacement Products

PRODUCT	STRENGTH PER DOSE	FORM	ACTIVE INGREDIENT	USUAL DOSAGE	TYPICAL QUANTITY	TYPICAL PRICE FOR 28-DAY SUPPLY	PRICE PER DOSE
Medroxyprogesterone	2.5mg	Tablet	Medroxyprogesterone	Take 1 tablet daily.	30	$15	50¢
Medroxyprogesterone	5mg	Tablet	Medroxyprogesterone	Take 1 tablet daily.	30	$16	53¢
Medroxyprogesterone	10mg	Tablet	Medroxyprogesterone	Take 1 tablet daily.	30	$17	57¢
Prempro	0.625/2.5mg	Tablet; combination product	Estrogen with medroxyprogesterone	Take 1 tablet daily.	28	$40	$1.43
Premphase	0.625/5mg	Tablet	Estrogen with medroxyprogesterone	Take 1 tablet daily.	28	$40	$1.43
Provera	2.5mg	Tablet	Medroxyprogesterone	Take 1 tablet daily.	30	$30	$1.00
Provera	5mg	Tablet	Medroxyprogesterone	Take 1 tablet daily.	30	$37	$1.23
Provera	10mg	Tablet	Medroxyprogesterone	Take 1 tablet daily.	30	$41	$1.37

flexibility in finding an effective dosage with the fewest side effects. For the greatest savings, your Smart Buy is the generic forms of these drugs in bulk quantities. And buy a tablet strength double the dose your doctor prescribes, so you can cut them in half. This can cut your costs to about 7 cents a dose for estradiol, 8 cents a dose for medroxyprogesterone.

ANDROGEN PRODUCTS

The last type of sex hormones used in humans are the androgens. These "male hormones" commonly are used to treat breast cancer in both women and men. They're also used to treat impotence, delayed puberty, and delayed testicular development in males. Some women find that androgen improves sex drive and energy levels following menopause, although it can be challenging to find a dose that provides the desired result without undesired side effects (such as developing male pattern facial and body hair). Because these side effects are less problematic with methyltestosterone and fluoxymesterone, these are usually chosen for use in women. Because fluoxymesterone can cause liver problems, start with methyltestosterone.

For men, usually the choice is made based on convenience. Androgens taken orally can cause nausea—not ideal. If this occurs for you, consider using topical products. Originally designed to apply to the scrotum, newer formulas may be applied to the arms, thighs, back, or buttocks for absorption through the skin.

> ## Government Halts Studies
>
> ---
>
> In August 2002, the federal government announced that it was discontinuing a major study of hormone replacement therapy in older men. This followed the discovery that testosterone can fuel the growth of prostate cancer. It also increases red blood cell production, possibly increasing the risk of clots that can cause heart attacks and strokes. According to news reports, doctors wrote 1.5 million prescriptions for testosterone and drugs like it in 2001, up from 806,000 in 1997.

$ SMART BUY
Androgen Products

Your Smart Buy for androgen products depends on whether you're a man or a woman. If you're a man, choose Androderm. These patches are a little more expensive than Testoderm, Halotestin, or Android, but they're far more convenient and have fewer potential side effects. Shop around for the best price; this product isn't yet available in a generic version.

If you're a woman, your Smart Buy is Android, because of its fewer potential side effects. For the greatest savings, buy the generic in bulk to pay just under $1.50 a dose.

OTHER DRUGS USED TO TREAT OSTEOPOROSIS

In addition to using estrogen, three other options are available to prevent osteoporosis. The first, Evista (generic name raloxifene), is known as an *estrogen receptor modulator*. Although it's not in the estrogen family, this drug works by binding to estrogen receptors in the bone to elicit estrogen-like effects. What's especially good about this drug is that it selects receptors in bone and not in the uterus or breasts, limiting the risk of breast or uterine cancer. Its most common side effects are hot flashes and leg cramps.

The second nonestrogen drug used to treat osteoporosis is Fosamax (generic name alendronate). This high-powered drug works by slowing the cells responsible for breaking down old bone so that new bone can gain ground. This means that alendronate can maintain and even increase bone mass, thwarting osteoporosis, and this makes alendronate unique.

Androgen Supplement Products

PRODUCT	STRENGTH PER DOSE	FORM	ACTIVE INGREDIENT	USUAL DOSAGE	TYPICAL QUANTITY	TYPICAL PRICE FOR 30-DAY SUPPLY	PRICE PER DAY
$ Androderm	2.5mg	Patch	Testosterone	Apply 2 patches daily.	60	$150	$5
$ Androderm	5mg	Patch	Testosterone	Apply 1 patch daily.	60	$150	$5
Androgel	2.5 grams	Gel	Testosterone	Apply once daily.	30	$175	$5.83
Androgel	5 grams	Gel	Testosterone	Apply once daily.	30	$175	$5.83
$ Android	10mg	Capsule	Methyltestosterone	Take 1-4 capsules daily.	100	$225	$9
Fluoxymesterone	10mg	Tablet	Fluoxymesterone	Take 1-2 tablets daily.	60	$110	$3.67
Halotestin	2mg	Tablet	Fluoxymesterone	Take 1-3 tablets daily.	90	$85	$2.83
Halotestin	5mg	Tablet	Fluoxymesterone	Take 1-3 tablets daily.	90	$85	$2.83
Halotestin	10mg	Tablet	Fluoxymesterone	Take 1-2 tablets daily.	60	$165	$5.50
Methyltestosterone	10mg	Tablet	Methyltestosterone	Take 1-4 tablets daily.	100	$140	$5.60
Testoderm	4mg	Patch	Testosterone	Apply 1 patch daily.	30	$120	$4
Testoderm	6mg	Patch	Testosterone	Apply 1 patch daily.	30	$120	$4

Although this drug helps a lot, don't think you can take your chances and avoid taking estrogen or calcium. Calcium and estrogen or raloxifene taken *before* osteoporosis occurs will make the task for alendronate much easier. If your doctor prescribes alendronate for you, it's crucial you take it correctly. For best absorption and effectiveness, take alendronate as soon as you awaken in the morning with a full glass of *plain water*. Then wait at least 30 minutes before taking any other food, drink, or medication. To prevent any indigestion symptoms, don't lie down during this time. Other side effects include headaches, muscle pain, and flatulence.

And don't be shocked when you see the price tag. Typical cost for one month of alendronate runs $70 to $80.

The third option for treating osteoporosis is a new drug called Actonel (generic name risedronate). Risedronate is in the same family as alendronate, and, as you might expect, it has the same actions and side effects. It's a bit more expensive than alendronate, so look for Fosamax to save money.

Drugs to Prevent or Treat Osteoporosis

PRODUCT	STRENGTH PER DOSE	FORM	ACTIVE INGREDIENT	USUAL DOSAGE	TYPICAL QUANTITY	TYPICAL PRICE	PRICE PER DAY
Actonel	5mg	Tablet	Risedronate	Take 1 tablet daily.	30	$85	$2.83
Actonel	30mg	Tablet	Risedronate	Take 1 tablet daily.	30	$450	$15
Evista	60mg	Tablet	Raloxifene	Take 1 tablet daily.	30	$77	$2.57
Fosamax	5mg	Tablet	Alendronate	Take 1 tablet daily.	30	$72	$2.40
Fosamax	10mg	Tablet	Alendronate	Take 1 tablet daily.	30	$72	$2.40
Fosamax	35mg	Tablet	Alendronate	Take 1 tablet weekly.	4	$75	$2.68
$ Fosamax	40mg	Tablet	Alendronate	Take 1 tablet weekly.	4	$35	$1.25
$ Fosamax	70mg	Tablet	Alendronate	Take 1 tablet weekly.	4	$70	$2.50

$ SMART BUY
Drugs to Prevent or Treat Osteoporosis

To prevent osteoporosis, the Smart Buy is generic Estrace and generic Provera, taken as separate drugs. Even though Evista does a good job and has fewer side effects, the high price of $77 a month isn't worth it. If you have osteoporosis already, Fosamax is the only way to go. A once-a-week version of Fosamax comes in 70mg and 35mg strengths, depending on the dose you need. It's much easier to take (once a week instead of every day), and it's cheaper, making it your Smart Buy (although they're still expensive at over $70 for a one-month supply).

By far the cheapest course of action is to begin your prevention efforts early and keep your bones strong and your calcium levels high: Include plenty of calcium in your diet (through foods and through supplements, if your doctor recommends them), and engage in regular "impact" exercise, such as walking or running.

ORAL DRUGS TO TREAT DIABETES

With diabetes, the body stops making insulin, or it becomes less able to use the insulin it does produce. Insulin is important for packaging glucose (sugar), the body's fuel source, so that the body can use it properly. When this doesn't happen, extra glucose remains in the bloodstream, where it can cause some very serious problems. People with diabetes are at risk for losing their eyesight (diabetes is the leading cause of blindness in the U.S.); developing kidney damage and kidney failure; losing limbs due to reduced circulation and nerve problems that allow severe infections to develop; and developing severe problems with their blood vessels and heart.

The American Diabetes Association reports that more than 16 million Americans live with diabetes; about half of them require some sort of treatment to control the condition. The first step in treating type 2 (adult onset) diabetes with medication is to increase the amount of insulin the body produces. The first drugs on the market that could do this were called *sulfonylureas*, which work by stimulating the pancreas to release insulin. For a long time, these were the only drugs that could be taken orally to help with diabetes. Anything else required an injection. Common older ("first-generation") sulfonylureas include Diabinese (generic name chlorpropamide), Dymelor (generic name acetohexamide), Tolinase (generic name tolazamide), and Orinase (generic name tolbutamide). The downside to using some of these older sulfonylureas is that they can cause weight gain, low blood-sugar levels (hypoglycemia), and other problems.

Newer (second-generation) sulfonylureas are much less apt to cause these problems. These include Diabeta (generic name glyburide), Micronase (generic name glyburide), Glucotrol (generic name glipizide), and Amaryl (generic name glimepiride). Of this group, glimepiride is your best choice for limited side effects. Much less weight gain and hypoglycemia occurs with this drug. But glimepiride is also more expensive than the other second-generation sulfonylureas. A 30-day supply of the 4mg strength typically will cost around $30. A therapeutically equivalent dose of glyburide, on the other hand, is available in a generic form that will cost around $15 for a 30-day supply, for a savings of 50 percent.

Bruce has been taking glyburide to treat his diabetes for the last two years. He knows that watching his diet and exercising are crucial to controlling his diabetes, so he's been vigilant about doing both. Despite this resolve, since he's been taking glyburide, he's gained about 25 pounds. Recently, Bruce asked me what he was doing wrong. We asked whether he'd be willing to pay a little more money for his medication if it controlled his weight better. He said yes, so we called his doctor to get the OK to try Bruce on Amaryl. Bruce's doctor agreed, and so far Bruce has lost 10 pounds.

More recent types of oral drugs used to treat diabetes work differently from sulfonylureas in that they don't stimulate the pancreas to release more insulin. Instead, they decrease glucose production in the liver, decrease intestinal absorption of glucose, improve insulin sensitivity and utilization, and increase glucose use in skeletal muscles. These new mechanisms make it far less likely that these newer drugs will cause hypoglycemia, so they're much safer drugs to take. These new drugs for diabetes break down into three groups—*thiazolidinediones*, *meglitinides*, and *biguanides*.

Thiazolidinediones are known as "insulin sensitizers." They work by reducing the amount of glucose the liver produces and by increasing the use of glucose in skeletal muscles. Members of this group include Avandia (generic name rosiglitazone), and

Actos (generic name rosiglitazone pioglitazone). A third drug in this class, Rezulin (generic name troglitazone), was pulled off the market after 60 deaths from liver failure associated with its use were reported to the FDA.

Despite the fact that rosiglitazone and pioglitazone are in the same family as troglitazone, there are far fewer incidences of liver problems with these two drugs. However, it may be prudent to have your doctor perform liver function tests every year as a precaution. Other side effects you might expect to see with each of these drugs include weight gain, edema, and headaches. One difference between these two drugs, however, is that they affect blood cholesterol levels in different ways. Pioglitazone increases HDL and decreases triglycerides. Rosiglitazone increases all types of cholesterol (good and bad). If your blood cholesterol levels concern you, steer your doctor toward pioglitazone. Finally, these drugs can cause a resumption of ovulation in women who take birth control pills. Ask your doctor about increasing the strength of your oral contraceptives, or use alternative methods of protection.

Meglitinides, like sulfonylureas, work on cells in the pancreas to increase insulin production. But unlike sulfonylureas, meglitinides are very short-acting, and so always should be taken with meals. The most commonly prescribed member of this group is Prandin (generic name repaglinide). Side effects to expect include mild hypoglycemia, weight gain, diarrhea, and joint pain.

Currently, the biguanide class of drugs has only one representative on the market—Glucophage (generic name metformin). Of all the oral drugs used for diabetes, this is, by far, the most commonly prescribed. Metformin works by decreasing glucose output from the liver and increasing tissue sensitivity to insulin. Although metformin rarely causes hypoglycemia and weight gain, you should be aware of its other side effects, including diarrhea, nausea, bloating, and flatulence. To limit these, take metformin with food. Don't take metformin if you have any degree of kidney or liver problems. Alcoholics should avoid this drug because of their increased risk of liver disease. Potential accumulation of this drug may lead to lactic acidosis, a buildup of lactic acid in the bloodstream. This results in malaise, muscle aches, respiratory distress, sleepiness, abdominal distress, hypothermia, low blood pressure, and slow and irregular heartbeats. It can be quite serious. Although it's exceedingly rare for metformin to cause this condition, it can be fatal if it does occur. Watch for early signs, such as malaise, muscle aches, hyperventilation, or unusual sleepiness.

> ### Alcohol and Diabetes: A Bad Combination
>
> If you have diabetes and take oral medications to control your blood sugar, avoid drinking alcohol.
>
> The combination, especially with sulfonylureas, can cause severe facial flushing.

One last type of drug for treating diabetes that's gaining popularity with doctors is Precose (generic name acarbose). This drug delays carbohydrate absorption from meals by inhibiting stomach enzymes responsible for breaking carbohydrates down. This reduces those pesky post-meal glucose peaks. For acarbose to work properly, it must be taken with the first bite of a meal, three times a day. Common side effects to expect include flatulence, diarrhea, and abdominal discomfort. Usually these occur during only the first few weeks you take the drug.

Products recently have become available that combine the two drugs used to treat diabetes. The most common of these is Glucovance. Combining glyburide and metformin has potential for treating diabetes, but, as with other combination products, we prefer using the two drugs in separate forms. Doing so allows for more dosage flexibility, which can be crucial in people with diabetes. Once you find the right dosage combination for you, however, switching to a combination product might save you some money. A 30-day supply of Glucovance 5/500 will cost you around $35, while the same amount of glyburide and metformin purchased separately will wind up costing about $60.

Like high blood pressure, diabetes often is treated using several types of medication. This protocol is so widely accepted that the American Diabetes Association recommends the following stepped approach:

Step 1: Diet and exercise
Step 2: Monotherapy (a single oral drug)
Step 3: Combination oral therapy
Step 4: Oral therapy plus insulin
Step 5: Insulin
Step 6: Insulin plus a thiazolidinedione

Because insulin is an over-the-counter drug, we discuss it in Chapter 21, "Other Over-the-Counter Products."

Oral Drugs to Treat Diabetes

PRODUCT	STRENGTH PER DOSE	TYPE	ACTIVE INGREDIENT	USUAL DOSAGE	TYPICAL QUANTITY	TYPICAL PRICE	PRICE PER DOSE
Actos (pioglitazone)	15mg	Thiazolidinedione (insulin sensitizer)	Pioglitazone	Take 1 tablet daily.	30	$105	$3.50
Actos (pioglitazone)	30mg	Thiazolidinedione (insulin sensitizer)	Pioglitazone	Take 1 tablet daily.	30	$155	$5.17
Actos (pioglitazone)	45mg	Thiazolidinedione (insulin sensitizer)	Pioglitazone	Take 1 tablet daily.	30	$170	$5.67
Amaryl (glimepiride)	1mg	Second-generation sulfonylurea	Glimepiride	Take 1 tablet daily.	30	$15	50¢
Amaryl (glimepiride)	2mg	Second-generation sulfonylurea	Glimepiride	Take 1 tablet daily.	30	$20	67¢
Amaryl (glimepiride)	4mg	Second-generation sulfonylurea	Glimepiride	Take 1 tablet daily.	30	$30	$1
Avandia (rosiglitazone)	2mg	Thiazolidinedione (insulin sensitizer)	Rosiglitazone	Take 1 tablet daily.	30	$65	$2.17
Avandia (rosiglitazone)	4mg	Thiazolidinedione (insulin sensitizer)	Rosiglitazone	Take 1 tablet daily.	30	$90	$3
Avandia (rosiglitazone)	8mg	Thiazolidinedione (insulin sensitizer)	Rosiglitazone	Take 1 tablet daily.	30	$145	$4.83
Chlorpropamide	100mg	First-generation sulfonylurea	Chlorpropamide	Take 1 tablet daily.	30	$15	50¢
Chlorpropamide	250mg	First-generation sulfonylurea	Chlorpropamide	Take 1 tablet daily.	30	$20	67¢
Diabeta (glyburide)	2.5mg	Second-generation sulfonylurea	Glyburide	Take 1 tablet daily.	30	$20	67¢
Diabeta (glyburide)	5mg	Second-generation sulfonylurea	Glyburide	Take 1 tablet daily.	30	$30	$1
Diabinese (chloropropamide)	250mg	First-generation sulfonylurea	Chlorpropamide	Take 1 tablet daily.	30	$45	$1.50
Diabinese (chloropropamide)	100mg	First-generation sulfonylurea	Chlorpropamide	Take 1 tablet daily.	30	$25	83¢
Glipizide	5mg	Second-generation sulfonylurea	Glipizide	Take 1 tablet daily.	30	$15	50¢

PRODUCT	STRENGTH PER DOSE	TYPE	ACTIVE INGREDIENT	USUAL DOSAGE	TYPICAL QUANTITY	TYPICAL PRICE	PRICE PER DOSE
Glipizide	10mg	Second-generation sulfonylurea	Glipizide	Take 1 tablet daily.	30	$20	67¢
Glucophage (metformin)	500mg	Biguanide	Metformin	Take 1 tablet twice a day.	60	$50	83¢
Glucophage (metformin)	850mg	Biguanide	Metformin	Take 1 tablet twice a day.	60	$90	$1.50
Glucophage (metformin)	1,000mg	Biguanide	Metformin	Take 1 tablet twice a day.	60	$100	$1.67
Glucophage XR (metformin)	500mg	Biguanide	Metformin	Take 1 tablet daily.	30	$30	$1
Glucotrol (glipizide)	5mg	Second-generation sulfonylurea	Glipizide	Take 1 tablet daily.	30	$20	67¢
Glucotrol (glipizide)	10mg	Second-generation sulfonylurea	Glipizide	Take 1 tablet daily.	30	$35	$1.17
Glucotrol XL (glipizide)	2.5mg	Second-generation sulfonylurea	Glipizide	Take 1 tablet daily.	30	$20	67¢
Glucotrol XL (glipizide)	5mg	Second-generation sulfonylurea	Glipizide	Take 1 tablet daily.	30	$20	67¢
Glucotrol XL (glipizide)	10mg	Second-generation sulfonylurea	Glipizide	Take 1 tablet daily.	30	$30	$1
Glucovance (glyburide and metformin)	1.25 /250mg	Second-generation sulfonylurea combined with a biguanide	Glyburide and metformin	Take 1 tablet daily.	30	$30	$1
Glucovance (glyburide and metformin)	2.5/500mg	Second-generation sulfonylurea combined with a biguanide	Glyburide and metformin	Take 1 tablet daily.	30	$35	$1.17
Glucovance (glyburide and metformin)	5/500mg	Second-generation sulfonylurea biguanide	Glyburide and metformin	Take 1 tablet daily.	30	$35	$1.17
Glyburide (glyburide and metformin)	2.5mg	Second-generation sulfonylurea	Glyburide	Take 1 tablet daily.	30	$15	50¢
Glyburide	5mg	Second-generation sulfonylurea	Glyburide	Take 1 tablet daily.	30	$20	67¢
Metformin	500mg	Biguanide	Metformin	Take 1 tablet twice a day.	60	$40	67¢
Metformin	850mg	Biguanide	Metformin	Take 1 tablet twice a day.	60	$80	$1.33
Metformin	1,000mg	Biguanide	Metformin	Take 1 tablet twice a day.	60	$90	$1.50

PRODUCT	STRENGTH PER DOSE	TYPE	ACTIVE INGREDIENT	USUAL DOSAGE	TYPICAL QUANTITY	TYPICAL PRICE	PRICE PER DOSE
Micronase (glyburide)	2.5mg	Second-generation sulfonylurea	Glyburide	Take 1 tablet daily.	30	$30	$1
Micronase (glyburide)	5mg	Second-generation sulfonylurea	Glyburide	Take 1 tablet daily.	30	$40	$1.33
Prandin (repaglinide)	0.5mg	Meglitinide	Repaglinide	Take 1 tablet with each meal.	90	$90	$1
Prandin (repaglinide)	1mg	Meglitinide	Repaglinide	Take 1 tablet with each meal.	90	$90	$1
Prandin (repaglinide)	2mg	Meglitinide	Repaglinide	Take 1 tablet with each meal.	90	$90	$1
Precose (acarbose)	25mg	Meglitinide	Acarbose	Take 1 tablet 3 times a day.	90	$70	78¢
Precose (acarbose)	50mg	Meglitinide	Acarbose	Take 1 tablet 3 times a day.	90	$70	78¢
Precose (acarbose)	100mg	Meglitinide	Acarbose	Take 1 tablet 3 times a day.	90	$85	94¢

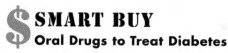

$ SMART BUY
Oral Drugs to Treat Diabetes

For type 2 diabetes, Glucophage is the Smart Buy. It presents far fewer potential side effects, and there's a less expensive generic version. To save even more money, buy in bulk. If your doctor wants to add 5mg of glyburide to the regimen, a common Step III treatment approach, buy the two drugs separately and avoid combination products such as Glucovance, which won't allow you to reduce the amount of glyburide if you need to. Once you're stable, though, consider buying the Glucovance to save some money. When buying metformin and glyburide, purchasing generic versions in bulk will drop your per-dose cost from $1 for the name brands to 75 cents, a savings of 25 percent, for the generics.

DRUGS TO TREAT HYPOTHYROIDISM

Hypothyroidism results when the thyroid gland produces too little thyroid hormone, which regulates your body's metabolism. Low thyroid levels usually slow metabolism and lower your energy level. You may feel tired all the time and could develop a problem with excessive weight gain. This is a frustrating condition for many people.

Drugs to treat hypothyroidism replenish the thyroid hormone. The original products developed to do this were desiccated (cleaned, dried, and powdered) animal thyroid glands, but at first, standardizing the active ingredients in these pills was a problem. Over the years, processing methods improved enough to allow for consistent dosages. You'll still find these early products on the market under names such as Thyroid USP and Armour Thyroid. The challenge of developing standardized products, though, led to the development of synthetic alternatives—that is, products made in the laboratory, rather than extracted from cow or pig thyroid glands. One of the more popular of these is Synthroid (generic name levothyroxine).

One of the difficulties in producing thyroid products, whether desiccated or synthetic, always has been getting accurate and consistent amounts of active thyroid into tablet form. This is especially important because the human body is so sensitive to this hormone. People who take thyroid supplements often can detect even the slightest variances. Synthroid, for example, comes in 11 different strengths to help pinpoint the optimum dose for each person who takes it. Because of this sensitivity, there has been considerable dispute about whether generic levothyroxine is, in fact, comparable to Synthroid. We consider all thyroid products to have narrow therapeutic indexes (NTIs).

Quality alternatives to Synthroid do exist. (To save some money, ask your doctor about Levoxyl.) But keep in mind that these substitutes aren't generically equivalent to Synthroid. Most doctors and pharmacists agree that if you're taking a thyroid replacement product and it works for you, you should stay with the same product. Don't change brands unless you're not getting acceptable results. And be aware that, because the body is so sensitive to thyroid, it might take some time for your doctor to pinpoint the right dose for you. To help things along, make sure you keep your appointments for blood work and report any unusual symptoms. If you feel tired and lack energy, your dose is probably too low. If you feel hot and hyperactive, or if your heart is racing, your dose is probably too high. Let your doctor know.

When long-time customer June came in for a refill of her Synthroid, she asked whether she could save money by switching to a generic version. We told her that no true generic equivalent to Synthroid exists, only alternative brands that are less expensive. If the Synthroid was working well for her, we said, she shouldn't mess with it. Determined to save money, June called her doctor and convinced him to allow her to try a cheaper thyroid supplement. It took several tries at different strengths of this new supplement to find the right dosage for June; this involved blood work and several months of feeling not-quite-right. June and her doctor finally found the right strength for her, but were the extra lab fees and discomfort worth the change?

Take Your Doses Correctly!

When you change manufacturers or thyroid supplement strength, it's very important to take every dose as directed. Missing even a single dose can lead to incorrect blood test results. The decisions your doctor makes about your dose depend on accurate laboratory measurements of the thyroid in your blood.

Drugs to Treat Hypothyroidism

PRODUCT	STRENGTH PER DOSE	ACTIVE INGREDIENT	USUAL DOSAGE	TYPICAL QUANTITY	TYPICAL PRICE	PRICE PER DAY
Armour Thyroid	15mg	Desiccated thyroid	Take 1 tablet daily.	100	$20	20¢
Armour Thyroid	30mg	Desiccated thyroid	Take 1 tablet daily.	100	$20	20¢
Armour Thyroid	60mg	Desiccated thyroid	Take 1 tablet daily.	100	$21	21¢
Armour Thyroid	90mg	Desiccated thyroid	Take 1 tablet daily.	100	$30	30¢
Armour Thyroid	120mg	Desiccated thyroid	Take 1 tablet daily.	100	$35	35¢
Armour Thyroid	180mg	Desiccated thyroid	Take 1 tablet daily.	100	$50	50¢
Levothroid (levothyroxine)	0.025mg	Levothyroxine	Take 1 tablet daily.	100	$30	30¢
Levothroid (levothyroxine)	0.05mg	Levothyroxine	Take 1 tablet daily.	100	$30	30¢
Levothroid (levothyroxine)	0.075mg	Levothyroxine	Take 1 tablet daily.	100	$30	30¢
Levothroid (levothyroxine)	0.088mg	Levothyroxine	Take 1 tablet daily.	100	$35	35¢
Levothroid (levothyroxine)	0.1mg	Levothyroxine	Take 1 tablet daily.	100	$35	35¢
Levothroid (levothyroxine)	0.112mg	Levothyroxine	Take 1 tablet daily.	100	$35	35¢
Levothroid (levothyroxine)	0.125mg	Levothyroxine	Take 1 tablet daily.	100	$37	37¢
Levothroid (levothyroxine)	0.137mg	Levothyroxine	Take 1 tablet daily.	100	$37	37¢

PRODUCT	STRENGTH PER DOSE	ACTIVE INGREDIENT	USUAL DOSAGE	TYPICAL QUANTITY	TYPICAL PRICE	PRICE PER DAY
Levothroid (levothyroxine)	0.15mg	Levothyroxine	Take 1 tablet daily.	100	$40	40¢
Levothroid (levothyroxine)	0.175mg	Levothyroxine	Take 1 tablet daily.	100	$40	40¢
Levothroid (levothyroxine)	0.2mg	Levothyroxine	Take 1 tablet daily.	100	$40	40¢
Levothyroxine	0.025mg	Levothyroxine	Take 1 tablet daily.	100	$28	28¢
Levothyroxine	0.05mg	Levothyroxine	Take 1 tablet daily.	100	$25	25¢
Levothyroxine	0.075mg	Levothyroxine	Take 1 tablet daily.	100	$25	25¢
Levothyroxine	0.088mg	Levothyroxine	Take 1 tablet daily.	100	$25	25¢
Levothyroxine	0.1mg	Levothyroxine	Take 1 tablet daily.	100	$30	30¢
Levothyroxine	0.112mg	Levothyroxine	Take 1 tablet daily.	100	$30	30¢
Levothyroxine	0.125mg	Levothyroxine	Take 1 tablet daily.	100	$30	30¢
Levothyroxine	0.15mg	Levothyroxine	Take 1 tablet daily.	100	$33	33¢
Levothyroxine	0.175mg	Levothyroxine	Take 1 tablet daily.	100	$35	35¢
Levothyroxine	0.2mg	Levothyroxine	Take 1 tablet daily.	100	$35	35¢
Levothyroxine	0.3mg	Levothyroxine	Take 1 tablet daily.	100	$35	35¢
$ Levoxyl(levothyroxine)	0.025mg	Levothyroxine	Take 1 tablet daily.	100	$25	25¢
$ Levoxyl(levothyroxine)	0.05mg	Levothyroxine	Take 1 tablet daily.	100	$25	25¢
$ Levoxyl(levothyroxine)	0.075mg	Levothyroxine	Take 1 tablet daily.	100	$25	25¢
$ Levoxyl(levothyroxine)	0.088mg	Levothyroxine	Take 1 tablet daily.	100	$25	25¢
$ Levoxyl(levothyroxine)	0.1mg	Levothyroxine	Take 1 tablet daily.	100	$25	25¢
$ Levoxyl(levothyroxine)	0.112mg	Levothyroxine	Take 1 tablet daily.	100	$30	30¢
$ Levoxyl(levothyroxine)	0.125mg	Levothyroxine	Take 1 tablet daily.	100	$30	30¢
$ Levoxyl(levothyroxine)	0.137mg	Levothyroxine	Take 1 tablet daily.	100	$35	35¢
$ Levoxyl(levothyroxine)	0.15mg	Levothyroxine	Take 1 tablet daily.	100	$35	35¢
$ Levoxyl(levothyroxine)	0.175mg	Levothyroxine	Take 1 tablet daily.	100	$35	35¢
$ Levoxyl(levothyroxine)	0.2mg	Levothyroxine	Take 1 tablet daily.	100	$35	35¢
Synthroid (levothyroxine)	0.025mg	Levothyroxine	Take 1 tablet daily.	100	$34	34¢
Synthroid (levothyroxine)	0.05mg	Levothyroxine	Take 1 tablet daily.	100	$34	34¢
Synthroid (levothyroxine)	0.075mg	Levothyroxine	Take 1 tablet daily.	100	$35	35¢
Synthroid (levothyroxine)	0.088mg	Levothyroxine	Take 1 tablet daily.	100	$36	36¢

PRODUCT	STRENGTH PER DOSE	ACTIVE INGREDIENT	USUAL DOSAGE	TYPICAL QUANTITY	TYPICAL PRICE	PRICE PER DAY
Synthroid (levothyroxine)	0.1mg	Levothyroxine	Take 1 tablet daily.	100	$36	36¢
Synthroid (levothyroxine)	0.112mg	Levothyroxine	Take 1 tablet daily.	100	$40	40¢
Synthroid (levothyroxine)	0.125mg	Levothyroxine	Take 1 tablet daily.	100	$40	40¢
Synthroid (levothyroxine)	0.15mg	Levothyroxine	Take 1 tablet daily.	100	$42	42¢
Synthroid (levothyroxine)	0.175mg	Levothyroxine	Take 1 tablet daily.	100	$50	50¢
Synthroid (levothyroxine)	0.2mg	Levothyroxine	Take 1 tablet daily.	100	$55	55¢
Synthroid (levothyroxine)	0.3mg	Levothyroxine	Take 1 tablet daily.	100	$70	70¢
Thyroid USP	15mg	Desiccated thyroid	Take 1 tablet daily.	100	$15	15¢
Thyroid USP	30mg	Desiccated thyroid	Take 1 tablet daily.	100	$15	15¢
Thyroid USP	60mg	Desiccated thyroid	Take 1 tablet daily.	100	$15	15¢
Thyroid USP	90mg	Desiccated thyroid	Take 1 tablet daily.	100	$15	15¢
Thyroid USP	120mg	Desiccated thyroid	Take 1 tablet daily.	100	$15	15¢
Thyroid USP	180mg	Desiccated thyroid	Take 1 tablet daily.	100	$20	20¢

 SMART BUY

Drugs to Treat Hypothyroidism

If you're just starting thyroid supplements, Levoxyl is your Smart Buy. This high-quality product is priced at about two-thirds the cost of the more expensive Synthroid ($10 compared to just over $15 for Synthroid). To increase your savings, buy in bulk. Thirty tablets of Levoxyl 0.1mg typically cost about $10, or 33 cents a dose, but buying a hundred at a time lowers this to around $25, or 25 cents a dose, for a savings of about 24 percent. Because this drug has a narrow therapeutic index (NTI), don't cut tablets. If you're already taking thyroid supplements, talk with your doctor or pharmacist about whether it makes sense to change to a different product on the basis of cost. Remember, if you choose to change, you'll need follow-up blood tests to make sure your dose is correct.

DRUGS TO TREAT GOUT

Gout can develop when uric acid builds up in the bloodstream. When uric acid levels get too high, crystals form that can accumulate near the nerves in the joints of toes and fingers and elsewhere, causing a tremendous amount of pain. Doctors generally treat this problem two ways. The first uses an anti-inflammatory drug called indomethacin to relieve the pain and inflammation. (See Chapter 13, "Prescription Drugs to Treat Pain and Inflammation," for full information about this drug.) The second approach involves taking a drug that limits uric acid production. Doctors commonly prescribe colchicine, probenecid, or allopurinol for this. (A third group of drugs sometimes is prescribed, but too rarely to warrant discussion here.)

Probenecid works in the kidneys to increase the urinary excretion of uric acid. Because of this, probenecid usually is reserved for patients whose kidneys don't excrete uric acid like they should (less than 800mg/day). Common side effects include nausea, anorexia, headaches, and urinary frequency. Take this drug with plenty of water (six to eight glasses per day) to avoid developing kidney stones. Finally, don't take aspirin while you're on probenecid. Aspirin can antagonize (decrease or block) the effects of this drug.

> ### Diet and Gout
>
> Gout usually occurs in people who have a diet rich in purines. One of the first things we tell people is to cut down on the amount of red meat, wine, and beer they consume. Ask your pharmacist for a complete list of foods to avoid.

Allopurinol works by blocking xanthine oxidase, an enzyme responsible for converting xanthine to uric acid. It's appropriate for treating excessive uric acid synthesis, not for inefficient urinary excretion of uric acid. Taking allopurinol usually results in a decline in uric acid blood levels within two or three days, but full benefits may take up to six weeks. Common side effects include headaches, skin rashes, nausea, and drowsiness. Allopurinol is better tolerated when taken with food. To avoid kidney stones, drink 10 to 12 glasses of fluids every day when taking allopurinol.

While the exact mechanism of colchicine is unknown, we do know that it rapidly reduces inflammation and relieves pain in gout sufferers. Although it doesn't affect the amount of uric acid in the body, it does play an important role in gout therapy—so much so that one drug, Co-Benemid, combines probenecid and colchicine. Colchicine's tendency to cause diarrhea is so predictable and severe that pharmacists usually tell people to stop taking it, regardless of whether their pain is relieved, at the very first sign of diarrhea. Inform your doctor if you develop a skin rash, sore throat, fever, weakness, or unusual bleeding or tingling.

Drugs to Treat Gout

PRODUCT	STRENGTH PER DOSE	TYPE	ACTIVE INGREDIENT	USUAL DOSAGE	TYPICAL QUANTITY	TYPICAL PRICE	PRICE PER DOSE
Allopurinol	100mg	Tablet	Allopurinol	Take 1 tablet daily.	30	$15	50¢
Allopurinol	300mg	Tablet	Allopurinol	Take 1 tablet daily.	30	$15	50¢
Colchicine	0.6mg	Tablet	Colchicine	Take 1 tablet daily.	100	$20	20¢
Probenecid	500mg	Tablet	Probenecid	Take 1 tablet twice a day.	60	$45	$1.50
Zyloprim (allopurinol)	100mg	Tablet	Allopurinol	Take 1 tablet daily.	30	$20	67¢
Zyloprim (allopurinol)	300mg	Tablet	Allopurinol	Take 1 tablet daily.	30	$35	$1.17

$ SMART BUY
Drugs to Treat Gout

The Smart Buy here is allopurinol. It has fewer side effects, and you can use aspirin or an NSAID to relieve your pain (see Chapter 13). You'll save the most money if you use the generic form and buy it in bulk, for a cost per dose of about 13 cents—a savings of 74 percent.

$ SMART OPTIONS FOR SAVINGS
Hormones

Hormones vary more from product to product than many other drugs. Even when they aren't NTIs, different brands can affect you in different ways. If you're already taking a hormone product, don't change brands just to save money. If you and your doctor choose to pursue hormone therapy, our Smart Buy recommendations will help you decide where to start. We recommend against buying most hormone products from alternative sources. Check our Web site at www.smartbuysdrugwise.com for the latest information and more ways to save money on these drugs.

Chapter 10

Prescription Drugs to Treat Genitourinary Conditions

Your urinary system removes waste products from your body and maintains its fluid and acid levels for healthy cell function. Every day, as much as 45 gallons of blood passes through your kidneys, which filter out and send potential toxins and excess fluid to be excreted in your urine.

Doctors prescribe drugs to alter the urine's chemical composition in treating a variety of health problems.

DRUGS THAT ALTER THE ACIDITY OF URINE

URINARY ALKALINIZERS

Urinary alkalinizers decrease the urine's acidity (increase its alkalinity). These drugs are used mostly to minimize uric acid crystallization in gout and to balance urine acidity in people who have kidney disorders. When uric acid levels in the bloodstream get too high—either from overproduction due to a diet high in purines or from reduced urinary secretion—crystals form that can accumulate near the nerves in the joints of toes and fingers and elsewhere to cause a tremendous amount of pain. Decreasing the acidity of the urine by taking one of these drugs helps to dissolve these crystals, reducing the pain and allowing more uric acid to be removed from the body. Drugs commonly used for this purpose include sodium bicarbonate, potassium citrate, and, less commonly, sodium citrate. Take these products with food to prevent stomach upset. Most people who have edema or congestive heart failure should take these drugs only under close medical supervision. If you have either of these health conditions, check with your doctor before you take a urinary alkalinizer.

URINARY ACIDIFIERS

Urinary acidifiers make the urine more acidic. Because higher urinary acidity makes it more difficult for bacteria to adhere to the walls of the bladder, these drugs are used to increase the antibacterial activity of methenamine, a drug used to fight urinary tract infections, and to reduce the odor and rash caused by excessive ammonia in the urine (often the result of a kidney abnormality). Drugs that increase acidity in urine include ammonium chloride, vitamin C, potassium acid phosphate, and sodium acid phosphate. Take these drugs with food to limit their potentially unpleasant side effects, which include abdominal pain, nausea, and vomiting. Because increased urinary acidity can lead to crystals forming in the urine, kidney stones are a potential risk of taking these drugs. Antacids containing aluminum, calcium, or magnesium interfere with the absorption of urinary acidifiers, so don't use these products if you're taking a drug to acidify your urine.

Ammonium Chloride Alters Ammonia

Although it might seem odd to use ammonium chloride to counter the problems of too much ammonia in the urine, from a chemical perspective it makes perfect sense. Ammonium chloride (one part nitrogen, four parts hydrogen, one part chlorine), when mixed with ammonia (one part nitrogen and three parts hydrogen), alters ammonia's chemical structure enough to change its physical properties, including the odor.

$ SMART BUY
Drugs that Alter the Acidity of Urine

For drugs that decrease the acidity of the urine, the Smart Buy is sodium bicarbonate. While this may not be quite as effective as some of the other products, this over-the-counter product could be a cheap and easy remedy. For the greatest savings, buy in bulk. Your cost per dose could be as low as 18 cents.

For drugs that increase the acidity of the urine, the Smart Buy is vitamin C. Although it might not be quite as effective as some of the other products, this over-the-counter product could be a cheap and easy remedy for the problem.

Drugs that Alter the Acidity of Urine

PRODUCT	STRENGTH PER DOSE	TYPE	ACTIVE INGREDIENT	USUAL DOSAGE	TYPICAL QUANTITY	TYPICAL PRICE	PRICE PER DOSE
K-Phos (potassium acid phosphate)	500mg	Acidifier	Potassium acid phosphate	Take 2 tablets 4 times a day.	100	$20	40¢
$ Sodium bicarbonate	325mg	Alkalinizer	Sodium bicarbonate	Take 6 tablets 1-4 times a day.	500	$25	30¢
$ Sodium bicarbonate	650mg	Alkalinizer	Sodium bicarbonate	Take 3 tablets 1-4 times a day.	500	$30	18¢
Urocit-K (potassium citrate)	540mg	Alkalinizer	Potassium citrate	Take 1-2 tablets 3 times a day.	100	$35	70¢
Urocit-K (potassium citrate)	1080mg	Alkalinizer	Potassium citrate	Take 1 tablet 3 times a day.	100	$40	40¢
$ Vitamin C	500mg	Acidifier	Vitamin C	Take 2 tablets 3 times a day.	100	$7	14¢

DRUGS THAT RELAX THE URINARY TRACT

Drugs known as *urinary antispasmodics* help relax the muscles of the bladder, easing the sensations of pressure in people who feel frequent urinary urgency. Some of the more commonly prescribed drugs in this group are Detrol (generic name tolterodine), Ditropan (generic name oxybutynin), and Urispas (generic name flavoxate).

Urispas was the first product in this group to come on the market. Although it does a good job in most cases, it does have some undesirable side effects, including nausea, dry mouth, drowsiness, blurred vision, and headaches. Urispas also can increase ocular pressure (the pressure of the fluid in your eyes), so don't take this drug if you have glaucoma.

The more recently developed drugs Ditropan and Detrol have far fewer problems with side effects, although some people do experience drowsiness, blurred vision, and constipation. Again, avoid these drugs if you have glaucoma. Although it's more expensive than Ditropan (because no generic version is available), the newer Detrol has the fewest side effects, which makes this drug more desirable. For greater convenience, ask your doctor about Detrol LA. You need to take this long-acting version only once a day.

Urgency Might Signal Infection

A frequent, intense urge to urinate can signal a bladder or urinary tract infection, especially when it produces only a few dribbles of urine with significant burning. Such an infection requires treatment with an antibiotic, so you must visit your doctor. It's important to begin treatment quickly to keep the infection from spreading into the kidneys. While bladder and lower urinary tract infections are common, particularly in women, kidney infections are more unusual and generally are a more serious problem.

Drugs to Relax the Urinary Tract

PRODUCT	STRENGTH PER DOSE	TYPE	ACTIVE INGREDIENT	USUAL DOSAGE	TYPICAL QUANTITY	TYPICAL PRICE	PRICE PER DOSE
Detrol (tolterodine)	1mg	Tablet	Tolterodine	Take 1-2 tablets twice a day.	60	$100	$3.33
Detrol (tolterodine)	2mg	Tablet	Tolterodine	Take 1 tablet twice a day.	60	$100	$1.67
Detrol LA (tolterodine)	2mg	Capsule	Tolterodine	Take 1 capsule daily.	30	$85	$2.83
Detrol LA (tolterodine)	4mg	Capsule	Tolterodine	Take 1 capsule daily.	30	$90	$3
Ditropan (oxybutynin)	5mg	Tablet	Oxybutynin	Take 1 tablet 3 times a day.	90	$90	$1
Ditropan XL (oxybutynin)	5mg	Tablet	Oxybutynin	Take 1 tablet daily.	30	$85	$2.83
Ditropan XL (oxybutynin)	10mg	Tablet	Oxybutynin	Take 1 tablet daily.	30	$95	$3.17
Ditropan XL (oxybutynin)	15mg	Tablet	Oxybutynin	Take 1 tablet daily.	30	$100	$3.33
Oxybutynin	5mg	Tablet	Oxybutynin	Take 1 tablet 3 times a day.	90	$30	33¢
Urispas (flavoxate)	100mg	Tablet	Flavoxate	Take 1-2 tablets 3-4 times a day.	100	$145	$2.90

$ SMART BUY
Drugs that Relax the Urinary Tract

For drugs that relax the urinary tract, our Smart Buy is Detrol. Although it's a bit more expensive than Ditropan, its fewer side effects make this product the better choice. For the best savings, stick with the regular, rather than the long-acting, tablets so you can buy a higher strength in bulk and cut the tablets. This can cut your per-dose cost in half.

DRUGS THAT STIMULATE THE URINARY TRACT

When the bladder muscle that must contract to initiate urination doesn't work properly, urination becomes difficult. The drug Urecholine (generic name bethanechol) acts to stimulate this muscle so you can urinate. Take this drug on an empty stomach to limit the potential side effects of nausea and vomiting. Other possible side effects include diarrhea, excess salivation, headaches, and tightening of the airway sufficient to trigger an asthma attack. Some people also experience lightheadedness or fainting, particularly when arising from a lying position. Getting up slowly can help relieve this problem.

Urecholine is your only choice here. In the past there has been a generic available, but unfortunately it isn't available at the time of this writing, so we can't really offer a Smart Buy. Ask your pharmacist if there is a generic version that has returned to the market. Then, shop around for the best price and buy in bulk. Consider buying tablets double the strength your doctor prescribes and cutting them in half. The savings will be small, but every little bit helps.

DRUGS TO TREAT INFECTIONS OF THE URINARY TRACT

Bladder infections, known medically as *cystitis*, are more common in women than in men. (When they do occur in men, they often signal the presence of a more serious problem.). Doctors detect a urinary tract infection by examining a urine sample, which will contain bacteria (and probably white cells) if an infection is present. Antibiotics are the standard course of treatment. (Refer to Chapter 7, "Prescription Drugs to Treat Infections.") Drugs that provide an anesthetic effect to relieve the discomfort of a bladder infection are available over the counter.

$ SMART BUY
Drugs to Treat Infections of the Urinary Tract

If you have a bladder or urinary tract infection and you've never had a problem with this

Drugs to Treat Infections of the Urinary Tract

PRODUCT	STRENGTH PER DOSE	TYPE	ACTIVE INGREDIENT	USUAL DOSAGE	TYPICAL QUANTITY	TYPICAL PRICE	PRICE PER DOSE
Bladder infections							
Cephalexin	500mg	Capsule	Cephalexin	Take 1 capsule 4 times a day.	40	$30	75¢
Cipro (ciprofloxacin)	500mg	Tablet	Ciprofloxacin	Take 1 tablet twice a day.	20	$102	$5.10
Floxin (ofloxacin)	400mg	Tablet	Ofloxacin	Take 1 tablet twice a day.	20	$119	$5.95
Levaquin(levofloxacin)	500mg	Tablet	Levofloxacin	Take 1 tablet daily.	10	$97	$9.70
SMZ/TMP DS	800/160mg	Tablet	Sulfamethox-azole with trimethoprim	Take 1 tablet twice a day.	20	$11	55¢
Kidney infections							
Augmentin (amoxicillin with clavulanic acid)	875mg	Tablet	Amoxicillin with clavulanic acid	Take 1 tablet twice a day.	28	$169	$6.04
Cipro (ciprofloxacin)	500mg	Tablet	Ciprofloxacin	Take 1 tablet twice a day.	14	$73	$5.21
SMZ/TMP DS	800/160mg	Tablet	Sulfamethox-azole with trimethoprim	Take 1 tablet twice a day.	28	$14	50¢
Tequin (gatifloxacin)	400mg	Tablet	Gatifloxacin	Take 1 tablet daily.	7	$62	$8.86
Prostate infections							
Cipro (ciprofloxacin)	500mg	Tablet	Ciprofloxacin	Take 1 tablet twice a day.	28	$142	$5.07
SMZ/TMP DS	800/160mg	Tablet	Sulfamethox-azole with trimethoprim	Take 1 tablet twice a day.	28	$14	50¢

before, your Smart Buy is the generic version of Septra DS or Bactrim DS to save money. At just 50 cents a dose, it's a far less expensive alternative to the "big gun" Cipro (generic name ciprofloxacin), which runs around $5 a pill. Of course, if you have a chronic problem with urinary tract infections, or if your doctor feels there's a good reason to prescribe Cipro, go with it. Just don't be shy about asking why Cipro is necessary.

DRUGS TO TREAT MALE ERECTILE DYSFUNCTION

For many years, all we had to treat male erectile dysfunction (sometimes called impotence) was a drug called yohimbine, an herb-based product that's been used for thousands of years. This drug works by increasing the flow of blood into the penis and decreasing the flow of blood out. It's available in prescription strength, as well as in over-the-counter herbal remedies. A few years ago, some breakthrough drugs began to come to market. Two products very good at causing erections became available. Muse (generic name alprostadil) and Caverject (generic name alprostadil) both created quite a stir. Despite their effectiveness, however, using these drugs met with considerable reluctance from many men: Muse is a tiny suppository inserted into the penis, and Caverject is a liquid injected into the base of the penis.

Then, in 1998, came the wonder drug Viagra (generic name sildenafil), manufactured in tablet form. When taken one-half to one hour before intercourse, this drug can aid men with existing erectile problems to obtain an erection. (It will *not* do anything to enhance or prolong erections in men who do not have erectile problems.) Viagra works by activating an enzyme that relaxes the smooth muscle of the corpus cavernosum, allowing inflow of penile blood. At about $8 a pill, Viagra is a very expensive prescription—and because this drug is still under patent, no generic version is available yet. Despite the steep price tag, Viagra became the fastest-selling drug in history within its first six months on the market, and it continues to lead pharmaceutical sales worldwide.

One effect of Viagra's action is that it allows a rise in nitric acid levels, which relaxes smooth muscle tissue. Nitroglycerin and other nitrate-containing heart drugs do the same. Because of this, taking Viagra if you're also taking one or more of these medications can cause dangerously low blood pressure; deaths have resulted. Likewise, Viagra's manufacturer recommends that men who experience cardiovascular symptoms (chest pain, nausea, dizziness) on initiating sexual activity stop the activity, and make an appointment to discuss the problem with their doctors. If this happens to you, don't continue to use Viagra without first checking with your doctor. Also, Tagamet (generic name cimetidine) and erythromycin antibiotics can increase the concentration of Viagra in your blood, so you might want to take a smaller dose of Viagra if you're taking either of those drugs.

$ SMART BUY
Drugs to Treat Male Erectile Dysfunction

Among the drugs to treat erectile dysfunction, your Smart Buy is Viagra (generic name sildenafil). The convenience of swallowing a pill instead of using a penile suppository or injection makes Viagra well worth its high price. For the greatest savings, buy in bulk, purchase a strength that's double what your doctor prescribes, and cut the tablets in half for each dose. This can cut your price per dose from over $8 to just over $4, a savings of 50 percent.

Drugs to Treat Male Erectile Dysfunction

PRODUCT	STRENGTH PER DOSE	FORM	ACTIVE INGREDIENT	USUAL DOSAGE	TYPICAL QUANTITY	TYPICAL PRICE	PRICE PER DOSE
Caverject (alprostadil)	5mcg	Injectable liquid	Alprostadil	Not to exceed 3 times a week.	6	$110	$18.33
Caverject (alprostadil)	10mcg	Injectable liquid	Alprostadil	Not to exceed 3 times a week.	6	$140	$23.33
Caverject (alprostadil)	20mcg	Injectable liquid	Alprostadil	Not to exceed 3 times a week.	6	$180	$30
Caverject (alprostadil)	40mcg	Injectable liquid	Alprostadil	Not to exceed 3 times a week.	6	$200	$33.33
Muse (alprostadil)	125mcg	Penile suppository	Alprostadil	Not to exceed 2 per day.	6	$125	$20.83
Muse (alprostadil)	250mcg	Penile suppository	Alprostadil	Not to exceed 2 per day.	6	$140	$23.33
Muse (alprostadil)	500mcg	Penile suppository	Alprostadil	Not to exceed 2 per day.	6	$150	$25
Muse (alprostadil)	1000mcg	Penile suppository	Alprostadil	Not to exceed 2 per day.	6	$160	$26.67
Viagra (sildenafil)	25mg	Oral tablet	Sildenafil	Not to exceed 1 per day.	6	$50	$8.33
Viagra (sildenafil)	50mg	Oral tablet	Sildenafil	Not to exceed 1 per day.	6	$50	$8.33
Viagra (sildenafil)	100mg	Oral tablet	Sildenafil	Not to exceed 1 per day.	6	$50	$8.33

Viagra Requires a Prescription ... Even Over the Internet

Have you seen Internet advertisements or received e-mail "spam" touting Viagra with no prescription, no medical exam, no questions asked? This is illegal in the U.S., because Viagra is a prescription-only drug. Legalities aside, however, consider whether you want to risk your health and your life by taking this drug without a doctor's evaluation and supervision. We urge you to avoid these offers!

DRUGS THAT INCREASE THE FLOW OF URINE THROUGH THE PROSTATE

Many men over the age of 50 have problems with an enlarged prostate gland, which inhibits the flow of urine from the bladder. A key symptom is dribbling after urination. Until recently, the medical approach was to wait until the prostate enlarged to the point of nearly cutting off the flow of urine altogether, and then surgically removing the prostate gland. This is a serious surgery with a high risk of impotence as a side effect. Fortunately, drugs are available now that can help shrink the prostate to improve urinary flow, delaying and often eliminating the need for surgery.

In 1997, a new drug that was targeted just for the problem of enlarged prostate became available. Flomax (generic name tamsulosin) is unique in that it relaxes the smooth muscles in the neck of the bladder and the prostate, but doesn't significantly affect other areas of the body, and thus reduces potential side effects. This is nice, especially when you take a look at some of the other drugs that have been used over the years to treat this condition. Both Hytrin (generic name terazosin) and Cardura (generic name doxazosin), two very potent drugs also used to reduce high blood pressure, while effective for improving urine flow, can cause intense headaches, dizziness, and low blood pressure. When compared to Flomax, these side effects can be enough of a drawback to offset any cost savings.

Drugs that Increase the Flow of Urine Through the Prostate

PRODUCT	STRENGTH PER DOSE	TYPE	ACTIVE INGREDIENT	USUAL DOSAGE	TYPICAL QUANTITY	TYPICAL PRICE	PRICE PER DOSE
Cardura (doxazosin)	1mg	Tablet	Doxazosin	Take 1 tablet daily.	30	$40	$1.33
Cardura (doxazosin)	2mg	Tablet	Doxazosin	Take 1 tablet daily.	30	$40	$1.33
Cardura (doxazosin)	4mg	Tablet	Doxazosin	Take 1 tablet daily.	30	$40	$1.33
Cardura (doxazosin)	8mg	Tablet	Doxazosin	Take 1 tablet daily.	30	$45	$1.50
Doxazosin	1mg	Tablet	Doxazosin	Take 1 tablet daily.	30	$20	67¢
Doxazosin	2mg	Tablet	Doxazosin	Take 1 tablet daily.	30	$20	67¢
Doxazosin	4mg	Tablet	Doxazosin	Take 1 tablet daily.	30	$25	83¢
Doxazosin	8mg	Tablet	Doxazosin	Take 1 tablet daily.	30	$25	83¢
Flomax (tamsulosin)	0.4mg	Capsule	Tamsulosin	Take 1 capsule daily.	30	$60	$2

PRODUCT	STRENGTH PER DOSE	TYPE	ACTIVE INGREDIENT	USUAL DOSAGE	TYPICAL QUANTITY	TYPICAL PRICE	PRICE PER DOSE
Hytrin (terazosin)	1mg	Capsule	Terazosin	Take 1 capsule daily.	30	$70	$2.33
Hytrin (terazosin)	2mg	Capsule	Terazosin	Take 1 capsule daily.	30	$70	$2.33
Hytrin (terazosin)	5mg	Capsule	Terazosin	Take 1 capsule daily.	30	$70	$2.33
Hytrin (terazosin)	10mg	Capsule	Terazosin	Take 1 capsule daily.	30	$70	$2.33
Terazosin	1mg	Capsule	Terazosin	Take 1 capsule daily.	30	$25	83
Terazosin	2mg	Capsule	Terazosin	Take 1 capsule daily.	30	$30	$1
Terazosin	5mg	Capsule	Terazosin	Take 1 capsule daily.	30	$35	$1.17
Terazosin	10mg	Capsule	Terazosin	Take 1 capsule daily.	30	$35	$1.17

SMART BUY
Drugs that Increase the Flow of Urine Through the Prostate

The Smart Buy here is not the least expensive drug, but rather the most expensive—Flomax. It has by far the fewest side effects, which means you're more likely to take it as prescribed—in the end, a savings of a different sort. Currently the only way to save money on Flomax is to buy it in bulk (no generic version is available), and even then the savings are minimal.

SMART OPTIONS FOR SAVINGS
Drugs to Treat Genitourinary Conditions

Whenever possible, buy generic versions and buy in quantity. This gives you the lowest cost per dose. For drugs that are new in the market, of course, your only option is to shop for the best prices. Internet pharmacies sometimes offer better prices than retail stores. Be sure a pharmacist is available for you to talk to about any concerns or questions you may have. If you live near the Canadian border, you're likely to find tremendous savings within easy travel distance. You'll first need a prescription, and quite possibly an examination, from a Canadian physician, and restrictions exist on the quantities of drugs you can bring back or have sent to you in the U.S. (See Chapter 4, "Savings on Drugs Across the Border.") Check our Web site at www.smartbuysdrugwise.com for the latest information about more ways to save money on these drugs.

Chapter 11

Prescription Drugs to Treat Allergies, Asthma, and Coughs

Allergies, asthma, or coughs plague most of us at one time or another. Allergies can cause a wide range of symptoms, from nasal congestion and irritated eyes to asthma-like breathing difficulties. Coughing can accompany either allergies or asthma, or indicate the presence of an unrelated condition. As widespread as such problems are, an equally wide range of prescription products exists to combat them—so many, in fact, that bargains aren't hard to find. And many of these drugs are available in generic versions that provide the greatest cost savings.

DRUGS TO TREAT ASTHMA

Asthma can be a serious and frightening disorder. During an asthma attack, the passages to the lungs spasm and tighten, creating the sensation that one is unable to breathe. In a severe attack the airways actually can close or collapse, a life-threatening situation that requires emergency medical attention.

Doctors prescribe three general kinds of medications to treat asthma:

1. Beta agonists, used to relax the muscles of the airways and help prevent asthma attacks
2. Steroids, which reduce inflammation and swelling
3. Mast cell stabilizers, which reduce the body's allergic response when allergies trigger asthma

A few drugs fit no general category, but instead, have a specific and targeted effect on certain tissues or functions. Drugs to treat asthma come in these three forms:

1. Metered-dose inhalers (MDIs) contain medications that "mist" into airways to ease spasms

2. Oral medication (tablets, capsules, liquids)

3. Inhalant solutions for use with nebulizers ("breathing machines" that fill the air with a very fine mist)

Many people with asthma use more than one drug or dosage form, depending on the severity of and triggers for their symptoms. A metered-dose inhaler (MDI) is a small pressurized canister that fits into a mouthpiece. It delivers a pre-measured amount of medication in a fine mist that helps the drug penetrate blocked airways. A person having an asthma attack might use an MDI to deliver a steroid or beta agonist to head off the attack, and also take the same drugs in pill or liquid form to continue treating inflammation or to help prevent future attacks. Some drugs are now available in long-acting formulas that provide relief for up to 12 hours per dose. Oral forms of the drugs that treat asthma have the highest risk of side effects and complications because they affect the entire body. Drugs delivered by MDIs and nebulizers, which travel directly to the airways and lungs, are far less likely to affect other body systems.

Using a Metered-Dose Inhaler

To use an MDI properly, follow these steps:

1. Shake the canister for five to 10 seconds.

2. Exhale to the end of a normal breath.

3. Place the upright MDI into your mouth and close your lips tightly around it.

4. As you press down on the canister, inhale slowly and deeply.

5. Hold your breath for about 10 seconds, and then exhale slowly.

6. Wait at least one minute between puffs.

Many of the asthma drugs that come in metered-dose inhalers also are available in inhalant solution forms for use in nebulizers. Because a nebulizer must contain a precise amount of liquid before it can deliver sufficient medication in aerosol form, many products that contain these drugs come mixed with saline (salt water or sodium chloride). This concentration of saline is easy on the lungs and allows the nebulizers to deliver the active drug effectively. Some products include only the drug, and you must add saline to the mix yourself. This extra step can be tedious, but doing it this way sometimes can save you money. Ask your pharmacist which form will be the least expensive for you.

BETA AGONISTS TO TREAT ASTHMA

The most common drugs that treat asthma are the beta agonists (also known as "sympathomimetics"). These drugs trigger sites in the bronchial tubes and lungs called beta-receptors. This causes tissues to relax, or dilate, which allows more air to enter the lungs. Beta-agonist products include:

1. Alupent (generic name metaproterenol)
2. Maxair (generic name pirbuterol)
3. Proventil (generic name albuterol)
4. Serevent (generic name salmeterol)
5. Ventolin (generic name albuterol)

Most of these are short-acting (lasting about four hours), and so are used only for breathing crises or just prior to exercise. Serevent, however, is a long-acting beta-agonist that can last for up to 12 hours; it's often used to prevent asthma attacks, rather than to thwart them once they start.

> ### ▶ New Propellants to Safeguard the Environment
>
> Newer types of MDIs have hit the market in recent years. Some of these employ propellants intended to be easier on the environment. (Replacing propellant chlorofluorocarbons with these alternatives is thought to help preserve the ozone layer.) If this is a concern for you, ask your doctor about Proventil HFA. You'll pay a higher price for this product, however. It usually retails for about $10 more than a generic version of plain Proventil. ◀

Of these drugs, those containing metaproterenol (such as Alupent) are the most potent, but they can take up to 30 minutes to work. Compared to the quick five minutes it takes to get relief with albuterol (found in products such as Ventolin and Proventil), 30 minutes can feel like a very long time to wait for an improvement in breathing. Like albuterol, pirbuterol (the active ingredient in Maxair) produces results in five minutes, but it's considerably more expensive. An MDI containing a generic version of albuterol typically costs about $20; you could expect to pay around $67 for a Maxair MDI.

Some beta agonists—albuterol and terbutaline for example—also are available in oral tablet and liquid forms. Used mostly to prevent attacks of wheezing and cough due to acute asthma attacks in children, these drugs often produce the same side effects experienced with the inhaled versions.

Alternative Use for Terbutaline

Terbutaline is more often used to control the contractions of premature delivery than to treat asthma. Scientists are unsure why this works, but a significant relaxation of uterine muscles occurs after a pregnant woman takes this drug.

Because they can trigger beta-receptors in the heart and blood vessels, beta agonists are poor choices for those with high blood pressure, arrhythmias, or other heart conditions. These drugs can cause shaking, nervousness, and tension even in users without such conditions (especially troublesome in children who are hyperactive or who have attention deficit disorder), and exceeding the recommended dosage can lead to serious side effects.

Beta Agonists Can Prevent Asthma Attacks

Asthma sufferers from schoolchildren to professional athletes find that using a short-acting beta agonist 15 minutes prior to exercise can prevent an exercise-induced asthma attack and dramatically improve performance.

Beta Agonists to Treat Asthma

PRODUCT	STRENGTH PER DOSE	FORM	ACTIVE INGREDIENT	USUAL DOSAGE	TYPICAL QUANTITY	TYPICAL PRICE	PRICE PER DOSE
$ Albuterol MDI	90mcg	MDI	Albuterol	Inhale 1 puff every 4-6 hrs.	1	$20	10¢
Albuterol nebulizer solution	0.083%	Inhalant solution	Albuterol	Use 1 vial in nebulizer every 4-6 hrs.	1 box of 25	$20	80¢
Alupent MDI (metaproterenol)	75mcg	MDI	Metaproterenol	Inhale 1 puff every 4-6 hrs.	1	$40	20¢
Maxair autohaler MDI (pirbuterol)	0.2mg	MDI	Pirbuterol	Inhale 1 puff every 4-6 hrs.	1	$70	18¢
Maxair MDI (pirbuterol)	0.2mg	MDI	Pirbuterol	Inhale 1 puff every 4-6 hrs.	1	$65	22¢
Proventil HFA MDI (albuterol)	90mcg	MDI	Albuterol	Inhale 1 puff every 4-6 hrs.	1	$30	15¢
Proventil MDI (albuterol)	90mcg	MDI	Albuterol	Inhale 1 puff every 4-6 hrs.	1	$35	18¢
Proventil nebulizer solution (albuterol)	0.083%	Inhalant solution	Albuterol	Use 1 vial in nebulizer every 4-6 hrs.	1 box of 25	$60	$2.40
$ Serevent MDI (salmeterol)	25mcg	MDI	Salmeterol	Inhale 1 puff every 12 hrs.	1	$79	66¢
Ventolin MDI (albuterol)	90mcg	MDI	Albuterol	Inhale 1 puff every 4-6 hrs.	1	$35	18¢
Ventolin nebulizer solution (albuterol)	0.083%	Inhalant solution	Albuterol	Use 1 vial in nebulizer every 4-6 hrs.	1 box of 25	$60	$2.40

$ SMART BUY

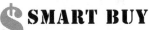

Beta Agonists to Treat Asthma

Buy the generic version of Proventil (albuterol) or Ventolin (albuterol). Albuterol gives you quick results and costs far less than any other beta agonist on the market, making it your Smart Buy. For longer-lasting action, we recommend Serevent (generic name salmeterol). It's expensive, but if you buy several inhalers at a time, you'll save money (one inhaler is about $79; three will cost around $215—a $22 savings.

STEROIDS TO TREAT ASTHMA

Other drugs commonly used for asthma work mostly to reduce the congestion that can accumulate in the airways. Lung congestion can irritate and narrow the air passages, triggering asthma attacks. Steroids are believed to decrease the number and activity of inflammatory cells in the airways, inhibit bronchoconstrictor (airway constriction) mechanisms, and relax the airway muscles.

Inhaled forms of steroids often are prescribed, including:

1. AeroBid (generic name flunisolide)
2. Azmacort (generic name triamcinolone)
3. Beclovent (generic name beclomethasone)
4. Flovent (generic name fluticasone)
5. Pulmicort (generic name budesonide)
6. Vanceril (generic name beclomethasone)

Of this group, Pulmicort and Flovent tend to require fewer inhalations to get the same results. These two products may cost more at the pharmacy, but overall, you'll save money and get better results because you don't need to use as much of the drug.

Pulmicort comes in a dry powder instead of an aerosol. Like some of the MDIs that use environmentally "friendly" propellants, this product doesn't affect the ozone layer. If you're accustomed to using a standard MDI, you'll find that Pulmicort feels very different the first time you use it. Because no "shot" of spray is involved, many people think at first that this product isn't delivering any drug; but it is. The powder is so fine, full doses are delivered with little sensation in the mouth.

Always rinse your mouth with a full glass of water after using any of these drugs to keep from developing a fungal infection that will coat your tongue with sores. Avoid exposure to contagious diseases, such as chickenpox or measles (especially relevant for children), because these drugs can hamper the immune system, making you less resistant to infection. And remember, inhaled steroids are designed to prevent asthma attacks, not to halt an attack in progress. If you have asthma, always carry an inhaler that has a beta agonist as the active ingredient.

An old remedy for asthma is oral prednisone, or a similar steroid. Like their inhaled counterparts, oral steroids can reduce lung inflammation dramatically to stop many asthma attacks. But oral steroids have more than a few side effects—so many, in fact, that doctors typically prescribe them only to stop an active asthma attack. Probably the most common complaint is that steroids are very hard on the stomach. They significantly reduce the mucus layer that protects the stomach lining, and this allows stomach acid to eat away at it. Over time this can result in stomach ulcers. To help limit this problem, always take oral steroids with food.

Other side effects that can occur over time include:

+ fluid retention
+ muscle weakness
+ osteoporosis
+ bone fractures
+ irregular heartbeats
+ thinning of the skin

+ convulsions
+ dizziness
+ headaches
+ menstrual irregularities
+ growth suppression in children

+ deposits of fat in the face and back
+ increased insulin requirements in diabetics

+ cataracts
+ glaucoma
+ insomnia

Steroids to Treat Asthma

PRODUCT	STRENGTH PER DOSE	FORM	ACTIVE INGREDIENT	USUAL DOSAGE	TYPICAL QUANTITY	TYPICAL PRICE	PRICE PER DOSE
AeroBid (flunisolide)	250mcg	MDI	Flunisolide	Inhale 2 puffs twice a day.	1	$80	$1.60
Azmacort (triamcinolone)	100mcg	MDI	Triamcinolone	Inhale 2 puffs 3 or 4 times a day.	1	$70	58¢
Beclovent (beclomethasone)	42mcg	MDI	Beclomethasone	Inhale 2 puffs 3 or 4 times a day.	1	$50	50¢
Flovent (fluticasone)	44mcg	MDI	Fluticasone	Inhale 1 puff 2 times a day.	1	$55	46¢
Flovent (fluticasone)	110mcg	MDI	Fluticasone	Inhale 1 puff 2 times a day.	1	$75	63¢
Flovent (fluticasone)	220mcg	MDI	Fluticasone	Inhale 1 puff 2 times a day.	1	$104	87¢
Pulmicort (budesonide)	200mcg	MDI	Budesonide	Inhale 1 puff 2 times a day.	1	$130	65¢
Vanceril (beclomethasone)	42mcg	MDI	Beclomethasone	Inhale 2 puffs 3 or 4 times a day.	1	$50	50¢

$ SMART BUY
Steroids to Treat Asthma

We recommend you try Flovent (generic name fluticasone) for your Smart Buy. It usually works better than most of the other inhaled steroids, it's cheaper than Pulmicort (generic name budesonide), and it comes in multiple strengths for dosage flexibility. To save money, buy in bulk: One MDI (220mcg) sells for around $104; buy three, and you'll pay around $300—a $12 savings!

MAST CELL STABILIZERS TO TREAT ASTHMA

Cromolyn can prevent the kinds of asthma attacks triggered by airborne allergens (substances the body is allergic to). It acts on specialized cells called mast cells. The most commonly prescribed inhaled product containing cromolyn is Intal. Cromolyn also comes in the form of nasal sprays and ophthalmic drops for those who develop allergic rhinitis (runny nose) or itchy eyes from pollen or other airborne allergens.

Cromolyn is effective only against allergen-triggered asthma, however—and only as a preventive measure, not a cure. It's important to use cromolyn regularly before you come in contact with allergens you know can trigger your attacks. For instance, if you know that in early spring certain blossoming trees will set off your allergies, start using Intal at least two weeks (and ideally four) before those trees begin to bloom, and continue until they're finished blooming. You'll need to take the cromolyn for the duration of the bloom, or allergy, season.

Intal is the only cromolyn option at this time. But if you buy just one inhaler at a time, you'll pay around $60 for the 8.1g size. Buying three of this size will cost around $160, for a savings of $20. Because one inhaler usually lasts about a month, this means an annual savings of around $80, or 13 percent.

OTHER KINDS OF DRUGS TO TREAT ASTHMA

Other inhaled drugs used to treat asthma act differently from steroids and beta agonists. Ipratropium, found in the brand Atrovent, blocks muscarinic receptors on the muscles of the air passages. When triggered, these receptors contribute to constriction of the lungs and increased secretions that can clog these passages. Blocking the receptors, then, relaxes the muscles and results in less fluid. Common side effects you might experience when using ipratropium include cough, dry throat, and nervousness. Avoid using ipratropium if you're allergic to soybeans or peanut butter. Researchers aren't sure why, but many people allergic to these foods also develop an allergy to ipratropium.

For years, the only asthma drugs available in oral form were xanthine derivatives. Scientists aren't sure why, but these drugs cause the muscles of the airways to relax and allow more air to enter. Drugs in this group include Theo-Dur (generic name theophylline), Slo-bid (generic name theophylline), and Theo-24 (generic name theophylline). These are taken daily to prevent asthma attacks. They won't work to stop an active attack. Your dose must maintain a stable blood level of the drug to achieve good results.

Xanthine derivatives are considered to have narrow therapeutic indexes (NTIs). Excessive blood levels can cause shaking, seizures, and even death. If you're taking a xanthine drug, notify your doctor immediately if you develop insomnia, jitters, convulsions, nausea, or irregular or rapid heartbeats. And because these drugs are so sensitive to changes in blood levels, don't change brands or products once you've reached a stable level.

If you're taking a xanthine derivative, check with your pharmacist before you take any over-the-counter medications. Many common drugs interact badly with such medications. Taking Tagamet (or any product containing cimetidine) for indigestion, for example, could land you in the hospital. Cimetidine slows a liver enzyme responsible for chemically altering theophylline so it can be removed from the body; this can result in elevated blood levels of this drug. Also avoid products that contain caffeine, from over-the-counter products to relieve menstrual discomfort to black tea, coffee, and cola drinks. Caffeine can amplify the side effects of xanthine drugs.

Leukotriene receptor antagonists are a new class of oral drugs for treating asthma. Leukotrienes are present naturally in the body, and increase in response to irritation or damage to create inflammation and edema. Leukotriene receptor antagonists work by blocking these effects to reduce swelling and relax the muscles in air passages. Drugs prescribed in this class include Accolate (zafirlukast) and Singulair (montelukast). These drugs are much safer than the xanthine derivatives, and have less severe potential side effects than the oral steroids, but they can cause problems, such as headaches and respiratory infections. As with the xanthine derivatives, you must take these drugs routinely to prevent asthma attacks. They aren't meant to stop an active attack. As is typically the case with new drugs, these are pricey. Singulair costs about $3 a day, Accolate around $2.30. No generics are available yet, and none are likely to become so in the near future.

Other Kinds of Drugs to Treat Asthma

PRODUCT	STRENGTH PER DOSE	FORM	ACTIVE INGREDIENT	USUAL DOSAGE	TYPICAL QUANTITY	TYPICAL PRICE	PRICE PER DOSE
Accolate (zafirlukast)	10mg	Tablet	Zafirlukast	Take 1 tablet 2 times a day.	60	$70	$1.17
Accolate (zafirlukast)	20mg	Tablet	Zafirlukast	Take 1 tablet 2 times a day.	60	$70	$1.17
Atrovent (ipratropium)	18mcg	MDI	Ipratropium	Inhale 2 puffs 4 times a day.	1	$45	45¢
Atrovent (ipratropium)	0.02%	Inhalant	Ipratropium	Use 1 vial in nebulizer solution 3-4 times a day.	1 box of 25	$75	$3
Ipratropium	0.02%	Inhalant	Ipratropium	Use 1 vial in nebulizer solution 3-4 times a day.	1 box of 25	$40	$1.60
Singulair (montelukast)	4mg	Tablet	Montelukast	Take 1 tablet daily.	30	$90	$3

PRODUCT	STRENGTH PER DOSE	FORM	ACTIVE INGREDIENT	USUAL DOSAGE	TYPICAL QUANTITY	TYPICAL PRICE	PRICE PER DOSE
Singulair (montelukast)	5mg	Tablet	Montelukast	Take 1 tablet daily.	30	$90	$3
Singulair (montelukast)	10mg	Tablet	Montelukast	Take 1 tablet daily.	30	$90	$3
Slo-Bid (theophylline)	100mg	Capsule	Theophylline	Take 1 capsule 2 times a day.	60	$20	33¢
Slo-Bid (theophylline)	125mg	Capsule	Theophylline	Take 1 capsule 2 times. a day.	60	$30	50¢
Slo-Bid (theophylline)	200mg	Capsule	Theophylline	Take 1 capsule 2 times a day.	60	$30	50¢
Slo-Bid (theophylline)	300mg	Capsule	Theophylline	Take 1 capsule 2 times a day.	60	$40	67¢
Theo-24 (theophylline)	100mg	Capsule	Theophylline	Take 1 capsule daily.	30	$15	50¢
Theo-24 (theophylline)	200mg	Capsule	Theophylline	Take 1 capsule daily.	30	$20	67¢
Theo-24 (theophylline)	300mg	Capsule	Theophylline	Take 1 capsule daily.	30	$25	83¢
Theo-24 (theophylline)	400mg	Capsule	Theophylline	Take 1 capsule daily.	30	$25	83¢
Theo-Dur (theophylline)	100mg	Tablet	Theophylline	Take 1 tablet 2 times a day.	60	$30	50¢
Theo-Dur (theophylline)	200mg	Tablet	Theophylline	Take 1 tablet 2 times a day.	60	$35	58¢
Theo-Dur (theophylline)	300mg	Tablet	Theophylline	Take 1 tablet 2 times a day.	60	$35	58¢
Theo-Dur (theophylline)	450mg	Tablet	Theophylline	Take 1 tablet 2 times a day.	60	$40	67¢
Theophylline	100mg	Tablet	Theophylline	Take 1 tablet 2 times a day.	60	$20	33¢
Theophylline	200mg	Tablet	Theophylline	Take 1 tablet 2 times a day.	60	$20	33¢
Theophylline	300mg	Tablet	Theophylline	Take 1 tablet 2 times a day.	60	$20	33¢
Theophylline	450mg	Tablet	Theophylline	Take 1 tablet 2 times a day.	60	$20	33¢
Theophylline	100mg	Capsule	Theophylline	Take 1 capsule 2 times a day.	60	$15	25¢
Theophylline	125mg	Capsule	Theophylline	Take 1 capsule 2 times a day.	60	$15	25¢
Theophylline	200mg	Capsule	Theophylline	Take 1 capsule 2 times a day.	60	$20	33¢
Theophylline	300mg	Capsule	Theophylline	Take 1 capsule 2 times a day.	60	$25	42¢

$ SMART BUY
Other Kinds of Drugs to Treat Asthma

We like Accolate for our Smart Buy. It's safer than the theophylline products, slightly less expensive than Singulair, and you can cut the tablets to save money. Consider buying in bulk to save even more! Where 30 tablets of Accolate 20mg sell for around $40, 90 typically will cost only $100, saving you 20 percent.

BETA AGONIST COMBINATION PRODUCTS TO TREAT ASTHMA

Doctors often prescribe inhalers that combine a beta agonist and a steroid or ipratropium. Common combination products include Advair (generic name salmeterol and fluticasone), DuoNeb (generic name ipratropium and albuterol), and Combivent (generic name ipratropium and albuterol). This is good for convenience and compliance, but we prefer using these drugs in separate inhalers. If you use the beta agonist first, wait about 15 minutes, and then use the steroid or ipratropium, the steroid or ipratropium will penetrate deeper into your lungs to provide greater relief. You can't control the timing of each drug like this with a combination product.

It's a little cheaper to buy the combination product, though. Combivent sells for around $55. Atrovent and albuterol MDIs (one of each equals one Combivent) sell for around $65. (Visit our Web site at www.smartdrugbuys.com for current information.) But you lose the flexibility of getting more of the Atrovent down into the lungs.

Beta Agonist Combination Products to Treat Asthma

PRODUCT	STRENGTH PER DOSE	FORM	ACTIVE INGREDIENT	USUAL DOSAGE	TYPICAL QUANTITY	TYPICAL PRICE	PRICE PER DOSE
Advair (salmeterol and fluticasone)	100mcg and 50mcg	Diskus	salmeterol and fluticasone	Use 1 unit twice daily.	60 units	$110	$1.83
Advair (salmeterol and fluticasone)	250mcg and 50mcg	Diskus	salmeterol and fluticasone	Use 1 unit twice daily.	60 units	$130	$2.17
Advair (salmeterol and fluticasone)	500mcg and 50mcg	Diskus	salmeterol and fluticasone	Use 1 unit twice daily.	60 units	$180	$3
Combivent (ipratropium and albuterol)	18mcg and 103mcg	MDI	ipratropium and albuterol	Inhale 2 puffs 4 times a day.	1	$55	55¢
DuoNeb (ipratropium and albuterol)	2.5mg and 0.5mg	Inhalant solution	ipratropium and albuterol	Use 1 vial in nebulizer 4 times a day.	30 vials	$70	$2.33

$ SMART BUY
Beta Agonist Combination Products to Treat Asthma

We recommend that you avoid combination products. This will cost you a bit more money, but you'll gain more flexibility and better results. Better results means you'll need fewer doses, and you'll get more for your money in the end. For your Smart Buy, see the tables for beta agonists and steroids.

ANTIHISTAMINES TO TREAT ALLERGIES

Antihistamines can prevent allergic responses throughout the body. Although they can prevent some forms of asthma, they're far more commonly used for hay fever and seasonal allergies. To benefit fully, you must have them in your bloodstream before you come in contact with allergens. Once histamine (your body's allergy response) has been released into the blood, the full benefit of taking an antihistamine probably won't kick in for several days or even a week. It can take that long for the effects of the already released histamine to wear off. If you know what you're allergic to and when it blooms or comes into season, plan to start taking your antihistamine one or two weeks before. You'll get much better results.

> ### ▶ Antihistamines Can Trigger Asthma
>
> Although antihistamines can be very effective for treating some forms of asthma, they can also cause problems. If antihistamines dry you out too much, they can actually trigger an asthma attack. ◀

The two main concerns people have when choosing an antihistamine are how much drowsiness can occur and how often they must take the drug. Most over-the-counter antihistamines, while effective, cause significant drowsiness. See Chapter 17, "Over-the-Counter Cold, Flu, Cough, and Allergy Preparations," for further information on these.

Three prescription-only antihistamines commonly prescribed for seasonal allergies cause little or no drowsiness. They are Claritin (generic name loratadine), Allegra (generic name fexofenadine), and Zyrtec (generic name cetirizine). Of these, we prefer Claritin and Allegra 180mg tablets. They need only be taken once a day and cause very limited drowsiness. Although Allegra 60mg in capsule form also causes few drowsiness problems, it must be taken twice a day. Zyrtec, too, is once-a-day, but it can cause more drowsiness than either Claritin or Allegra. Other side effects to watch for in all antihistamines include a worsening of glaucoma, urinary retention, and possibly birth defects. Talk with your doctor before taking any antihistamine.

Prescription antihistamines share one non-medical side effect—sticker shock. These drugs are so expensive that some insurance companies try to steer doctors toward Zyrtec, the lower cost one, first. A typical 30-day supply of Zyrtec will cost about $72, compared to $77 for a 30-day supply of Allegra and $80 for a 30-day supply of Claritin. If Zyrtec works for you and doesn't cause drowsiness, then save yourself some money and go with that.

But not everyone gets the same results with these drugs. Some people say Claritin works best, while others swear by Zyrtec or Allegra. We suggest you find what works best for you and pay whatever it costs. If your insurance company doesn't want to pay for the product you prefer, ask your doctor to write a letter explaining why you need the particular drug. We rarely see an insurance company deny a claim with such documentation (for these products, at least!). It might take time and effort to jump through all the hoops, but you should prevail. Claritin is due to become available in a generic version in the near future, so ask about it if your doctor prescribes this drug for you.

Antihistamines to Treat Allergies

PRODUCT	STRENGTH PER DOSE	ACTIVE INGREDIENT	USUAL DOSAGE	TYPICAL PRICE	TYPICAL QUANTITY	PRICE PER DOSE
Allegra (fexofenadine)	60mg	Fexofenadine	Take 1 capsule 2 times a day.	60	$77	$2.57
Allegra (fexofenadine)	180mg	Fexofenadine	Take 1 tablet daily.	30	$77	$2.57
Claritin (loratadine)	10mg	Loratadine	Take 1 tablet daily.	30	$80	$2.67
Zyrtec (cetirizine)	5mg	Cetirizine	Take 1 tablet daily.	30	$72	$2.40
Zyrtec (cetirizine)	10mg	Cetirizine	Take 1 tablet daily.	30	$72	$2.40

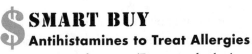

$ SMART BUY
Antihistamines to Treat Allergies

We recommend you try Zyrtec and take it at bedtime. This will save you a little money when compared to Allegra and Claritin. We consider it your Smart Buy. If you wake up drowsy, switch to Claritin (look for a new generic to arrive soon) or Allegra 180mg tablets. These cost a little more but don't cause drowsiness and need only be taken once a day.

COUGH PRODUCTS

A cough can be a real nuisance, whether it's due to allergies, viral or bacterial infection, or is simply a nagging tickle that won't go away. A variety of drugs are commonly prescribed to treat a cough, most frequently codeine—yes, the same codeine used to relieve pain. Cough preparations contain a smaller amount, usually in an oral liquid form, which calms the brain's "cough center." Many cough products combine codeine with either an antihistamine to dry up drainage that may be irritating the throat, an expectorant to loosen phlegm in the chest, or a decongestant to relieve sinus congestion.

While codeine is extremely effective, it can cause considerable drowsiness, and in some people, quite a bit of nausea. And because it's a narcotic, the potential exists for addiction and abuse. A very good nonnarcotic alternative is benzonatate; although it can cause some drowsiness, it's less pronounced than with codeine. This drug works directly on the stretch receptors in the throat and lungs. Numbing these areas limits their response to the irritations that normally generate a cough. Because it can numb the areas it comes in contact with, take care to swallow this drug whole and follow it with a full glass of water. Chewing these capsules may result in difficulty swallowing, which can lead to a dangerous situation. To save money on this drug, buy a generic version. Thirty "perles" (soft capsules) of Tessalon, a common brand of benzonatate, will make you cough up around $40, while the same amount of the generic usually runs around $20, a savings of 50 percent. Our Web site at www.smartbuysdrugwise.com, will provide you with updates on prescription and over-the-counter drugs.

Numerous over-the-counter products are available to treat coughs. See Chapter 17, "Over-the-Counter Cold, Flu, Cough, and Allergy Preparations," for further information on these.

$ SMART OPTIONS FOR SAVINGS
Prescription Drugs to Treat Allergies, Asthma, and Coughs

When it comes to these drugs, either it's been on the market for a very long time or it's brand-new! Older drugs, of course, are available in generic versions that offer significant savings. For new drugs still under patent, your best option is to shop for the best price.

1. Because many of these drugs are taken long-term, buying in bulk makes sense and can be an effective way to cut your costs.
2. If you live near Canada, you'll find the savings on many of these drugs are worth the drive across the border and the cost of an exam from a Canadian physician. This remains the most reliable way to take advantage of low drug prices in Canada.

Check Internet and mail-order pharmacies to compare prices, but remember to factor in shipping charges and the length of time it takes for the drugs to reach you. Be especially cautious about using Internet pharmacies located in Canada. Although the savings can be tremendous, there's also the risk that your order might not be allowed through if regulations change on either side of the border. Check our Web site at www.smartbuysdrugwise.com for the latest information on this and other cost-saving approaches.

Chapter 12

Prescription Drugs that Affect the Central
Nervous System

This group of drugs covers an enormous number of products. From sleeping pills to muscle relaxants, it includes more than 20 subcategories. Here we focus on drugs used for common chronic problems.

DRUGS TO TREAT ANXIETY AND INSOMNIA

Most of us have experienced anxiety at some point in our lives. But when anxiety becomes a constant presence, it interferes with virtually every aspect of living. Chronic anxiety can be debilitating, and many drugs are available to treat it. Products commonly prescribed to treat anxiety include these:

1. Ativan (generic name lorazepam)
2. Buspar (generic name buspirone)
3. Librium (generic name chlordiazepoxide)
4. Serax (generic name oxazepam)
5. Tranxene (generic name clorazepate)
6. Valium (generic name diazepam)
7. Xanax (generic name alprazolam)

The best-known drug by far for calming anxiety is Valium, which belongs to the class of drugs known as the benzodiazepines. It's no longer the most commonly prescribed antianxiety drug, however, because it can last so long in the body that more than half the drug may still be active when it's time to take the next dose! That can be a problem if you must get up and go to work in the morning, and is especially troublesome in the elderly, whose metabolisms are slower.

Some of these drugs take longer to work than others. If you're having an anxiety attack, a slow-working drug isn't what you want. Ativan and Xanax are most commonly used to treat anxiety. Both start to work fairly quickly and won't linger in your system. Valium and Tranxene take effect slightly faster, but their "half-lives" can be as long as 50 hours.

To save great amounts of money on these drugs, buy the generic versions. For example, 30 tablets of Valium 5mg typically cost $40, while 30 tablets of diazepam 5mg (the generic version) cost around $10, for a savings of 75 percent. Likewise, 30 tablets of Xanax 0.5mg cost $44, while its generic version, alprazolam, is just $15—a savings of 66 percent. To save even more, consider splitting higher strength tablets: Fifteen tablets of diazepam 10mg cost around $5 and 15 tablets of alprazolam 1mg around $7, giving a savings over time of 30 percent.

A drawback to the benzodiazepines is that they can be addictive. If you think you'll need medication for a long period, talk with your doctor about this potential problem. A nonaddictive drug such as Buspar might be a better choice. There are tradeoffs, of course. Although Buspar is nonaddictive, you may have to take it for as long as four weeks before you feel any effects. Valium, on the other hand, starts to work in about half an hour. Common side effects from buspirone (Buspar's active ingredient and generic form) include dizziness, drowsiness, nausea, and headaches. And Buspar hits your pocketbook a bit harder: Thirty 10mg tablets of its generic, buspirone, cost around $40— the same as name-brand Valium. At this writing, name-brand Buspar costs about $50 for the same quantity. (See our Web site, www.smartbuysdrugwise.com, for updates on prescription and over-the-counter drugs.)

Antianxiety drugs sometimes are prescribed to treat insomnia (sleeplessness), as well. Other drugs in the same chemical family (the benzodiazepines) are used almost exclusively to induce sleep. Drugs commonly prescribed to treat chronic insomnia are:

1. Ambien (generic name zolpidem)
2. Dalmane (generic name flurazepam)
3. Doral (generic name quazepam)
4. Halcion (generic name triazolam)
5. ProSom (generic name estazolam)
6. Restoril (generic name temazepam)
7. Sonata (generic name zaleplon)

Addiction is a risk here, as well. Ambien and Sonata are slightly less addictive than the benzodiazepines and their action is of relatively short duration (most people won't feel "hungover" in the morning)—although headache is a common complaint with them. And Ambien and Sonata provide more time in stages three and four of the sleep cycle than the benzodiazepines, so you'll feel more rested. You'll pay more for these, though. A 30-day supply of the generic versions of Restoril or Halcion will cost around $25, while for Ambien or Sonata, you can expect to pay as much as $80 for a month's supply.

Drugs to Treat Anxiety and Insomnia

PRODUCT	STRENGTH PER DOSE	ACTIVE INGREDIENT	USUAL DOSAGE	TYPICAL QUANTITY	TYPICAL PRICE	PRICE PER DAY
$ Alprazolam	0.25mg	Alprazolam	Take 1 tablet 3 times a day as needed.	90	$20	67¢
$ Alprazolam	0.5mg	Alprazolam	Take 1 tablet 3 times a day as needed.	90	$20	67¢
$ Alprazolam	1mg	Alprazolam	Take 1 tablet 3 times a day as needed.	90	$20	67¢
$ Alprazolam	2mg	Alprazolam	Take 1 tablet 3 times a day as needed.	90	$25	83¢
Ambien (zolpidem)	5mg	Zolpidem	Take 1 tablet at bedtime.	30	$65	$2.17
Ambien (zolpidem)	10mg	Zolpidem	Take 1 tablet at bedtime.	30	$80	$2.67
Ativan (lorazepam)	0.5mg	Lorazepam	Take 1 tablet 3 times a day as needed.	90	$85	$2.83
Ativan (lorazepam)	1mg	Lorazepam	Take 1 tablet 3 times a day as needed.	90	$110	$3.67
Ativan (lorazepam)	2mg	Lorazepam	Take 1 tablet 3 times a day as needed.	90	$155	$5.17
Buspar (buspirone)	5mg	Buspirone	Take 1 tablet 3 times daily.	90	$90	$3
Buspar (buspirone)	10mg	Buspirone	Take 1 tablet 3 times daily.	90	$145	$4.83
Buspar (buspirone)	15mg	Buspirone	Take 1 tablet 3 times daily.	90	$270	$9
$ Buspirone	5mg	Buspirone	Take 1 tablet 3 times daily.	90	$65	$2.17
$ Buspirone	10mg	Buspirone	Take 1 tablet 3 times daily.	90	$110	$3.67
$ Buspirone	15mg	Buspirone	Take 1 tablet 3 times daily.	90	$150	$5
Chlordiazepoxide	5mg	Chlordia- zepoxide	Take 1 capsule 3 times daily as needed.	90	$25	83¢
Chlordiazepoxide	10mg	Chlordia- zepoxide	Take 1 capsule 3 times daily as needed.	90	$25	83¢
Chlordiazepoxide	25mg	Chlordia- zepoxide	Take 1 capsule 3 times daily as needed.	90	$30	$1
Clorazepate	3.75mg	Clorazepate	Take 1 capsule 3 times daily as needed.	90	$70	$2.33
Clorazepate	7.5mg	Clorazepate	Take 1 capsule 3 times daily as needed.	90	$85	$2.83
Clorazepate	15mg	Clorazepate	Take 1 tablet 3 times a day as needed.	90	$110	$3.67
Dalmane (flurazepam)	15mg	Flurazepam	Take 1 capsule 3 times daily as needed.	30	$50	$1.67

PRODUCT	STRENGTH PER DOSE	ACTIVE INGREDIENT	USUAL DOSAGE	TYPICAL QUANTITY	TYPICAL PRICE	PRICE PER DAY
Dalmane (flurazepam)	30mg	Flurazepam	Take 1 capsule at bedtime.	30	$55	$1.83
Diazepam	2mg	Diazepam	Take 1 tablet 3 times a day as needed.	90	$20	67¢
Diazepam	5mg	Diazepam	Take 1 tablet 3 times a day as needed.	90	$20	67¢
Diazepam	10mg	Diazepam	Take 1 tablet 3 times a day as needed.	90	$20	67¢
Doral (quazepam)	7.5mg	Quazepam	Take 1 tablet at bedtime.	30	$90	$3
Doral (quazepam)	15mg	Quazepam	Take 1 tablet at bedtime.	30	$100	$3.33
Estazolam	1mg	Estazolam	Take 1 tablet at bedtime.	30	$25	83¢
Estazolam	2mg	Estazolam	Take 1 tablet at bedtime.	30	$25	83¢
Flurazepam	15mg	Flurazepam	Take 1 capsule at bedtime.	30	$15	50¢
Flurazepam	30mg	Flurazepam	Take 1 capsule at bedtime.	30	$15	50¢
Halcion (triazolam)	0.125mg	Triazolam	Take 1 tablet at bedtime.	30	$45	$1.50
Halcion (triazolam)	0.25mg	Triazolam	Take 1 tablet at bedtime.	30	$50	$1.67
Librium (chlordiazepoxide)	5mg	Chlordiazepoxide	Take 1 capsule 3 times daily as needed.	90	$75	$2.50
Librium (chlordiazepoxide)	10mg	Chlordiazepoxide	Take 1 capsule 3 times daily as needed.	90	$100	$3.33
Librium (chlordiazepoxide)	25mg	Chlordiazepoxide	Take 1 capsule 3 times daily as needed.	90	$145	$4.83
Lorazepam	0.5mg	Lorazepam	Take 1 tablet 3 times a day as needed.	90	$40	$1.33
Lorazepam	1mg	Lorazepam	Take 1 tablet 3 times a day as needed.	90	$50	$1.67
Lorazepam	2mg	Lorazepam	Take 1 tablet 3 times a day as needed.	90	$60	$2
Oxazepam	10mg	Oxazepam	Take 1 capsule 3 times daily as needed.	90	$35	$1.17
Oxazepam	15mg	Oxazepam	Take 1 capsule 3 times daily as needed.	90	$50	$1.67
Oxazepam	30mg	Oxazepam	Take 1 capsule 3 times daily as needed.	90	$50	$1.67
ProSom (estazolam)	1mg	Estazolam	Take 1 tablet at bedtime.	30	$45	$1.50
ProSom (estazolam)	2mg	Estazolam	Take 1 tablet at bedtime.	30	$50	$1.67
Restoril (temazepam)	15mg	Temazepam	Take 1 capsule at bedtime.	30	$50	$1.67
Restoril (temazepam)	30mg	Temazepam	Take 1 capsule at bedtime.	30	$55	$1.83
Serax (oxazepam)	10mg	Oxazepam	Take 1 capsule 3 times daily as needed.	90	$95	$3.17
Serax (oxazepam)	15mg	Oxazepam	Take 1 capsule 3 times daily as needed.	90	$115	$3.83
Serax (oxazepam)	30mg	Oxazepam	Take 1 capsule 3 times daily as needed.	90	$165	$5.50
Sonata (zaleplon)	5mg	Zaleplon	Take 1 capsule at bedtime.	30	$60	$2
Sonata (zaleplon)	10mg	Zaleplon	Take 1 capsule at bedtime.	30	$80	$2.67

PRODUCT	STRENGTH PER DOSE	ACTIVE INGREDIENT	USUAL DOSAGE	TYPICAL QUANTITY	TYPICAL PRICE	PRICE PER DAY
Temazepam	15mg	Temazepam	Take 1 capsule at bedtime.	30	$25	83¢
Temazepam	30mg	Temazepam	Take 1 capsule at bedtime.	30	$25	83¢
Tranxene (clorazepate)	3.75mg	Clorazepate	Take 1 tablet 3 times a day as needed.	90	$170	$5.67
Tranxene (clorazepate)	7.5mg	Clorazepate	Take 1 tablet 3 times a day as needed.	90	$210	$7
Tranxene (clorazepate)	15mg	Clorazepate	Take 1 tablet 3 times a day as needed.	90	$265	$8.83
Triazolam	0.125mg	Triazolam	Take 1 tablet at bedtime.	30	$25	83¢
Triazolam	0.25mg	Triazolam	Take 1 tablet at bedtime.	30	$25	83¢
Valium (diazepam)	2mg	Diazepam	Take 1 tablet 3 times a day as needed.	90	$70	$2.33
Valium (diazepam)	5mg	Diazepam	Take 1 tablet 3 times a day as needed.	90	$100	$3.33
Valium (diazepam)	10mg	Diazepam	Take 1 tablet 3 times a day as needed.	90	$160	$5.33
Xanax (alprazolam)	0.25mg	Alprazolam	Take 1 tablet 3 times a day as needed.	90	$95	$3.17
Xanax (alprazolam)	0.5mg	Alprazolam	Take 1 tablet 3 times a day as needed.	90	$110	$3.67
Xanax (alprazolam)	1mg	Alprazolam	Take 1 tablet 3 times a day as needed.	90	$150	$5
Xanax (alprazolam)	2mg	Alprazolam	Take 1 tablet 3 times a day as needed.	90	$235	$7.83

$ SMART BUY
Drugs to Treat Anxiety and Insomnia

For short-term anxiety, your Smart Buys are Ativan and Xanax. Buy generic versions of either for the best savings. For long-term problems, we prefer Buspar. It's not addictive and doesn't cause much drowsiness. To lower your costs by better than half, buy the generic version (buspirone) in the largest quantity possible, and consider buying a strength that's twice what your doctor prescribes and cutting the tablets in half.

For insomnia that occurs only occasionally, your Smart Buys are either Restoril or Halcion. These drugs will save you about $55 a month compared to Ambien or Sonata. Use the generic and buy in bulk. For Halcion (triazolam), see if you can cut the tablets. For long-term problems, the increased amount of time in stages three and four of the sleep cycle makes the more expensive drugs worthwhile.

DRUGS TO TREAT DEPRESSION

Depression is a potentially serious condition that affects millions of people at some point in their lives. The development of medications called antidepressants has made it possible to treat depression successfully and has made life far more enjoyable for those who suffer from it. Researchers have yet to develop the "perfect" antidepressant—one that can help everyone, with few side effects—but the quest to do so has resulted in numerous products. All the antidepressants currently in use can cause undesirable and unpleasant side effects, and can take up to six weeks to become effective. Often an individual must try two or three or more different drugs before finding one that works. And some people never get adequate results.

Three major classifications of drugs exist for treating depression:

1. Monoamine oxidase inhibitors (MAOIs)
2. Tricyclic and tetracyclic antidepressants
3. Serotonin reuptake inhibitors (SSRIs)

Four drugs we discuss fit none of these categories. (We call them "other.") Because many people must try more than one antidepressant before they find one that provides an appropriate balance between desired therapeutic effects and undesired side effects, we cover each drug group first, and then provide a summary table and our Smart Buy recommendations for antidepressant drugs overall.

MAO Inhibitors

Among the first drugs to become available for treating depression were monoamine oxidase inhibitors (MAOIs). These are very good at increasing the brain's levels of norepinephrine and serotonin (natural substances your body manufactures that help you "feel good"). Studies correlate low levels of these chemicals with depression.

Drugs commonly prescribed in this group include the following:

1. Nardil (generic name phenelzine)
2. Parnate (generic name tranylcypromine)
3. Marplan (generic name isocarboxazid)

The problem with MAO inhibitors is that they can cause severe increases in blood pressure—sometimes to the extent of causing strokes and heart attacks. If you're taking an MAO inhibitor, it's critical you avoid any drugs or substances that can elevate blood pressure, such as over-the-counter decongestants containing pseudoephedrine. And avoid foods and drinks that contain the ingredient tyramine, often present in fermented foods. These include:

1. Alcoholic beverages, including beer (especially imports), red wine, sherry, and liqueurs
2. Fermented dairy products, including American, blue, Boursault, Brie, Camem-

bert, cheddar, Emmenthaler, Gruyere, mozzarella, Parmesan, Romano, Stilton, Swiss, and Roquefort cheeses, sour cream, and yogurt

3. Certain fruits, vegetables, and bean products, including avocados, bananas, bean curd (tofu), figs (canned), prunes, raisins, raspberries, sauerkraut, soy sauce, and yeast extracts

4. Smoked, dried, pickled, or fermented meats and fish, including anchovies, bologna, caviar, pepperoni, salami, shrimp paste, summer sausage, and dry sausage

Ask your doctor or pharmacist for a complete list of food restrictions.

TRICYCLIC AND TETRACYCLIC ANTIDEPRESSANTS

The next group of antidepressants to hit the market were the tricyclic and tetracyclic antidepressants. This group contains a lot of drugs, but they all elevate norepinephrine and some serotonin levels in the brain.

Members of this group include:

1. Anafranil (generic name clomipramine)
2. Elavil (generic name amitriptyline)
3. Norpramin (generic name desipramine)
4. Pamelor (generic name nortriptyline)
5. Remeron (generic name mirtazapine)
6. Sinequan (generic name doxepin)
7. Surmontil (generic name trimipramine)
8. Tofranil (generic name imipramine)

These drugs are a big improvement over the MAOIs because they involve no food restrictions, and you're far less likely to develop high blood pressure when you take them. On the downside, though, they can cause significant drowsiness. Some people who take them also experience blurred vision, dry mouth, constipation, and irregular heartbeats; often they stop taking the drug because of these side effects.

To save money on these products, do three things:

1. Buy generic.
2. Buy in bulk.
3. Ask whether tablets can be cut.

For example, 30 tablets of Elavil 25mg sells for around $25 (cost per day 83 cents). A hundred tablets of its generic, amitriptyline 50mg, sells for around $20 (cost per day 20 cents)—a savings of nearly 76 percent.

> ### Dry Mouth Can Lead to Dental Problems
>
> ---
>
> The dry mouth people get from taking tricyclic antidepressants isn't only annoying, but can also lead
>
> to cavities in the teeth. Dentists will tell you that an adequate supply of saliva in the mouth is essential
>
> to prevent tooth decay. If you're taking a tricyclic antidepressant, rinse your mouth frequently with
>
> water and visit your dentist regularly.

SEROTONIN REUPTAKE INHIBITORS (SSRIs)

A new group of antidepressants emerged in the 1990s—serotonin reuptake inhibitors. These drugs, known as SSRIs, work by elevating serotonin levels in the brain. Of all the types of antidepressants on the market, these are by far the most commonly prescribed. They include:

1. Celexa (generic name citalopram)
2. Luvox (generic name fluvoxamine)
3. Paxil (generic name paroxetine)
4. Prozac (generic name fluoxetine)
5. Zoloft (generic name sertraline)

If these drugs sound familiar, yet you've never taken one of them, pay closer attention to television commercials. Drug companies heavily promote SSRIs, which have been a true blessing for millions of people. A large-scale study reported in 2002, however, that among the three top-prescribed name-brand SSRIs—Paxil, Prozac, and Zoloft—no one has clinically distinctive attributes rendering it more effective than the others. In other words, they all work the same!

SSRIs are very good at alleviating depression in most people, and also are used to treat obsessive-compulsive disorder (OCD) and social anxiety disorder (SAD). They also tend to have far fewer side effects than other types of antidepressants. Common side effects include headaches, insomnia, nausea, diarrhea, and anxiety or nervousness. Some of these drugs also can cause sexual difficulties and erectile dysfunction. Another downside is that it can take up to six weeks before the drugs start to relieve your symptoms. People who are severely depressed will find this a long time to wait.

To save money, buy the higher strength and cut the pills. Thirty tablets of Zoloft 50mg cost around $80; 15 tablets of the 100mg strength cost just $40. Cut these pills to cut your costs in half!

OTHER DRUGS USED TO TREAT DEPRESSION

Four other products commonly used to treat depression fit into none of the aforementioned categories. These are:

1. Desyrel (generic name trazodone)
2. Effexor (generic name venlafaxine)
3. Serzone (generic name nefazodone)
4. Wellbutrin (generic name bupropion)

Effexor and Serzone produce similar elevation and activity of both norepinephrine and serotonin and have side effects similar to those of both SSRI drugs and the tricyclic antidepressants. Desyrel and Wellbutrin are unique. Researchers don't fully understand how either of these drugs work, but they clearly reduce the symptoms of depression. Because these two drugs have potentially serious side effects, however, doctors generally prescribe them only after SSRIs fail to have the desired effect.

Desyrel can be a strong sedative. In fact, it's so good at inducing sleep that it's often prescribed for that purpose alone. Desyrel's one rather notorious, and fortunately unique, side effect—priapism, an irreversible erection of the penis. Priapism is extremely painful and usually requires a trip to the emergency room. Wellbutrin, on the other hand, can cause seizures. Although this side effect is rare—less than one in 200—just the possibility is enough to steer people away from this drug. More common side effects include headaches, dizziness, sweating, tremor, sedation, agitation, weight loss, blurred vision, and dry mouth.

▶ Bupropion to Reduce Nicotine Cravings

Zyban, a new prescription drug used to help relieve the symptoms of nicotine withdrawal, contains bupropion. Many ex-smokers swear by its effectiveness. For some reason, it reduces withdrawal symptoms (cravings). Researchers aren't sure why. ◀

Drugs to Treat Depression

PRODUCT	STRENGTH PER DOSE	ACTIVE INGREDIENT	USUAL DOSAGE	TYPICAL QUANTITY	TYPICAL PRICE	PRICE PER DAY
Amitriptyline	10mg	Amitriptyline	Take 1 tablet daily.	30	$10	33¢
Amitriptyline	25mg	Amitriptyline	Take 1 tablet daily.	30	$10	33¢
Amitriptyline	50mg	Amitriptyline	Take 1 tablet daily.	30	$10	33¢
Amitriptyline	75mg	Amitriptyline	Take 1 tablet daily.	30	$10	33¢
Amitriptyline	100mg	Amitriptyline	Take 1 tablet daily.	30	$10	33¢
Anafranil (clomipramine)	25mg	Clomipramine	Take 1 capsule daily.	30	$55	$1.83
Anafranil (clomipramine)	50mg	Clomipramine	Take 1 capsule daily.	30	$75	$2.50
Anafranil (clomipramine)	75mg	Clomipramine	Take 1 capsule daily.	30	$95	$3.17
Bupropion	75mg	Bupropion	Take 1 tablet 3 times a day.	90	$25	83¢
Bupropion	100mg	Bupropion	Take 1 tablet 3 times a day.	90	$30	$1
Celexa (citalopram)	10mg	Citalopram	Take 1 tablet daily.	30	$70	$2.33
Celexa (citalopram)	20mg	Citalopram	Take 1 tablet daily.	30	$70	$2.33
Celexa (citalopram)	40mg	Citalopram	Take 1 tablet daily.	30	$75	$2.50
Clomipramine	25mg	Clomipramine	Take 1 capsule daily.	30	$20	67¢
Clomipramine	50mg	Clomipramine	Take 1 capsule daily.	30	$25	83¢
Clomipramine	75mg	Clomipramine	Take 1 capsule daily.	30	$30	$1
Desipramine	10mg	Desipramine	Take 1 tablet daily.	30	$10	33¢
Desipramine	25mg	Desipramine	Take 1 tablet daily.	30	$10	33¢
Desipramine	50mg	Desipramine	Take 1 tablet daily.	30	$10	33¢
Desipramine	75mg	Desipramine	Take 1 tablet daily.	30	$15	50¢
Desipramine	100mg	Desipramine	Take 1 tablet daily.	30	$20	67¢
Desyrel (trazodone)	50mg	Trazodone	Take 1 tablet daily.	30	$65	$2.17
Desyrel (trazodone)	100mg	Trazodone	Take 1 tablet daily.	30	$120	$4
Desyrel (trazodone)	150mg	Trazodone	Take 1 tablet daily.	30	$100	$3.33
Desyrel (trazodone)	300mg	Trazodone	Take 1 tablet daily.	30	$175	$5.83
Doxepin	10mg	Doxepin	Take 1 capsule daily.	30	$15	50¢
Doxepin	25mg	Doxepin	Take 1 capsule daily.	30	$15	50¢
Doxepin	50mg	Doxepin	Take 1 capsule daily.	30	$15	50¢

PRODUCT	STRENGTH PER DOSE	ACTIVE INGREDIENT	USUAL DOSAGE	TYPICAL QUANTITY	TYPICAL PRICE	PRICE PER DAY
Doxepin	75mg	Doxepin	Take 1 capsule daily.	30	$15	50¢
Doxepin	100mg	Doxepin	Take 1 capsule daily.	30	$15	50¢
Effexor (venlafaxine)	25mg	Venlafaxine	Take 1 tablet daily.	30	$45	$1.50
Effexor (venlafaxine)	37.5mg	Venlafaxine	Take 1 tablet daily.	30	$50	$1.67
Effexor (venlafaxine)	50mg	Venlafaxine	Take 1 tablet daily.	30	$50	$1.67
Effexor (venlafaxine)	75mg	Venlafaxine	Take 1 tablet daily.	30	$50	$1.67
Effexor (venlafaxine)	100mg	Venlafaxine	Take 1 tablet daily.	30	$55	$1.83
Effexor XR (venlafaxine)	37.5mg	Venlafaxine	Take 1 capsule daily.	30	$75	$2.50
Effexor XR (venlafaxine)	75mg	Venlafaxine	Take 1 capsule daily.	30	$80	$2.67
Effexor XR (venlafaxine)	150mg	Venlafaxine	Take 1 capsule daily.	30	$85	$2.83
Elavil (amitriptyline)	10mg	Amitriptyline	Take 1 tablet daily.	30	$15	50¢
Elavil (amitriptyline)	25mg	Amitriptyline	Take 1 tablet daily.	30	$25	83¢
Elavil (amitriptyline)	50mg	Amitriptyline	Take 1 tablet daily.	30	$35	$1.17
Elavil (amitriptyline)	75mg	Amitriptyline	Take 1 tablet daily.	30	$50	$1.67
Elavil (amitriptyline)	100mg	Amitriptyline	Take 1 tablet daily.	30	$65	$2.17
Fluoxetine	10mg	Fluoxetine	Take 1 tablet daily.	30	$30	$1
Fluoxetine	10mg	Fluoxetine	Take 1 capsule daily.	30	$30	$1
Fluoxetine	20mg	Fluoxetine	Take 1 capsule daily.	30	$30	$1
Fluoxetine	40mg	Fluoxetine	Take 1 capsule daily.	30	$100	$3.33
Fluvoxamine	25mg	Fluvoxamine	Take 1 tablet daily.	30	$55	$1.83
Fluvoxamine	50mg	Fluvoxamine	Take 1 tablet daily.	30	$60	$2
Fluvoxamine	100mg	Fluvoxamine	Take 1 tablet daily.	30	$65	$2.17
Imipramine	10mg	Imipramine	Take 1 tablet daily.	30	$15	50¢
Imipramine	25mg	Imipramine	Take 1 tablet daily.	30	$15	50¢
Imipramine	50mg	Imipramine	Take 1 tablet daily.	30	$15	50¢
Luvox (fluvoxamine)	25mg	Fluvoxamine	Take 1 tablet daily.	30	$95	$3.17
Luvox (fluvoxamine)	50mg	Fluvoxamine	Take 1 tablet daily.	30	$105	$3.50
Luvox (fluvoxamine)	100mg	Fluvoxamine	Take 1 tablet daily.	30	$105	$3.50
Nardil (phenelzine)	15mg	Phenelzine	Take 1 tablet 3 times a day.	90	$60	$2
Norpramin (desipramine)	10mg	Desipramine	Take 1 tablet daily.	30	$25	83¢

PRODUCT	STRENGTH PER DOSE	ACTIVE INGREDIENT	USUAL DOSAGE	TYPICAL QUANTITY	TYPICAL PRICE	PRICE PER DAY
Norpramin (desipramine)	25mg	Desipramine	Take 1 tablet daily.	30	$30	$1
Norpramin (desipramine)	50mg	Desipramine	Take 1 tablet daily.	30	$50	$1.67
Norpramin (desipramine)	75mg	Desipramine	Take 1 tablet daily.	30	$60	$2
Norpramin (desipramine)	100mg	Desipramine	Take 1 tablet daily.	30	$90	$3
Nortriptyline	10mg	Nortriptyline	Take 1 capsule daily.	30	$15	50¢
Nortriptyline	25mg	Nortriptyline	Take 1 capsule daily.	30	$15	50¢
Nortriptyline	50mg	Nortriptyline	Take 1 capsule daily.	30	$15	50¢
Nortriptyline	75mg	Nortriptyline	Take 1 capsule daily.	30	$17	57¢
Pamelor (nortriptyline)	10mg	Nortriptyline	Take 1 capsule daily.	30	$30	$1
Pamelor (nortriptyline)	25mg	Nortriptyline	Take 1 capsule daily.	30	$65	$2.17
Pamelor (nortriptyline)	50mg	Nortriptyline	Take 1 capsule daily.	30	$105	$1.75
Pamelor (nortriptyline)	75mg	Nortriptyline	Take 1 capsule daily.	30	$150	$5
Parnate (tranylcypromine)	10mg	Tranylcypromine	Take 1 tablet 3 times a day.	90	$70	$2.33
Paxil (paroxetine)	10mg	Paroxetine	Take 1 tablet daily.	30	$85	$2.83
Paxil (paroxetine)	20mg	Paroxetine	Take 1 tablet daily.	30	$85	$2.83
Paxil (paroxetine)	30mg	Paroxetine	Take 1 tablet daily.	30	$90	$3
Paxil (paroxetine)	40mg	Paroxetine	Take 1 tablet daily.	30	$90	$3
Prozac (fluoxetine)	10mg	Fluoxetine	Take 1 tablet daily.	30	$85	$2.83
Prozac (fluoxetine)	10mg	Fluoxetine	Take 1 capsule daily.	30	$85	$2.83
Prozac (fluoxetine)	20mg	Fluoxetine	Take 1 capsule daily.	30	$87	$2.90
Prozac (fluoxetine)	40mg	Fluoxetine	Take 1 capsule daily.	30	$172	$5.73
Prozac Weekly (fluoxetine)	90mg	Fluoxetine	Take 1 capsule weekly.	4	$80	$2.67
Remeron (mirtazapine)	15mg	Mirtazapine	Take 1 tablet daily.	30	$90	$3
Remeron (mirtazapine)	30mg	Mirtazapine	Take 1 tablet daily.	30	$95	$3.17
Remeron (mirtazapine)	45mg	Mirtazapine	Take 1 tablet daily.	30	$100	$3.33
Serzone (nefazodone)	50mg	Nefazodone	Take 1 tablet twice a day.	60	$50	$1.67
Serzone (nefazodone)	100mg	Nefazodone	Take 1 tablet twice a day.	60	$55	$1.83
Serzone (nefazodone)	150mg	Nefazodone	Take 1 tablet twice a day.	60	$55	$1.83
Serzone (nefazodone)	200mg	Nefazodone	Take 1 tablet twice a day.	60	$55	$1.83
Serzone (nefazodone)	250mg	Nefazodone	Take 1 tablet twice a day.	60	$60	$2

PRODUCT	STRENGTH PER DOSE	ACTIVE INGREDIENT	USUAL DOSAGE	TYPICAL QUANTITY	TYPICAL PRICE	PRICE PER DAY
Sinequan (doxepin)	10mg	Doxepin	Take 1 capsule daily.	30	$25	83¢
Sinequan (doxepin)	25mg	Doxepin	Take 1 capsule daily.	30	$25	83¢
Sinequan (doxepin)	50mg	Doxepin	Take 1 capsule daily.	30	$30	$1
Sinequan (doxepin)	75mg	Doxepin	Take 1 capsule daily.	30	$40	$1.33
Sinequan (doxepin)	100mg	Doxepin	Take 1 capsule daily.	30	$50	$1.67
Surmontil (trimipramine)	25mg	Trimipramine	Take 1 capsule daily.	30	$35	$1.17
Surmontil (trimipramine)	50mg	Trimipramine	Take 1 capsule daily.	30	$50	$1.67
Surmontil (trimipramine)	100mg	Trimipramine	Take 1 capsule daily.	30	$70	$2.33
Tofranil (imipramine)	10mg	Imipramine	Take 1 tablet daily.	30	$25	83¢
Tofranil (imipramine)	25mg	Imipramine	Take 1 tablet daily.	30	$35	$1.17
Tofranil (imipramine)	50mg	Imipramine	Take 1 tablet daily.	30	$55	$1.83
Trazodone	50mg	Trazodone	Take 1 tablet daily.	30	$15	50¢
Trazodone	100mg	Trazodone	Take 1 tablet daily.	30	$15	50¢
Trazodone	150mg	Trazodone	Take 1 tablet daily.	30	$20	67¢
Trazodone	300mg	Trazodone	Take 1 tablet daily.	30	$100	$3.33
Wellbutrin (bupropion)	75mg	Bupropion	Take 1 tablet 3 times a day.	90	$35	$1.17
Wellbutrin (bupropion)	100mg	Bupropion	Take 1 tablet 3 times a day.	90	$45	$1.50
Wellbutrin SR (bupropion)	100mg	Bupropion	Take 1 tablet twice a day.	60	$60	$2
Wellbutrin SR (bupropion)	150mg	Bupropion	Take 1 tablet twice a day.	60	$104	$3.47
$ Zoloft (sertraline)	25mg	Sertraline	Take 1 tablet daily.	30	$82	$2.73
$ Zoloft (sertraline)	50mg	Sertraline	Take 1 tablet daily.	30	$82	$2.73
$ Zoloft (sertraline)	100mg	Sertraline	Take 1 tablet daily.	30	$82	$2.73

$ SMART BUY
Drugs to Treat Depression

For depression, the Smart Buys are the SSRI drugs. Good results with comparatively few side effects make this group an excellent choice. Results of a comprehensive study conducted in 2001 showed that these drugs all work equally well. Of this group, fluoxetine, the generic form of Prozac, purchased in large quantities offers the best savings.

If you're taking Zoloft, Paxil, Luvox, or Celexa, cut the higher strength tablets for big savings. Prozac and its generic versions come in capsules, which you can't cut.

DRUGS TO TREAT PSYCHOTIC DISORDERS

Psychotic disorders such as schizophrenia and bipolar disorder (formerly called manic-depressive disorder) typically keep their sufferers from living normal and productive lives. The drugs doctors use to treat psychoses are powerful and work by blocking the effects of the brain chemical dopamine, which plays a key role in the expression of numerous psychotic conditions, including schizophrenia. Reducing its activity provides some relief of these conditions.

The three types of antipsychotic drugs are:

1. Phenothiazines, which have many potential side effects
2. Nonphenothiazines, which affect the brain in much the same way as phenothiazines but with far fewer side effects
3. Atypical antipsychotics, a new type of drug that seems to work in up to 30 percent of those who do not respond to phenothiazines and nonphenothiazines

The most commonly prescribed antipsychotic drugs are the phenothiazines, which include:

1. Mellaril (generic name thioridazine)
2. Thorazine (generic name chlorpromazine)
3. Trilafon (generic name perphenazine)

These drugs have been on the market for a very long time so generic versions are available for them all. This is where you'll save the most money.

Phenothiazine drugs have many side effects. Like antidepressants, they can cause severe sedation, blurred vision, constipation, and dry mouth. They also can trigger very undesirable body movements, such as akathisia (fidgeting, pacing, and an inability to sit quietly), bradykinesia (slowing of voluntary movements), and tardive dyskinesia (involuntary movements of the face, lips, and tongue that include grimacing, smacking of the lips, rolling of the tongue, and puffing of the cheeks). Unfortunately, some of these side effects become permanent (they don't go away when the medication is stopped). And because phenothiazine drugs can worsen Parkinson's disease, most physicians avoid prescribing them for people with this disorder.

Nonphenothiazine drugs similar in activity to the phenothiazines include:

1. Haldol (generic name haloperidol)
2. Loxitane (generic name loxapine)

3. Navane (generic name thiothixene)

4. Orap (generic name pimozide)

Although nonphenothiazines tend to be less sedating and cause fewer problems with blurred vision, dry mouth, and constipation, they do seem to be more prone to causing akathisia, bradykinesia, and dyskinesia. Because such side effects can be permanent, these drugs generally are reserved for those suffering from severe psychosis that doesn't respond to other medications. These drugs, too, have been around for a while. Ask about a generic to save big money.

Four new drugs became available recently. Classified as atypical antipsychotics, these are effective in treating people who don't respond to traditional antipsychotics:

1. Clozaril (generic name clozapine)

2. Risperdal (generic name risperidone)

3. Seroquel (generic name quetiapine)

4. Zyprexa (generic name olanzapine)

These drugs cause far fewer problems with involuntary-movement side effects, but still can cause sedation, blurred vision, dry mouth, and constipation. Of this group, Clozaril seems to cause the most problems with side effects.

Clozapine's Dangerous Side Effect

The atypical antipsychotic drug clozapine can cause a dangerous condition called agranulocytosis (low white blood cell count). Left untreated, this condition is fatal in 1 to 2 percent of those afflicted. If it's going to occur at all, agranulocytosis usually will manifest within the first six months of therapy. Blood cell counts should be performed weekly during that time.

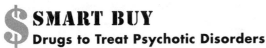

$ SMART BUY
Drugs to Treat Psychotic Disorders

The new atypical antipsychotics are the Smart Buys among drugs to treat psychotic disorders. Although these new drugs cost a lot more than traditional options, they cause

Drugs to Treat Psychotic Disorders

PRODUCT	STRENGTH PER DOSE	ACTIVE INGREDIENT	USUAL DOSAGE	TYPICAL QUANTITY	TYPICAL PRICE	PRICE PER DAY
Chlorpromazine	25mg	Chlorpromazine	Take 1 tablet 3 times a day.	90	$20	67¢
Chlorpromazine	100mg	Chlorpromazine	Take 1 tablet 3 times a day.	90	$25	83¢
Clozapine	25mg	Clozapine	Take 1 tablet daily.	30	$45	$1.50
Clozapine	100mg	Clozapine	Take 1 tablet daily.	30	$80	$2.67
Clozaril (clozapine)	25mg	Clozapine	Take 1 tablet daily.	30	$60	$2
Clozaril (clozapine)	100mg	Clozapine	Take 1 tablet daily.	30	$140	$4.67
Haldol (haloperidol)	0.5mg	Haloperidol	Take 1 tablet 3 times a day.	90	$55	$1.83
Haldol (haloperidol)	1mg	Haloperidol	Take 1 tablet 3 times a day.	90	$70	$2.33
Haldol (haloperidol)	2mg	Haloperidol	Take 1 tablet 3 times a day.	90	$95	$3.17
Haldol (haloperidol)	5mg	Haloperidol	Take 1 tablet 3 times a day.	90	$150	$5
Haldol (haloperidol)	10mg	Haloperidol	Take 1 tablet 3 times a day.	90	$195	$6.50
Haloperidol	0.5mg	Haloperidol	Take 1 tablet 3 times a day.	90	$15	50¢
Haloperidol	1mg	Haloperidol	Take 1 tablet 3 times a day.	90	$15	50¢
Haloperidol	2mg	Haloperidol	Take 1 tablet 3 times a day.	90	$20	67¢
Haloperidol	5mg	Haloperidol	Take 1 tablet 3 times a day.	90	$25	83¢
Haloperidol	10mg	Haloperidol	Take 1 tablet 3 times a day.	90	$35	$1.17
Loxapine	5mg	Loxapine	Take 1 capsule 3 times a day.	90	$75	$2.50
Loxapine	10mg	Loxapine	Take 1 capsule 3 times a day.	90	$75	$2.50
Loxapine	25mg	Loxapine	Take 1 capsule 3 times a day.	90	$120	$4
Loxitane (loxapine)	5mg	Loxapine	Take 1 capsule 3 times a day.	90	$100	$3.33
Loxitane (loxapine)	10mg	Loxapine	Take 1 capsule 3 times a day.	90	$140	$4.67
Loxitane (loxapine)	25mg	Loxapine	Take 1 capsule 3 times a day.	90	$200	$6.67
Mellaril (thioridazine)	10mg	Thioridazine	Take 1 tablet 3 times a day.	90	$25	83¢
Mellaril (thioridazine)	25mg	Thioridazine	Take 1 tablet 3 times a day.	90	$30	$1
Mellaril (thioridazine)	50mg	Thioridazine	Take 1 tablet 3 times a day.	90	$35	$1.17
Mellaril (thioridazine)	100mg	Thioridazine	Take 1 tablet 3 times a day.	90	$35	$1.17
Navane (thiothixene)	1mg	Thiothixene	Take 1 capsule 3 times a day.	90	$55	$1.83
Navane (thiothixene)	2mg	Thiothixene	Take 1 capsule 3 times a day.	90	$65	$2.17
Navane (thiothixene)	5mg	Thiothixene	Take 1 capsule 3 times a day.	90	$130	$4.33

PRODUCT	STRENGTH PER DOSE	ACTIVE INGREDIENT	USUAL DOSAGE	TYPICAL QUANTITY	TYPICAL PRICE	PRICE PER DAY
Navane (thiothixene)	10mg	Thiothixene	Take 1 capsule 3 times a day.	90	$155	$5.17
Orap (pimozide)	1mg	Pimozide	Take 1 tablet daily.	30	$30	$1
Orap (pimozide)	2mg	Pimozide	Take 1 tablet daily.	30	$35	$1.17
Perphenazine	2mg	Perphenazine	Take 1 tablet 3 times a day.	90	$25	83¢
Perphenazine	4mg	Perphenazine	Take 1 tablet 3 times a day.	90	$30	$1
Risperdal (risperidone)	0.5mg	Risperidone	Take 1 tablet twice a day.	60	$85	$2.83
Risperdal (risperidone)	1mg	Risperidone	Take 1 tablet twice a day.	60	$85	$2.83
Risperdal (risperidone)	2mg	Risperidone	Take 1 tablet twice a day.	60	$140	$4.67
Risperdal (risperidone)	3mg	Risperidone	Take 1 tablet twice a day.	60	$160	$5.33
Risperdal (risperidone)	4mg	Risperidone	Take 1 tablet twice a day.	60	$210	$7
Seroquel (quetiapine)	25mg	Quetiapine	Take 1 tablet twice a day.	60	$95	$3.17
Seroquel (quetiapine)	100mg	Quetiapine	Take 1 tablet twice a day.	60	$165	$5.50
Seroquel (quetiapine)	200mg	Quetiapine	Take 1 tablet twice a day.	60	$315	$10.50
Seroquel (quetiapine)	300mg	Quetiapine	Take 1 tablet twice a day.	60	$420	$14
Thioridazine	10mg	Thioridazine	Take 1 tablet 3 times a day.	90	$10	33¢
Thioridazine	25mg	Thioridazine	Take 1 tablet 3 times a day.	90	$15	50¢
Thioridazine	50mg	Thioridazine	Take 1 tablet 3 times a day.	90	$15	50¢
Thioridazine	100mg	Thioridazine	Take 1 tablet 3 times a day.	90	$20	67¢
Thiothixene	1mg	Thiothixene	Take 1 capsule 3 times a day.	90	$20	67¢
Thiothixene	2mg	Thiothixene	Take 1 capsule 3 times a day.	90	$20	67¢
Thiothixene	5mg	Thiothixene	Take 1 capsule 3 times a day.	90	$30	$1
Thiothixene	10mg	Thiothixene	Take 1 capsule 3 times a day.	90	$35	$1.17
Thorazine (chlorpromazine)	25mg	Chlorpromazine	Take 1 tablet 3 times a day.	90	$70	$2.33
Thorazine (chlorpromazine)	100mg	Chlorpromazine	Take 1 tablet 3 times a day.	90	$105	$3.50
Trilafon (perphenazine)	2mg	Perphenazine	Take 1 tablet 3 times a day.	90	$85	$2.83
Trilafon (perphenazine)	4mg	Perphenazine	Take 1 tablet 3 times a day.	90	$110	$3.67
$ Zyprexa (olanzapine)	2.5mg	Olanzapine	Take 1 tablet daily.	30	$150	$5
$ Zyprexa (olanzapine)	5mg	Olanzapine	Take 1 tablet daily.	30	$180	$6
$ Zyprexa (olanzapine)	7.5mg	Olanzapine	Take 1 tablet daily.	30	$260	$7
$ Zyprexa (olanzapine)	10mg	Olanzapine	Take 1 tablet daily.	30	$210	$8.67
$ Zyprexa (olanzapine)	20mg	Olanzapine	Take 1 tablet daily.	30	$380	$12.67

far fewer serious side effects. Most people will find this improvement well worth the money. Zyprexa is your best choice for the smartest savings. Buy in bulk—30 tablets of Zyprexa 5mg cost about $180 ($6 a dose) and 90 tablets of the same strength cost about $485 (a little over $5 a dose), to give you a savings of about $1 a day, or 17 percent.

DRUGS TO TREAT SEIZURE DISORDERS

When most people hear the words "seizure disorder" or "epilepsy," they think of fits or convulsions that cause people to writhe uncontrollably on the ground. But many people with epilepsy don't develop such "typical" seizures. Instead, they may simply become unresponsive or experience out-of-place sense phenomena, such as the smell of something that's not there. It depends on the area of the brain the seizure affects.

When a seizure disorder exists, the brain is abnormally sensitive to electrical stimulation. Healthcare professionals call this a lower threshold of activity. The drugs doctors use to treat seizure disorders work by slowing electrical activity or by raising the brain's threshold of activity so it's less affected. Doctors use many different groups of drugs to treat epilepsy. Sometimes these drugs are called "anticonvulsants," but that's not an entirely accurate description. Doctors consider the type and severity of the patient's seizures, as well as the patient's age, when choosing a treatment from among these medications. Often it takes some trial and error to find the drug best suited to an individual. Some of these drugs have potentially serious side effects, and all share the side effects of dizziness, drowsiness, confusion, and headaches.

Drugs commonly prescribed for seizure disorders include:

1. Depakene (generic name valproic acid), which can cause potentially fatal liver failure especially in children under age 16
2. Depakote (generic name divalproex)
3. Dilantin (generic name phenytoin)
4. Felbatol (generic name felbamate; because it can cause anemia—low numbers of red blood cells—severe enough to be fatal, this drug should only be used when seizures fail to respond to other medications)
5. Lamictal (generic name lamotrigine; can cause severe rash, especially in children under age 16)
6. Mysoline (generic name primidone)
7. Neurontin (generic name gabapentin)
8. Phenobarbital (on the market so long there's no price difference between name-brand and generic versions)
9. Tegretol (generic name carbamazepine)

10. Topamax (generic name topiramate)
11. Valium (generic name diazepam)

▶ Antiseizure Drugs Also Relieve Nerve Pain

Drugs to treat seizures also are used to treat neuralgias (nerve pain). Researchers aren't sure why they work, but they do. In fact, some of these drugs are prescribed more often for this affliction than for epilepsy. Neurontin, in particular, is commonly prescribed to help relieve pain in people with diabetes, people who've had surgery, and people with pinched nerves.

Drug interactions pose problems common to antiseizure drugs. Phenytoin, phenobarbital, and carbamazepine are notorious for interfering with other drugs: After being absorbed into the bloodstream, many drugs are altered by chemicals and enzymes in the liver. This allows the kidneys to filter them out more easily so they can pass from the body in urine. But the liver doesn't make one clean sweep of the blood; it often takes many cycles through the liver for certain substances to be removed. Drug doses are calculated to take advantage of the length of time this takes. Phenytoin, phenobarbital, and carbamazepine, known as "enzyme inducers," cause the liver to produce more enzymes, which speeds up the processing of other substances. Dilantin (phenytoin), for example, accelerates the liver's metabolism of oral contraceptives (birth control pills); this causes the concentration of contraceptive in your blood to drop precipitously, hampering its effectiveness at preventing pregnancy.

$ SMART BUY
Drugs to Treat Seizure Disorders

Generic versions of Dilantin and Tegretol are two good Smart Buy options to start with for many people, because they have fewer potential side effects than other antiseizure products. If you're already taking any product to treat seizures, don't switch just to save money! Antiseizure drugs have narrow therapeutic indexes (NTIs), so don't change if

Drugs to Treat Seizure Disorders

PRODUCT	STRENGTH PER DOSE	ACTIVE INGREDIENT	USUAL DOSAGE	TYPICAL QUANTITY	TYPICAL PRICE	PRICE PER DAY
$ Carbamazepine	100mg	Carbamazepine	Take 1 tablet twice a day.	60	$20	67¢
$ Carbamazepine	200mg	Carbamazepine	Take 1 tablet twice a day.	60	$20	67¢
Depakene (valproic acid)	250mg	Valproic acid	Take 1 capsule 3 times a day.	90	$175	$5.83
Depakote (divalproex)	125mg	Divalproex	Take 1 tablet 3 times a day.	90	$55	$1.83
Depakote (divalproex)	250mg	Divalproex	Take 1 tablet 3 times a day.	90	$95	$3.17
Depakote (divalproex)	500mg	Divalproex	Take 1 tablet 3 times a day.	90	$175	$5.83
Dilantin (phenytoin)	30mg	Phenytoin	Take 1 capsule 3 times a day.	90	$30	$1
Dilantin (phenytoin)	50mg	Phenytoin	Take 1 tablet 3 times a day.	90	$30	$1
Dilantin (phenytoin)	100mg	Phenytoin	Take 1 capsule 3 times a day.	90	$35	$1.17
Felbatol (felbamate)	400mg	Felbamate	Take 1 tablet 3 times a day.	90	$140	$4.67
Felbatol (felbamate)	600mg	Felbamate	Take 1 tablet 3 times a day.	90	$160	$5.33
Lamictal (lamotrigine)	25mg	Lamotrigine	Take 1 tablet twice a day.	60	$150	$5
Lamictal (lamotrigine)	100mg	Lamotrigine	Take 1 tablet twice a day.	60	$160	$5.33
Lamictal (lamotrigine)	150mg	Lamotrigine	Take 1 tablet twice a day.	60	$170	$5.67
Lamictal (lamotrigine)	200mg	Lamotrigine	Take 1 tablet twice a day.	60	$185	$6.17
Mysoline (primidone)	50mg	Primidone	Take 1 tablet 3 times a day.	90	$30	$1
Mysoline (primidone)	250mg	Primidone	Take 1 tablet 3 times a day.	90	$100	$3.33
Neurontin (gabapentin)	100mg	Gabapentin	Take 1 capsule 3 times a day.	90	$60	$2
Neurontin (gabapentin)	300mg	Gabapentin	Take 1 capsule 3 times a day.	90	$115	$3.83
Neurontin (gabapentin)	400mg	Gabapentin	Take 1 capsule 3 times a day.	90	$130	$4.33
Neurontin (gabapentin)	600mg	Gabapentin	Take 1 tablet 3 times a day.	90	$200	$6.67
Neurontin (gabapentin)	800mg	Gabapentin	Take 1 tablet 3 times a day.	90	$230	$7.67
Phenobarbital	15mg	Phenobarbital	Take 1 tablet twice a day.	60	$10	33¢
Phenobarbital	30mg	Phenobarbital	Take 1 tablet twice a day.	60	$15	50¢
Phenobarbital	60mg	Phenobarbital	Take 1 tablet twice a day.	60	$15	50¢
Phenobarbital	100mg	Phenobarbital	Take 1 tablet twice a day.	60	$15	50¢
$ Phenytoin	100mg	Phenytoin	Take 1 capsule 3 times a day.	90	$25	83¢
Primidone	250mg	Primidone	Take 1 tablet 3 times a day.	90	$50	$1.67
Tegretol (carbamazepine)	100mg	Carbamazepine	Take 1 tablet twice a day.	60	$30	$1

PRODUCT	STRENGTH PER DOSE	ACTIVE INGREDIENT	USUAL DOSAGE	TYPICAL QUANTITY	TYPICAL PRICE	PRICE PER DAY
Tegretol (carbamazepine)	200mg	Carbamazepine	Take 1 tablet twice a day.	60	$40	$1.33
Tegretol XR (carbamazepine)	100mg	Carbamazepine	Take 1 tablet twice a day.	60	$25	83¢
Tegretol XR (carbamazepine)	200mg	Carbamazepine	Take 1 tablet twice a day.	60	$40	$1.33
Tegretol XR (carbamazepine)	400mg	Carbamazepine	Take 1 tablet twice a day.	60	$70	$2.33
Topamax (topiramate)	25mg	Topiramate	Take 1 tablet twice a day.	60	$90	$3
Topamax (topiramate)	100mg	Topiramate	Take 1 tablet twice a day.	60	$190	$6.33
Topamax (topiramate)	200mg	Topiramate	Take 1 tablet twice a day.	60	$225	$7.50
Valproic acid	250mg	Valproic acid	Take 1 capsule 3 times a day.	90	$25	83¢

you're already stable on one of these products. And don't cut the tablets! Instead, consider buying a larger quantity to lower your cost per dose.

DRUGS TO TREAT PARKINSON'S DISEASE

Parkinson's disease is a progressive, debilitating brain disorder characterized by tremors, slowed mobility, stooped posture, expressionless (mask-like) face, and increasingly severe rigidity. It affects mostly people over age 60, although early onset Parkinson's disease can strike people who are in their thirties. Former U.S. Attorney General Janet Reno, boxing legend Muhammad Ali, and actor Michael J. Fox, all of whom have Parkinson's, have brought this disease to the forefront of public awareness. About 50,000 new cases of Parkinson's disease are diagnosed each year in the U.S.

Researchers believe Parkinson's disease occurs when there's a reduction in the number of brain cells that produce a chemical called dopamine. Dopamine is responsible for fine-tuning the control of the movements of many skeletal muscles. Drugs used to treat Parkinson's attempt to replenish the brain's dopamine supply in one of three ways:

1. By increasing production from the cells that remain active in the brain
2. By slowing the elimination of dopamine from the body
3. By binding to and stimulating the brain's dopamine receptors

In addition to replenishing dopamine, researchers have found that drugs that block acetylcholine (another chemical involved in controlling muscles throughout the body) also improve symptoms of Parkinson's disease. Acetylcholine-blocking drugs (also known as anticholinergic drugs) commonly prescribed to treat Parkinson's disease include Artane (generic name trihexyphenidyl) and Cogentin (generic name benztropine).

Drugs used to treat Parkinson's disease either by supplying dopamine or stimulating dopamine receptors in the brain include:

1. Eldepryl (generic name selegiline)
2. Mirapex (generic name pramipexole)
3. Parlodel (generic name bromocriptine)
4. Permax (generic name pergolide)
5. Requip (generic name ropinirole)
6. Sinemet (a combination of levodopa and carbidopa)
7. Symmetrel (generic name amantadine)
8. Tasmar (generic name tolcapone)

With Parkinson's disease, typically there's a window of time when the drugs that stimulate dopamine receptors and/or replenish dopamine to the brain are effective. When this time frame occurs and how long it lasts vary from person to person. Because Parkinson's disease generally takes 15 years or longer to run its course, the stronger drugs usually are reserved for use after the weaker ones lose their effectiveness. Because of the relatively brief window of opportunity with dopamine agonists/supplements, therapy usually starts with one of the anticholinergic drugs. Artane is a good choice for the newly diagnosed, because it tends to have fewer side effects than other anticholinergic drugs. These side effects include dizziness, drowsiness, blurred vision, dry mouth, and constipation.

Tasmar should be reserved for use later in the course of the disease, because it can cause liver failure that can be fatal. The drug's manufacturer recommends that liver function tests be performed every two weeks for the first year of treatment, every four weeks for the next six months, and every eight weeks thereafter. If Parkinson's symptoms don't improve substantially within three weeks of initiating Tasmar therapy, it's recommended the drug be discontinued. Severe liver failure isn't worth the risk.

Between the time when anticholinergic drugs lose their effectiveness and Tasmar is initiated, doctors usually will prescribe one or more of the other dopamine agonists. These may work for a short period of time or for several years. Often there's a "wearing-off" effect when response to these drugs deteriorates: Increasingly higher doses produce briefer and briefer effects, until the drug itself begins to cause more intense abnormal movements than the disease. This problem is seen most commonly with levodopa. To help prevent this problem, sometimes doctors will have patients take drug "holidays," withdrawing completely from levodopa for five to 14 days, and then reintroduce the drug slowly at a lower strength. Check with your doctor before doing this.

Side effects common to dopamine agonist drugs include nausea, dizziness, light-headedness, blurred vision, diarrhea, and uncontrollable abnormal movements. You'll want to take most of these drugs with food to lessen nausea. Finally, don't take levodopa with vitamin B6, which limits its effectiveness.

Drugs to Treat Parkinson's Disease

PRODUCT	STRENGTH PER DOSE	ACTIVE INGREDIENT	USUAL DOSAGE	TYPICAL QUANTITY	TYPICAL PRICE	PRICE PER DAY
Amantadine	100mg	Amantadine	Take 1 capsule twice a day.	60	$20	67¢
Artane (trihexyphenidyl)	2mg	Trihexyphenidyl	Take 1 tablet 3 times a day.	90	$25	83¢
Benztropine	0.5mg	Benztropine	Take 1 tablet daily.	30	$10	33¢
Benztropine	1mg	Benztropine	Take 1 tablet daily.	30	$10	33¢
Benztropine	2mg	Benztropine	Take 1 tablet daily.	30	$10	33¢
Bromocriptine	2.5mg	Bromocriptine	Take 1 tablet twice a day.	60	$115	$3.83
Bromocriptine	5mg	Bromocriptine	Take 1 capsule twice a day.	60	$140	$4.67
Carbidopa with levodopa	10/100	Carbidopa with levodopa	Take 1 tablet 3 times a day.	90	$45	$1.50
Carbidopa with levodopa	25/100	Carbidopa with levodopa	Take 1 tablet 3 times a day.	90	$50	$1.67
Carbidopa with levodopa	25/250	Carbidopa with levodopa	Take 1 tablet 3 times a day.	90	$55	$1.83
Carbidopa with levodopa CR	25/100	Carbidopa with levodopa	Take 1 tablet twice a day.	60	$75	$2.50
Carbidopa with levodopa CR	50/200	Carbidopa with levodopa	Take 1 tablet twice a day.	60	$130	$4.33
Cogentin (benztropine)	0.5mg	Benztropine	Take 1 tablet daily.	30	$20	67¢
Cogentin (benztropine)	1mg	Benztropine	Take 1 tablet daily.	30	$20	67¢
Cogentin (benztropine)	2mg	Benztropine	Take 1 tablet daily.	30	$25	83¢
Eldepryl (selegiline)	5mg	Selegiline	Take 1 capsule twice a day.	60	$170	$5.67
Mirapex (pramipexole)	0.125mg	Pramipexole	Take 1 tablet 3 times a day.	90	$85	$2.83
Mirapex (pramipexole)	0.25mg	Pramipexole	Take 1 tablet 3 times a day.	90	$100	$3.33
Mirapex (pramipexole)	0.5mg	Pramipexole	Take 1 tablet 3 times a day.	90	$170	$5.67

PRODUCT	STRENGTH PER DOSE	ACTIVE INGREDIENT	USUAL DOSAGE	TYPICAL QUANTITY	TYPICAL PRICE	PRICE PER DAY
Mirapex (pramipexole)	1mg	Pramipexole	Take 1 tablet 3 times a day.	90	$170	$5.67
Mirapex (pramipexole)	1.5mg	Pramipexole	Take 1 tablet 3 times a day.	90	$175	$5.83
Parlodel (bromocriptine)	2.5mg	Bromocriptine	Take 1 tablet twice a day.	60	$155	$5.17
Parlodel (bromocriptine)	5mg	Bromocriptine	Take 1 capsule twice a day.	60	$225	$7.50
Permax (pergolide)	0.05mg	Pergolide	Take 1 tablet 3 times a day.	90	$110	$3.67
Permax (pergolide)	0.25mg	Pergolide	Take 1 tablet 3 times a day.	90	$170	$5.67
Permax (pergolide)	1mg	Pergolide	Take 1 tablet 3 times a day.	90	$350	$11.67
Requip (ropinirole)	0.25mg	Ropinirole	Take 1 tablet 3 times a day.	90	$110	$3.67
Requip (ropinirole)	0.5mg	Ropinirole	Take 1 tablet 3 times a day.	90	$110	$3.67
Requip (ropinirole)	1mg	Ropinirole	Take 1 tablet 3 times a day.	90	$110	$3.67
Requip (ropinirole)	3mg	Ropinirole	Take 1 tablet 3 times a day.	90	$200	$6.67
Requip (ropinirole)	4mg	Ropinirole	Take 1 tablet 3 times a day.	90	$200	$6.67
Requip (ropinirole)	5mg	Ropinirole	Take 1 tablet 3 times a day.	90	$200	$6.67
Selegiline	5mg	Selegiline	Take 1 capsule twice a day.	60	$75	$2.50
Sinemet (carbidopa with levodopa)	10/100	Carbidopa with levodopa	Take 1 tablet 3 times a day.	90	$85	$2.83
Sinemet (carbidopa with levodopa)	25/100	Carbidopa with levodopa	Take 1 tablet 3 times a day.	90	$90	$3
Sinemet (carbidopa with levodopa)	25/250	Carbidopa with levodopa	Take 1 tablet 3 times a day.	90	$115	$3.83
Sinemet CR (carbidopa with levodopa)	25/100	Carbidopa with levodopa	Take 1 tablet twice a day.	60	$100	$3.33
Sinemet CR (carbidopa with levodopa)	50/200	Carbidopa with levodopa	Take 1 tablet twice a day.	60	$185	$6.17
Tasmar (tolcapone)	100mg	Tolcapone	Take 1 tablet 3 times a day.	90	$225	$7.50
Tasmar (tolcapone)	200mg	Tolcapone	Take 1 tablet 3 times a day.	90	$235	$7.83
Trihexyphenidyl	2mg	Trihexyphenidyl	Take 1 tablet 3 times a day.	90	$20	67¢

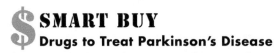

$ SMART BUY
Drugs to Treat Parkinson's Disease

Artane is the Smart Buy among drugs used to treat Parkinson's disease. Taking it in the early stages reserves the stronger drugs for use later on. To save money, use a generic version and increase the quantity to drop your cost from 28 cents a dose to nine cents a dose, a savings of 68 percent. When Artane is no longer enough to control the symptoms, go to the Smart Buy of Sinemet (a combination of levodopa and carbidopa). The generic form of this dopamine replacement product is considerably cheaper than most of the others. For the biggest savings, buy generic in bulk, and consider purchasing a strength twice what your doctor prescribes and cutting the tablets in half. This can lower your cost to about 40 cents a dose.

DRUGS TO TREAT ALZHEIMER'S DISEASE

Two drugs currently on the market are prescribed to delay symptoms of Alzheimer's disease. These drugs—Cognex (generic name tacrine) and Aricept (generic name donepezil)—are known as cholinesterase inhibitors: They work by blocking a brain enzyme that breaks down acetylcholine. This results in an increase in acetylcholine that, for reasons researchers don't fully understand, results in improved cognitive abilities in people with Alzheimer's disease.

Side effects of these drugs include a slowed heart rate, an increased risk of stomach ulcers (from increased acid production), and liver abnormalities and damage. If you already have one of these problems, cholinesterase inhibitors probably aren't appropriate for you. These drugs also can cause headaches, dizziness, nausea, and vomiting.

Drugs to Treat Alzheimer's Disease

PRODUCT	STRENGTH PER DOSE	ACTIVE INGREDIENT	USUAL DOSAGE	TYPICAL QUANTITY	TYPICAL PRICE	PRICE PER DAY
$ Aricept (donepezil)	5mg	Donepezil	Take 1 tablet daily.	30	$140	$4.67
$ Aricept (donepezil)	10mg	Donepezil	Take 1 tablet daily.	30	$140	$4.67
Cognex (tacrine)	10mg	Tacrine	Take 1 capsule 4 times a day.	120	$150	$5
Cognex (tacrine)	20mg	Tacrine	Take 1 capsule 4 times a day.	120	$150	$5
Cognex (tacrine)	30mg	Tacrine	Take 1 capsule 4 times a day.	120	$150	$5
Cognex (tacrine)	40mg	Tacrine	Take 1 capsule 4 times a day.	120	$150	$5

$ SMART BUY
Drugs to Treat Alzheimer's Disease

Aricept is slightly less expensive than Cognex, making it your Smart Buy. For more savings, buy Aricept in bulk and see whether the tablets can be cut. This will cost you about $2 a dose, half the cost of the higher strength tablet.

DRUGS TO TREAT ATTENTION DEFICIT DISORDER (ADD)

Attention deficit disorder (ADD) once was called "hyperactivity." It primarily affects children and can be challenging to diagnose. Children with ADD often have difficulty focusing on one task at a time. Because they're easily distracted, their behavior can become disruptive.

Many parents and health experts worry that many children who are just active and difficult for harried teachers to cope with are being misdiagnosed and treated for ADD. Because no definitive diagnostic test exists for this problem—an accurate diagnosis may require many examinations by pediatric neurologists and psychologists—no doubt children who don't really need them are taking medications for ADD.

But for the thousands of children who do need them, the drugs to treat ADD are truly a blessing, allowing them to focus and learn. Commonly prescribed drugs in this group include:

1. Adderall (amphetamine mixtures)
2. Catapress (generic name clonidine)
3. Concerta (extended-release methylphenidate)
4. Cylert (generic name pemoline)
5. Dexedrine (generic name dextroamphetamine)
6. Ritalin (generic name methylphenidate)
7. Tenex (generic name guanfacine)

These drugs' various mechanisms of action aren't completely understood; what works in one child might not work in another. It's believed that Tenex and Catapress reduce the activity of the brain chemical norepinephrine. These two drugs are particularly helpful for children who have problems with aggression or insomnia. Of the two, Tenex often is preferred, because its effects last longer and it's slightly less sedating. The downside to both drugs is that they're simply not as effective as the other products, and they can cause depression in some children.

More commonly used are the stimulant drugs. It seems odd that these have a calming effect in these cases; you'd think they would make children even more hyperactive. In children with ADD, however, stimulants have the opposite effect, calming them down.

> ## Do You Need a Written Prescription?
>
> Most stimulants (such as Ritalin, Dexedrine, and Adderall) are controlled substances that require a written prescription from the doctor every time you need more pills. Drugs that aren't stimulants (such as Tenex and Catapress) aren't controlled substances; your doctor can authorize refills on the original prescription or over the phone.

One downside to this group of drugs is that they can reduce the appetite dramatically. This might be a good thing in some adults, but in most children it's not. Reduced growth rates have been seen in children taking these types of drugs. If your child takes a stimulant to treat ADD, make sure he or she eats balanced meals. Other potential side effects include dizziness, headaches, rapid heartbeat, increased blood pressure, nervousness, and insomnia. To avoid insomnia, the last daily dose should be taken early in the evening (prior to 6 p.m.). Also, stimulants can intensify anxiety and tension. If your child experiences either or both of these, consider using a nonstimulant product such as Tenex or Catapress first.

Drugs to Treat Attention Deficit Disorder (ADD)

PRODUCT	STRENGTH PER DOSE	ACTIVE INGREDIENT	USUAL DOSAGE	TYPICAL QUANTITY	TYPICAL PRICE	PRICE PER DAY
Adderall (amphetamine)	5mg mixtures	Amphetamine	Take 1 tablet in the morning and 1 at noon.	60	$90	$3
Adderall (amphetamine)	7.5mg mixtures	Amphetamine	Take 1 tablet in the morning and 1 at noon.	60	$90	$3
Adderall (amphetamine)	10mg mixtures	Amphetamine	Take 1 tablet in the morning and 1 at noon.	60	$90	$3
Adderall (amphetamine)	12.5mg mixtures	Amphetamine	Take 1 tablet in the morning and 1 at noon.	60	$90	$3
Adderall (amphetamine)	15mg mixtures	Amphetamine	Take 1 tablet in the morning and 1 at noon.	60	$90	$3

PRODUCT	STRENGTH PER DOSE	ACTIVE INGREDIENT	USUAL DOSAGE	TYPICAL QUANTITY	TYPICAL PRICE	PRICE PER DAY
Adderall (amphetamine)	20mg	Amphetamine mixtures	Take 1 tablet in the morning and 1 at noon.	60	$90	$3
Adderall (amphetamine)	30mg	Amphetamine mixtures	Take 1 tablet in the morning and 1 at noon.	60	$90	$3
Adderall XR (amphetamine)	10mg	Amphetamine mixtures	Take 1 tablet in the morning and 1 at noon.	30	$75	$2.50
Adderall XR (amphetamine)	20mg	Amphetamine mixtures	Take 1 tablet in the morning and 1 at noon.	30	$75	$2.50
Adderall XR (amphetamine)	30mg	Amphetamine mixtures	Take 1 tablet in the morning and 1 at noon.	30	$75	$2.50
Catapress (clonidine)	0.1mg	Clonidine	Take 1 tablet twice a day.	60	$50	$1.67
Catapress (clonidine)	0.2mg	Clonidine	Take 1 tablet twice a day.	60	$80	$2.67
Catapress (clonidine)	0.3mg	Clonidine	Take 1 tablet twice a day.	60	$100	$3.33
Clonidine	0.1mg	Clonidine	Take 1 tablet twice a day.	60	$15	50¢
Clonidine	0.2mg	Clonidine	Take 1 tablet twice a day.	60	$15	50¢
Clonidine	0.3mg	Clonidine	Take 1 tablet twice a day.	60	$25	83¢
Concerta (methylphenidate)	18mg	Methylphenidate	Take 1 tablet daily.	30	$80	$2.67
Concerta (methylphenidate)	36mg	Methylphenidate	Take 1 tablet daily.	30	$85	$2.83
Concerta (methylphenidate)	54mg	Methylphenidate	Take 1 tablet daily.	30	$90	$3
Cylert (pemoline)	18.75mg	Pemoline	Take 1 tablet daily.	30	$40	$1.33
Cylert (pemoline)	37.5mg	Pemoline	Take 1 tablet daily.	30	$55	$1.83
Cylert (pemoline)	75mg	Pemoline	Take 1 tablet daily.	30	$100	$3.33
Dexedrine (dextroamphetamine)	5mg	Dextro-amphetamine	Take 1 tablet in the morning and 1 at noon.	60	$30	$1
Dexedrine spansules) (dextroamphetamine)	5mg	Dextro-amphetamine	Take 1 capsule daily.	30	$30	$1
Dexedrine spansules (dextroamphetamine)	10mg	Dextro-amphetamine	Take 1 capsule daily.	30	$40	$1.33
Dexedrine spansules (dextroamphetamine)	15mg	Dextro-amphetamine	Take 1 capsule daily.	30	$45	$1.50
Dextrostat (dextroamphetamine)	5mg	Dextro-amphetamine	Take 1 tablet in the morning and 1 at noon.	60	$25	83¢
Guanfacine	1mg	Guanfacine	Take 1 tablet daily.	30	$15	50¢

PRODUCT	STRENGTH PER DOSE	ACTIVE INGREDIENT	USUAL DOSAGE	TYPICAL QUANTITY	TYPICAL PRICE	PRICE PER DAY
Guanfacine	2mg	Guanfacine	Take 1 tablet daily.	30	$20	67¢
Methylphenidate	5mg	Methylphenidate	Take 1 tablet in the morning and 1 at noon.	60	$30	$1
Methylphenidate	10mg	Methylphenidate	Take 1 tablet in the morning and 1 at noon.	60	$30	$1
Methylphenidate	20mg	Methylphenidate	Take 1 tablet in the morning and 1 at noon.	60	$40	$1.33
Methylphenidate ER	20mg	Methylphenidate	Take 1 tablet daily.	30	$30	$1
Pemoline	18.75mg	Pemoline	Take 1 tablet daily.	30	$25	83¢
Pemoline	37.5mg	Pemoline	Take 1 tablet daily.	30	$40	$1.33
Pemoline	75mg	Pemoline	Take 1 tablet daily.	30	$75	$2.50
Ritalin (methylphenidate)	5mg	Methylphenidate	Take 1 tablet in the morning and 1 at noon.	60	$40	$1.33
Ritalin (methylphenidate)	10mg	Methylphenidate	Take 1 tablet in the morning and 1 at noon.	60	$40	$1.33
Ritalin (methylphenidate)	20mg	Methylphenidate	Take 1 tablet in the morning and 1 at noon.	60	$60	$2
Ritalin SR (methylphenidate)	20mg	Methylphenidate	Take 1 tablet daily.	30	$45	$1.50
Tenex (guanfacine)	1mg	Guanfacine	Take 1 tablet daily.	30	$40	$1.33
Tenex (guanfacine)	2mg	Guanfacine	Take 1 tablet daily.	30	$50	$1.67

 # SMART BUY
Drugs to Treat Attention Deficit Disorder (ADD)

Of the choices available for stimulant drugs, Concerta (extended-release methyl-phenidate) is the smartest buy. This long-acting product comes in a unique dosage form that produces a quick release of some of the drug to initiate an immediate response, followed by a continual release of the balance of the drug that produces results for up to 12 hours. The advantage of this over drugs such as Ritalin and Dexedrine is that only one morning dose needs to be taken, and results will last until much later in the day. Concerta is more expensive than, say, a generic version of Ritalin (methylphenidate). Sixty tablets of methylphenidate 5mg typically sell for around $30 and 30 tablets of Concerta 18mg for around $80. If money is a major concern, methylphenidate is the way to go. But be aware that your child will have the extra hassle of remembering to take a second pill at school, and he or she probably will experience a little "dip" in its effectiveness. With Concerta you pay more, but you certainly get your money's worth. To convert dosages from methylphenidate to Concerta, two doses of methylphenidate 5mg (one in the morning and one at noon) are "equivalent" to 18mg of Concerta. Likewise, two doses of methylphenidate 10mg equals one of Concerta 36mg, and two doses of methylphenidate 15mg equal one of Concerta 54mg. Finally, Concerta's advantage over Cylert is that children seem to respond better to Concerta's active ingredient, methylphenidate. Adults being treated for ADD receive the same drugs.

$ SMART OPTIONS FOR SAVINGS
Prescription Drugs that Affect the Central Nervous System

Whenever possible, buy generic versions of these drugs. Newer drugs are unavailable in generic forms, which makes them much more expensive. The expense is sometimes worth it, however, because they can be far more effective than older and cheaper alternatives.

1. Buy in the largest quantities possible, to get your per-dose costs down.
2. Check with your pharmacist before cutting tablets. Many of these drugs are NTIs or must be taken intact at the correct dose for other reasons.
3. We don't recommend alternative sources for most of these drugs, unless you're confident of quality and can order them far enough in advance that you don't run out while waiting for them. Those that contain amphetamines are Schedule II drugs, which means you need a new written prescription each time you buy more and must pick up your prescription in person. (Schedule II drugs can't be sent through the mail.)
4. Because the conditions for which these drugs are prescribed require close medical supervision, we don't recommend going to Canada to buy them. However, you might find Internet or mail-order pharmacies located in Canada offer better prices; review Chapter 4, "Saving on Drugs Across the Border," for cautions about using this approach.

And be sure to check our Web site at www.smartbuysdrugwise.com for the latest information about more ways to save money on these drugs.

Chapter 13

Prescription Drugs to Treat Pain and Inflammation

Each year, U.S. doctors write more than 122 million prescriptions for drugs to relieve pain and inflammation—more than 10 percent of all drugs prescribed in this country. Prescription-only pain relievers are more powerful than those available over the counter, which means they also have potentially more severe side effects. Some of these drugs, such as ibuprofen and naproxen, also are available in nonprescription products. (See Chapter 18, "Over-the-Counter Pain Relief.") Prescription-strength versions can be 2 to 4 times more potent than nonprescription preparations. Over-the-counter ibuprofen comes in 200mg tablets, for example, while prescription ibuprofen tablets come in 400mg, 600mg, and 800mg strengths.

Pain medications fall into two broad categories, narcotic and non-narcotic. Narcotic pain relievers derive from opium and are potentially addictive; federal regulations classify these as "controlled substances" or "scheduled" drugs. The most potent of these are the Schedule II narcotics, which may not be refilled. Each time you receive a supply of a Schedule II drug, you must have a new, written, signed prescription from your doctor. Doctors prescribe narcotic pain relievers for pain that's severe but short-term (such as during recovery from an injury or following surgery) or severe and terminal (end-stage cancer, for example).

Non-narcotic pain medications aren't addictive, but this doesn't mean using them is without risk. Kidney and liver failure are potentially serious consequences of long-term use of nonsteroidal anti-inflammatory drugs (NSAIDs), for example. Your doctor may choose to permit refills of a non-narcotic pain medication. If you have a chronic condition that causes pain, such as arthritis, your doctor might authorize long-term refills and specify a time for you to come back for a checkup or to have lab tests run. (More on this later in this chapter.) Your doctor also may authorize refills of these drugs by telephone.

DRUGS THAT TREAT ARTHRITIS

More than 33 million Americans suffer from either osteo- or rheumatoid arthritis. Most have osteoarthritis, an irritation and degeneration of the joints brought about by wear and tear. The older you get, the more likely you are to suffer from some degree of this often painful problem. Reducing the resulting inflammation typically reduces or eliminates the pain, although it doesn't make the osteoarthritis go away.

Rheumatoid arthritis is a beast of a different nature. It occurs when, for reasons researchers don't fully understand, the body's immune system attacks the tissues of its joints. This results in very painful stiffness, inflammation, and deformity. Although more common in the elderly, rheumatoid arthritis can strike at any age and sometimes afflicts even children. Rheumatoid arthritis is progressive and incurable, although drugs relieve the symptoms (except deformity) for many people.

DRUGS THAT RELIEVE PAIN AND INFLAMMATION

Many drugs provide relief from the pain and swelling common with either kind of arthritis, although neither form is curable. Doctors consider rheumatoid arthritis the more severe form, because it's relentlessly progressive and deforms the joints. Certain drugs, called disease-modifying antirheumatic drugs (DMARDs), can slow the progression of rheumatoid arthritis.

Until a few years ago, about the only drugs that were effective for arthritis were steroids and nonsteroidal anti-inflammatory drugs (NSAIDs), because they reduce swelling. (See Chapter 18, "Over-the-Counter Pain Relief," for discussion of over-the-counter NSAIDs.) This, in turn, lessens stiffness and reduces pain. These drugs remain at the forefront of pain-relief treatment. They include the steroid prednisone, available in many generic versions, and the following prescription NSAIDs:

1. Ansaid (generic name flurbiprofen)
2. Celebrex (generic name celecoxib)
3. Clinoril (generic name sulindac)
4. Daypro (generic name oxaprozin)
5. Dolobid (generic name diflunisal)
6. Feldene (generic name piroxicam)
7. Indocin (generic name indomethacin)
8. Lodine (generic name etodolac)
9. Mobic (generic name meloxicam)
10. Motrin (generic name ibuprofen)
11. Naprosyn (generic name naproxen)

12. Orudis (generic name ketoprofen)
13. Relafen (generic name nabumetone)
14. Toradol (generic name ketorolac)
15. Vioxx (generic name rofecoxib)
16. Voltaren (generic name diclofenac)

Among these drugs, Indocin, Toradol, and Feldene are notorious for causing stomach irritation, including bleeding ulcers that can become life-threatening. Given the many newer drugs available that can provide comparable relief with far fewer side effects, we recommend you avoid taking these three drugs unless nothing else works. The other NSAIDs in this list are equally effective at reducing joint inflammation, but are much easier on the stomach. For most people, these are the way to go.

▶ COX-1 and COX-2 Inhibitors

Want the technical details? NSAIDs are divided into two classes, based on how they work in the body—COX-1 inhibitors and COX-2 inhibitors. "COX" is shorthand for the enzyme *cyclo-oxygenase*, which plays a key role in initiating the sequence of events you feel as pain. Inhibiting, or stopping, this action greatly reduces or even ends your pain. COX-1 receptors (the cells that produce COX) are present throughout the body, including the stomach lining. COX-2 receptors are present everywhere, *except* the stomach lining. This is why NSAIDs that are selective COX-2 inhibitors cause fewer stomach-irritation problems than COX-1-inhibiting NSAIDs.

The newest NSAIDs to hit the market are called COX-2 inhibitors. (See sidebar.) These drugs are the least likely to cause stomach irritation. As you might expect, however, this benefit comes with a price tag: These drugs are very expensive. A typical cost for a 30-day supply of Celebrex 200mg will cost you around $83, and Vioxx 25mg will set you back $87.

Although the potential for stomach problems with NSAIDs gets much attention, other problems pose even more serious risks. Prolonged use of NSAIDs can result in kidney and or liver damage that can be life-threatening if not detected early. If you're taking an NSAID regularly, make sure your doctor does blood tests to check your liver and kidney functions at least once a year.

Another side effect common with NSAIDs is fluid retention. For most people, this isn't a big deal. If you have high blood pressure, however, it can be significant. If you're taking an NSAID and you also have high blood pressure, ask your doctor about this side effect. And NSAIDs can cause some thinning of the blood. If you're taking blood thinners already, or if you're about to undergo surgery, talk with your doctor before taking an NSAID.

In several situations, you should avoid taking NSAIDs altogether. Don't take an NSAID if you:

...have an allergy to aspirin, because it's highly likely you'll also be allergic to NSAIDs ("cross-sensitivity").

...are allergic to sulfa drugs, again because of potential cross-sensitivity.

...are in the last trimester of pregnancy, because NSAIDs can cause premature closure of the ductus arteriosis in the fetus, shutting down the oxygen supply and leading to very serious problems.

Drugs that Relieve Pain and Inflammation

PRODUCT	STRENGTH PER DOSE	ACTIVE INGREDIENT	USUAL DOSAGE	TYPICAL QUANTITY	TYPICAL PRICE	PRICE PER DOSE
Ansaid (flurbiprofen)	50mg	Flurbiprofen	Take 1 tablet 3 times a day.	90	$130	$1.44
Ansaid (flurbiprofen)	100mg	Flurbiprofen	Take 1 tablet 3 times a day.	90	$180	$2
Celebrex (celecoxib)	100mg	Celecoxib	Take 1 capsule daily.	30	$55	$1.83
Celebrex (celecoxib)	200mg	Celecoxib	Take 1 capsule daily.	30	$83	$2.77
Clinoril (sulindac)	150mg	Sulindac	Take 1 tablet 2 times a day.	60	$80	$1.33
Clinoril (sulindac)	200mg	Sulindac	Take 1 tablet 2 times a day.	60	$95	$1.58
Daypro (oxaprozin)	600mg	Oxaprozin	Take 1 or 2 tablets once daily.	60	$115	$1.92
Diflunisal	250mg	Diflunisal	Take 1 tablet 2 times a day.	60	$40	67¢
Diflunisal	500mg	Diflunisal	Take 1 tablet 2 times a day.	60	$60	$1
Dolobid (diflunisal)	250mg	Diflunisal	Take 1 tablet 2 times a day.	60	$85	$1.42
Dolobid (diflunisal)	500mg	Diflunisal	Take 1 tablet 2 times a day.	60	$100	$1.67
Etodolac	200mg	Etodolac	Take 1 capsule 3 times a day.	90	$40	44¢
Etodolac	300mg	Etodolac	Take 1 capsule 3 times a day.	90	$60	67¢

PRODUCT	STRENGTH PER DOSE	ACTIVE INGREDIENT	USUAL DOSAGE	TYPICAL QUANTITY	TYPICAL PRICE	PRICE PER DOSE
Etodolac	400mg	Etodolac	Take 1 tablet 3 times a day.	90	$65	72¢
Etodolac	500mg	Etodolac	Take 1 tablet 3 times a day.	90	$90	$1
Etodolac ER	400mg	Etodolac	Take 1 tablet daily.	30	$45	$1.50
Etodolac ER	500mg	Etodolac	Take 1 tablet daily.	30	$45	$1.50
Etodolac ER	600mg	Etodolac	Take 1 tablet daily.	30	$75	$2.50
Feldene (piroxicam)	10mg	Piroxicam	Take 1 capsule daily.	30	$65	$2.17
Feldene (piroxicam)	20mg	Piroxicam	Take 1 capsule daily.	30	$95	$3.17
Flurbiprofen	50mg	Flurbiprofen	Take 1 tablet 3 times a day.	90	$40	44¢
Flurbiprofen	100mg	Flurbiprofen	Take 1 tablet 3 times a day.	90	$75	83¢
Ibuprofen	400mg	Ibuprofen	Take 1 tablet 3 times a day.	90	$20	22¢
Ibuprofen	600mg	Ibuprofen	Take 1 tablet 3 times a day.	90	$20	22¢
Ibuprofen	800mg	Ibuprofen	Take 1 tablet 3 times a day.	90	$20	22¢
Indocin (indomethacin)	25mg	Indomethacin	Take 1 capsule 3 times a day.	90	$65	72¢
Indocin (indomethacin)	50mg	Indomethacin	Take 1 capsule 3 times a day.	90	$110	$1.22
Indocin SR (indomethacin)	75mg	Indomethacin	Take 1 capsule daily.	30	$65	$2.17
Indomethacin	25mg	Indomethacin	Take 1 capsule 3 times a day.	90	$20	22¢
Indomethacin	50mg	Indomethacin	Take 1 capsule 3 times a day.	90	$20	22¢
Indomethacin ER	75mg	Indomethacin	Take 1 capsule daily.	30	$25	83¢
Ketoprofen	75mg	Ketoprofen	Take 1 capsule 3 times a day.	90	$50	56¢
Lodine (etodolac)	200mg	Etodolac	Take 1 capsule 3 times a day.	90	$130	$1.44
Lodine (etodolac)	300mg	Etodolac	Take 1 capsule 3 times a day.	90	$150	$1.67
Lodine (etodolac)	400mg	Etodolac	Take 1 tablet 3 times a day.	90	$155	$1.72
Lodine (etodolac)	500mg	Etodolac	Take 1 tablet 3 times a day.	90	$155	$1.72
Lodine XL (etodolac)	400mg	Etodolac	Take 1 tablet daily.	30	$50	$1.67
Lodine XL (etodolac)	500mg	Etodolac	Take 1 tablet daily.	30	$55	$1.83
Lodine XL (etodolac)	600mg	Etodolac	Take 1 tablet daily.	30	$90	$3
Mobic (meloxicam)	7.5mg	Meloxicam	Take 1 tablet daily.	30	$70	$2.33
Mobic (meloxicam)	15mg	Meloxicam	Take 1 tablet daily.	30	$75	$2.50
Motrin (ibuprofen)	400mg	Ibuprofen	Take 1 tablet 3 times a day.	90	$35	39¢
Motrin (ibuprofen)	600mg	Ibuprofen	Take 1 tablet 3 times a day.	90	$35	39¢

PRODUCT	STRENGTH PER DOSE	ACTIVE INGREDIENT	USUAL DOSAGE	TYPICAL QUANTITY	TYPICAL PRICE	PRICE PER DOSE
Motrin (ibuprofen)	800mg	Ibuprofen	Take 1 tablet 3 times a day.	90	$40	44¢
Naprosyn (naproxen)	375mg	Naproxen	Take 1 tablet 2 times a day.	60	$75	$1.25
Naprosyn (naproxen)	500mg	Naproxen	Take 1 tablet 2 times a day.	60	$100	$1.67
Naproxen	375mg	Naproxen	Take 1 tablet 2 times a day.	60	$20	33¢
Naproxen	500mg	Naproxen	Take 1 tablet 2 times a day.	60	$25	42¢
Orudis (ketoprofen)	75mg	Ketoprofen	Take 1 capsule 3 times a day.	90	$125	$1.39
Oxaprozin	600mg	Oxaprozin	Take 1 or 2 tablets once daily.	60	$50	83¢
Piroxicam	10mg	Piroxicam	Take 1 capsule daily.	30	$15	50¢
Piroxicam	20mg	Piroxicam	Take 1 capsule daily.	30	$15	50¢
Sulindac	150mg	Sulindac	Take 1 tablet 2 times a day.	60	$30	50¢
Sulindac	200mg	Sulindac	Take 1 tablet 2 times a day.	60	$30	50¢
Vioxx (rofecoxib)	12.5mg	Rofecoxib	Take 1 tablet daily.	30	$80	$2.67
Vioxx (rofecoxib)	25mg	Rofecoxib	Take 1 tablet daily.	30	$87	$2.90
Vioxx (rofecoxib)	50mg	Rofecoxib	Take 1 tablet daily.	30	$115	$3.83

 SMART BUY

Drugs that Relieve Pain and Inflammation

For a 30-day supply of ibuprofen 800mg (a generic version of Motrin or Advil) you'll pay only about $30, making it your Smart Buy. Also, compare the cost of over-the-counter generic ibuprofen products. Remember to calculate the correct dose. Over-the-counter ibuprofen comes in 200mg strength, so you'll need to take 4 tablets to get an 800mg dose. If you buy over-the-counter ibuprofen in bulk (500-count bottles), you should be able to find prices of around $20. A 30-day supply going this route will wind up costing you around $14—$6 less than the prescription strength. If ibuprofen is too hard on your stomach, try a generic version of Daypro (oxaprozin), for which you can expect to pay about $50 for a 30-day supply.

Among the new COX-2 inhibitors, Celebrex and Vioxx are equally effective, but Vioxx is your Smart Buy. It comes in a tablet form that can be cut for further savings, especially if you buy in bulk. Ninety Vioxx 50mg tablets will cost you about $300 but give you a per-dose cost of about $1.70—over $1 a dose less than the 30-tablet bottle of Vioxx 25mg (at about $87), giving you a savings of 41 percent. Neither of these drugs is available yet in a generic version. Check out the www.smartbuysdrugwise.com Web site for current information.

DRUGS THAT SLOW THE PROGRESS OF RHEUMATOID ARTHRITIS

Rheumatoid arthritis is a progressive autoimmune disease. Although NSAIDs excel at reducing inflammation and the symptoms of rheumatoid arthritis, they can't do anything about the progression of the disease. Other drugs are needed to do this. For years doctors have prescribed Rheumatrex (generic name methotrexate), a drug better known for its use (at much higher doses) to fight cancer, to slow the progress of rheumatoid arthritis. Researchers don't entirely understand why it's effective here. Methotrexate has some strong potential side effects that limit its use to severe cases. Liver, kidney, and bone-marrow problems in people taking this drug have resulted in deaths.

New drugs now available offer amazing results with far fewer side effects. These drugs, called disease-modifying antirheumatic drugs (DMARDs), modify the disease process of rheumatoid arthritis, giving most people who take them nearly complete relief from pain and inflammation. Again, as you might expect, these new drugs are very expensive. Probably the most exciting new product we've seen is Enbrel. This comes only in liquid form and is injected beneath the skin. These shots aren't very painful and most people can do it, but Enbrel's price tag hurts—typically around $1,100 a month! Before trying Enbrel, ask your doctor about Arava (generic name leflunomide). This drug comes in a tablet form for the more reasonable price of around $250 a month.

Drugs that Slow the Progress of Rheumatoid Arthritis

PRODUCT	STRENGTH PER DOSE	ACTIVE INGREDIENT	USUAL DOSAGE	TYPICAL QUANTITY	TYPICAL PRICE	PRICE PER DOSE
Arava (leflunomide)	10mg	Leflunomide	Take 1 tablet daily.	30	$250	$8.33
Arava (leflunomide)	20mg	Leflunomide	Take 1 tablet daily.	30	$250	$8.33
Arava (leflunomide)	100mg	Leflunomide	Take 1 tablet daily for 3 days.	3	$140	$46.67
Enbrel (etanercept)	25mg	Etanercept	Inject twice a week.	1 box	$600	$42.86
Methotrexate	2.5mg	Methotrexate	Take 3 tablets once a week.	3	$10	$1.43
Rheumatrex Dose Pack (methotrexate)	2.5mg	Methotrexate	Take 3 tablets once a week.	1 pack of 3	$60	$8.57

$ SMART BUY
Drugs that Slow the Progress of Rheumatoid Arthritis

To slow down the progression of rheumatoid arthritis, we recommend you ask your doctor about Arava (leflunomide), our suggestion for your Smart Buy. It's quite a bit more expensive than methotrexate, but it tends to have fewer side effects. And it's much less expensive then Enbrel. To save money with Arava, ask whether the tablets can be cut. For example, if your dose should be 10mg a day, buy the 20mg tablets and cut them in half. Doing so can cut your costs in half, too, dropping your monthly bill from around $250 to $125, a savings of 50 percent.

NARCOTIC PAIN RELIEVERS

When deciding how to treat pain, doctors often will consider several factors. First, because pain is a normal response that forces us to limit our use of a damaged body part, doctors first must consider whether blocking the pain will be beneficial. Second, once treatment is deemed necessary, the doctor must determine which type of medication will best treat the pain with the fewest side effects. In most cases, doctors first will try an NSAID, but if this isn't effective (or if it's unlikely to be effective), or if you can't tolerate an NSAID (particularly if you have stomach ulcers or limited kidney function), the next type of drug to try is one that blocks the pain receptors found throughout the body. Most of these drugs are narcotics.

Commonly known as opiate derivatives, narcotic drugs vary considerably in effectiveness. The word "narcotic" means "to sleep," a strong clue to one common effect of these drugs! Opiate derivatives bind to opioid receptors, or "buttons," on nerve cells that influence the perception of pain. A narcotic pain reliever's effectiveness depends on which of these receptors the drug affects; this can differ from person to person. Drugs in the morphine family are most effective: Strong opiates such as morphine and Demerol are far more likely to work than codeine or propoxyphene. But, as is usually the case with pharmaceuticals, with the good comes the bad. These stronger drugs also have far more incidences of drowsiness, nausea, and constipation, and far greater potential for causing addiction.

Commonly prescribed opiate derivatives, or narcotics, are:

1. Codeine (usually combined with acetaminophen; a common brand name is Tylenol with Codeine)
2. Darvocet (combination of propoxyphene and acetaminophen)
3. Darvon (generic name propoxyphene)
4. Demerol (generic name meperidine)
5. Dilaudid (generic name hydromorphone)
6. Dolophine (generic name methadone)
7. Duragesic patches (generic name fentanyl)

8. Hydrocodone (usually combined with acetaminophen; a common brand name is Vicodin)
9. MS Contin (generic name morphine)
10. MSIR (generic name morphine)
11. Oxycontin (generic name oxycodone)
12. Percocet (combination of oxycodone and acetaminophen)
13. Stadol nasal spray (generic name butorphanol)

Because of the potential for addiction, narcotic pain relievers are controlled substances. This means that for some of them, you need a written prescription. Prescriptions for Tylenol with codeine, Vicodin, Darvon, Darvocet, and Stadol can be phoned in. The strongest narcotics have the strongest restriction—Schedule II. Schedule II prescriptions can't be refilled; you must get a new written prescription from your doctor each time you need a refill. Narcotics classified as Schedule II are codeine (when not combined with acetaminophen or aspirin), Demerol, Dilaudid, Duragesic, Dolophine, morphine, and Oxycontin.

Narcotics and Constipation

If you anticipate that you'll be taking narcotic pain relievers for longer than a month, talk with your doctor or pharmacist about things you can do to prevent constipation. (And check out Chapter 19, "Over-the-Counter Gastrointestinal Remedies," for more ideas.)

Stadol nasal spray is up to 7 times stronger than morphine and 40 times stronger than Demerol. Stadol affects opiate receptors differently from other narcotics, however, so despite its strength, it has significantly less potential for addiction. Talwin, which is comparable to codeine in strength, is another narcotic pain reliever with a similar action in the body. Doctors often prescribe Talwin for people who need a fairly strong pain reliever but who might have potential drug-abuse problems.

The quest for strong pain relief without the risk of addiction has led to the development of a synthetic drug called Ultram (generic name tramadol). Created entirely in the laboratory, Ultram is neither a narcotic nor a controlled substance. Known as a central analgesic, Ultram works by affecting the pain center in the brain, where it's believed to increase norepinephrine and serotonin levels.

Narcotic Pain Relievers

PRODUCT	STRENGTH PER DOSE	ACTIVE INGREDIENT	USUAL DOSAGE	TYPICAL QUANTITY	TYPICAL PRICE	PRICE PER DOSE
Acetaminophen with codeine	300/30	Acetaminophen with codeine	Take 1 tablet every 4-6 hrs. as needed.	30	$15	50¢
Darvocet N-100 (propoxyphene with acetaminophen)	100/650	Propoxyphene with acetaminophen	Take 1 tablet every 4-6 hrs. as needed.	30	$30	$1
Darvon (propoxyphene)	65mg	Propoxyphene	Take 1 capsule every 4-6 hrs. as needed.	30	$20	67¢
Demerol (meperidine)	50mg	Meperidine	Take 1 tablet every 4-6 hrs. as needed.	30	$35	$1.17
Dilaudid (hydromorphone)	2mg	Hydromorphone	Take 1 tablet every 4-6 hrs. as needed.	30	$20	67¢
Dilaudid (hydromorphone)	4mg	Hydromorphone	Take 1 tablet every 4-6 hrs. as needed.	30	$30	$1
Duragesic patches (fentanyl)	25mcg	Fentanyl	Apply 1 patch every 72 hours.	5	$75	$15
Duragesic patches (fentanyl)	50mcg	Fentanyl	Apply 1 patch every 72 hours.	5	$110	$22
Duragesic patches (fentanyl)	75mcg	Fentanyl	Apply 1 patch every 72 hours.	5	$175	$35
Duragesic patches (fentanyl)	100mcg	Fentanyl	Apply 1 patch every 72 hours.	5	$220	$44
Hydrocodone with acetaminophen	5/500	Hydrocodone with acetaminophen	Take 1 tablet every 4-6 hrs. as needed.	30	$15	50¢
Hydrocodone with acetaminophen E.S.	7.5/750	Hydrocodone with acetaminophen	Take 1 tablet every 4-6 hrs. as needed.	30	$15	50¢
Hydromorphone	2mg	Hydromorphone	Take 1 tablet every 4-6 hrs. as needed.	30	$15	50¢
Hydromorphone	4mg	Hydromorphone	Take 1 tablet every 4-6 hrs. as needed.	30	$20	67¢
Meperidine	50mg	Meperidine	Take 1 tablet every 4-6 hrs. as needed.	30	$25	83¢
Methadone	5mg	Methadone	Take 1 tablet every 4-6 hrs. as needed.	30	$10	33¢
Methadone	10mg	Methadone	Take 1 tablet every 4-6 hrs. as needed.	30	$10	33¢
Morphine sulfate	10mg	Morphine sulfate	Take 1 tablet every 4-6 hrs. as needed.	30	$10	33¢
Morphine sulfate	15mg	Morphine sulfate	Take 1 tablet every 4-6 hrs. as needed.	30	$10	33¢

PRODUCT	STRENGTH PER DOSE	ACTIVE INGREDIENT	USUAL DOSAGE	TYPICAL QUANTITY	TYPICAL PRICE	PRICE PER DOSE
Morphine sulfate	30mg	Morphine sulfate	Take 1 tablet every 4-6 hrs. as needed.	30	$10	33¢
Morphine sulfate ER	15mg	Morphine sulfate	Take 1 tablet 2 times a day.	60	$55	92¢
Morphine sulfate ER	30mg	Morphine sulfate	Take 1 tablet 2 times a day.	60	$90	$1.50
Morphine sulfate ER	60mg	Morphine sulfate	Take 1 tablet 2 times a day.	60	$165	$2.75
Morphine sulfate ER	100mg	Morphine sulfate	Take 1 tablet 2 times a day.	60	$310	$5.17
MS Contin (morphine sulfate ER)	15mg	Morphine sulfate	Take 1 tablet 2 times a day.	60	$65	$1.08
MS Contin (morphine sulfate ER)	30mg	Morphine sulfate	Take 1 tablet 2 times a day.	60	$120	$2
MS Contin (morphine sulfate ER)	60mg	Morphine sulfate	Take 1 tablet 2 times a day.	60	$225	$3.75
MS Contin (morphine sulfate ER)	100mg	Morphine sulfate	Take 1 tablet 2 times a day.	60	$325	$5.42
MSIR (morphine sulfate)	15mg	Morphine sulfate	Take 1 tablet every 4-6 hrs. as needed.	30	$15	50¢
MSIR (morphine sulfate)	30mg	Morphine sulfate	Take 1 tablet every 4-6 hrs. as needed.	30	$15	50¢
Oxycodone with acetaminophen	5/325	Oxycodone with acetaminophen	Take 1 tablet every 4-6 hrs. as needed.	30	$20	67¢
Oxycodone with acetaminophen	5/500	Oxycodone with acetaminophen	Take 1 capsule every 4-6 hrs. as needed.	30	$20	67¢
Oxycodone with aspirin	5/325	Oxycodone with aspirin	Take 1 tablet every 4-6 hrs. as needed.	30	$20	67¢
Oxycontin (oxycodone)	10mg	Oxycodone	Take 1 tablet 2 times a day.	60	$80	$1.33
Oxycontin (oxycodone)	20mg	Oxycodone	Take 1 tablet 2 times a day.	60	$150	$2.50
Oxycontin (oxycodone)	40mg	Oxycodone	Take 1 tablet 2 times a day.	60	$260	$4.33
Oxycontin (oxycodone)	80mg	Oxycodone	Take 1 tablet 2 times a day.	60	$475	$7.92
Percocet (oxycodone with acetaminophen)	5/325	Oxycodone with acetaminophen	Take 1 tablet every 4-6 hrs. as needed.	30	$40	$1.33
Percocet (oxycodone with acetaminophen)	7.5/500	Oxycodone with acetaminophen	Take 1 tablet every 4-6 hrs. as needed.	30	$45	$1.50
Percocet (oxycodone with acetaminophen)	10/650	Oxycodone with acetaminophen	Take 1 tablet every 4-6 hrs. as needed.	30	$50	$1.67
Percodan (oxycodone with aspirin)	5/325	Oxycodone with aspirin	Take 1 tablet every 4-6 hrs. as needed.	30	$40	$1.33
Propoxyphene	65mg	Propoxyphene	Take 1 capsule every 4-6 hrs. as needed.	30	$15	50¢
Propoxyphene with acetaminophen	100/650	Propoxyphene with acetaminophen	Take 1 tablet every 4-6 hrs. as needed.	30	$15	50¢

PRODUCT	STRENGTH PER DOSE	ACTIVE INGREDIENT	USUAL DOSAGE	TYPICAL QUANTITY	TYPICAL PRICE	PRICE PER DOSE
Roxicodone (oxycodone)	5mg	Oxycodone	Take 1 tablet every 4-6 hrs. as needed.	30	$20	67¢
Stadol Nasal Spray (butorphanol)	10mg/ml	Butorphanol	Spray once in 1 nostril every 3-4 hrs. as needed.	1 bottle	$110	$7.33
Tylenol #3 (acetaminophen with codeine)	300/30	Acetaminophen with codeine	Take 1 tablet every 4-6 hrs. as needed.	30	$20	67¢
Tylox (oxycodone with acetaminophen)	5/500	Oxycodone with acetaminophen	Take 1 capsule every 4-6 hrs. as needed.	30	$40	$1.33
Vicodin (hydrocodone with acetaminophen)	5/500	Hydrocodone with acetaminophen	Take 1 tablet every 4-6 hrs. as needed.	30	$25	83¢
Vicodin ES (hydrocodone with acetaminophen)	7.5/750	Hydrocodone with acetaminophen	Take 1 tablet every 4-6 hrs. as needed.	30	$25	83¢

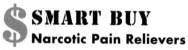

$ SMART BUY
Narcotic Pain Relievers

For mild to moderate pain relievers, your Smart Buy is a generic version of hydrocodone. This drug tends to cause less of a problem with nausea than codeine and does a better job of relieving pain than the Darvon (propoxyphene) products. Also, it doesn't cause the constipation, dry mouth, and blurred vision seen with many tricyclic antidepressants (see the following section). Buy the generic version for the best savings. Because this drug is a controlled substance, quantities typically are limited.

For severe pain relief, your Smart Buy is Oxycontin. This long-acting form of oxy-codone does a very good job and causes less drowsiness and constipation than some of the other strong narcotics. Because this drug is still under patent, there's not much you can do to save money other than shop around for the best price. Be sure to visit www.smartbuysdrugwise.com for the latest information.

OTHER DRUGS USED TO RELIEVE PAIN

More and more physicians are reaching outside the realm of conventional pain medica-tions to drugs that target pain in other ways. Antidepressants and anticonvulsants have proven quite effective in blocking the pain of pinched nerves and the nerve pain caused by diabetic neuropathies. Drugs prescribed for specialized pain relief include the anti-seizure drug Neurontin (generic name gabapentin), and these tricyclic antidepressants:

1. Elavil (generic name amitriptyline)

2. Sinequan (generic name doxepin)
3. Tofranil (generic name imipramine)
4. Norpramin (generic name desipramine)
5. Pamelor (generic name nortriptyline)

These drugs aren't addictive, but they can cause considerable drowsiness and constipation. (For more specific information about each of these drugs, see Chapter 12, "Prescription Drugs that Affect the Central Nervous System.")

Skeletal muscle relaxers comprise another class of drugs that can be helpful in relieving pain. Often tight muscles (from overworking a muscle group or otherwise injuring muscle tissue, for example) can cause pain. Relaxing the muscles can help. Currently, doctors may choose from eight muscle relaxers when prescribing on an outpatient basis. These are:

1. Flexeril (generic name cyclobenzaprine)
2. Lioresal (generic name baclofen)
3. Norflex (generic name orphenadrine)
4. Parafon (generic name chlorzoxazone)
5. Robaxin (generic name methocarbamol)
6. Skelaxin (generic name metaxalone)
7. Soma (generic name carisoprodol)
8. Zanaflex (generic name tizanidine)

Most muscle relaxers work on the spinal cord and areas of the brain stem to limit nerves from stimulating spasming muscles. The results can be quite impressive, but because they work in the brain, undesirable side effects often occur. Drowsiness, lightheadedness, and dizziness can limit your ability to perform certain tasks. Use caution when taking these medications, and don't drink alcohol; this can intensify these side effects.

Although no huge differences exist among members of this group, two are closely related to other drugs and could have some of the same side effects.

1. Soma is metabolized in the liver to a barbiturate called meprobamate, a mildly addictive drug. However, no extra restrictions are in place for prescribing products that contain carisoprodol, unlike other drugs with addictive potential.
2. Flexeril is so closely related to tricyclic antidepressants that taking both at once could lead to serious side effects, such as irregular heartbeats. If you're taking a tricyclic antidepressant, talk with your doctor before starting a drug containing cyclobenzaprine to treat pain.

Other Drugs that Relieve Pain

PRODUCT	STRENGTH PER DOSE	ACTIVE INGREDIENT	USUAL DOSAGE	TYPICAL QUANTITY	TYPICAL PRICE	PRICE PER DAY
Amitriptyline	10mg	Amitriptyline	Take 1 tablet daily.	30	$10	33¢
Amitriptyline	25mg	Amitriptyline	Take 1 tablet daily.	30	$10	33¢
Amitriptyline	50mg	Amitriptyline	Take 1 tablet daily.	30	$10	33¢
Amitriptyline	75mg	Amitriptyline	Take 1 tablet daily.	30	$10	33¢
Amitriptyline	100mg	Amitriptyline	Take 1 tablet daily.	30	$10	33¢
Baclofen	10mg	Baclofen	Take 1 tablet 3 times a day.	90	$20	67¢
Baclofen	20mg	Baclofen	Take 1 tablet 3 times a day.	90	$25	83¢
Carisoprodol	350mg	Carisoprodol	Take 1 tablet 3 times a day.	90	$35	$1.17
Chlorzoxazone	500mg	Chlorzoxazone	Take 1 tablet 3 times a day.	90	$30	$1
Cyclobenzaprine	10mg	Cyclobenzaprine	Take 1 tablet 3 times a day.	90	$30	$1
Desipramine	10mg	Desipramine	Take 1 tablet daily.	30	$10	33¢
Desipramine	25mg	Desipramine	Take 1 tablet daily.	30	$10	33¢
Desipramine	50mg	Desipramine	Take 1 tablet daily.	30	$10	33¢
Desipramine	75mg	Desipramine	Take 1 tablet daily.	30	$15	50¢
Desipramine	100mg	Desipramine	Take 1 tablet daily.	30	$20	67¢
Doxepin	10mg	Doxepin	Take 1 capsule daily.	30	$15	50¢
Doxepin	25mg	Doxepin	Take 1 capsule daily.	30	$15	50¢
Doxepin	50mg	Doxepin	Take 1 capsule daily.	30	$15	50¢
Doxepin	75mg	Doxepin	Take 1 capsule daily.	30	$15	50¢
Doxepin	100mg	Doxepin	Take 1 capsule daily.	30	$15	50¢
Elavil (amitriptyline)	10mg	Amitriptyline	Take 1 tablet daily.	30	$15	50¢
Elavil (amitriptyline)	25mg	Amitriptyline	Take 1 tablet daily.	30	$25	83¢
Elavil (amitriptyline)	50mg	Amitriptyline	Take 1 tablet daily.	30	$35	$1.17
Elavil (amitriptyline)	75mg	Amitriptyline	Take 1 tablet daily.	30	$50	$1.67
Elavil (amitriptyline)	100mg	Amitriptyline	Take 1 tablet daily.	30	$65	$2.17
Flexeril (cyclobenzaprine)	10mg	Cyclobenzaprine	Take 1 tablet 3 times a day.	90	$110	$3.67
Imipramine	10mg	Imipramine	Take 1 tablet daily.	30	$15	50¢
Imipramine	25mg	Imipramine	Take 1 tablet daily.	30	$15	50¢
Imipramine	50mg	Imipramine	Take 1 tablet daily.	30	$15	50¢

PRODUCT	STRENGTH PER DOSE	ACTIVE INGREDIENT	USUAL DOSAGE	TYPICAL QUANTITY	TYPICAL PRICE	PRICE PER DAY
Lioresal (baclofen)	10mg	Baclofen	Take 1 tablet 3 times a day.	90	$75	$2.50
Lioresal (baclofen)	20mg	Baclofen	Take 1 tablet 3 times a day.	90	$125	$4.17
$ Methocarbamol	500mg	Methocarbamol	Take 1 tablet 3 times a day.	90	$25	83¢
$ Methocarbamol	750mg	Methocarbamol	Take 1 tablet 3 times a day.	90	$30	$1
$ Neurontin (gabapentin)	100mg	Gabapentin	Take 1 capsule 3 times a day.	90	$60	$2
$ Neurontin (gabapentin)	300mg	Gabapentin	Take 1 capsule 3 times a day.	90	$115	$3.83
$ Neurontin (gabapentin)	400mg	Gabapentin	Take 1 capsule 3 times a day.	90	$130	$4.33
$ Neurontin (gabapentin)	600mg	Gabapentin	Take 1 tablet 3 times a day.	90	$200	$6.67
$ Neurontin (gabapentin)	800mg	Gabapentin	Take 1 tablet 3 times a day.	90	$230	$7.67
Norflex (orphenadrine)	100mg	Orphenadrine	Take 1 tablet 3 times a day.	90	$200	$6.67
Norpramin (desipramine)	10mg	Desipramine	Take 1 tablet daily.	30	$25	83¢
Norpramin (desipramine)	25mg	Desipramine	Take 1 tablet daily.	30	$30	$1
Norpramin (desipramine)	50mg	Desipramine	Take 1 tablet daily.	30	$50	$1.67
Norpramin (desipramine)	75mg	Desipramine	Take 1 tablet daily.	30	$60	$2
Norpramin (desipramine)	100mg	Desipramine	Take 1 tablet daily.	30	$90	$3
Nortriptyline	10mg	Nortriptyline	Take 1 capsule daily.	30	$15	50¢
Nortriptyline	25mg	Nortriptyline	Take 1 capsule daily.	30	$15	50¢
Nortriptyline	50mg	Nortriptyline	Take 1 capsule daily.	30	$15	50¢
Nortriptyline	75mg	Nortriptyline	Take 1 capsule daily.	30	$17	57¢
Orphenadrine	100mg	Orphenadrine	Take 1 tablet 3 times a day.	90	$110	$3.67
Pamelor (nortriptyline)	10mg	Nortriptyline	Take 1 capsule daily.	30	$30	$1
Pamelor (nortriptyline)	25mg	Nortriptyline	Take 1 capsule daily.	30	$65	$2.17
Pamelor (nortriptyline)	50mg	Nortriptyline	Take 1 capsule daily.	30	$105	$3.50
Pamelor (nortriptyline)	75mg	Nortriptyline	Take 1 capsule daily.	30	$150	$5
Parafon Forte DSC (chlorzoxazone)	500mg	Chlorzoxazone	Take 1 tablet 3 times a day.	90	$130	$4.33
$ Robaxin (methocarbamol)	500mg	Methocarbamol	Take 1 tablet 3 times a day.	90	$70	$2.33
$ Robaxin (methocarbamol)	750mg	Methocarbamol	Take 1 tablet 3 times a day.	90	$100	$3.33
Sinequan (doxepin)	10mg	Doxepin	Take 1 capsule daily.	30	$25	83¢
Sinequan (doxepin)	25mg	Doxepin	Take 1 capsule daily.	30	$25	83¢
Sinequan (doxepin)	50mg	Doxepin	Take 1 capsule daily.	30	$30	$1

PRODUCT	STRENGTH PER DOSE	ACTIVE INGREDIENT	USUAL DOSAGE	TYPICAL QUANTITY	TYPICAL PRICE	PRICE PER DAY
Sinequan (doxepin)	75mg	Doxepin	Take 1 capsule daily.	30	$40	$1.33
Sinequan (doxepin)	100mg	Doxepin	Take 1 capsule daily.	30	$50	$1.67
Skelaxin (metaxalone)	400mg	Metaxalone	Take 1 tablet 3 times a day.	90	$85	$2.83
Soma (carisoprodol)	350mg	Carisoprodol	Take 1 tablet 3 times a day.	90	$275	$9.17
Tofranil (imipramine)	10mg	Imipramine	Take 1 tablet daily.	30	$25	83¢
Tofranil (imipramine)	25mg	Imipramine	Take 1 tablet daily.	30	$35	$1.17
Tofranil (imipramine)	50mg	Imipramine	Take 1 tablet daily.	30	$55	$1.83
Zanaflex (tizanidine)	2mg	Tizanidine	Take 1 tablet 3 times a day.	90	$125	$4.17
Zanaflex (tizanidine)	4mg	Tizanidine	Take 1 tablet 3 times a day.	90	$125	$4.17

$ SMART BUY
Other Drugs that Relieve Pain

Among the muscle relaxers, we prefer Robaxin. It lacks Flexeril's potential cardiac side effects, there's no risk of addiction, and it causes less drowsiness than some of the other muscle relaxers. To save money with this drug, purchase its generic version, methocarbamol, in bulk if you'll be taking it for some time.

For pinched nerves or diabetic neuropathy, we recommend you first try Neurontin. It's more expensive than the tricyclic antidepressants, especially because no generic is available, but it does a very good job at slowing nerve-generated pain, and it has fewer anticholinergic side effects. If Neurontin's price is too steep, try amitriptyline (the generic version of Elavil); it works a little better than the other tricyclic antidepressants and produces a little less drowsiness.

DRUGS TO TREAT MIGRAINE HEADACHES

Recent years have seen major breakthroughs in treatments for migraine headaches. Before 1992, people who suffered from migraines were limited to NSAIDs, narcotic pain relievers, beta-blockers, and ergotamine with caffeine combinations (which had rather unpleasant side effects). Although these provided moderate relief, they did nothing to end the migraine. Today, several drugs are available that actually interrupt and stop migraines. These potent drugs work by stimulating serotonin receptors in the brain, which constricts the blood vessels there and interrupts the migraine. These drugs are:

1. Axert (generic name almotriptan)
2. Imitrex (generic name sumatriptan)
3. Maxalt (generic name rizatriptan)
4. Zomig (generic name zolmitriptan)

These drugs are very effective, but they have drawbacks. First, they aren't cheap. In fact, they're quite expensive. Just one Imitrex 50mg tablet costs around $17. This is far more expensive than a dose of codeine. But most migraine sufferers find it far more effective—and it's considerably cheaper than a trip to the emergency room for a shot of Demerol. Second, you must take these drugs at the onset of a migraine. They're less effective once the migraine is underway.

Further, you shouldn't take these drugs if you have high blood pressure, high cholesterol, are obese, have diabetes, are a smoker, or have a strong family history of heart

Drugs to Treat Migraine Headaches

PRODUCT	STRENGTH PER DOSE	ACTIVE INGREDIENT	USUAL DOSAGE	TYPICAL QUANTITY	TYPICAL PRICE	PRICE PER DAY
Axert (almotriptan)	12.5mg	Almotriptan	Take 1 tablet at onset of headache.	6	$70	$11.67
Imitrex (sumatriptan)	25mg	Sumatriptan	Take 1 tablet at onset of headache.	9	$150	$16.67
Imitrex (sumatriptan)	50mg	Sumatriptan	Take 1 tablet at onset of headache.	9	$150	$16.67
Imitrex (sumatriptan)	100mg	Sumatriptan	Take 1 tablet at onset of headache.	9	$150	$16.67
Imitrex injection (sumatriptan)	6mg	Sumatriptan	Inject once at onset of headache.	1 box	$90	$45
Imitrex Nasal Spray (sumatriptan)	20mg	Sumatriptan	Spray once in one nostril at onset of headache.	1 box	$140	$23.33
Imitrex Nasal Spray (sumatriptan)	5mg	Sumatriptan	Spray once in one nostril at onset of headache.	1 box	$140	$23.33
Maxalt (rizatriptan)	5mg	Rizatriptan	Take 1 tablet at onset of headache.	6	$95	$15.83
Maxalt (rizatriptan)	10mg	Rizatriptan	Take 1 tablet at onset of headache.	6	$95	$15.83
Maxalt MLT (rizatriptan)	5mg	Rizatriptan	Take 1 tablet at onset of headache.	3	$95	$31.67
Maxalt MLT (rizatriptan)	10mg	Rizatriptan	Take 1 tablet at onset of headache.	3	$95	$31.67
Zomig (zolmitriptan)	2.5mg	Zolmitriptan	Take 1 tablet at onset of headache.	6	$100	$16.67
Zomig (zolmitriptan)	5mg	Zolmitriptan	Take 1 tablet at onset of headache.	3	$100	$33.33

disease. Heart attacks and deaths have resulted among people with these conditions who also use these drugs. If your doctor is considering prescribing one of these drugs for you and you have any of these cardiovascular problems, discuss the risks with him or her. Finally, if you're taking any of the SSRI antidepressants (Zoloft, Prozac, Paxil, Celexa, or Luvox), don't take one of these drugs to treat a migraine. SSRI antidepressants, you might remember from Chapter 12, work by increasing the levels of serotonin in your brain. Further increasing serotonin levels can result in a very serious situation.

 ## SMART BUY
Drugs to Treat Migraine Headaches

For migraine headaches, your Smart Buy is Maxalt. We think it works as well as the other drugs that relieve migraine pain by acting on serotonin receptors, and it usually costs just a little less. For the best savings, ask whether the tablets can be cut, and buy in bulk to cut your per-dose cost from $16 to less than $8—a savings of over 50 percent.

 ## SMART OPTIONS FOR SAVINGS
Prescription Drugs to Treat Pain and Inflammation

As always, check our Web site, www.smartbuysdrugwise.com, for updates on prescription and over-the-counter drugs.

And keep in mind the following points:

+ Buying a generic version here can save you big bucks. If your doctor prescribes an NSAID that's also available in an over-the-counter version, compare prices to see whether it would be cheaper to buy the nonprescription form.
+ Because of their addictive potential, narcotics are considerably restricted. Although checking on the price of a generic version is always a good idea, usually you can't purchase narcotics in bulk.
+ You can't buy some of these drugs legally from Internet or mail-order pharmacies, or in other countries for use in the U.S.

Chapter 14

Prescription Drugs to Treat Gastrointestinal Conditions

Digestive disorders account for 45 million doctor visits each year in the U.S. In today's fast-paced and stressful world, one of the more common ailments is a buildup of acid in the stomach. This can result in health problems such as indigestion, heartburn, and gastroesophageal reflux disorder (GERD), and it can contribute to the discomfort of ulcers and colitis.

DRUGS THAT REDUCE STOMACH ACID

When it comes to treating excess stomach acid or ulcers, the most common approach is to prescribe drugs that reduce the amount of acid in the stomach. Two groups of drugs are used to do this—H_2 blockers and proton pump inhibitors. A third group of drugs takes a different approach, creating a protective physical barrier over stomach ulcers that allows them to heal.

Bacteria Causes Most Ulcers

The vast majority of stomach ulcers are caused by the bacteria known as *Helicobacter pylori*. Treatment often involves a two-pronged approach, with antibiotics to kill the bacteria and a drug that lowers the amount of acid in the stomach to reduce irritation.

HISTAMINE H$_2$ BLOCKERS

Histamine H$_2$ blockers have been on the market for many years. These specialized anti-histamines block histamine receptors in the stomach. (They have no effect on allergic histamine responses.) When triggered, these receptors cause the stomach to secrete acid; blocking them inhibits this response. Common side effects of some H$_2$ blockers include headaches, dizziness, confusion (especially in the elderly), and diarrhea. Drugs in this group include:

1. Axid (generic name nizatidine)
2. Pepcid (generic name famotidine)
3. Tagamet (generic name cimetidine)
4. Zantac (generic name ranitidine)

▶ Different Kinds of Antihistamines

You may wonder why other antihistamines, such as Benadryl, aren't helpful for the stomach. Those antihistamines block H$_1$ receptors, which aren't located in the stomach. Likewise, H$_2$ blockers are ineffective for treating hay fever, because there are no H$_2$ receptors in the nose.

The H$_2$ blockers have become very popular. They're effective and very safe—so safe, in fact, that the FDA allows lower strength formulas to be sold over the counter. You sometimes can save huge amounts of money by buying the over-the-counter versions. To make sure you get the dose your doctor has prescribed, ask your pharmacist how many tablets of the over-the-counter product you must take. Even though you might have to take 2 or 3 pills of nonprescription product compared to one of the prescription form, the savings can be worth the inconvenience.

There's an exception if your insurance plan covers the prescription-strength product. Say your doctor prescribes Pepcid 20mg, the prescription-strength formula. You can expect to pay around $65 for 30 tablets. With a typical 20 percent insurance co-payment, your out-of-pocket cost will be $13. To buy 60 tablets of Pepcid-AC 10mg, the nonprescription-strength formula, you'll pay $17. (You must take 2 tablets to match the 20mg dose.) Buying the prescription strength through your insurance plan will save you $4. If you have no insurance, or if your health insurance plan doesn't cover either prescription drugs or this drug in particular, then the over-the-counter product is clearly the better choice; you'll save nearly 74 percent. Other than strength, there's no difference between prescription-strength and over-the-counter products.

No Insurance for OTC Versions

Insurance plans rarely, if ever, pay for the over-the-counter forms of H_2 blockers. And some won't pay for a prescription-strength product, either, if an over-the-counter version is available. Check your policy, or ask your pharmacist, before you decide which choice is the better deal.

Among the H2 blockers, cimetidine, found in Tagamet, is notorious for causing adverse drug interactions. Because it's an enzyme inhibitor, it slows the elimination of many other drugs from the body. For example, if you have asthma and take theophylline to keep your airways open, and then you take a product that contains cimetidine (such as Tagamet) for heartburn, the cimetidine will slow the action of the liver enzymes involved in removing theophylline from your blood. If you continue to take the same amount of theophylline you took before you started taking the cimetidine product, the amount of theophylline in your blood could elevate to dangerous levels. Many deaths have resulted from this combination. This is of extra concern for pharmacists, now that Tagamet and other cimetidine products are available over the counter.

Don't Mix Antacids and H_2 Blockers

Over-the-counter antacids such as Maalox and Mylanta often are used to neutralize acid in the stomach. For more information on these products, see Chapter 19, "Over-the-Counter Gastrointestinal Remedies." These should not be taken at the same time as an H_2 blocker. Antacids can limit the absorption, and thus the effectiveness, of several H_2 blockers. To avoid this problem, separate these doses by at least 2 hours.

PROTON PUMP INHIBITORS

Proton pumps are acid-making cells in the stomach walls. As the name implies, these cells pump acid into the stomach. Slowing or blocking these pumps reduces the amount of acid that makes it into the stomach. Proton pump inhibitors tend to be more effective than the H_2 blockers at reducing stomach acid, but they're more expensive. A 30-day supply of Prilosec 20mg normally will cost around $125; compare this to the $60 you'd expect to pay for a 30-day supply of famotidine 40mg (generic for Pepcid). Doctors usually will begin treatment with an H_2 blocker. If that doesn't quite do the job, then they prescribe one of these stronger drugs. Common side effects for these drugs include headaches, diarrhea, nausea, and abdominal pain.

Commonly prescribed drugs in this group include:

1. Aciphex (generic name rabeprazole)
2. Prevacid (generic name lansoprazole)
3. Prilosec (generic name omeprazole)
4. Protonix (generic name pantoprazole)

▶ Have a Cola Drink!

Proton pump inhibitors are so good at reducing acid levels in the stomach that drugs that *need* some acid in the stomach before they can be absorbed into the blood may not be effective when you take them. If you must take Nizoral, ampicillin, Lanoxin, cyanocobalamin (vitamin B_{12}), or iron, take your dose with a can of Coca-Cola or other cola soda. Colas are acidic enough to help you absorb these drugs even in the presence of a proton pump inhibitor.

DRUGS THAT FORM A PHYSICAL BARRIER OVER ULCERS

Imagine that you have a stomach ulcer. Wouldn't it make sense to cover that ulcer with some kind of shield to prevent acid from reaching it? A third approach to treating conditions caused by excess stomach acid is to provide a physical barrier that shields stomach ulcers from stomach acid, giving them time to heal. Two products currently on the market do just that.

Carafate (generic name sucralfate) binds to certain protein areas present in ulcers. The complex that forms as a result creates a shield that blocks acid, forming a chemical "bandage." This allows the ulcer time to heal without receiving further damage. Very few side effects are associated with taking sucralfate. The most common is constipation. Take sucralfate at least one hour before each meal and at bedtime. Don't take antacids less than half an hour before or after you take sucralfate.

The other drug that provides a physical barrier to stomach acid is Cytotec (generic name misoprostol). The barrier this drug creates doesn't result from a binding complex. Instead, it works by stimulating mucous production to form a more "natural" acid barrier. It's a very good choice for most people. Women who are pregnant or who think they may become pregnant should never take Cytotec. Fetal fatalities are so common with this drug that, before they can get a prescription for Cytotec, women of childbearing age must sign a statement confirming that they have received written and verbal information about the risks of using this drug during pregnancy. Furthermore, a woman must have a pregnancy test that shows a negative result no later than two weeks before beginning therapy, and she should begin therapy only on the second or third day of her next normal menstrual period. Other side effects of misoprostol include diarrhea, abdominal pain, nausea, and flatulence. To limit side effects, take Cytotec (misoprostol) with food.

Drugs to Reduce the Effects of Stomach Acid

PRODUCT	STRENGTH PER DOSE	TYPE	ACTIVE INGREDIENT	USUAL DOSAGE	TYPICAL QUANTITY	TYPICAL PRICE	PRICE PER DAY
Aciphex (rabeprazole)	20mg	Proton pump inhibitor	Rabeprazole	Take 1 tablet daily.	30	$130	$4.33
Carafate (sucralfate)	1g	Barrier	Sucralfate	Take 1 tablet 4 times a day.	120	$125	$4.17
Cimetidine	300mg	H2 blocker	Cimetidine	Take 1 tablet 3 times a day.	90	$40	$1.33
Cimetidine	400mg	H2 blocker	Cimetidine	Take 1 tablet 2 times a day.	60	$35	$1.17
Cimetidine	800mg	H2 blocker	Cimetidine	Take 1 tablet daily.	30	$30	$1
Cytotec (misoprostol)	100 mcg	Barrier	Misoprostol	Take 1 tablet 4 times a day.	60	$55	$3.67
Cytotec (misoprostol)	200 mcg	Barrier	Misoprostol	Take 1 tablet 4 times a day.	60	$80	$5.33
Famotidine	20mg	H2 blocker	Famotidine	Take 1 tablet 2 times a day.	60	$60	$2

PRODUCT	STRENGTH PER DOSE	TYPE	ACTIVE INGREDIENT	USUAL DOSAGE	TYPICAL QUANTITY	TYPICAL PRICE	PRICE PER DAY
Famotidine	40mg	H2 blocker	Famotidine	Take 1 tablet daily.	30	$60	$2
$ Pepcid (famotidine)	20mg	H2 blocker	Famotidine	Take 1 tablet 2 times a day.	60	$130	$4.33
$ Pepcid (famotidine)	40mg	H2 blocker	Famotidine	Take 1 tablet daily.	30	$120	$4
Prevacid (lansoprazole)	15mg	Proton pump inhibitor	Lansoprazole	Take 1 capsule daily.	30	$129	$4.30
Prevacid (lansoprazole)	30mg	Proton pump inhibitor	Lansoprazole	Take 1 capsule daily.	30	$129	$4.30
Prilosec (omeprazole)	10mg	Proton pump inhibitor	Omeprazole	Take 1 capsule daily.	30	$125	$4.17
Prilosec (omeprazole)	20 mg	Proton pump inhibitor	Omeprazole	Take 1 capsule daily.	30	$125	$4.17
$ Protonix (pantoprazole)	40mg	Proton pump inhibitor	Pantoprazole	Take 1 tablet daily.	30	$90	$3
Ranitidine	150mg	H2 blocker	Ranitidine	Take 1 tablet 2 times a day.	60	$30	$1
Ranitidine	300mg	H2 blocker	Ranitidine	Take 1 tablet daily.	30	$50	$1.67
Sucralfate	1g	Barrier	Sucralfate	Take 1 tablet 4 times a day.	120	$60	$2
Tagamet (cimetidine)	300mg	H2 blocker	Cimetidine	Take 1 tablet 3 times a day.	90	$115	$3.83
Tagamet (cimetidine)	400mg	H2 blocker	Cimetidine	Take 1 tablet 2 times a day.	60	$125	$4.17
Tagamet (cimetidine)	800mg	H2 blocker	Cimetidine	Take 1 tablet daily.	30	$100	$3.33
Zantac (ranitidine)	150mg	H2 blocker	Ranitidine	Take 1 tablet 2 times a day.	60	$125	$4.17
Zantac (ranitidine)	300mg	H2 blocker	Ranitidine	Take 1 tablet daily.	30	$300	$10
Tagamet (cimetidine)	400mg	H2 blocker	Cimetidine	Take 1 tablet 2 times a day.	60	$125	$4.17
Tagamet (cimetidine)	800mg	H2 blocker	Cimetidine	Take 1 tablet daily.	30	$100	$3.33
$ Zantac (ranitidine)	150mg	H2 blocker	Ranitidine	Take 1 tablet 2 times a day.	60	$125	$4.17
$ Zantac (ranitidine)	300mg	H2 blocker	Ranitidine	Take 1 tablet daily.	30	$300	$10

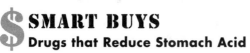

$ SMART BUYS
Drugs that Reduce Stomach Acid

If your insurance doesn't cover H_2 blockers because over-the-counter versions are available (even though they come in weaker strengths), or if you have no insurance (and sometimes if you do, depending on your co-pay), your Smart Buy is one of the over-the-counter versions, and increase the dose. You'll save huge amounts of money. If you have insurance that pays for H_2 blockers, your Smart Buy is either Zantac or Pepcid. These two products cause no drug interaction problems, as Tagamet does, and they're usually less expensive than Axid. Whether you choose Zantac or Pepcid really doesn't matter. To save money, though, we suggest you ask whether the tablets can be cut, buy the generic version, and purchase in bulk quantities. Also, ask your pharmacist for coupons the drug manufacturer may have available.

For proton pump inhibitors, the Smart Buy is Protonix. All of these drugs are fairly equivalent, but this drug is a little less expensive. To save money when purchasing Protonix, consider buying in bulk—but prepare for sticker shock. A 3-month supply of Protonix (90 tablets) will cost about $250, but it affords you a per-dose cost of about $2.77, an percent savings. Buying a 30-day supply (30 tablets) will cost around $90, or about $3 a dose.

For drugs that produce a barrier to acid when treating ulcers, your Smart Buy is Carafate. It has, by far, the fewest side effects and does a good job. To save money with Carafate, purchase the generic in large quantities to reduce your per-dose cost by two-thirds.

DRUGS TO TREAT INTESTINAL CRAMPING AND RELATED PROBLEMS

If you have, or ever have had, intestinal cramping, you know how miserable it makes you feel. This problem can keep you from going to work or school. Several conditions can be responsible for these potentially debilitating symptoms.

DRUGS TO TREAT IRRITABLE BOWEL SYNDROME (IBS)

This common condition affects an estimated 35 million Americans, 75 percent of them female. Researchers are unsure why this condition afflicts women more than men, but some believe that because the symptoms seem to coincide with a woman's menstrual cycle, a hormonal component may be involved.

The first step in bringing IBS under control is to increase physical activity, eliminate certain foods from your diet—especially those to which you may be allergic—and to use certain relaxation techniques. Heating pads, hot baths, and warm drinks to slow abdominal contractions also can help.

Many drugs used to treat IBS work by relaxing the intestinal muscles. The following products are among those often prescribed for this purpose:

1. Bellergal-S (belladonna alkaloids with phenobarbital and ergotamine)

2. Bentyl (generic name dicyclomine)
3. Donnatal (belladonna alkaloids with phenobarbital)
4. Levsin (generic name hyoscyamine)
5. Levsinex (generic name hyoscyamine)
6. Librax (chlordiazepoxide with clidinium)

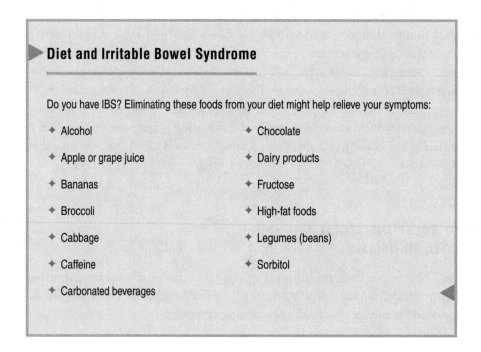

Diet and Irritable Bowel Syndrome

Do you have IBS? Eliminating these foods from your diet might help relieve your symptoms:

✦ Alcohol	✦ Chocolate
✦ Apple or grape juice	✦ Dairy products
✦ Bananas	✦ Fructose
✦ Broccoli	✦ High-fat foods
✦ Cabbage	✦ Legumes (beans)
✦ Caffeine	✦ Sorbitol
✦ Carbonated beverages	

We really don't prefer one product over another here. Although doctors seem to choose those with fewer ingredients (Levsin and Bentyl), we recommend using whatever works. Intestinal cramping can be such an uncomfortable ailment that if it takes a product that has ingredients in it to do the job, take it. Potential side effects for these drugs include drowsiness, blurred vision, constipation, and dry mouth.

Other drugs often used to relieve IBS symptoms target diarrhea and constipation; still others are antidepressants. Probably the most commonly used antidiarrheal drug is Imodium (generic name loperamide). Related somewhat to opiate derivatives, this drug does a fantastic job of reducing diarrhea. Despite its opiate connection, drowsiness and physical dependence usually aren't a concern, because so little of this drug reaches the brain. Instead, its effects are produced at specific problem sites in the intestines. Another product that provides relief from diarrhea for some people is cholestyramine powder. Usually used to lower cholesterol, this powder works by absorbing excess fluid in the intestines. Take care, though, to maintain proper fluid intake. Too much of this powder without enough fluid can lead to some serious constipation problems.

Some people who have IBS have trouble with constipation. If you're one of them, try a bulk-forming laxative. Metamucil and Citrucel are two very good brands available in generic form, and they usually work better than simply adding bran to your diet. Bran can cause abdominal pain and bloating in people who have IBS. (For more information about bulk-forming laxatives, see Chapter 19, "Over-the-Counter Gastrointestinal Remedies.")

Because antidepressants have analgesic (pain-relieving) properties, doctors often prescribe them to treat IBS. Those used most commonly are the tricyclic antidepressants, such as amitriptyline and desipramine, to help relieve abdominal pain and mild diarrhea. These drugs relieve pain by slowing the transmission of pain signals from nerves to brain. They also work to reduce diarrhea by relaxing the muscles of the intestines. Side effects to watch for include constipation, dry mouth, blurred vision, and drowsiness.

On the horizon are drugs known as 5-HT3 receptor antagonists. Serotonin triggers 5-HT3 receptors located in the intestines, which causes intestinal muscles to contract. Blocking (or "antagonizing") these receptors decreases abdominal pain, flatulence, and diarrhea. The only 5-HT3 receptor antagonist that's been tried for IBS is Lotronex (generic name alosetron). This drug was very effective at reducing IBS symptoms, but its side effects included a high rate of constipation and intestinal blockage severe enough to cause several deaths; the manufacturer pulled the product off the market. In those instances when it didn't cause severe constipation, though, the drug's success was remarkable. We expect to see Lotronex become available again in the near future for severe cases of IBS that don't respond to other treatment.

DRUGS TO TREAT ULCERATIVE COLITIS AND CROHN'S DISEASE

Ulcerative colitis and Crohn's disease are other long-term ailments characterized by inflammation and irritation of the intestines. Bloody stools are the most common symptom. The drugs used to treat the diarrhea and intestinal cramping common with IBS provide some relief, but doctors usually add drugs to relieve inflammation to the treatment regimen. In ulcerative colitis and Crohn's disease, it's the inflammation that sets the stage for the unpleasant symptoms. Reducing the inflammation usually lessens irritation, diarrhea, and cramping. Anti-inflammatory drugs commonly prescribed for this group of ailments include:

1. Asacol (generic name mesalamine)
2. Azulfidine (generic name sulfasalazine)

3. Dipentum (generic name olsalazine)
4. Pentasa (generic name mesalamine)
5. Rowasa (generic name mesalamine) suppositories and enemas

Of these drugs, Dipentum usually is preferred. It causes much less severe side effects than Asacol or Azulfidine. Side effects to watch for with any of these drugs include headaches, diarrhea, abdominal pain or cramping, and nausea.

▶ Getting the Drug to the Problem

Why aren't regular NSAIDs used to treat ulcerative colitis and Crohn's disease? To be effective, a sufficient amount of the drug must reach the colon. Before regular NSAIDs reach the colon, however, most of them are absorbed into the bloodstream and are removed from the body by the kidneys. This isn't the case with the other drugs used for these conditions. For example, about 99 percent of olsalazine taken orally reaches the colon.

Drugs to Treat Intestinal Cramping and Related Problems

PRODUCT	STRENGTH PER DOSE	USED TO TREAT	ACTIVE INGREDIENT	USUAL DOSAGE	TYPICAL QUANTITY	TYPICAL PRICE	PRICE PER DAY
Asacol (mesalamine)	400mg	Ulcerative colitis, Crohn's disease	Mesalamine	Take 2 tablets 3 times a day.	90	$90	$2
Azulfidine (sulfasalazine)	500mg	Ulcerative colitis, Crohn's disease	Sulfasalazine	Take 4 tablets a day.	120	$50	$1.67
Azulfidine Entabs (sulfasalazine)	500mg	Ulcerative colitis, Crohn's disease	Sulfasalazine	Take 4 tablets a day.	120	$50	$1.67
Belladonna with phenobarbit	N/A	IBS	Belladonna alalkaloids with phenobarbital	Take 3–8 tablets a day.	90	$15	50¢
Bentyl (dicyclomine)	10mg	IBS	Dicyclomine	Take 1 capsule 4 times a day.	120	$50	42¢

PRODUCT	STRENGTH PER DOSE	USED TO TREAT	ACTIVE INGREDIENT	USUAL DOSAGE	TYPICAL QUANTITY	TYPICAL PRICE	PRICE PER DAY
$ Bentyl (dicyclomine)	20mg	IBS	Dicyclomine	Take 1 tablet 4 times a day.	120	$65	54¢
Chlordiazepoxide with clidinium	5/2.5mg	IBS	Chlordiazepoxide with clidinium	Take 3–8 capsules a day.	90	$25	83¢
Dicyclomine	10mg	IBS	Dicyclomine	Take 1 capsule 4 times a day.	120	$33	28¢
Dicyclomine	20mg	IBS	Dicyclomine	Take 1 tablet 4 times a day.	120	$40	33¢
$ Dipentum (olsalazine)	250mg	Ulcerative colitis, Crohn's disease	Olsalazine	Take 4 capsules 2 times a day.	100	$135	$5.40
Donnatal (belladonna alkaloids with phenobarbital)	N/A	IBS	Belladonna alkaloids with phenobarbital	Take 3–8 tablets a day.	90	$40	$1.33
Hyoscyamine	0.125mg	IBS	Hyoscyamine	Take 3–8 tablets a day.	90	$35	$1.17
Hyoscyamine	0.375mg	IBS	Hyoscyamine	Take 1 capsule twice a day.	60	$35	58¢
$ Levsin(hyoscyamine)	0.125mg	IBS	Hyoscyamine	Take 3–8 tablets a day.	90	$70	$2.33
$ Levsinex(hyoscyamine)	0.375mg	IBS	Hyoscyamine	Take 1 capsule twice a day.	60	$77	$1.28
Librax(chlordiazepoxide with clidinium)	5/2.5mg	IBS	Chlordiazepoxide with clidinium	Take 3–8 capsules a day.	90	$175	$5.83
Pentasa(mesalamine)	250mg	Ulcerative colitis, Crohn's disease	Mesalamine	Take 4 capsules 4 times a day.	240	$145	$2.42
Rowasa (mesalamine enemas)	4 grams	Ulcerative colitis, Crohn's disease	Mesalamine	Use 1 enema a day.	7 bottles	$115	$16.43
Sulfasalazine	500mg	Ulcerative colitis, Crohn's disease	Sulfasalazine	Take 4 tablets a day.	120	$30	$1

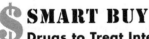

$ SMART BUY
Drugs to Treat Intestinal Cramping and Related Problems

For drugs used to relieve intestinal cramping due to IBS, your Smart Buys are Levsin or Bentyl. All the products work fairly well, but these two contain fewer ingredients and tend to produce fewer side effects. Of these two, we recommend you try Bentyl first; it's considerably less expensive. For the greatest savings, ask whether the tablets can be cut, buy the generic version, and buy in larger quantities.

For drugs used to relieve diarrhea that occurs with IBS, the Smart Buy is Imodium. This drug does a good job and produces few side effects. It's also much more palatable than the cholestyramine powder that's sometimes used. To save money with Imodium, purchase the generic form (loperamide) and buy it in large quantities. And be sure to check the price of over-the-counter loperamide. You may find that buying it that way will save you even more money.

For ulcerative colitis and Crohn's disease, your Smart Buy is Dipentum. This is a good drug that has far fewer side effects than some of the other drugs used for these conditions. To save money on Dipentum, about all you can do is purchase it in larger quantities. Your savings won't be great, though—only about a nickel a dose.

$ SMART OPTIONS FOR SAVINGS
Drugs that Treat Gastrointestinal Conditions

For many gastrointestinal problems, the same drugs are available in prescription and over-the-counter versions. Although the prescription version is stronger, it's also more expensive. It's worth checking out the over-the-counter versions to see whether buying those instead would save you money. Just remember to calculate the amount of the over-the-counter form you must take to equal the dose your doctor wants you to take. Here are some other Smart Options for Savings that might reduce your expenses for these drugs:

1. Buy generic versions. Of course, the newer drugs will still be under patent and consequently unavailable in generic versions. But always ask!
2. Buy in quantity. Even though buying more costs more at the cash register, the savings per dose can really add up.
3. If you live near the Canadian border and it's convenient for you to see a doctor and get your prescriptions filled in Canada, doing so could save you money on some of these drugs.
4. Mail-order and Internet pharmacies are an option if you're taking these drugs regularly and can order them far enough in advance that you don't run out before your new supply arrives. Canadian Web sites might offer the best prices, but they carry the risk that your order might not make it to you (depending on changes in Canadian and U.S. legislative and regulatory actions). Remember to factor in shipping charges when calculating your costs to be sure these options are really saving you money.

Don't forget to check our Web site at www.smartbuysdrugwise.com for the latest information about more ways to save money on these drugs.

Chapter 15

Prescription Drugs to Treat Conditions of the Eyes and Skin

M ost drugs to treat conditions of the eyes and the skin are delivered topically, rather than taken internally. This puts the medication where it's needed quickly and directly, and at the same time avoids side effects that can result from taking drugs systemically (into your bloodstream). Sometimes it's necessary to use both topical and internal drugs, as for some cases of glaucoma or kinds of skin problems. Always ask your doctor whether this is medically necessary to treat your specific condition; there's no point in paying for two drugs if one will do the job.

DRUGS TO TREAT GLAUCOMA

Your eye continually adds new fluid to and drains old fluid from the space between the lens and cornea, maintaining a steady volume and pressure. This fluid is called aqueous humor. When more new fluid is produced than old fluid being drained, the pressure inside the eye increases. This results in a condition called glaucoma, which, left untreated, can lead to damage of the optic nerve and eventually blindness. To restore the aqueous humor to its normal level and pressure, current drug therapies can either reduce fluid production or increase fluid drainage rate. Some drugs do both.

Drops for the eyes that only increase drainage include Isopto Carbachol (generic name carbachol), Isopto Carpine (generic name pilocarpine), and Xalatan (generic name latanoprost).

Of these, we prefer Xalatan, for two reasons. First, it doesn't cause a problem with night vision, as some drugs do. Because carbachol and pilocarpine both cause the pupil to constrict, products that contain these drugs (Isopto Carbachol and Isopto Carpine) can hamper night vision significantly. Second, Xalatan's effects last much longer. Products containing carbachol and pilocarpine can last 8 hours at best, while products that contain latanoprost (such as Xalatan) are good for a full twenty-four.

The following eye-drop products only decrease the production of aqueous humor:

1. Azopt (generic name brinzolamide)
2. Betagan (generic name levobunolol)
3. Betoptic (generic name betaxolol)
4. Ocupres (generic name carteolol)
5. Trusopt (generic name dorzolamide)

Of these, you'll get the best results and the biggest savings with either Betagan or Betoptic. Although both of these drugs provide similar results, the effects of products that contain levobunolol (such as Betagan) last longer. Side effects of Azopt include fatigue and drowsiness. Because Betoptic, Ocupres, and Betagan are beta-blockers (see Chapter 8), common side effects include lowered blood pressure and heart rate, and possibly asthma attacks.

These eye-drop products both increase drainage and decrease production of aqueous humor:

1. Alphagan (generic name brimonidine)
2. Cosopt (combination of dorzolamide and timolol)
3. OptiPranolol (generic name metipranolol)
4. Propine (generic name dipivefrin)
5. Timoptic (generic name timolol)

Propine can sting quite a bit and may also cause rapid heartbeat, arrhythmias, and high blood pressure. Because of this, we prefer either OptiPranolol or Timoptic. These have fewer potential side effects than Propine and last longer than Alphagan. But if you really need to reduce the pressure in your eyes, ask your doctor about the combination product Cosopt.

Some drugs taken orally provide similar results in reducing pressure within the eye. These drugs are good for people who have difficulty using eye drops, but they produce more side effects. Nausea, drowsiness, and an increased sensitivity to sunlight are fairly common. Products we commonly see prescribed are Diamox (generic name acetazolamide) and Neptazane (generic name methazolamide).

Eye Drops Can Affect Your Whole Body

Although systemic (whole-body) side effects from eye drops aren't overly common, they can occur. To minimize this possibility, ask your doctor or pharmacist to show you how to block the channel through which drops can drain—a duct that connects the eye to the nasal cavity. From there, drugs can reach the bloodstream and thus the rest of the body. To limit such absorption, use your index finger to press the ducts in the inside corners of your eyes against the bridge of your nose. Continue applying pressure for about a minute after using eye drops to limit drainage through the duct.

Drugs to Treat Glaucoma

PRODUCT	STRENGTH PER DOSE	TYPE	ACTIVE INGREDIENT	USUAL DOSAGE	TYPICAL QUANTITY	TYPICAL PRICE	PRICE PER ML
Alphagan (brimonidine)	0.2%	Alpha adronergic agonist	Brimonidine	Use 1 drop 3 times a day.	10ml	$70	$7
Azopt (brinzolamide)	1%	Carbonic	Brinzolamide anhydrase inhibitor	Use 1 drop 3 times a day.	15ml	$85	$5.67
Betagan (levobunolol)	0.25%	Beta-blocker	Levobunolol	Use 1-2 drops 2 times a day.	5ml	$29	$5.80
Betagan (levobunolol)	0.5%	Beta-blocker	Levobunolol	Use 1-2 drops once a day.	15ml	$87	$5.80
Betaxolol	0.5%	Beta-blocker	Betaxolol	Use 1-2 drops twice a day.	15ml	$60	$4
Betoptic (betaxolol)	0.5%	Beta-blocker	Betaxolol	Use 1–2 drops 2 times a day.	15ml	$79	$5.27
Betoptic S (betaxolol)	0.25%	Beta-blocker	Betaxolol	Use 1-2 drops twice a day.	15ml	$85	$5.67
Carteolol	1%	Beta-blocker	Carteolol	Use 1 drop 2 times a day.	15ml	$55	$3.67
Cosopt (dorzolamide and timolol)	2% and 0.5%	Carbonic anhydrase inhibitor and beta-blocker	Dorzolamide and timolol	Use 1 drop 2 times a day.	10ml	$93	$9.30

PRODUCT	STRENGTH PER DOSE	TYPE	ACTIVE INGREDIENT	USUAL DOSAGE	TYPICAL QUANTITY	TYPICAL PRICE	PRICE PER ML
Dipivefrin	0.1%	Sympathomimetics	Dipivefrin	Use 1 drop every 12 hrs.	15ml	$27	$1.80
Isopto Carbachol (carbachol)	0.075%	Increases drainage (direct-acting miotic)	Carbachol	Use 2 drops up to 3 times a day.	15ml	$30	$2
Isopto Carbachol (carbachol)	1.5%	Direct-acting miotic	Carbachol	Use 2 drops up to 3 times a day.	15ml	$33	$2.20
Isopto Carbachol (carbachol)	2.25%	Direct-acting miotic	Carbachol	Use 2 drops up to 3 times a day.	15ml	$33	$2.20
Isopto Carbachol (carbachol)	3%	Direct-acting miotic	Carbachol	Use 2 drops up to 3 times a day.	15ml	$38	$2.53
Isopto Carpine (pilocarpine)	0.5%	Direct-acting miotic	Pilocarpine HCl	Use 1-2 drops 3–4 times a day.	15ml	$20	$1.33
Isopto Carpine (pilocarpine	1%	Direct-acting miotic	Pilocarpine HCl	Use 1-2 drops 3-4 times a day.	15ml	$25	$1.67
Isopto Carpine (pilocarpine)	2%	Direct-acting miotic	Pilocarpine HCl	Use 1-2 drops 3-4 times a day.	15ml	$25	$1.67
Isopto Carpine (pilocarpine)	3%	Direct-acting miotic	Pilocarpine HCl	Use 1-2 drops 3-4 times a day.	15ml	$20	$1.33
Isopto Carpine (pilocarpine)	4%	Direct-acting miotic	Pilocarpine HCl	Use 1-2 drops 3-4 times a day.	15ml	$26	$1.73
Isopto Carpine (pilocarpine)	6%	Direct-acting miotic	Pilocarpine HCl	Use 1-2 drops 3-4 times a day.	15ml	$26	$1.73
Levobunolol	0.25%	Beta-blocker	Levobunolol	Use 1-2 drops 2 times a day.	5ml	$15	$3
Levobunolol	0.5%	Beta-blocker	Levobunolol	Use 1-2 drops once a day.	15ml	$20	$1.33
Ocupress (carteolol)	1%	Beta-blocker	Carteolol	Use 1 drop 2 times a day.	15ml	$75	$5
OptiPranolol (metipranolol)	0.3%	Beta-blocker	Metipranolol	Use 1 drop 2 times a day.	10ml	$37	$3.70
Pilocarpine	0.5%	Direct-acting miotic	Pilocarpine HCl	Use 1-2 drops 3-4 times a day.	15ml	$10	67¢
Pilocarpine	1%	Direct-acting miotic	Pilocarpine HCl	Use 1-2 drops 3-4 times a day.	15ml	$7	47¢
Pilocarpine	2%	Direct-acting miotic	Pilocarpine HCl	Use 1-2 drops 3-4 times a day.	15ml	$9	60¢
Pilocarpine	3%	Direct-acting miotic	Pilocarpine HCl	Use 1-2 drops 3-4 times a day.	15ml	$9	60¢
Pilocarpine	4%	Direct-acting miotic	Pilocarpine HCl	Use 1-2 drops 3-4 times a day.	15ml	$11	73¢

PRODUCT	STRENGTH PER DOSE	TYPE	ACTIVE INGREDIENT	USUAL DOSAGE	TYPICAL QUANTITY	TYPICAL PRICE	PRICE PER ML
Pilocarpine	6%	Direct-acting miotic	Pilocarpine HCl	Use 1-2 drops 3-4 times a day.	15ml	$17	$1.13
Propine (dipivefrin)	0.1%	Sympathomimetics	Dipivefrin	Use 1 drop every 12 hrs.	15ml	$75	$5
Timolol	0.25%	Beta-blocker	Timolol	Use 1 drop 2 times a day.	15ml	$26	$1.73
Timolol	0.5%	Beta-blocker	Timolol	Use 1 drop 2 times a day.	15ml	$26	$1.73
Timolol gel forming solution	0.25%	Beta-blocker	Timolol	Use 1 drop 2 times a day.	5ml	$30	$6
Timolol gel forming solution	0.5%	Beta-blocker	Timolol	Use 1 drop 2 times a day.	5ml	$32	$6.40
Timoptic (timolol)	0.25%	Beta-blocker	Timolol	Use 1 drop 2 times a day.	15ml	$57	$3.80
Timoptic (timolol)	0.5%	Beta-blocker	Timolol	Use 1 drop 2 times a day.	15ml	$68	$4.53
Timoptic XE (timolol)	0.25%	Beta-blocker	Timolol	Use 1 drop 2 times a day.	5ml	$40	$8
Timoptic XE (timolol)	0.5%	Beta-blocker	Timolol	Use 1 drop 2 times a day.	5ml	$42	$8.40
Trusopt (dorzolamide) anhydrase inhibitor	2%	Carbonic	Dorzolamide	Use 1 drop 3 times a day.	10ml	$60	$6
Xalatan (latanoprost)	05%	Prostaglandin tagonis	Latanoprost	Use 1 drop once a day.	2.5ml	$60	$24

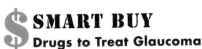

$ SMART BUY
Drugs to Treat Glaucoma

For drugs to treat glaucoma, your Smart Buys are Xalatan, Betagan, and Cosopt. Xalatan doesn't cause the problems with night vision that similar products do, and it lasts for a full 24 hours. No generic is available yet, however, and buying in larger volumes will do little good, so there's not much you can do to save money beyond comparing prices. Buying several bottles at a time usually will help. Typically, one bottle will cost around $60 and three bottles around $160, saving you about 11 percent. Betagan does a good job of decreasing aqueous humor production and its effects tend to last longer than comparable products. To cut your cost by better than half, use the generic version. Again, buy several bottles at a time. Cosopt is more expensive than most glaucoma medications, but it's also one of the best. It strongly reduces fluid production and increases drainage. Use this if other combinations aren't doing the job. One 10ml bottle typically will last about 30 days. Yet again, buy more than one bottle at a time.

DRUGS TO TREAT INFLAMMATION, ALLERGIES, CONGESTION, AND INFECTIONS OF THE EYES

A variety of ophthalmic drops are available to treat eye irritations. Which ones your doctor prescribes for you will depend on the reason for the irritation. The most common causes of eye irritation that requires medical treatment are inflammation, allergies, and infections.

DRUGS TO TREAT INFLAMED EYES

To simply reduce inflammation, several NSAID drugs in drop form are available. Common products in this category include Acular (generic name ketorolac), Ocufen (generic name flurbiprofen), and Voltaren (generic name diclofenac).

There's not a huge difference in effectiveness or side effects among these products, but there's quite a difference in price. Ask for a generic version of Ocufen (flurbiprofen) to save big money. Usually this will cost you around $15, as opposed to $30 for Voltaren or $35 for Acular. Common side effects of NSAID eye drops include burning and stinging, dryness of the eyes, blurred vision, and increased ocular pressure. Oddly, using these products isn't contraindicated for people with glaucoma. The increase in pressure is said to be mild and occurs mostly with Voltaren.

Although NSAIDs are used primarily for inflammation due to surgery (laser to correct vision or cataract removal), steroids are indicated for all inflamed areas of the eye. They include these products:

1. Alrex (generic name loteprednol)
2. Econopred (generic name prednisolone)
3. FML (generic name fluorometholone)
4. Lotemax (generic name loteprednol)
5. Pred Forte (generic name prednisolone)
6. Vexol (generic name rimexolone)

Your doctor may steer you toward Lotemax, Alrex, or Vexol—especially if the drug rep has just been to visit—but ask if you can try FML, Pred Forte, or Econopred, instead. These have been on the market much longer and their generic versions are available. Unless the inflammation is extreme, these should work just fine for you. Potential side effects that can occur with continued use include glaucoma, cataract formation, thinning of the cornea, stinging and burning, dry eyes, and blurred vision. Ask your doctor about the risks of using these drugs for extended periods.

DRUGS TO TREAT ALLERGIC REACTIONS INVOLVING THE EYES

For years, all that was available to treat eye irritations caused by allergies was Crolom (generic name cromolyn). This drug prevents the release of histamine (the substance the body produces that generates an allergic response), and it does a good job of preventing allergy symptoms. Recently, though, several new comparable products have arrived on the market. The first in this new group is Alomide (generic name lodoxamide), another drug that prevents histamine release. Although people have very good things to say about this product, we suggest first giving cromolyn a try. It's about half the price, so significant savings will add up over the long term. Also, lodoxamide can cause some erosion of the cornea, scales on the eyelids, and eye discomfort not seen with cromolyn.

> ### ▶ Just One Drop is Enough!
>
> The normal eye holds 10mcl of fluid. The average eyedropper delivers 25mcl to 50mcl per drop. So you gain nothing by using more than one drop at a time. Most of the second drop will be wasted. Instead, wait 5 minutes between drops.

Two of the few true antihistamine products now available in a drop form are Livostin (generic name levocabastine) and Patanol (generic name olopatadine). These groundbreaking products are well worth a try, but they're expensive. They affect the eyes the same as oral antihistamines—a breakthrough in treatment for allergies affecting the eyes. Expect to pay around $60 for a 5ml bottle. These products are appropriate only for temporary relief of seasonal allergies. The most common side effects include stinging eyes and headaches.

Another product, Zaditor (generic name ketotifen), is impressive in that it is both a mast cell stabilizer (blocks the release of histamine) and an antihistamine (blocks histamine from producing its effects). It's extremely effective at preventing allergy symptoms in the eyes. Ketotifen costs around $50 for 5ml, saving you $10. And it's a better buy than Livostin because you need only use it twice a day, compared to the 4 times a day Livostin requires.

DRUGS TO TREAT CONGESTION IN THE EYE

Usually found in over-the-counter products such as Visine and Murine, drugs that relieve congestion in the eyes eliminate redness by causing blood vessels in the eyes to constrict. These products can be hard on the eyes, so use them only when absolutely necessary. Two commonly prescribed drugs in this group are Albalon (generic name naphazoline) and Vasocon (generic name naphazoline). Side effects can include blurred vision, dizziness, drowsiness, pain with exposure to light, headaches, a rapid heartbeat, and irregular heartbeats. Don't use these products if you have glaucoma.

DRUGS TO TREAT INFECTIONS OF THE EYE

To gain a working knowledge of the different classes of antibiotics and the types of bacteria they cover, you may first want to read Chapter 7, "Prescription Drugs to Treat Infections." The following nine antibiotics are commonly used to treat eye infections:

1. Ciloxan (generic name ciprofloxacin)
2. Garamycin (generic name gentamicin)
3. Ilotycin (generic name erythromycin)
4. Neosporin (combination product that includes generic names for gramicidin, polymyxin B, and neomycin)
5. Ocuflox (generic name ofloxacin)
6. Polysporin (combination product that includes generic names of bacitracin and polymyxin B)
7. Polytrim (combination product that includes generic names for trimethoprim and polymyxin B)
8. Sulamyd (generic name sulfacetamide)
9. Tobrex (generic name tobramycin)

Trimethoprim, polymyxin B, neomycin, bacitracin, and gramicidin usually are grouped together to provide a fairly broad coverage of bacteria. These products include Polysporin (bacitracin and polymyxin B) and Neosporin (gramicidin, polymyxin B, and neomycin). Despite this blending of antibiotics, these products still fail to cover some key gram-negative bacteria. Gentamicin and tobramycin often are better choices, because they cover more bacteria, including gram-negative ones—more, in fact, than sulfacetamide, erythromycin, Polysporin, and Neosporin—and they're far less expensive than Ciloxan and Ocuflox.

An infection often causes inflammation in the eyes, so doctors also will prescribe some kind of steroid drop to reduce this. Some products combine a steroid with an antibiotic. Doctors often prescribe one such product—Tobradex—because it contains both tobramycin and dexamethasone. Although this is a very good product, consider asking your doctor to write two prescriptions for you, instead. Tobramycin drops usually sell for around $15 and dexamethasone for around $10. This is much cheaper than the $45 you're likely to pay for Tobradex.

If you wear contact lenses, it's a good idea to stop wearing them until your infection is gone and you've completed the course of treatment. Many antibiotics can stain lenses permanently. And wearing lenses when fighting an infection can reinfect the eye with bacteria. When using eye drops for an infected eye, be extremely careful to avoid touching the tip of the bottle to any part of the eye or lid. Bacteria easily can get into the bottle and reinfect the eye in future doses.

Contact Lenses Can Absorb Preservatives

Soft contact lenses can absorb some preservatives found in various eye drops. Remove your contact lenses to put drops in your eyes, and wait at least 15 minutes before putting your contact lenses back in.

Drugs to Treat Inflammation, Allergies, Congestion, and Infections of the Eyes

PRODUCT	STRENGTH PER DOSE	USED TO TREAT	ACTIVE INGREDIENT	USUAL DOSAGE	TYPICAL QUANTITY	TYPICAL PRICE	PRICE PER ML OR G
Acular (ketorolac)	0.5%	Inflammation	Ketorolac	Use 1 drop 4 times a day.	3ml	$35	$11.67
Albalon (naphazoline)	0.1%	Congestion	Naphazoline	Use 1-2 drops every 3-4 hrs.	15ml	$29	$1.93
Alomide (lodoxamide)	0.1%	Allergies	Lodoxamide	Use 1-2 drops 4 times a day.	10ml	$70	$7
Alrex (loteprednol)	0.2%	Inflammation	Loteprednol	Use 1 drop 4 times a day.	5ml	$41	$8.20
Bacitracin and polymyxin B	500 units and 10,000 units	Infections	Bacitracin and polymyxin B	Apply 2-3 times a day.	3.5g	$15	$4.29

PRODUCT	STRENGTH PER DOSE	USED TO TREAT	ACTIVE INGREDIENT	USUAL DOSAGE	TYPICAL QUANTITY	TYPICAL PRICE	PRICE PER ML OR G
Ciloxan (ciprofloxacin)	0.3%	Infections	Ciprofloxacin	Use 1-2 drops every 4 hrs.	5ml	$43	$8.60
Crolom (cromolyn)	4%	Allergies	Cromolyn	Use 1-2 drops 4-6 times a day.	10ml	$45	$4.50
Cromolyn	4%	Allergies	Cromolyn	Use 1-2 drops 4-6 times a day.	10ml	$35	$3.50
Diclofenac	0.1%	Inflammation	Diclofenac	Use 1 drop 4 times a day.	2.5ml	$29	$11.60
Econopred (prednisolone)	0.125%	Inflammation	Prednisolone	Use 1 drop every 4 hrs.	5ml	$30	$6
Econopred Plus (prednisolone)	1%	Inflammation	Prednisolone	Use 1 drop every 4 hrs.	5ml	$36	$7.20
Erythromycin	5%	Infections	Erythromycin	Apply up to 6 times a day.	3.5g	$5	$1.43
Fluorometholone	0.1%	Inflammation	Fluorometholone	Use 1-2 drops 2-4 times a day.	5ml	$14	$2.80
Flurbiprofen	0.03%	Inflammation	Flurbiprofen	Use 1 drop every 30 mins. beginning 2 hrs. prior to surgery.	2.5ml	$15	$6
FML (fluorometholone)	0.1%	Inflammation	Fluorometholone	Use 1-2 drops 2-4 times a day.	5ml	$32	$6.40
FML Forte (fluorometholone)	0.25%	Inflammation	Fluorometholone	Use 1-2 drops 2-4 times a day.	5ml	$26	$5.20
Garamycin (gentamicin)	0.3%	Infections	Gentamicin	Use 1-2 drops every 4 hrs.	5ml	$27	$5.40
Gentamicin	0.3%	Infections	Gentamicin	Use 1-2 drops every 4 hrs.	5ml	$15	$3
Gramicidin, polymyxin B, and neomycin	0.025mg, 10,000 units and 1.75mg	Infections	Gramicidin, polymyxin B, and neomycin	Use 1-2 drops every 4-6 hrs.	10ml	$25	$2.50
Lotemax (loteprednol)	0.5%	Inflammation	Loteprednol	Use 1 drop 4 times a day.	5ml	$34	$6.80
Neosporin (gramicidin, polymyxin B, and neomycin)	0.025mg, 10,000 mg units and 1.75mg	Infections	Gramicidin, polymyxin B, and neomycin	Use 1-2 drops every 4-6 hrs.	10ml	$37	$3.70
Ocufen (flurbiprofen)	0.03%	Inflammation	Flurbiprofen	Use 1 drop every 30 mins. beginning 2 hrs. prior to surgery.	2.5ml	$25	$10
Ocuflox (ofloxacin)	0.3%	Infections	Ofloxacin	Use 1-2 drops every 4 hrs. for 2 days, then 4 times a day.	5ml	$43	$8.60
Patanol (olopatadine)	0.1%	Allergies	Olopatadine	Use 1-2 drops 2 times a day.	5ml	$65	$13
Polysporin (bacitracin and polymyxin B)	500 units and 10,000 units	Infections	Bacitracin and polymyxin B	Apply 2-3 times a day.	3.5g	$33	$9.43

PRODUCT	STRENGTH PER DOSE	USED TO TREAT	ACTIVE INGREDIENT	USUAL DOSAGE	TYPICAL QUANTITY	TYPICAL PRICE	PRICE PER ML OR G
Polytrim (trimethoprim and polymyxin B)	1mg and 10,000 units	Infections	Trimethoprim and polymyxin B	Use 1 drop every 3 hrs.	10ml	$39	$3.90
Pred Forte (prednisolone)	1%	Inflammation	Prednisolone	Use 1 drop every 4 hrs.	5ml	$30	$6
Pred Mild (prednisolone)	0.12%	Inflammation	Prednisolone	Use 1 drop every 4 hrs.	5ml	$30	$6
Prednisolone	0.125%	Inflammation	Prednisolone	Use 1 drop every 4 hrs.	5ml	$8	$1.60
Prednisolone	1%	Inflammation	Prednisolone	Use 1 drop every 4 hrs.	5ml	$17	$3.40
Prednisolone	1%	Inflammation	Prednisolone	Use 1 drop every 4 hrs.	5ml	$18	$3.60
Sulamyd (sulfacetamide)	10%	Infections	Sulfacetamide	Use 1-2 drops every 2-3 hrs.	15ml	$30	$2
Sulfacetamide	10%	Infections	Sulfacetamide	Use 1-2 drops every 2-3 hrs.	15ml	$10	67¢
Tobramycin	0.3%	Infections	Tobramycin	Use 1-2 drops every 4 hrs.	5ml	$15	$3
Tobrex (tobramycin)	0.3%	Infections	Tobramycin	Use 1-2 drops every 4 hrs.	5ml	$44	$8.80
Trimethoprim and polymyxin B	1mg and 10,000 units	Infections	Trimethoprim and polymyxin B	Use 1 drop every 3 hrs.	10ml	$20	$2
Vasocon (naphazoline)	0.1%	Congestion	Naphazoline	Use 1-2 drops every 3-4 hrs.	15ml	$23	$1.53
Vexol (rimexolone)	1%	Inflammation	Rimexolone	Use 1-2 drops 4 times a day.	5ml	$30	$6
Voltaren (diclofenac)	0.1%	Inflammation	Diclofenac	Use 1 drop 4 times a day.	2.5ml	$35	$14
Zaditor (ketotifen)	0.025%	Allergies	Ketotifen	Use 1 drop every 8-12 hrs.	5ml	$52	$10.40

$ SMART BUY
Drugs to Treat Inflammation, Irritation, and Allergies of the Eyes

When choosing an NSAID eye drop after surgery, ask your doctor to consider Ocufen. The generic form, flurbiprofen, will save you about 25 percent. For other kinds of eye inflammation, take a look at either Pred Forte or Econopred; both contain the steroid prednisolone. These two products cost considerably less than the newer options. For maximum savings that could be more than half, buy generic for either of these drugs.

To treat allergic reactions that affect the eyes, your Smart Buy is a generic version of cromolyn. It costs about half as much as Alomide and will do a good job. If this isn't quite strong enough to take care of the problem, consider Zaditor.

For infections in the eyes, consider gentamicin (generic for Garamycin) or tobramycin (generic for Tobrex). These two drugs offer fairly broad coverage of bacteria and cost around $15, about a third as much as Ciloxan or Ocuflox. Of course, keep in mind that you actually may need the Ciloxan, but it's usually worthwhile to try gentamicin first. Because these drugs are used to treat acute (short-term) problems, we don't recommend that you buy more than one bottle at a time to save money.

DRUGS TO TREAT CONDITIONS OF THE SKIN

It's easy to feel overwhelmed when you look at the multitude of drugs available to treat skin conditions. More drugs exist for treating skin conditions than for probably any other part of the body. This is mostly because so many problems can occur with the skin. Our largest organ is vulnerable to a vast number and variety of conditions, from acne to athlete's foot. Many skin conditions are quite difficult to diagnose.

Beth had a rash on the back of her neck that was driving her crazy. The more she scratched, the more it itched, and soon the rash began to spread. After a couple of days of this, she decided to visit her doctor. Her physician, a general practitioner, took one look at Beth's neck and said it was some kind of eczema, and that she'd probably have to deal with off and on for the rest of her life. Not happy with this diagnosis, Beth made an appointment with a dermatologist (a specialist in conditions of the skin). This was a good move: The dermatologist diagnosed the specific type of eczema, and gave Beth a prescription for a cream and oral prednisone that made the rash go away within a couple of days. The rash has never returned.

DRUGS TO TREAT ACNE

Acne most commonly affects teenagers, but some continue to confront this problem into adulthood. The usual way to treat acne is to dry the oils on the surface of the skin. Over-the-counter products such as Clearasil and Stridex can be quite effective for this. When these products don't work, a prescription product is in order. Probably the most common topical product used to treat acne is Retin-A (generic name tretinoin), a form of vitamin A. This cream is very effective at drying out the skin—so effective, in fact, that people often end up with red, dry, irritated skin that can be quite painful. The key when using Retin-A is to find the lowest strength possible that works for you. Also, avoid exposure to the sun. Retin-A can make you far more vulnerable to sunburn, so apply it just before bedtime, and use a good sunscreen during the day.

> ## Doctor Can Affirm Retin-A is for Acne, Not Wrinkles
>
> Retin-A also is used to eliminate wrinkles. It's so drying that the skin responds by tightening up, so the wrinkles disappear. Because this use is cosmetic rather than therapeutic, many insurance companies refuse to pay for Retin-A for patients older than 35. A letter from your doctor affirming that your problem is acne might convince your insurance company to cover your Retin-A prescription, but you'll have no luck if you're just smoothing your face.

Another vitamin A product often used to treat acne is Accutane. This drug taken by mouth is extremely effective at reducing acne conditions. It does have a couple of drawbacks, however. First, it's very expensive. A 30-day supply of the 40mg capsules will run you around $620. (Yes, that's right—*$620!*) Second, this product is notorious for causing severe birth defects, and women should be absolutely sure they won't become pregnant while taking it. *If you're a woman of childbearing age, do not use Accutane unless you also use two forms of birth control.*

Several of the antibiotics also are commonly used to treat acne. In both topical and oral forms, antibiotics are effective at treating acne because many times the pores that become clogged with excessive oils become infected, worsening the skin condition. Three commonly prescribed antibiotics include Cleocin (clindamycin; various topical forms); A/T/S (erythromycin) and Ery-Tab (erythromycin) both orally and topically; and several members of the tetracycline family—Minocin (minocycline), Vibramycin (doxycycline), and Sumycin (tetracycline). Of these products, we mostly tend to see prescriptions for Benzamycin (a topical product that combines erythromycin with benzoyl peroxide to provide drying), and minocycline. Benzamycin, of course, is good because it works by killing bacteria and drying out the oils. Minocycline is a good choice because it doesn't cause the stomach irritation erythromycin and doxycycline can produce, and it doesn't have the food and dairy restrictions for which tetracycline is notorious. (Chapter 7, "Prescription Drugs to Treat Infections," provides a complete discussion of side effects and warnings for the oral antibiotics mentioned here.)

Drugs to Treat Acne

PRODUCT	STRENGTH PER DOSE	FORM	ACTIVE INGREDIENT	USUAL DOSAGE	TYPICAL QUANTITY	TYPICAL PRICE	PRICE PER G, ML, DOSE
A/T/S (erythromycin)	2%	Solution	Erythromycin	Apply 2 times a day.	60ml	$26	43¢
Accutane (Isotretinoin)	10mg	Capsule	Isotretinoin	Take 1 capsule 2 times a day.	60	$425	$7.08
Accutane (Isotretinoin)	20mg	Capsule	Isotretinoin	Take 1 capsule 2 times a day.	60	$499	$8.32
Accutane (Isotretinoin)	40mg	Capsule	Isotretinoin	Take 1 capsule 2 times a day.	60	$620	$10.33
Achromycin (tetracycline)	250mg	Capsule	Tetracycline	Take 1 capsule 2 times a day.	100	$10	10¢
Achromycin (tetracycline)	500mg	Capsule	Tetracycline	Take 1 capsule 2 times a day.	100	$10	10¢
Benzamycin (erythromycin with benzoyl peroxide)	3% and 5%	Gel	Erythromycin with benzoyl peroxide	Apply 2 times a day.	23.3g	$55	$2.36
Benzamycin (erythromycin with benzoyl peroxide)	3% and 5%	Gel	Erythromycin with benzoyl peroxide	Apply 2 times a day.	46.6g	$95	$2.04
Cleocin T (clindamycin)	1%	Gel	Clindamycin	Apply 2 times a day.	30g	$42	$1.40
Cleocin T (clindamycin)	1%	Lotion	Clindamycin	Apply 2 times a day.	60ml	$56	93¢
Cleocin T (clindamycin)	1%	Solution	Clindamycin	Apply 2 times a day.	60ml	$45	75¢
Clindamycin topical	1%	Gel	Clindamycin	Apply 2 times a day.	30g	$33	$1.10
Clindamycin topical	1%	Solution	Clindamycin	Apply 2 times a day.	60ml	$25	42¢
Doxycycline	100mg	Tablet	Doxycycline	Take 1 tablet 2 times a day.	20	$12	60¢
Erygel (erythromycin)	2%	Gel	Erythromycin	Apply 2 times a day.	30g	$42	$1.40
Erythromycin	2%	Gel	Erythromycin	Apply 2 times a day.	30g	$27	90¢
Erythromycin	250mg	Tablet	Erythromycin	Take 1 tablet 2 times a day.	60	$19	32¢
Erythromycin topical	2%	Solution	Erythromycin	Apply 2 times a day.	60ml	$10	17¢
Minocin (minocycline)	50mg	Capsule	Minocycline	Take 1 capsule daily.	100	$200	$2
Minocin (minocycline)	100mg	Capsule	Minocycline	Take 1 capsule daily.	100	$320	$3.20
Minocycline	50mg	Capsule	Minocycline	Take 1 capsule daily.	100	$55	55¢
Minocycline	100mg	Capsule	Minocycline	Take 1 capsule daily.	100	$70	70¢
Retin-A (tretinoin)	0.025%	Cream	Tretinoin	Apply once a day.	20g	$40	$2

PRODUCT	STRENGTH PER DOSE	FORM	ACTIVE INGREDIENT	USUAL DOSAGE	TYPICAL QUANTITY	TYPICAL PRICE	PRICE PER G, ML, DOSE
Retin-A (tretinoin)	0.05%	Cream	Tretinoin	Apply once a day.	20g	$45	$2.25
Retin-A (tretinoin)	0.1%	Cream	Tretinoin	Apply once a day.	20g	$52	$2.60
Retin-A (tretinoin)	0.025%	Gel	Tretinoin	Apply once a day.	15g	$36	$2.40
Retin-A (tretinoin)	0.01%	Gel	Tretinoin	Apply once a day.	15g	$36	$2.40
Retin-A Micro (tretinoin)	0.1%	Gel	Tretinoin	Apply once a day.	20g	$44	$2.20
Sumycin (tetracycline)	250mg	Capsule	Tetracycline	Take 1 capsule 2 times a day.	100	$15	15¢
Sumycin (tetracycline)	500mg	Capsule	Tetracycline	Take 1 capsule 2 times a day.	100	$15	15¢
Tretinoin	0.025%	Cream	Tretinoin	Apply once a day.	20g	$28	$1.40
Tretinoin	0.05%	Cream	Tretinoin	Apply once a day.	20g	$28	$1.40
Tretinoin	0.1%	Cream	Tretinoin	Apply once a day.	20g	$28	$1.40
Tretinoin	0.025%	Gel	Tretinoin	Apply once a day.	15g	$31	$2.07

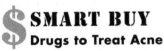

$ SMART BUY
Drugs to Treat Acne

For acne, we recommend you ask your doctor about Benzamycin and minocycline. Benzamycin is cost effective because it both dries the skin and kills bacteria. To save money on Benzamycin, buy in bulk. A 23g jar typically will cost around $55; a jar of the 46g size will cost around $95, saving you 14 percent. Also consider buying three jars of the 46g size for about $270 to save an additional 5 percent—about $15. Minocycline is good because it's easier on the stomach. Again, consider buying the generic form in bulk. Buying just 30 capsules of the name-brand product Minocin 50mg will cost you around $80 a month, and 90 of the generic form just $50 a month, a 38 percent savings! (Be sure to check our Web site, www.smartbuysdrugwise.com, for updates on prescription and over-the-counter drugs.)

DRUGS TO TREAT BACTERIAL AND VIRAL SKIN INFECTIONS

Staphylococcus causes most bacterial infections of the skin. Doctors usually treat these types of infections with oral antibiotics (see Chapter 7). Sometimes topical creams or ointments are appropriate, however. Probably the most common such condition is impetigo. This crusting of the skin generally affects the area below the nostrils down to the lips and chin and is usually seen in young children. It's a staph infection usually treated with a topical cream or ointment called Bactroban (generic name mupirocin), which is very effective. Just be sure to cover the affected areas well and continue to use the product until all symptoms are gone.

You can also develop viral infections of the skin. By far the most common of these is the unsightly and unpleasant cold sore, caused by a virus in the herpes family. Viral infections can also occur in other areas, too. From genital herpes to plantar warts, viruses can attack the skin relentlessly and are extremely contagious. For many years, the old standby for viral skin infections was Zovirax (generic name acyclovir) ointment. It's quite effective for clearing the symptoms of both cold sores and genital herpes. Recently, though, a new product has emerged that's been quite effective at treating cold sores. Denavir (generic name penciclovir) cream seems to work even better than Zovirax, and is well worth a try. For genital herpes, Zovirax (acyclovir) ointment, along with an antiviral medication taken orally, is still the way to go. Several other antiviral products also are available that can be taken orally.

To get the most for your money, though, stick with the generic version of Zovirax. Significant savings more than offset the inconvenience of having to take it more often than some other antivirals. A course of acyclovir (generic Zovirax) 800mg (50 tablets) typically costs in the neighborhood of $75. An equivalent course of therapy of Famvir (famciclovir) 500mg (21 tablets) sells for around $167, and Valtrex (valacyclovir) 500mg (42 tablets) moves to a very pricey $164.

Antiviral Drugs Relieve Pain of Shingles

Shingles is a painful condition of the skin that usually appears later in life in those who had chickenpox as children. It's caused by the same virus, which has hidden itself in the nerves of the body waiting to come out during times of stress. To treat this painful condition, many times doctors will prescribe oral anti-viral drugs, such as acyclovir, to put the virus back into remission.

Prescription Drugs to Treat Bacterial and Viral Skin Infections

PRODUCT	STRENGTH PER DOSE	FORM	ACTIVE INGREDIENT	USUAL DOSAGE	TYPICAL QUANTITY	TYPICAL PRICE	PRICE PER G, OR DOSE
Acyclovir	200mg	Capsule	Acyclovir	Take 1 capsule 5 times a day.	50	$40	80¢
Acyclovir	400mg	Tablet	Acyclovir	Take 1 tablet 2 times a day.	20	$27	$1.35
Acyclovir	800mg	Tablet	Acyclovir	Take 1 tablet 5 times a day.	50	$75	$1.50
Bactroban (mupirocin)	2%	Ointment	Mupirocin	Apply 3 times a day.	30g	$44	$1.47
Bactroban (mupirocin)	2%	Cream	Mupirocin	Apply 3 times a day.	30g	$55	$1.83
Denavir (penciclovir)	1%	Cream	Penciclovir	Apply every 2 hrs.	1.5g	$28	$18.67
Famvir (famciclovir)	125mg	Tablet	Famciclovir	Take 1 tablet 2 times a day.	10	$39	$3.90
Famvir (famciclovir)	250mg	Tablet	Famciclovir	Take 1 tablet 2 times a day.	10	$42	$4.20
Famvir (famciclovir)	500mg	Tablet	Famciclovir	Take 1 tablet 3 times a day.	21	$167	$7.95
Valtrex (valacyclovir)	500mg	Tablet	Valacyclovir	Take 1 tablet 2 times a day.	42	$164	$3.90
Valtrex (valacyclovir)	1g	Tablet	Valacyclovir	Take 1 tablet 3 times a day.	21	$145	$6.90
Zovirax (acyclovir)	200mg	Capsule	Acyclovir	Take 1 capsule 5 times a day.	50	$75	$1.50
Zovirax (acyclovir)	400mg	Tablet	Acyclovir	Take 1 tablet 2 times a day.	20	$60	$3
Zovirax (acyclovir)	800mg	Tablet	Acyclovir	Take 1 tablet 5 times a day.	50	$275	$5.50
Zovirax (acyclovir)	5%	Ointment	Acyclovir	Apply 6 times a day.	3g	$31	$10.33
Zovirax (acyclovir)	5%	Ointment	Acyclovir	Apply 6 times a day.	15g	$85	$5.67

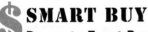

$ SMART BUY
Drugs to Treat Bacterial and Viral Skin Infections

For viral infections of the skin, we recommend Denavir cream for the lips and Zovirax (acyclovir) for all other areas. For savings of up to 73 percent, buy generic oral versions of Zovirax (acyclovir). If you have frequent problems with cold sores, buy Denavir in more than one tube at a time. One tube typically will cost around $30 and three tubes around $75, for a $15 (17 percent) savings.

For bacterial skin infections, about your only choice of creams or ointments is Bactroban. No generic is available yet, so you can't save money that way. And because skin infections are an acute condition, it doesn't make sense to buy more than one tube at a time. Instead, about your only way to save money is to shop around for the cheapest price in town. Alternative sources aren't a good idea because you'll want to begin treatment as quickly as possible.

DRUGS TO TREAT BURNS

One common injury-related skin condition that can become very dangerous is a burn. The treatment of choice depends on the burn's area and severity. Over-the-counter pain relievers usually suffice to treat small first-degree (unblistered) burns. (See Chapter 18, "Over-the-Counter Pain Relief," for more information.) For second-degree (blistered) burns, particularly large ones, and any third-degree (blackened skin) burn, a trip to the doctor's office is in order.

While your primary concern likely will be relief from the pain, one of your doctor's goals will be to prevent the burn from becoming infected and to provide healing. Probably the best product on the market for this is Silvadene (silver sulfadiazine). This product, now available in a generic form, is truly miraculous at healing most burns. If you have a second- or third-degree burn, see a doctor immediately. Silvadene will improve the situation greatly. A potential cross-sensitivity exists between Silvadene and other sulfa drugs. If you have a sulfa allergy, use Silvadene with caution. Odds are you'll have no problems, but the possibility of an allergic response exists.

DRUGS TO TREAT FUNGAL INFECTIONS

Fungal skin infections have different names depending on the area affected. Whether you have athlete's foot, jock itch, nail fungus, or diaper rash, you need an antifungal product to cure the infection. Dozens of products are available over the counter, from gentian violet to Lamisil. Predictably, they have varying degrees of effectiveness. (Chapter 20, "Over-the-Counter Treatments for Eyes, Ears, Mouth, and Skin," covers these products in detail.) Prescription drugs to treat fungal infections exhibit the same variable effectiveness. Your doctor probably knows which products are stronger than others, but ask his or her opinion of Nizoral (generic name ketoconazole) cream. This is a broad-spectrum antifungal product that comes in a generic version. As you know by now, that's a prescription for significant savings! The exception is for children with diaper rash. For this, your doctor probably will want to try Mycostatin (generic name nystatin), which is a good choice. This is a little safer in children than other products and a generic version is available.

Don't waste your money on topical products for bad cases of nail fungus. Topical medication rarely penetrates the nail sufficiently to kill all the fungus. To achieve this, you need to take an oral antifungal product. Those usually prescribed, such as Sporanox (generic name itraconazole), are very expensive and can cause side effects in your liver. Watch for unusual fatigue, anorexia, nausea, vomiting, jaundice, dark urine, and/or pale stool.

Keep Skin Dry

When treating fungal infections, it's important to limit the amount of moisture on the skin. Fungal infections thrive in a moist environment. If you have athlete's foot, wear cotton socks and change them throughout the day, and use powders to keep your feet dry. If your child has diaper rash, avoid diapers that trap moisture without absorbing, and let your child go without a diaper as much as possible throughout the day.

Drugs to Treat Fungal Infections

PRODUCT	STRENGTH PER DOSE	FORM	ACTIVE INGREDIENT	USUAL DOSAGE	TYPICAL QUANTITY	TYPICAL PRICE	PRICE PER G,ML,DOSE
Ketoconazole	2%	Cream	Ketoconazole	Apply once a day.	30g	$28	93¢
Naftin (naftifine)	1%	Cream	Naftifine	Apply once a day.	30g	$45	$1.50
Naftin (naftifine)	1%	Gel	Naftifine	Apply twice a day.	40g	$60	$1.50
Nizoral (ketoconazole)	2%	Cream	Ketoconazole	Apply once a day.	30g	$55	$1.83
Nizoral (ketoconazole)	2%	Shampoo	Ketoconazole	Apply once a day.	120ml	$28	23¢
Nystatin units	100,000	Cream	Nystatin	Apply 3 times a day.	30g	$10	33¢
Nystatin units	100,000	Ointment	Nystatin	Apply 3 times a day.	30g	$10	33¢
Oxistat (oxiconazole)	1%	Cream	Oxiconazole	Apply once a day.	30g	$35	$1.17
Oxistat (oxiconazole)	1%	Lotion	Oxiconazole	Apply once a day.	30ml	$35	$1.17

PRODUCT	STRENGTH PER DOSE	FORM	ACTIVE INGREDIENT	USUAL DOSAGE	TYPICAL QUANTITY	TYPICAL PRICE	PRICE PER G, ML, DOSE
Silvadene (silver sulfadiazine)	1%	Cream	Silver sulfadiazine	Apply 1 or 2 times a day.	50g	$15	30¢
Silver sulfadiazine	1%	Cream	Silver sulfadiazine	Apply 1 or 2 times a day.	50g	$12	24¢
Sporanox PulsePak (itraconazole)	100mg	Capsule	Itraconazole	Take 2 capsules a day.	1 PulsePak (28 capsules)	$220	$15.71

$ SMART BUY
Drugs to Treat Fungal Infections

To treat fungal infections of the skin, we like Nizoral (ketoconazole) cream. It's a fairly strong antifungal product that's reasonably priced, and buying the generic version can save you half. When you buy ketoconazole cream, see if you can purchase the larger tube. If you go with the 15g size, you'll pay around $15, while the 60g size (4 times as much) runs around $40. This means a savings of about $20, or 33 percent, and will ensure that you have enough cream to treat the often stubborn fungal infection.

DRUGS TO TREAT PSORIASIS, ITCHING, IRRITATION, AND RASH

Psoriasis is an irritating condition that can affect all areas of the skin, including the scalp. Characterized by scaling, burning, and itching skin, psoriasis can be very uncomfortable. The most common treatment for psoriasis is coal tar. Applied topically, this dark-brown liquid can provide considerable relief, despite its strong odor and tendency to stain. Some over-the-counter products contain coal tar (Neutrogena T-gel shampoo is a good one to try on the scalp), but often coal tar alone is not enough. Psoriasis can cause significant inflammation of the skin at involved areas, and topical steroids can improve this symptom greatly. Most cases of psoriasis will need to be treated with a prescription-strength steroid. Ointment forms generally are more effective than creams, even though they have a Vaseline-like, greasy feel to them. Ointments tend to increase moisture levels in the skin. This is important with psoriasis, because the dry, scaly skin it causes is quite irritating.

Doctors are unable to diagnose many cases of skin rash and itching. There's even a five-dollar word for these—idiopathic, which is medicalese for "We don't know!" Sometimes even skin specialists (dermatologists) simply don't know what's causing the problem. Don't be alarmed if this is the case with you. Even though your doctor may not know exactly what the problem is, any of a large number of topical steroids more than likely will solve it. And when a topical steroid doesn't do the job, oral versions, such as prednisone, quickly come to the rescue. Steroids must come in contact with the affected area to work, so to avoid internal side effects, doctors first will attempt to treat a skin condition topically, using weaker to middle-of-the-road strengths. If these don't work, they'll try stronger topical drugs. If they don't do the job, then they'll turn to oral steroids. Because oral versions absorb into the bloodstream, they have improved access to all levels of the skin, and thus greater success.

> ### Custom Compound Effective But Takes Time to Prepare

For many patients with psoriasis, doctors prescribe an ointment called Lidex (a steroid), to which the pharmacist adds salicylic acid (aspirin powder) and coal tar. This will take the pharmacist a while to mix for you, so expect to wait at least a day to get your prescription.

Whether it's due to eczema, psoriasis, or poison oak, if you experience inflammation and itching, try using a topical steroid. Over-the-counter options are limited to hydrocortisone products. These may work for mild inflammation, itching, and irritations, but they have limitations. Topical steroids available only with a prescription are abundant and vary greatly in strength. For most rashes, ask your doctor about Kenalog (generic name triamcinolone). This middle-of-the-road steroid does a good job, and its generic version will save you money. Remember, too, that in most cases ointments will work better than creams, but they'll feel greasy. (When dry, irritated skin is involved, ointments are preferred.)

> ▶ **Cellophane Wrap Increases Absorption**
>
> Ask your doctor about covering the applied steroid with a cellophane wrap. For severe conditions,
>
> this allows more of the steroid to absorb into the skin and produce better results. ◀

Keep a few precautions in mind when applying topical steroids. First, avoid contact with your eyes. Getting a steroid in your eye can cause serious burning and irritation. Ophthalmic steroid preparations are isotonic; that is, they have the same salt balance as the fluid in your eyes. Putting something in your eyes that isn't isotonic will, quite simply, hurt, just as if you were putting salt in your eye. Some steroids aren't meant to be applied to the facial skin, anyway, so check with your doctor before doing so. Second, steroids needn't be applied in a thick layer; a little bit goes a long way. Most pharmacists will advise you to apply a thin film and rub it in well. Third, steroids should rarely be applied to infants. Never apply a topical steroid to a baby without first checking with a pediatrician. Babies have very thin skin that a steroid can penetrate easily to reach the bloodstream and cause potentially serious effects on various organs.

$ SMART BUY
Drugs to Treat Psoriasis, Skin Inflammation, and Rashes

To treat inflammation, itching, and general rashes, your Smart Buy is Kenalog in either the cream or the ointment. This product has good activity and a great price when you purchase its generic version (triamcinolone): An 80g tube of Kenalog 0.1% cream costs about $50, compared to $15 for the same quantity of the generic form. In this case, the generic saves you 70 percent!

Drugs to Treat Dry Skin

One of the best things you can do to prevent or treat skin conditions is keep your skin healthy. This starts with providing adequate moisture. Drink plenty of water throughout the day; 8 to 10 glasses a day do wonders. If this isn't enough for your skin, try a moisturizing cream. For the most part, over-the-counter products such as Eucerin

Drugs to Treat Psoriasis, Skin Inflammation, and Rashes

PRODUCT	STRENGTH PER DOSE	FORM	ACTIVE INGREDIENT	USUAL DOSAGE	TYPICAL QUANTITY	TYPICAL PRICE	PRICE PER G, OR ML
Aclovate (alclometasone)	0.05%	Ointment	Alclometasone	Apply 2-4 times a day.	45g	$37	82¢
Aclovate (alclometasone)	0.05%	Cream	Alclometasone	Apply 2-4 times a day.	45g	$37	82¢
Betamethasone dipropionate	0.05%	Ointment	Betamethasone dipropionate	Apply 2-4 times a day.	50g	$35	70¢
Betamethasone dipropionate	0.05%	Ointment	Betamethasone dipropionate	Apply 2-4 times a day.	45g	$15	33¢
Betamethasone dipropionate	0.05%	Cream	Betamethasone dipropionate	Apply 2-4 times a day.	45g	$15	33¢
Clobetasol	0.05%	Ointment	Clobetasol	Apply 2-4 times a day.	45g	$29	64¢
Clobetasol	0.05%	Cream	Clobetasol	Apply 2-4 times a day.	45g	$29	64¢
Cutivate (fluticasone)	0.05%	Ointment	Fluticasone	Apply 2-4 times a day.	60g	$52	87¢
Cutivate (fluticasone)	0.05%	Cream	Fluticasone	Apply 2-4 times a day.	60g	$52	87¢
Desonide	0.05%	Ointment	Desonide	Apply 2-4 times a day.	60g	$26	43¢
Desonide	0.05%	Cream	Desonide	Apply 2-4 times a day.	60g	$25	42¢
DesOwen (desonide)	0.05%	Ointment	Desonide	Apply 2-4 times a day.	60g	$55	92¢
DesOwen (desonide)	0.05%	Cream	Desonide	Apply 2-4 times a day.	60g	$55	92¢
Desoximetasone	0.05%	Cream	Desoximetasone	Apply 2-4 times a day.	60g	$35	58¢
Diprolene (betamethasone dipropionate)	0.05%	Ointment	Betamethasone dipropionate	Apply 2-4 times a day.	50g	$79	$1.58
Diprolene AF (beta-methasone dipropionate)	0.05%	Cream	Betamethasone dipropionate	Apply 2-4 times a day.	50g	$79	$1.58
Diprosone (beta-methasone dipropionate)	0.05%	Ointment	Betamethasone dipropionate	Apply 2-4 times a day.	45g	$59	$1.31
Diprosone (beta-methasone dipropionate)	0.05%	Cream	Betamethasone dipropionate	Apply 2-4 times a day.	45g	$59	$1.31
Dovonex (anthralin)	0.005%	Ointment	Anthralin	Apply 2 times a day.	100g	$170	$1.70
Dovonex (anthralin)	0.005%	Cream	Anthralin	Apply 2 times a day.	100g	$170	$1.70
Fluocinolone	0.025%	Ointment	Fluocinolone	Apply 2-4 times a day.	60g	$20	33¢
Fluocinolone	0.025%	Cream	Fluocinolone	Apply 2-4 times a day.	60g	$20	33¢
Fluocinonide	0.05%	Ointment	Fluocinonide	Apply 2-4 times a day.	60g	$26	43¢
Fluocinonide	0.05%	Cream	Fluocinonide	Apply 2-4 times a day.	60g	$26	43¢

PRODUCT	STRENGTH PER DOSE	FORM	ACTIVE INGREDIENT	USUAL DOSAGE	TYPICAL QUANTITY	TYPICAL PRICE	PRICE PER G, OR ML
Hydrocortisone valerate	0.2%	Ointment valerate	Hydrocortisone	Apply 2-4 times a day.	45g	$34	76¢
Hydrocortisone valerate	0.2%	Cream valerate	Hydrocortisone	Apply 2-4 times a day.	45g	$34	76¢
Kenalog (triamcinolone)	0.025%	Ointment	Triamcinolone	Apply 2-4 times a day.	80g	$55	69¢
Kenalog (triamcinolone)	0.1%	Ointment	Triamcinolone	Apply 2-4 times a day.	80g	$50	63¢
Kenalog (triamcinolone)	0.5%	Ointment	Triamcinolone	Apply 2-4 times a day.	80g	$55	69¢
Kenalog (triamcinolone)	0.025%	Cream	Triamcinolone	Apply 2-4 times a day.	80g	$55	69¢
Kenalog (triamcinolone)	0.1%	Cream	Triamcinolone	Apply 2-4 times a day.	80g	$50	63¢
Kenalog (triamcinolone)	0.5%	Cream	Triamcinolone	Apply 2-4 times a day.	15g	$50	$3.33
Kenalog (triamcinolone)	0.1%	Lotion	Triamcinolone	Apply 2-4 times a day.	60ml	$55	92¢
Kenalog (triamcinolone)	N/A	Aerosol spray	Triamcinolone	Spray 2-4 times a day.	63g	$40	63¢
Lidex (fluocinonide)	0.05%	Ointment	Fluocinonide	Apply 2-4 times a day.	60g	$65	$1.08
Lidex (fluocinonide)	0.05%	Cream	Fluocinonide	Apply 2-4 times a day.	60g	$65	$1.08
Synalar (fluocinolone)	0.025%	Ointment	Fluocinolone	Apply 2-4 times a day.	60g	$55	92¢
Synalar (fluocinolone)	0.025%	Cream	Fluocinolone	Apply 2-4 times a day.	60g	$55	92¢
Temovate (clobetasol)	0.05%	Ointment	Clobetasol	Apply 2-4 times a day.	45g	$60	$1.33
Temovate (clobetasol)	0.05%	Cream	Clobetasol	Apply 2-4 times a day.	45g	$60	$1.33
Topicort (desoximetasone)	0.25%	Ointment	Desoximetasone	Apply 2-4 times a day.	60g	$71	$1.18
Topicort (desoximetasone)	0.05%	Cream	Desoximetasone	Apply 2-4 times a day.	60g	$71	$1.18
$ Triamcinolone	0.025%	Ointment	Triamcinolone	Apply 2-4 times a day.	80g	$15	19¢
$ Triamcinolone	0.1%	Ointment	Triamcinolone	Apply 2-4 times a day.	80g	$15	19¢
$ Triamcinolone	0.5%	Ointment	Triamcinolone	Apply 2-4 times a day.	15g	$10	67¢
$ Triamcinolone	0.025%	Cream	Triamcinolone	Apply 2-4 times a day.	80g	$15	19¢
$ Triamcinolone	0.1%	Cream	Triamcinolone	Apply 2-4 times a day.	80g	$15	19¢
$ Triamcinolone	0.5%	Cream	Triamcinolone	Apply 2-4 times a day.	15g	$8	53¢
$ Triamcinolone	0.1%	Lotion	Triamcinolone	Apply 2-4 times a day.	60ml	$15	25¢
Westcort (hydrocortisone valerate)	0.2%	Ointment	Hydrocortisone valerate	Apply 2-4 times a day.	45g	$42	93¢
Westcort (hydrocortisone valerate)	0.2%	Cream	Hydrocortisone valerate	Apply 2-4 times a day.	45g	$42	93¢

cream and Keri-lotion do an outstanding job. Rarely is it necessary to obtain a prescription drug for dry skin. When it is, a couple of products are available only with a prescription. Of these, Lac-Hydrin (lactic acid) is probably the most commonly prescribed. We doubt that it's worth the money and time to go to the doctor to obtain it, though. Over-the-counter products, applied properly, will provide nearly equivalent results for far less money.

► Apply Moisturizer When Skin is Damp

The most effective way to apply moisturizing cream or lotion is to first moisten the affected area, pat it gently with a towel just to remove excess water, and then apply the moisturizer. Doing so allows the moisturizer to trap the water, forcing the skin to absorb it.

Prescription Drugs to Treat Dry Skin

PRODUCT	STRENGTH PER DOSE	ACTIVE INGREDIENT	USUAL DOSAGE	TYPICAL QUANTITY	TYPICAL PRICE	PRICE PER G, OR ML
Amlactin (ammonium lactate) lotion	12%	Ammonium lactate	Apply 2 times a day.	225g	$15	7¢
Lac-Hydrin (ammonium lactate) lotion	12%	Ammonium lactate	Apply 2 times a day.	225g	$45	20¢
Lactinol (lactic acid) lotion	10%	Lactic acid	Apply 2 times a day.	237ml	$30	13¢
Lactinol-E (lactic acid and vitamin E) cream	10% and 3500 IU	Lactic acid and vitamin E	Apply 2 times a day.	56.7g	$30	53¢

$ SMART BUY
Drugs that Treat Dry Skin

Save yourself some money and stick with the over-the-counter products. Eucerin comes in a generic form that will save you even more money. Apply it properly, drink plenty of water, and your dry skin should become a thing of the past.

$ SMART OPTIONS FOR SAVINGS
Drugs for the Eyes and Skin

When it comes to these products, you can save money in a number of ways:

1. Buy generic versions whenever they're available. (Ask your doctor to authorize them and your pharmacist to use them to fill your prescription.)
2. Look for quantity discounts. Often you'll get significant price breaks if you buy 2 or 3 bottles of eye drops at a time, for example. A larger quantity nearly always results in a lower per-dose cost, even if your initial expense is higher than for a smaller quantity.
3. Look for, and ask your doctor and pharmacist about, manufacturer's coupons, especially for eye drops to treat glaucoma.
4. If you're a senior using glaucoma medications, compare prices on the Internet at www.AARP.com. Be sure to factor in fees and shipping charges.
5. If you use these products regularly and can wait up to two weeks for them to arrive, often you can find deep discounts through mail-order sources. Canadian Internet pharmacies typically offer the greatest savings, although regulatory changes by either the Canadian or the U.S. government might curtail or eliminate this option. Check our Web site at www.smartbuysdrugwise.com for the latest information.
6. If you live near the Canadian border, or near an American physician who is licensed to practice medicine in Canada, buying these prescription products there might save you 50 percent or more. Just be sure to consider the cost of the medical examination or service fee you'll have to pay.
7. For skin problems, over-the-counter products can be as effective as prescription ones, at significantly less expense.

PART 3

Saving Money on Over-the-Counter Drugs

Chapter 16

SOS Over-the-Counter: Smart Options for Saving Money on Over-the-Counter Drugs

How familiar is this: You wake up in the morning with a screaming sore throat, or you come home from work with a splitting headache. You want relief—now. So you zip over to the local supermarket or drugstore to pick something up. But what confronts you there is row upon row upon row of choices—clearly not what you want! You don't want to read labels and compare ingredients or shop around for the best price. You just want to feel better. So instead of making an informed decision, you scan the shelves for something, anything, you recognize. You grab a product you saw in a TV commercial last night and head for the checkout line.

The myriad of options available to treat minor aches, pains, and annoyances without first making a trip to the doctor's office is one of the more impressive elements of American healthcare, but it's also one of the most perplexing. How do you know what to buy, where to buy it, and whether it will really do what its label or advertising claims?

Making the right over-the-counter choices isn't difficult once you understand how the industry works. As with anything else, knowledge is power when it comes to choosing and buying over-the-counter drugs. And selecting the right kind of drug is just the start. Once you know how to shop for the appropriate remedy, often you'll find amazing savings sure to help you feel better, no matter what ails you! Our SOS approach—Smart Options for Savings—will show you the best ways to get the best deals.

THE GROWING OVER-THE-COUNTER LIST

Since 1972, more than 80 drugs once available only by prescription have become available over the counter. The result: more than 700 new products have hit the market. These drugs multiplied faster than rabbits! What's going on? Well, the high cost and inconvenience of going to the doctor has fueled the American public's demand for self-treatment options. Researchers estimate that six out of 10 medications purchased by consumers are available over-the-counter. Yet most of these are variations on a theme—different products and combinations that contain similar ingredients.

Before the FDA will approve a drug's transition from prescription to over-the-counter status, drug manufacturers must prove certain criteria. This includes evidence that the drug is safe and effective, and that the manufacturer can develop clear and understandable labeling that allows self-medication without the help of a healthcare professional. Also, the drug must have no addictive potential. Because the drug already has been tested and approved for use (in prescription-only form), the process of meeting these criteria is much easier and faster than getting FDA approval for a completely new drug. The FDA need only determine the safe and effective over-the-counter dosage, and whether consumers can understand the label and follow the instructions.

► Once Prescription, Now Over-the-Counter

Some of the big over-the-counter sellers that used to be prescription-only include:

- Actifed
- Advil
- Afrin
- Aleve
- Axid
- Benadryl
- Cortaid
- Dimetapp
- Drixoral
- Excedrin PM
- Gyne-Lotrimin

- Imodium
- Lotrimin AF
- Micatin
- Monistat-7
- Motrin IB
- Neosporin Ointment
- Nicoderm CQ
- Nicorette
- Nuprin
- Nytol

- Pamprin IB
- Pepcid AC
- Rogaine
- Sudafed
- Tagamet HB
- Tavist
- Tinactin
- Tylenol
- Unisom
- Zantac 75

Clear and understandable labeling is crucial to ensure the proper use of a medication and to warn people about potential side effects. Although the FDA does attempt to prevent unsafe drugs from entering the marketplace, its approval of a medication for over-the-counter use doesn't mean the drug is free of potential side effects or is 100 percent safe for all people to take. Consider over-the-counter antihistamines (products that treat allergies), for example. For most people, the only concern is that the drug might cause drowsiness. Read the labels of these products, though, and you'll learn that antihistamines can be dangerous to people who have glaucoma, enlarged prostate, or asthma. If you have one of the conditions listed in a "Do not use this product if you have" warning on a product's label, check with your doctor before taking the drug.

Sometimes label information isn't enough to base your choice on. For example, the only potential side effects noted in the warnings section on a box of over-the-counter Motrin IB are severe allergic reactions and stomach bleeding. The label also cautions consumers to report unusual symptoms to their doctor and avoid using an ibuprofen product during the last three months of pregnancy. Sounds pretty safe, right? Well, the list of side effects included in the references for pharmacists and doctors is much longer. From stomach ulcers to kidney and liver problems, the list of potential side effects from ibuprofen or similar drugs includes more than 200 problems! For most people, ibuprofen is a safe and effective drug. For some people, however, the drug can cause serious side effects. When in doubt, discuss your concerns with your pharmacist or doctor.

Possible Drug Interactions

If you're taking any prescription medications, herbal remedies, or other over-the-counter drugs,

check with the pharmacist about possible interactions before trying a new over-the-counter product.

KNOW WHEN TO SEEK MEDICAL CARE

Always use sound judgment when deciding to treat your symptoms on your own. Certain symptoms indicate potentially serious medical problems. If you have any of these symptoms, seek medical attention before you shop for over-the-counter remedies:

+ Chest pain
+ Head injuries
+ Eye injuries and problems, including any discharge
+ Pain severe enough to keep you from using an extremity

+ Wounds that bleed heavily or develop a discharge (pus)
  Also see a health care professional when you have

...a sore throat that lasts longer than three days, is accompanied by a fever, or interferes with your ability to swallow.

...diarrhea that continues for longer than three days or is bloody.

...indigestion that continues for longer than two weeks.

...a muscle sprain or strain that isn't significantly better in two weeks.

...any health problem that continues beyond two weeks.

And, of course, anytime you're not sure what the problem is, at least call your doctor's office or health clinic to talk with a nurse who can help you determine whether you
should receive medical attention.

▶ Even "Natural" Products Have Risks

Just because a drug or product is available without a prescription or is a "natural" herbal product
doesn't mean you can take it without risk. All drugs carry the potential of side effects. Always read
package labels and informational inserts carefully and completely before taking or using an over-the-
counter product. If you experience any unusual effects, stop taking the product immediately and contact your pharmacist or doctor.

"SOS" FOR OVER-THE-COUNTER DRUG COSTS: WAYS TO SAVE MONEY

One of the most significant advantages to having so many drugs available without a
doctor's prescription is cost: Over-the-counter drugs often are priced competitively—
if you know what you're comparing. Based on our many years of experience in retail
pharmacies, we've developed the following Smart Options for Savings—your SOS
approach to saving money on over-the-counter drugs:

1. Choose the right kind of drug.
2. Go generic.
3. Buy in bulk.
4. Shop around.
5. Watch for coupons and store sales.
6. Resist advertising claims.
7. Take advantage of manufacturers' rebates.

Not every option will work for every over-the-counter product you need, but at least one option will apply for just about anything. The "SOS Worksheet" at the end of this chapter gives you a fast and easy way to determine which options work for the products you need to buy so you can save as much money as possible. Photocopy this worksheet as many times as you like, so you have copies you can carry with you.

OVER-THE-COUNTER SOS #1:
CHOOSE THE RIGHT KIND OF DRUG

First you must determine the kind of drug you need. What's bothering you? Do you have a headache, a sore throat, sore muscles from your weekend of activity? Before you can know which remedy to buy, you need to know what's ailing you. In more technical terms, you need to identify your symptoms so you can select appropriate treatment. Sometimes this process is simple and straightforward, as when you have a headache or an upset stomach. Other times, as with a cold or the flu, you may experience a combination of discomforts, including headache, cough, stuffy or runny nose, achy muscles, and fever.

Over-the-counter drugs fall into eight general categories. Chapters 17-22 provide detailed discussions of these.

+ Cold, flu, cough, and allergy preparations (Chapter 17)
+ Pain relief (Chapter 18)
+ Gastrointestinal remedies (Chapter 19)
+ Treatments for eyes, ears, mouth, and skin (Chapter 20)
+ Other over-the-counter products (Chapter 21)
+ Over-the-counter drugs for children (Chapter 22)

To know which over-the-counter product will best relieve your symptoms, first identify all the symptoms bothering you. Then turn to the appropriate chapter to read more about over-the-counter preparations to treat those symptoms. Taking a product that doesn't target your symptoms is unlikely to make you feel better. Nor will taking multi-symptom products if you have only one or two of the symptoms the drug treats, or experimenting with various single-component drugs until you find the right one. These approaches generally result in your spending more money than you need to before you find a product that works. The most effective strategy—the one that gets you feeling better fastest and saves you money—is to identify your specific symptoms, and then identify the products that treat them.

For example, say you have a sore throat. That's one symptom. Do you have a cough? Is your nose runny? Is your nose plugged? Do you have other aches and pains? Each of these is another symptom that might require different treatment. A pain reliever might relieve your sore throat. If you also have a headache or other aches and pains, those might feel better, too. But if you have a cough, that could be causing your sore throat. Taking a preparation to ease your coughing could reduce or end your sore throat. A stuffy nose can make your throat dry, while a runny nose can cause throat-irritating postnasal drainage. A pain reliever alone won't alleviate any of these symptoms. But taking a decongestant to relieve a stuffy nose or an antihistamine to dry up a runny nose could, and eliminate the source of your sore throat in the process. You'll feel better faster, and you'll save money because you buy only the products you really need!

SINGLE-COMPONENT PRODUCTS

Single-component products treat one specific kind of discomfort, such as pain, cough, itching, athlete's foot, bad breath, or any of dozens of other symptoms. Unless you have multiple symptoms, it's best to take a product that targets your discomfort. If you have a runny nose but not a cough, fever, sore throat, or other cold and flu symptoms, take a product that contains only an antihistamine; don't take a combination product, such as those for cold and flu symptoms. You might as well throw your money out the window, because taking something you don't need won't help you feel any better.

Some single-ingredient products relieve multiple or various symptoms. Ibuprofen, for example, can relieve pain, reduce swelling, and reduce fever, while acetaminophen can relieve pain and reduce fever. An antihistamine can relieve your runny nose due to allergies and reduce the itching and swelling of poison ivy, hives, or chickenpox. Some antihistamines also are effective as sleep aids—so effective, in fact, that you're better off to buy them in allergy-product form than to spend extra money on products touted as sleep aids. (See Chapter 21.)

MULTI-COMPONENT OR COMBINATION PRODUCTS

Products to treat multiple ailments include several active ingredients that target different symptoms. For example, many cold and flu preparations contain substances to relieve headache and muscle aches, reduce fever, relieve coughing, unplug your nose, and dry up your nose. Allergy products might include both an antihistamine and a decongestant. Other products combine ingredients for common discomforts—for example, those that blend a pain reliever with a sleep aid, such as Tylenol PM. Always read the label to learn what the product contains and how the manufacturer recommends that you take or use the product. If you're unsure whether a multi-ingredient product is right for your symptoms, ask the pharmacist.

Many people like combination products because they're convenient: One pill can relieve a host of symptoms. But combination products are often pricey. Before settling on a one-dose-treats-all preparation, price the individual ingredients. It's sometimes more cost-effective per dose to buy several products—such as an antihistamine, a cough suppressant, and a pain reliever—than to purchase one preparation that includes multiple ingredients. Be sure to compare dose-for-dose. A combination product might contain enough tablets for, say, four days' worth of treatment (24 tablets, with instructions to take one tablet every four hours). A single-ingredient product might contain 30, 60, or 100 tablets—far more doses. Buy generic and you can save even more.

As you can see, the savings per dose can be significant. You could spend a dollar for the recommended dose of two Nyquil Liqui-gels, for example, or take separate doses of the four generic-equivalent products in the chart and spend about 40 cents. You'll save 60 cents, or 60 percent, for each dose. Many people look at the overall cost of buying the combination product compared to buying the separate products, and at first glance feel this is hardly a bargain. But buying the separate products affords you numerous options for taking these drugs to treat other problems, such as seasonal allergies.

Sample Comparisons: Combination and Single-Ingredient Products

PRODUCT	STRENGTH	ACTIVE INGREDIENT	TYPICAL QUANTITY	TYPICAL PRICE	COST PER DOSE
Nyquil Multi-Symptom Cold/Flu Relief Liqui-Gels	6.25mg, 10mg, 250mg,30mg	Doxylamine succinate, dextromethorphan Hbr, acetaminophen, pseudoephedrine	12	$5.99	$1
Taking these four products gives you the same result as taking NYQUIL, for a savings of 60 cents or 60 percent per dose:					
Aller-Chlor, Chlortabs, or Chlorpheniramine 4-hr Tablets(generic version of Chlor-Trimeton)	4mg	Chlorpheniramine	100	$5.99	$0.06
Rite Aid, Wal-Mart, or Walgreens Tussin DM (generic for Robitussin DM Syrup)	100mg, 10mg, (in 5ml)	Guaifenesin, dextromethorphan	12oz	$6.49	$0.186

PRODUCT	STRENGTH	ACTIVE INGREDIENT	TYPICAL QUANTITY	TYPICAL PRICE	COST PER DOSE
Genapap, "No-Aspirin," Acetaminophen or "Non-aspirin"Extra-strength non-aspirin tablets	500mg	Acetaminophen	500	$14.99	$0.03
Walgreens or Wal-Mart Pseudoephedrine Decongestant tablets(generic-version of Sudafed)	30 mg	Pseudoephedrine	100	$5.99	$0.12
Contac Severe Cold/Flu Caplets OR Theraflu Nighttime Cold, Flu, & Cough Caplets	500mg, 15mg, 30mg, 2mg	Acetaminophen, dextromethorphan, pseudoephedrine chlorpheniramine	16 24	$ 4.99 $6.99	$0.625 Contac $0.583 Theraflu

Taking these four products gives you the same result as taking Contac or TheraFlu for a savings of 11 cents or 17.7 percent per dose:

PRODUCT	STRENGTH	ACTIVE INGREDIENT	TYPICAL QUANTITY	TYPICAL PRICE	COST PER DOSE
Aller-Chlor, Chlortabs, or Chlorpheniramine 4hr Tablets(generic version of Chlor-Trimeton)	4mg	Chlorpheniramine	100	$5.99	$0.06
Rite Aid, Wal-Mart, or Walgreens Tussin DM (generic version of Robitussin DM Syrup)	100mg, 10mg, (in 5ml)	Guaifenesin,dextromethorphan	12oz	$6.49	$0.274
Genapap, "No-Aspirin," Acetaminiophen or "Non-aspirin"Extra-strength nonaspirin tablets	500mg	Acetaminophen	500	$14.99	$0.06
Walgreens or Wal-Mart Pseudoephedrine Decongestant tablets (generic version of Sudafed)	30 mg	Pseudoephedrine	100	$5.99	$0.12
Tylenol Maximum Strength Allergy Sinus Caplets	2mg 500mg 30mg	Chlorphenirame Acetaminophen Pseudoephedrine	24	$6.99	$0.282

Taking these three products gives you the same result as taking Tylenol Maximum Strength Allergy Sinus Caplets, for a savings of 4.2 cents or 14.9 percent per dose

PRODUCT	STRENGTH	ACTIVE INGREDIENT	TYPICAL QUANTITY	TYPICAL PRICE	COST PER DOSE
Aller-Chlor, Chlortabs, or Chlorpheniramine 4hr Tablets(generic version of Chlor-Trimeton)	4mg	Chlorpheniramine	100	$5.99	$0.06
Genapap, "No-Aspirin," Acetaminophen or "Non-aspirin"Extra-strength nonaspirin tablets	500mg	Acetaminophen	500	$14.99	$0.06

PRODUCT	STRENGTH	ACTIVE INGREDIENT	TYPICAL QUANTITY	TYPICAL PRICE	COST PER DOSE
Walgreens or Wal-Mart Pseudoephedrine Decongestant tablets (generic version of Sudafed)	30 mg	Pseudoephedrine	100	$5.99	$0.12

OVER-THE-COUNTER SOS #2: GO GENERIC

Not only prescription drugs are available in generic forms. Most over-the-counter drugs also have name-brand and generic alternatives. Large pharmacy and supermarket chains often produce "generic brand names"—generic forms of over-the-counter products with the store's name on the label (and sometimes a unique name for the product). As with prescription drugs, you can save tremendous amounts of money by buying generic over-the-counter products.

When you buy a generic version of a prescription drug, you don't have to know what products to look for because the pharmacist does that for you. Finding generic alternatives to name-brand over-the-counter products is another experience entirely. Of course, you can always ask the pharmacist for assistance, but often it's faster and easier if you can do this yourself. Here are some tips.

- ✦ Look for sound-alike names. People go with what's familiar, and manufacturers try to take advantage of that. Generic products containing diphenhydramine, the antihistamine ingredient in the popular name-brand product Benadryl, might be called Benahist, Diphenhist, Hydramine, Genahist, or Banophen.
- ✦ Look for labels that say "Compare to the active ingredient in…," and then give a popular brand name. For example, generic cimetidine packaging might proclaim, "Same active ingredient as Tagamet!" Sometimes these comparisons mention economy or savings, hoping to catch your attention with the promise of a bargain.
- ✦ Look to the right of the name-brand product on the shelf. Many retailers organize their shelf displays in this sequence, with generic versions to the right of their name-brand counterparts.

Although some prescription drugs have narrow therapeutic indexes (NTIs) that make it important to stay with the same (generic or name-brand) product, over-the-counter drugs aren't so sensitive. Seldom does it matter, from a therapeutic perspective, whether you use a name-brand or generic over-the-counter product. Because each formulation differs a little, however, you might notice variations among brands of the same drug. One manufacturer's version of the product might have soft tablets that break easily; another product's tablets are so hard you wonder if they'll even dis-

Name-Brand and Generic Over-the-Counter Product Comparisons

BRAND NAME PRODUCT	TAKEN TO TREAT	TYPICAL QUANTITY	TYPICAL RETAIL COST	COST PER DOSE	GENERIC VERSION	TYPICAL RETAIL	COST PER DOSE
Actifed Cold & Allergy Tablets	Cold, allergy symptoms	24	$7.49	$0.31	Wal-Act Cold & Allergy Tabs	$5.29	$0.22
Advil 200mg Tablets	Pain, fever, inflammation	100	$8.49	$0.085	Ibuprofen, Genpril, Ibu-200, Menadol	$6.99	$0.07
Afrin 12-hr Original Decongestant Nasal Spray, Pump Mist	Nasal congestion	0.5oz	6.29	$12.58/ oz.	"12-Hour" Nasal Pump Mist(Generic for Afrin 12-hr) original formula pump mist	4.99	$9.98/ oz.
Aleve 220mg Tablets	Pain, fever, inflammation	100	$8.99	$0.09	Naproxen Sodium,Wal-Pro-xen(Generic version of Aleve)	$6.99	$0.07
Benadryl Allergy Relief Kapseals	Cold and allergy symptoms	24	$4.69	$0.19	Diphenhist, Wal-Dryl or Benahist store brand versions of Benadryl	$3.49	$0.15
Chlor-Trimeton 4-hour Tablets	Cold and allergy symptoms	24	$5.99	$0.25	Aller-Chlor, Chlor-Tabs, Chlorphenira-mine, or 4-hour Allergy Tablets	$3.99	$0.16
Dimetapp Children's Cold & Allergy Liquid	Cold and allergy symptoms	8oz	$8.99	$0.19 (per 5ml)	DiBromm, Wal-Tap or Bromphen Cold & Allergy Liquid	$6.99	$0.15 (per 5ml)
Robitussin DM Cough Suppressant	Cough	8oz	$9.99	$0.21	Rite Aid, Wal-Mart, or Walgreens Tussin DM	$5.99	$0.13
Tylenol Maximum Strength Allergy Sinus Caplets	Cold, allergy, sinus symptoms	24	$6.99	$0.29	Non-Aspirin Sinus Allergy Aspirin Free or No Aspirin Allergy Sinus Caplets	$4.99	$0.21
Tylenol PM Gelcaps	Sleep aid	50	$8.99	$0.18	Non-Aspirin PM or Aspirin-Free NiteTime or No-Aspirin Headache Relief PM	$5.99	$0.12

solve after you take them. Or one brand of a cream rubs in smoothly and quickly, while another remains on the surface of your skin after minutes of rubbing. Although the active ingredients of these products are the same, the *inactive* ingredients can differ, and that can result in subtle differences in how the drug works for you. If you notice such differences, experiment with various brands until you find the one that works best for you.

OVER-THE-COUNTER SOS #3: BUY IN BULK

You'll find big savings when you buy in quantity (especially when you combine quantity with generics). It's important to calculate the per-dose cost before going for the big bottle, however—sometimes the big bottle simply costs more than the small one. Many retail stores include the per-unit price on the shelf tags to help you determine which size is the better deal. Packaging also can influence price. Generally, blister packs and other forms of single-dose packaging cost more than bottles that contain loose tablets. This is in part because products packaged by the dose generally contain fewer tablets (or caplets or whatever the form of the product is), and in part because single-dose packaging is more expensive to make, period. Look also at the product strength. You'd think that less product would mean less cost, but it doesn't often work this way. Nearly always, it's cheaper per dose to buy larger quantities.

Sometimes it's more cost-effective to buy a greater quantity of a lesser strength and take two tablets instead of one. (Be sure to calculate per-dose cost.) Sometimes a pharmacy will order common over-the-counter products, such as ibuprofen (a generic version of Motrin or Advil) or diphenhydramine (a generic version of Benadryl), in bulk sizes or packaging for you if it doesn't carry them already. Some retail stores with limited shelf space might stock just the 24- or 36-count package because these are the sizes most people buy. If you ask, however, the pharmacist can order a 100-count bottle for you (for most products) at a substantial savings.

There's a practical reason many over-the-counter products come in limited dose sizes: It limits the number of doses you can take. In general, you shouldn't take over-the-counter drugs for longer than the label or insert recommends unless your doctor instructs you otherwise. Some drugs can accumulate in your body, while others become less effective as your body becomes used to them. And if your symptoms continue beyond the recommended treatment period, see a doctor to identify and receive appropriate treatment for the underlying problem. Let's not overlook the reality that limited quantities also benefit the manufacturer and the drugstore. You need to buy more of the product if you want to continue taking it, which increases sales.

> ## Whose Loss is It?
>
> Beware the "loss leader." This is a product a store advertises for a price at or below its cost simply to draw customers into the store. Once there, you can buy your bargain and leave—or, if you're like the typical consumer, you might pick up a few other items you need while you're there. The store might take a small loss on the advertised item, but it gains big on those other purchases. Go for the good deal on the advertised special, but remain a cautious consumer on those other purchases!

OVER-THE-COUNTER SOS #4: SHOP AROUND

Just about every kind of store carries at least a few over-the-counter products. Even service stations and convenience stores usually have travel-size packages of pain relievers, antacids, and other such commonly used drugs. These products are no longer the domain of the drugstore. In fact, major supermarkets often have large pharmacy departments that sell prescription and over-the-counter drugs (just as many drugstores also sell food items). And just as the selling locations vary widely, so do the prices. Often certain stores offer lower prices on particular products, so get to know the stores in your area. Do you have a membership at a retail or warehouse store that carries the over-the-counter products you need? Membership stores typically offer lower costs, although it's important to factor in the cost of the membership considering how often you'll shop there.

Stores are free to charge what they think they can get people to pay. Although most stores try to remain close to the prices their competitors charge for the same products, some consistently charge more or less. You're likely to pay more for an over-the-counter product when the store is the only retailer within a reasonable distance. When several stores are in close proximity, prices are likely to be lower as each store jockeys to be the favorite. Prices can vary widely even within a small community or neighborhood, though, so it pays to shop around and compare. Check stores near your home, near your workplace, and in between. Just be sure you compare the same products. Sometimes store brands differ slightly, making it more challenging for you to determine whether the

Sample Savings When Buying Larger Quantities

OVER-THE-COUNTER PRODUCT	RETAIL COST FOR SMALLER PACKAGE SIZE	RETAIL COST FOR LARGER PACKAGE SIZE	SAVINGS OF LARGE OVER SMALL PACKAGE SIZE
Sudafed 30mg tablets	$5.99 for 24	$14.29 for 96	$9.67/40%
Pseudoephedrine 30mg tablets	$2.99 for 24	$4.99 for 100	$7.47/60%
Ibuprofen 200mg Tabs	$2.59 for 24	$6.49 for 100	$4.30/40%
Robitussin DM Cough Supressant	$5.79 for 4oz	$9.99 for 12oz	$7.38/42%
Chlorpheniramine 4-hr tablets	$4.49 for 24	$9.99 for 100	$8.72/47%
Bayer Genuine Aspirin Pain Reliever	$1.99 for 12	$10.99 for 200	$22.18/71%
Diphenhydramine 25mg capsules	$3.49 for 24	$5.99 for 100	$8.55/59%
Tylenol Extra Strength Caplets	$4.99 for 24	$16.99 for 250	$34.99/67%
Pepcid AC Tablets	$8.29 for 18	$22.99 for 90	$18.50/45%

products are the same. Read labels carefully. If you have questions, ask a pharmacist to explain the differences between products.

It's a good idea to get your prescription drugs at the same store where you buy most of your over-the-counter drugs, because pharmacies keep records of the medications they dispense to you. This helps the pharmacist and your doctor stay informed about what you're taking, and to be on the alert for potential interactions or other problems. But stores don't keep track of over-the-counter drug purchases, so buying all your over-the-counter drugs at the same store offers little advantage to you unless the store always has the best prices.

OVER-THE-COUNTER SOS #5: WATCH FOR COUPONS AND STORE SALES

You might think coupons and store sales offer great ways for you to save money—and they can. But from the store's point of view, the real reason to offer discounts is to get you into the store. It's human nature to feel more inclined to buy other items (even items you don't really need) when the item you need costs less than you'd expected to spend. Instead of pocketing your savings, the store hopes you'll spend it—and more.

Many retail stores feature specials that change every few days, or weekly. Often these sales are seasonal: When winter rolls around, cold and flu products typically go on sale; in the spring, stores might discount allergy products. It pays to read the ads in the newspapers and circulars that come in the mail, and even to keep a file of coupons for products you routinely use. Some stores will honor competitors' coupons. "Buy one, get one free" ads often run prominently in local newspapers. Always compare prices, however, especially when the advertised product is a name brand.

Many chain stores offer discounted prices—either consistently or for defined periods of time—for customers who participate in the chain's "membership" program. Generally, you must fill out an application form and receive a bar-coded card or key-chain tag the clerk scans every time you make a purchase. In exchange, the chain tracks your spending habits, which helps it target its marketing campaigns. Sometimes the discounts are significant, so it's worth at least looking into these programs. Before you sign up, though, be sure you fully understand what information the chain collects when you use your card.

OVER-THE-COUNTER SOS #6: RESIST ADVERTISING CLAIMS

The young woman in the television commercial clearly hurts. She sits with her head in her hands, oblivious to what's going on around her. She takes a pill and—immediate relief! Just that fast, her debilitating headache disappears and life is grand.

To believe all the advertising hype and marketing claims that bombard you, you'd have to believe that there was never any reason for anyone to feel the slightest discomfort. While we might like this to be true, it simply isn't. What is true is that numerous products exist that can make you feel better, but none that can make your life picture-perfect.

The role of advertising is to sell, not to inform. Most advertising is not intentionally misleading, but instead, emphasizes the aspects of the product that are most likely to generate sales. Actors in TV commercials and magazine ads play characters who find relief by using a particular product—"people just like you" presenting a picture of what your life, were it ideal, would be like. If the ad can get you to identify with these portrayals, it's likely that the next time you confront that wall of indecision in the drugstore or grocery store, you'll choose that particular product, even if it's priced higher than another, equally effective, product.

Manufacturers—and to some extent, retailers—count on brand loyalty. They want you to feel such a strong connection to their products that you won't even look at other labels. Seldom does this benefit you. Ibuprofen is ibuprofen, cimetidine is cimetidine, and diphenhydramine is diphenhydramine—no matter how clever the brand name or advertising campaign. Buy the product that's most cost effective, not the promotion!

> ### Special Displays Offer Special Savings
>
> When you shop, check out the special displays at the ends of the aisles or in kiosks at the front of the store. Items receiving special promotion often are on sale or come with manufacturer rebates.

OVER-THE-COUNTER SOS #7: TAKE ADVANTAGE OF MANUFACTURER REBATES

Manufacturer rebates can save you a lot of money. Some pay a percentage of the cost of the product; others pay a flat amount, usually at least a dollar and sometimes as much as $5 or $10, depending on the product. Sometimes the store provides the rebate coupon, or you may find a coupon inside the packaging. Send in your rebate coupon and any required proof of purchase (usually your receipt or the bar code from the product package) promptly. Pay attention to rebate expiration dates; if you send in your rebate request after the offer has expired, you won't get the rebate (and often no notice explaining why).

As with coupons and sales, these rebates aren't exactly offers of altruistic generosity. Manufacturers want you to buy their brands, hoping that once you do, you'll continue buying them. They know humans are creatures of habit. Manufacturers also use the information you provide when filling out your rebate coupon to refine their marketing and advertising strategies. Some put you on their mailing lists; others compile information anonymously into databases.

> ▶ **Get Your Rebate Coupons**
>
> Membership warehouse stores and large retail stores often have designated locations in the stores, usually near the exit, where you can pick up rebate coupons. These stores may automatically generate "rebate receipts" for you to send in for your proof-of-purchase, so you can keep your real receipt in case you need it for your records. ◀

OVER-THE-COUNTER SOS:
IDENTIFY *YOUR* SAVINGS OPTIONS

We've created an "SOS" Worksheet to help you determine which Smart Options for Savings can save you money on over-the-counter drugs. Photocopy this worksheet as many times as you like, and use it to help you find the best prices for the over-the-counter products you need to use.

The filled-in worksheet provides an example of how it might be used. Photocopy the blank one to take with you when you shop. Use a separate worksheet for each drug.

SAMPLE: SOS WORKSHEET FOR SAVING MONEY ON OVER-THE-COUNTER DRUGS

SYMPTOMS	LIST YOUR MAJOR SYMPTOMS.		
	Sore muscles after weekend of doing yard work		

SOS #1	SELECT ALL THAT APPLY.		
The Right Kind of Drug	❏ Cold, flu, cough, and allergy preparations ❏ Pain relief ❏ Gastrointestinal remedies ❏ Treatments for eyes, ears, mouth, and skin ❏ Other over-the-counter products	❏ Herbal substitutes ❏ Vitamins and minerals ❏ Single-component Product ❏ Multicomponent or Combination Product	

SOS #2	NAME-BRAND PRODUCTS	STORE BRAND PRODUCTS	GENERIC PRODUCTS
Go Generic	*Motrin IB 200mg* *Advil 200mg*	*MorProfen 200mg* *(Save More)*	*Ibuprofen 200mg*

SOS #3	AVAILABLE QUANTITY	COST PER DOSE (PRICE DIVIDED BY AMOUNT)	
Buy in Bulk	*24 (blister pack), 100, 250*	*65 cents, 12 cents, 4 cents*	

SOS #4	STORE 1	STORE 2	STORE 3
Shop Around	*Save More Pharmacy* *$9.99*	*Get More Drugstore* *$12.79*	*Best Buy Bargains* *$10.89*

SOS #5	LIST VALUE AND RESTRICTIONS OF ANY STORE COUPONS.		
Coupons and Sales	*50 cents off at Save More Pharmacy, expires in 5 days*		

SOS #6	LIST ANY PRODUCTS THAT CURRENTLY APPEAR IN PRINT, TELEVISION, OR RADIO ADVERTISING.		
Ignore Advertising	*Motrin IB on television commercial*		

SOS #7	LIST VALUE OF ANY MANUFACTURERS' REBATES.		
Use Rebates	*None*		

SMART BUYS	LIST THE SMART BUYS IN EACH CHAPTER FOR THE CATEGORIES OF PRODUCTS THAT YOU NEED.		
$	*Generic ibuprofen 200mg*		

YOUR BEST CHOICE(S)	PRODUCT	QUANTITY	PRICE	STORE
	MorProfen 200mg	*250*	*$9.99*	*Save More Pharmacy*

SOS WORKSHEET FOR SAVING MONEY ON OVER-THE-COUNTER DRUGS

SYMPTOMS	LIST YOUR MAJOR SYMPTOMS.
	_____

SOS #1	SELECT ALL THAT APPLY.	
The Right Kind of Drug	❏ Cold, flu, cough, and allergy preparations ❏ Pain relief ❏ Gastrointestinal remedies ❏ Treatments for eyes, ears, mouth, and skin ❏ Other over-the-counter products	❏ Herbal substitutes ❏ Vitamins and minerals ❏ Single-component Product ❏ Multicomponent or Combination Product

SOS #2	NAME-BRAND PRODUCTS	STORE BRAND PRODUCTS	GENERIC PRODUCTS
Go Generic	_____	_____	_____
	_____	_____	_____

SOS #3	AVAILABLE QUANTITY	COST PER DOSE (PRICE DIVIDED BY AMOUNT)
Buy in Bulk		

SOS #4	STORE 1	STORE 2	STORE 3
Shop Around	_____	_____	_____
	_____	_____	_____

SOS #5	LIST VALUE AND RESTRICTIONS OF ANY STORE COUPONS.
Coupons and Sales	_____ _____

SOS #6	LIST ANY PRODUCTS THAT CURRENTLY APPEAR IN PRINT, TELEVISION, OR RADIO ADVERTISING.
Ignore Advertising	_____ _____

SOS #7	LIST VALUE OF ANY MANUFACTURERS' REBATES.
Use Rebates	_____

SMART BUYS	LIST THE SMART BUYS IN EACH CHAPTER FOR THE CATEGORIES OF PRODUCTS THAT YOU NEED.
[$]	_____ _____

YOUR BEST CHOICE(S)	PRODUCT	QUANTITY	PRICE	STORE
	_____	_____	_____	_____
	_____	_____	_____	_____

Chapter 17

Over-the-Counter Cold, Flu, Cough, and Allergy Preparations

When Claire's pharmacist suggested she try the decongestant pseudoephedrine to relieve her stuffy nose, Claire thought her misery would finally end. But when she stood in the drugstore aisle looking over the bewildering number of product variations on this seemingly simple suggestion, she wondered whether her misery was instead just beginning. There were nine different kinds of the name-brand product Sudafed alone, and dozens of generic versions! Claire had to ask the pharmacist to help her make an appropriate selection. Had the pharmacist been unable to assist her, Claire might have just closed her eyes and pointed!

Sadly, Claire's predicament was small-scale compared to the myriad of choices available within the category of over-the-counter products for colds, flu, coughs, and allergies. At the time of this writing, there are 474 different such products on the U.S. market. This isn't surprising. A 2001 study conducted by the National Institutes for Health revealed that cold symptoms are the leading reason Americans miss work. The good news is that these hundreds of products break down into only five broad categories:

1. Antihistamines
2. Antitussives
3. Decongestants
4. Expectorants
5. Fever and pain relievers

And within these five categories are just drugs, found in cold and allergy remedies. So how do so few ingredients account for so many products? Two words—duplication and combination.

For a good example of duplication, let's look at ibuprofen, a common pain and fever reliever. Ibuprofen is available in eight different name-brand products:

- ✦ Motrin
- ✦ Motrin IB
- ✦ Advil
- ✦ Bayer Select Pain Relief

- ✦ Haltran
- ✦ Midol IB
- ✦ Arthritis Foundation
- ✦ Saleto-200

Numerous store-brand and generic versions are available, as well. As you can see, it doesn't take long for the numbers to add up!

It also doesn't take long for the numbers to become exponentially large. In the battle for market share, manufacturers always look for new ways to snare more customers. One effective way for them to do this is to create combination products that treat multiple symptoms. Comtrex Maximum Strength Multi-Symptom Cold and Flu Relief, MediFlu, and Nyquil are all examples of combination products that treat the variety of symptoms common with upper respiratory viral infections.

Which product is right for you? Yet again, it depends on your symptoms. Our overarching recommendation is simple: Just treat the symptoms you have. If you just have a stuffy nose, you don't need medication for cough or fever. Not only is there no therapeutic benefit in taking extra drugs (they don't prevent you from getting other symptoms!), but it's a waste of money.

PHENYLPROPANOLAMINE (PPA) ALERT

In 2001, the FDA withdrew approval for the over-the-counter decongestant drug phenylpropranolamine, also known as PPA. This was a request to manufacturers to recall and reformulate all products containing PPA, which they have done. The FDA made this request based on Yale University's School of Medicine study showing PPA may increase the risk of hemorrhagic stroke (bleeding into the brain and tissue around the brain). Because many people keep leftover cold remedies in the medicine cabinet for the next round of viral infections, we include here a list of common products that contained PPA. If any of these still lurk on your shelves, throw them away. If you're not sure, look for "PPA" or "phenylpropanolamine" in the list of ingredients.

PRODUCTS CONTAINING PHENYLPROPANOLAMINE (PPA)

- ✦ 4-Way Cold Tablets
- ✦ Alka Seltzer Plus Cold Tablets
- ✦ Alka Seltzer Plus Night-Time Cold Tablets
- ✦ Allerest 12-hr. Caplets

- ✦ Allerest Headache Strength Tablets
- ✦ Allerest Sinus Pain Formula Tablets
- ✦ Allerest Tablets
- ✦ Bayer Children's Cough Syrup
- ✦ Bromotap Elixir
- ✦ Cheracol Plus Syrup

- Children's Allerest Tablets
- Comtrex Liquid
- Comtrex Tablets And Caplets
- Conar-A Tablets
- Congesprin Cold Tablets For Children
- Contac 12-hour Capsules
- Contac Maximum Strength and 12 Hour Caplets
- Contac Severe Cold Formula Caplets
- Coricidin D Decongestant Tablets
- Coricidin Demilets Tablets
- Coricidin Extra Strength Sinus Headache Tablets
- Dimetapp Elixir
- Dimetapp Extentabs
- Dimetapp Tablets
- Halls Mentho-Lyptus Decongestant Liquid
- Hold Children's Formula Lozenges
- Naldecon Dx Adult Liquid
- Naldecon Dx Children's Syrup
- Naldecon Dx Pediatric Drops
- Naldecon Ex Pediatric Drops
- Naldecon Ex Syrup
- Poly-Histine Expectorant Syrup
- Robitussin-CF Syrup
- Sinapils Tablets
- Sinarest Extra Strength Tablets
- Sinarest Tablets
- Sine-Off Sinus Medicine Tablets
- Spec-T Sore Throat/ Decongestant Lozenges
- St. Joseph's Cold Tablets For Children
- Tavist-D Tablets
- Triaminic Allergy Tablets
- Triaminic Chewable
- Triaminic Cold Tablets
- Triaminic Expectorant
- Triaminic-12 Tablets
- Triaminic-DM Liquid
- Triaminicin Tablets
- Triaminicol Multi-Symptom Cold Liquid
- Triaminicol Multi-Symptom Cold Tablets
- Triaminic Cold Syrup
- Vicks Head and Chest Liquid

RELIEVING A STUFFY NOSE: ORAL DECONGESTANTS

To relieve sinus congestion and a stuffy nose, you need a decongestant. There are only two active ingredients in oral over-the-counter products (substances you take by mouth) in this category—pseudoephedrine and phenylephrine. In terms of function, these two decongestants differ very little. However, you should be aware of some general concerns when using decongestants. First, if you have diabetes, high blood pressure, prostate problems, glaucoma, an overactive thyroid, or an irregular heartbeat, you may want to avoid using these drugs without your doctor's supervision. Oral decongestants can act as stimulants, raising your heart rate and blood pressure and affecting your body systems in various ways. If you have one of these conditions, a nasal spray may be a good alternative. (See the next section, "Topical Decongestants.")

The vast majority of decongestant products have pseudoephedrine as their active ingredient. So is there really any difference among these products? The short answer is no. But don't stop there. What does matter is the product's strength. Buying the strength that's right for you will help you get the most for your money. Many people like the 12-hour products because they last all day; they needn't carry the bottle with them and stop what they're doing to take their next dose. But for some people, the 12-hour products can be too strong, drying them out to the point of discomfort and sometimes even keeping them awake at night. If you don't take decongestants very often, start with a lower dose (30mg pseudoephedrine).

> ### Limits on Pseudoephedrine Sales
>
> Most U.S. pharmacies restrict the sales of the 60mg strength of pseudoephedrine (Sudafed and its generic counterparts). This drug has become a major ingredient in illegal methamphetamine manufacturing. As a result, some manufacturers have even stopped making this strength. Usually you can still purchase the 60mg-strength product in some version, although you might need to ask the pharmacist for it and sign a statement affirming that it's for your personal use. (This requirement varies from place to place.)

Purchasing the stronger version is usually more cost-effective. Using a generic or store-brand product (such as Susphrine, Pseudogest, Pseudotabs, or Genaphed) can save you considerable money, and buying larger quantities of a generic product can save you even more. These options make sense for you if

...you use or take the product daily.
...you'll use up the product before it expires.
...several people in your household will use or take the product.

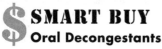

$ SMART BUY
Oral Decongestants

When it comes to an oral decongestant, let these three Smart Options for Savings guide your purchasing decision:

Oral Decongestants

Product	Strength	Active Ingredient	Usual Dosage	Typical Quantity	Typical Price	Cost per Dose
Alka-Seltzer Plus Cold & Cough Medicine, Effervescent Tablets	20mg	Phenylephrine (and other ingredients	Take 2 tablets but no more every 4 hrsthan 8 in 24 hrs.	20	$5.49	27¢
Allermed Tablets	60mg	Pseudoephedrine	Take 1-2 every 6 hrs.	24	$4.50	18¢
Congestion Relief Tablets	30mg	Pseudoephedrine	Take 1-2 every 6 hrs.	24	$5.50	23¢
Dimetapp Cold & Allergy Tabs	5mg	Phenylephrine + other ingredients	Take 2 tabs every 4 hrs. with no more than 12 tabs in 24 hrs.	20	$4.99	25¢
Dristan Multi-Symptom Decongestant Tabs	5mg	Phenylephrine + other ingredients	Take 2 tabs every 4 hrs. with no more than 12 tabs in 24 hrs.	20	$4.99	25¢
Drixoral Non-Drowsy Tabs	120mg	Pseudoephedrine	Take 1 every 12 hrs.	20	$7.99	40¢
Pseudoephedrine Syrup	30mg/5ml	Pseudoephedrine	Take 1 tsp every 6 hrs.	8oz	$1.50	3¢/tsp
Pseudoephedrine Tablets	60mg	Pseudoephedrine	Take 1-2 every 6 hrs.	100	$8	8¢
Seudotabs Tablets	30mg	Pseudoephedrine	Take 1-2 every 6 hrs.	24	$4.40	18¢
Sinustop Pro Tablets	60mg	Pseudoephedrine	Take 1-2 every 6 hrs.	24	$5.40	23¢
Suda-Tabs, Pseudo-Tabs (Wal-Mart, Walgreens, Rite Aid)Pseudoephedrine tablets	30mg	Pseudoephedrine	Take 1-2 every 6 hrs.	100	$6	6¢
Sudafed 12 Hour Caplets	120mg	Pseudoephedrine	Take 1 every 12 hrs.	20	$6.44	32¢
Sudafed Tablets	30mg	Pseudoephedrine	Take 1-2 every 6 hrs.	24	$4	17¢
Sudafed Tablets	60mg	Pseudoephedrine	Take 1-2 every 6 hrs.	24	$4.69	20¢
Sufafed 12-Hour Caplets	120mg	Pseudoephedrine	Take 1 every 12 hrs.	100	$24	24¢

1. Buy generic (or store brand).
2. Buy in bulk (quantity of 100, if possible).
3. Buy a single-ingredient product (not a combination product).

Generic products containing pseudoephedrine often use comparisons to brand name products for quick name recognition, and might say on the label, for example,

"Same active ingredient as Sudafed." The product that's least expensive in your location might be a regional store brand, such as Safeway, Rite Aid, Wal-Mart, Kmart or Walgreens. The Smart Buy is a bottle of 100 generic pseudoephedrine 30mg tablets made by United Research Laboratories (URL), which will cost you about $6, or 6 cents a dose. You might have to ask your pharmacist to order it for you. Buying a name-brand product in the handy but pricey 24-count package will set you back about $4, or 17 cents a dose. Buying generic pseudoephedrine in bulk quantity (such as the URL product) saves you 11 cents for every dose—a 35 percent savings!

But don't purchase a decongestant in a combination product. Most of these products contain ingredients you probably don't need—and if you do need them, you're better off buying them as separate products (as we explain elsewhere in this chapter), so you can mix and match to cover only the symptoms you actually have.

TOPICAL NASAL DECONGESTANTS

Nasal decongestant sprays offer an effective alternative to oral decongestants for many people. They're much less apt to cause problems with existing health conditions than their oral counterparts, and they're equally effective in relieving sinus congestion. Just take care not to use a nasal spray for longer than three days in a row. If you do, you run the risk of getting what health professionals call "rebound congestion"—the original cause of your stuffy nose, such as a cold, goes away, but the stuffiness returns with a vengeance. Your nose has become accustomed to assistance from the spray to keep its passages from swelling. When you stop using the spray, your nasal passages swell again, even though the virus that originally caused the problem is no longer present. This very uncomfortable ailment can be worse than the original problem (and might send you rushing to the drugstore or medicine cabinet for a pain reliever). If your congestion continues beyond three days of using a nasal decongestant, check with your doctor.

Over-the-counter topical or nasal decongestants contain one of the two active ingredients oxymetazoline or phenylephrine. Products containing oxymetazoline are long-acting and can relieve symptoms for up to 12 hours. The most common name-brand product containing oxymetazoline product is Afrin. As with most cold and flu products, numerous store brands and generic formulations are available. Products containing phenylephrine are short-acting, with their effectiveness generally lasting 4 to 6 hours. There's no advantage to taking the short-acting formulas, and taking the medication more often is less convenient.

We suggest a generic original formula Afrin (oxymetazoline). Often you'll find a store-brand generic right next to the name-brand with some mention of "12-hour

Nasal Spray" on the label. Because these products last about 12 hours, you may use them before school or work and won't need another dose until you're home again, so you needn't carry the medication with you.

Topical Nasal Decongestants

PRODUCT	ACTIVE INGREDIENT	USUAL DOSAGE	TYPICAL QUANTITY	TYPICAL PRICE	COST PER OZ
4-way 12 hour Nasal Decongestant Spray	Oxymetazoline 0.05%	Spray 2 or 3 times in each nostril no more often than every 10-12 hrs.	0.5oz	$4.99	$9.98
4-way 1% Nasal Decongestant Spray Fast-Acting	Phenylephrine1%	Spray 2 or 3 times in each nostril no more often than every 4 hrs.	0.5oz	$4.99	$9.98
4-way 1% Nasal Decongestant Spray Fast-Acting	Phenylephrine1%	Spray 2 or 3 times in each nostril no more often than every 4 hrs.	1oz	$7.99	$7.99
"12-Hour" Nasal Pump Mist(Generic for Afrin 12-hr) original formula pump mist (Walgreens, Rite Aid, Wal-Mart)	Oxymetazoline 0.05%	Spray 2 or 3 times in each nostril no more often than every 10-12 hrs.	1oz	$4.99	$4.99
Afrin 12-hour Original Decongestant Nasal Spray	Oxymetazoline 0.05%	Spray 2 or 3 times in each nostril no more often than every 10-12 hrs.	0.5oz	$5.99	$11.98
Afrin 12-hour Original Decongestant Nasal Spray	Oxymetazoline 0.05%	Spray 2 or 3 times in each nostril no more often than every 10-12 hrs.	1oz	$8.49	$8.49
Afrin 12 hr Original Decongestant Nasal Spray, Pump Mist	Oxymetazoline 0.05%	Spray 2 or 3 times in each nostril no more often than every 10-12 hrs.	0.5oz	$6.29	$12.58
Afrin Allergy 0.5% Nasal Decongestant	Phenylephrine 0.5%	Spray 2 or 3 times in each nostril no more often than every 4 hrs.	0.5oz	$5.99	$11.98
Afrin Extra Moisturizing Nasal Spray	Oxymetazoline 0.05%	Spray 2 or 3 times in each nostril no more often than every 10-12 hrs.	0.5oz	$5.99	$11.98
Afrin No Drip Severe Congestion Nasal Spray w/Menthol	Oxymetazoline 0.05%	Spray 2 or 3 times in each nostril no more often than every 10-12 hrs.	0.5oz	$6.49	$12.98
Afrin Severe Congestion Nasal Spray w/Menthol	Oxymetazoline 0.05%	Spray 2 or 3 times in each nostril no more often than every 10-12 hrs.	0.5oz	$5.99	$11.98

PRODUCT	ACTIVE INGREDIENT	USUAL DOSAGE	TYPICAL QUANTITY	TYPICAL PRICE	COST PER OZ
Afrin Sinus w/Vapornase Decongestant Nasal Spray	Oxymetazoline 0.05%	Spray 2 or 3 times in each nostril no more often than every 10–12 hrs.	0.5oz	$5.99	$11.98
Dristan 12 hr Decongestant Nasal Spray	Oxymetazoline 0.05%	Spray 2 or 3 times in each nostril no more often than every 10-12 hrs.	0.5oz	$5.99	$11.98
Dristan 0.5% Nasal Mist Spray	Phenylephrine 0.5%	Spray 2 or 3 times in each nostril no more often than every 4 hrs.	1oz	$7.99	$7.99
Neo-Synephrine 12-hour Decongestant Nasal Spray	Oxymetazoline 0.05%	Spray 2 or 3 times in each nostril no more often than every 10-12 hrs.	0.5oz	$6.49	$12.98
Neo-Synephrine 12-hour Extra-Moisturizing Nasal Spray	Oxymetazoline 0.05%	Spray 2 or 3 times in each nostril no more often than every 10-12 hrs.	0.5oz	$5.49	$10.98
Neo-Synephrine 1% Extra Strength Nasal Spray	Phenylephrine 1%	Spray 2 or 3 times in each nostril no more often than every 4 hrs.	0.5oz	$5.49	$10.98
Neo-Synephrine 0.25% Mild Nasal Spray	Phenylephrine 0.25%	Spray 2 or 3 times in each nostril no more often than every 4 hrs.	0.5oz	$4.99	$9.98
Nostrilla 12-Hour Nasal Decongestant Spray	Oxymetazoline 0.05%	Spray 2 or 3 times in each nostril no more often than every 10-12 hrs.	0.5oz	$6.59	$13.18
Otrivin Nasal Drops	Xylometazoline 0.1%	Spray 1-3 times in each nostril no more often than every 8-10 hrs.	0.83oz	$9.99	$12.04
Otrivin Nasal Spray	Xylometazoline 0.1%	Spray 1-3 times in each nostril no more often than every 8-10 hrs.	0.83oz	$8.49	$10.22
Vicks Sinex 12-Hour Nasal Spray	Oxymetazoline 0.05%	Spray 2 or 3 times in each nostril no more often than every 10-12 hrs.	0.5oz	$5.79	$11.58
Vicks Sinex 12-Hour Ultra Fine Mist for Sinus Relief	Oxymetazoline 0.05%	Spray 2 or 3 times in each nostril no more often than every 10-12 hrs.	0.5oz	$5.99	$11.98

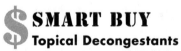

$ SMART BUY
Topical Decongestants

Almost every store carries a generic version of Afrin. ("12-Hour Nasal Spray" is the most common labeling.) Read the label's active ingredients list to be sure the product contains oxymetazoline. Do you think all the "extras" mean you'll get more for your money? Not usually! "No Drip," "with menthol," and "extra moisturizing" are all enticements to get you to write a bigger check. They add nothing to the product's ability to unstuff your nose. And such extras typically aren't available in generic formulas, forcing you to buy more expensive name-brand products. Name-brand Afrin will cost you about $5.99 for a 0.5-fluid-ounce pump. (We recommend the pump because it atomizes the spray into a finer mist, which allows for better absorption and less dripping.) Your Smart Buy is a typical store-brand 12-hour nasal spray. It's likely to cost you about the same per bottle, but you'll get twice as much. If your mind thinks in terms of bargains, think of this as "buy one, get one free!"

SQUELCHING THE ITCH: ANTIHISTAMINES

Antihistamines block the body's histamine, or allergic, reaction. They can provide relief for runny noses due to allergies and colds. One common complaint about antihistamine products is that they can cause intense drowsiness—so much so, in fact, that antihistamines show up as the main ingredients in a number of over-the-counter sleep-aid products. There's little you can do about this; it's the nature of the drug. The only nondrowsy antihistamine product available over the counter is Tavist (clemestine). In general, you shouldn't take over-the-counter antihistamine products if you must stay awake and alert!

You'll find the following four active ingredients in over-the-counter antihistamine products:

1. Brompheniramine
2. Chlorpheniramine
3. Clemestine
4. Diphenhydramine

Clemestine is the weakest but longest acting—a great combination for people who need some relief but are sensitive to some of the adverse effects of antihistamine, such as drowsiness. Of the four antihistamines, clemestine (found in the name-brand product Tavist) gives 12 hours of relief from allergy symptoms and causes the least drowsiness. Brompheniramine (brand name Dimetapp) and chlorpheniramine (brand name Chlor-Trimeton) are stronger-acting than clemestine but cause more drowsiness. Products containing brompheniramine and chlorpheniramine come in 4-hour, 8-hour, and 12-hour tablets, allowing you to take as few as 2 doses a day. Diphenhydramine (brand name Benadryl) is the strongest over-the-counter antihistamine; it also causes the greatest drowsiness. It's the least expensive, however, if you buy the generic or store-brand formulations.

Oral Antihistamines

PRODUCT	STRENGTH	ACTIVE INGREDIENT	USUAL DOSAGE	TYPICAL QUANTITY	TYPICAL PRICE	COST PER DOSE
Aller-Chlor, Chlortabs, or Chlorpheniramine 4 hr Tablets(Generic Chlor-Trimeton)Wal-Mart, Walgreens, Rite Aid	4mg	Chlorpheniramine	Ages 6-under 12 yrs = 2mg (1/2 tablet) every 4-6 hrs (NMT 6 tablets/24 hrs)	100	$5.99	6¢
Benadryl Allergy Relief, Kapseals	25mg	Diphenhydramine	Take 1 capsule every 4-6 hrs.	24	$4.69	20¢
Benadryl Allergy Relief, Ultratab Tablets	25mg	Diphenhydramine	Take 1 capsule every 4-6 hrs.	24	$4.69	20¢
Benadryl Dye-Free Allergy Relief, Liqui-gels	25mg	Diphenhydramine	Take 1 capsule every 4-6 hrs.	24	$5.49	23¢
Chlor-Trimeton 12-hr tablets	12mg	Chlorpheniramine	Take 1 tablet every 12 hrs.	24	$10.99	46¢
Chlor-Trimeton 4-hr tablets	4mg	Chlorpheniramine	Take 1 tablet every 4 hrs.	24	$5.99	25¢
Chlor-Trimeton 8-hr tablets	8mg	Chlorpheniramine	Take 1 tablet every 8 hrs.	15	$5.99	40¢
Comtrex Acute Head Cold & Sinus Pressure Relief Tablets (in combination with other ingredients)	2mg 500mg 30mg	Brompheniramine, acetaminophen, pseudoephedrine	Take 2 tablets every 6 hrs while symptoms persist, not to exceed 8 tablets in 24 hrs.	24	$8.29	69¢
Dimetapp Cold & Allergy Elixir	1mg 15mg	Brompheniramine, pseudoephedrine	Take 4 tsp. every 4 hrs.	12oz	$12.99	72¢/dose
Diphenhist or Benahist (Store brand versions of benadryl)	25mg	Diphenhydramine	Take 1 capsule every 4-6 hrs.	100	$7.49	8¢
Generic Store Brand 4-hr tabs of Chlor-Trimeton	4mg	Chlorpheniramine	Take 1 tablet every 4 hrs.	100	$4.99	5¢
Store Brand versions of Tavist (such as Dayhist-1)	1.34mg	Clemestine	Take 1 tablet every 12 hrs.	16	$4.99	31¢
Tavist 12-hr Relief of Allergy and Hay Fever Symptoms	1.34mg	Clemestine	Take 1 tablet every 12 hrs.	16	$8.99	56¢

$ SMART BUY
Oral Antihistamines

When choosing an antihistamine, consider its cost, effectiveness, and potential side effects. For most people, the Smart Buy is a store-brand version of Chlor-Trimeton (chlorpheniramine) 4-hour product. This good middle-of-the-road antihistamine should give you reasonable relief with few side effects. Store-brand equivalents are often sound-alikes that suggest a brand name, something like "Aller-chlor" or "Chlortabs," for example. Some generic products simply go by the drug's generic name—in this example, chlorpheniramine—on the package label. A bottle of 100 tablets of the store's generic version will cost about $6, or 6 cents a dose . This is a con-siderable savings over a name-brand product, which might cost you $5 for a package of just 24 tablets. This savings quickly adds up: For every hundred tablets you buy, going with the store or generic brand saves you $15 or so—72 percent.

Long-acting products are popular because you need take them less often, but this convenience comes at a cost. The 12-hour Chlor-Trimeton name-brand product costs about $12 for 24 tablets, or about a dollar a day. By comparison, 5 doses of the 4-hour product (taken every 4 hours while you're awake) will cost just 25 cents a day. Over the three months of the typical spring allergy season, the savings adds up to 75 percent per day, or about $70!

COMBINATION PRODUCTS

Clarence came into the pharmacy one afternoon and said, "My wife wants some Benadryl Allergy for Sinuses medicine." What should have been an easy purchase quickly became instead an unwieldy challenge. The allergy aisle contained a number of Benadryl products, including Benadryl Allergy, Benadryl Allergy Congestion, Benadryl Allergy/Sinus + Headache, and Benadryl Dye-Free. Clarence was confused and con-cerned. He wanted to get what his wife sent him to get, but he really didn't know what it was. Some questions elicited the information that Clarence's wife had high blood pressure, which meant she shouldn't take decongestants. But being the good husband he was, Clarence finally located and purchased just what his wife had asked him to— Benadryl Allergy/Sinus + Headache, which contains the active ingredients diphenhy-dramine (antihistamine), pseudoephedrine (decongestant), and acetaminophen (pain and fever relief). It wasn't the ideal choice, given her high blood pressure. Clarence would have done better to buy a diphenhydramine product, an acetaminophen prod-uct (which most people already have at home), and a topical nasal decongestant, instead.

Clarence had a reason for choosing a multi-ingredient product (doing as his wife had asked because she had runny nose, sneezing, congestion, and a headache), but most people pick one simply because they want to cover all possibilities. In reality, though, you'll rarely have all the symptoms a combination product treats. Taking a combination product increases the likelihood that you'll experience adverse side effects, and you'll spend more than you need to. Buying single-ingredient products separately is almost always more cost-effective than buying a combination product. (Remember to consider the per-dose cost, not just the per-item price.)

When it comes to cough, cold, and allergy symptoms, everyone is a little different. The best buy for you is the drug or drugs that relieve your specific symptoms. (Use our handy SOS worksheet from Chapter 16 to help you identify appropriate products and approaches.) Odds are, you won't have every symptom the all-in-one products claim to cover.

▶ What to Buy for Your Cough, Cold, or Allergy Symptoms

If you have these symptoms...	Then buy...
Runny nose, sneezing, watery eyes	An antihistamine
Stuffy head and nose	A decongestant
Aches, pains, and fever	Acetaminophen
Dry cough	Product with dextromethorphan
Tight chest, feel like you need to "cough up" something	Product with guaifenesin

Combination cough products, which are common, also waste your money. If you have a dry cough, you need a product with dextromethorphan to suppress it. If you have a "tight chest," or feel you need to cough something up, you need an expectorant, such as guaifenesin. Most combination cough products contain both of these ingredients. What sense does it make to put both ingredients in the same product? They cancel each other out!

And forget the "nighttime" preparations, advertised to last longer and help you sleep. Combining ingredients doesn't make them last any longer. And liquid forms of these products typically contain substantial amounts of alcohol—up to 25 percent, or what you'd order as 50 proof at a bar! Not surprisingly, these preparations are also quite expensive. Vicks Nyquil, for example, costs about 55 cents a dose. Yet if you bought its ingredients separately (except the alcohol, which serves only to help keep the combination product's ingredients dissolved), according to our SOS guidelines, you'd spend only about 20 cents a dose—a savings of 64 percent—and have the flexibility to forgo ingredients that treat symptoms you don't have.

Combination Products

PRODUCT	ACTIVE INGREDIENT	USUAL DOSAGE	TYPICAL QUANTITY	TYPICAL PRICE	COST PER DOSE
Actifed Maximum Cold/Sinus Caplet	Acetaminophen 500mg, pseudoephedrine30mg, chlorpheniramine 2mg	Take 2 tabs every 6 hrs., no more than 8 per 24 hrs.	20	$5.99	60¢
Alka-Seltzer Plus Cold & Cough Medicine Liqu-Gels	Dextromethorphan 10mg, chlorpheniramine 2mg, acetaminophen 325mg, pseudoephedrine 30mg	Take 2 gels every 4 hrs., no more than 4 doses per 24 hrs.	20	$5.99	60¢
Alka-Seltzer Plus Cold Medicine Liqu-Gels	Chlorpheniramine 2mg, pseudoephedrine 30mg, acetaminophen 325mg	Take 2 gels every 4 hrs., no more than 4 doses per 24 hrs.	20	$5.99	60¢
Alka-Seltzer PM Pain Reliever & Sleep Aid, Effervescent Tablets	Each effervescent tablet contains aspirin 325mg, diphenhydramine citrate 38mg	Dissolve 2 tabs in water and take at bedtime.	24	$4.99	42¢
Allerest Maximum Strength Allergy & Hay Fever Reducer Tablets	Pseudoephedrine 30mg, chlorpheniramine 2mg	Take 2 tabs every 6 hrs, no more than 8 per 24 hrs.	24	$5.49	46¢
Benadryl Allergy Cold Tablets	Acetaminophen 500mg, diphenhydramine 12.5mg, pseudoephedrine 30mg	Take 2 tabs every 6 hrs., no more than 8 per 24 hrs.	24	$5.49	46¢
Benadryl Allergy/Sinus Tablets	Diphenhydramine 25mg, pseudoephedrine 60mg	Take 2 tabs every 6 hrs., no more than 8 per 24 hrs.	24	$4.99	42¢
Benadryl Allergy & Sinus FastMelt, Dissolving Tablets	Diphenhydramine citrate 19mg (equivalent to 12.5mg of diphenhydramine HCl)	Take 2 tabs every 6 hrs., no more than 8 per 24 hrs.	20	$4.99	50¢
Benadryl Allergy & Sinus Headache Gelcaps	Acetaminophen 500mg, diphenhydramine 12.5mg, pseudoephedrine 30mg.	Take 2 tabs every 6 hrs., no more than 8 per 24 hrs.	24	5.50	46¢
Benadryl Maximum Strength Severe Allergy & Sinus Headache, Caplets	Acetaminophen 500mg, diphenhydramine 25mg, pseudoephedrine 30mg	Take 2 tabs every 6 hrs., no more than 8 per 24 hrs.	20	$5.50	56¢

PRODUCT	ACTIVE INGREDIENT	USUAL DOSAGE	TYPICAL QUANTITY	TYPICAL PRICE	COST PER DOSE
Chlor-Trimeton Allergy-D 4-hour Tablets	Chlorpheniramine 4mg, pseudoephedrine 60mg	Take 1 tablet every 4 hrs.	24	$4.99	21¢
Chlor-Trimeton Allergy-D 4-hour Tablets	Chlorpheniramine 4mg, pseudoephedrine 60mg	Take 1 tablet every 4 hrs.	24	$4.99	21¢
Chlor-Trimeton Allergy-D 12-hour Tablets	Chlorpheniramine 8mg, pseudoephedrine 120mg	Take 1 tablet every 12 hrs.	24	$10.99	46¢
Contac Severe Cold and Flu, Caplets	Acetaminophen 500mg, dextromethorphan 15mg, pseudoephedrine 30mg, chlorpheniramine 2mg	Take 2 caplets every 6 hrs., no more than 8 per 24 hrs.	16	$4.99	62¢
Contac Day & Night Allergy/Sinus Relief, Caplets	Acetaminophen 650mg, pseudoephedrine 60mg, diphenhydramine 50mg (night caplet only)	Day dose: Take 1 caplet every 6 hrs. Night dose: Take 1 caplet at bedtime, no more than 4 doses in 24 hrs.	20	$6.99	35¢
Contac Day & Night, Cold And Flu Relief, Caplets	Acetaminophen 650mg, pseudoephedrine 60mg, dextromethorphan 30mg, (day caplet only) diphenhydramine 50mg (night caplet only)	Day dose: Take 1 caplet every 6 hrs. Night dose: Take 1 caplet at bedtime, no more than 4 doses in 24 hrs.	20	$6.99	35¢
Coricidin 'D' Cold, Flu & Sinus, Tablets	Acetaminophen 325mg, chlorpheniramine 2mg, pseudoephedrine 30mg	Take 2 tabs every 4-6 hrs., no more than 8 per 24 hrs.	24	$5.99	50 ¢
Coricidin HBP Anti-histamine Cough Suppressant, for People with High Blood Pressure, Tablets	Chlorpheniramine 4mg, dextromethorphan 30mg	Take 1 tab every 6 hrs., no more than 4 doses per 24 hrs.	16	$5.99	37¢
Coricidin HBP Cold & Flu Relief for People with High Blood Pressure, Tablets	Acetaminophen 325mg, chlorpheniramine 2mg	Take 2 tabs every 4-6 hrs., no more than 12 doses per 24 hrs.	12	$4.19	70¢
Coricidin HBP Decon-gestant Free Cold Relief for People with High Blood Pressure, Tablets	Acetaminophen 325mg, chlorpheniramine 2mg	Take 2 tabs every 4-6 hrs., no more than 12 doses per 24 hrs.	24	$6.99	58¢
Dimetapp Cold & Allergy Tablets, Coated	Acetaminophen 325mg, chlorpheniramine 2mg, phenylephrine 5mg	Take 2 tabs every 4 hrs., no more than 12 doses per 24 hrs.	20	$5.50	55¢
Dristan Multi-Symptom Nasal Decongestant, Coated Tablets	Acetaminophen 325mg, phenylephrine 5mg, chlorpheniramine 2mg	Take 2 tabs every 4 hrs., no more than 12 doses per 24 hrs.	20	$5.99	60¢
Robitussin Honey Flu Nighttime Hot Syrup Pouches	Each pouch = 15ml: dextromethorphan 20mg, pseudoephedrine 60mg, acetaminophen 500mg, chlorpheniramine 4mg	Take contents of 1 pouch every 4 hrs.	6 pouches	$5.99	$1

PRODUCT	ACTIVE INGREDIENT	USUAL DOSAGE	TYPICAL QUANTITY	TYPICAL PRICE	COST PER DOSE
Sinutab Maximum Strength Sinus Allergy, Caplets	Acetaminophen 500mg, chlorpheniramine 2mg, pseudoephedrine 30mg	Take 2 caplets every 6 hrs., no more than 8 per 24 hrs.	24	$5.99	50¢
Sudafed Maximum Strength Dose Cold & Allergy Tablets	Pseudoephedrine 60mg, chlorpheniramine 4mg	Take 1 tab every 4–6 hrs., no more than 4 per 24 hrs.	24	$5.99	25¢
TheraFlu Flu, Cold, & Cough Medicine, Lemon Flavor Packets	Each packet contains: acetaminophen 650mg, pseudoephedrine 60mg, dextromethorphan 20mg, chlorpheniramine 4mg	Take contents of 1 packet every 4–6 hrs., no more than 4 per 24 hrs.	12	$8.99	75¢
TheraFlu Maximum Nighttime, Flu, Cold, & Cough Medicine Packets	Each packet contains: acetaminophen 1000mg, pseudoephedrine 60mg, dextromethorphan 30mg, chlorpheniramine 4mg	Take contents of 1 packet every 4-6 hrs., no more than 4 per 24 hrs.	12	$8.99	75¢
TheraFlu Night-time, Flu, Cold & Cough Formula Caplets	Acetaminophen 500mg, pseudoephedrine 30mg, dextromethorphan 15mg, chlorpheniramine 2mg	Take 2 caplets every 6 hrs., no more than 8 per 24 hrs.	12	$3.50	58¢
TheraFlu Nighttime, Flu, Cold & Cough Medicine Caplets	Acetaminophen 500mg, pseudoephedrine 30mg, dextromethorphan 15mg, chlorpheniramine 2mg	Take 2 caplets every 6 hrs., no more than 8 per 24 hrs.	24	$6.99	58¢
Tylenol Allergy Sinus Antihistamine Nasal Decongestant Caplets	Acetaminophen 500mg, chlorpheniramine 2mg, pseudoephedrine 30mg	Take 2 caplets every 6 hrs., no more than 8 per 24 hrs.	24	$5.99	50¢
Tylenol Allergy Sinus Antihistamine Nasal Decongestant Caplets	Acetaminophen 500mg, chlorpheniramine 2mg, pseudoephedrine 30mg	Take 2 caplets every 6 hrs., no more than 8 per 24 hrs.	48	$7.99	33¢
Tylenol Allergy Sinus Maximum Strength Gelcaps, Multi-Symptom Relief	Acetaminophen 500mg, chlorpheniramine 2mg, pseudoephedrine 30mg	Take 2 gelcaps every 4-6 hrs., no more than 8 doses per 24 hrs.	48	$7.99	33¢
Tylenol Cold Multi-Symptom Complete Formula, Caplets	Acetaminophen 325mg, chlorpheniramine 2mg, dextromethorphan 15mg, pseudoephedrine 30mg	Take 2 caplets every 4-6 hrs., no more than 8 doses per 24 hrs.	48	$8.99	38¢
Vicks 44M Cough, Cold & Flu Relief Liquid	Per 4 tsps. (20mls): dextromethorphan 30mg, pseudoephedrine 60mg, chlorpheniramine 4mg, acetaminophen 650mg	Take 2 tbsp. every 4 hrs., no more than 6 doses per 24 hrs.	4oz	$4.99	$1.25

$ SMART BUYS
Combination Products

As you know by now, we tend not to recommend multidrug combinations because of the cost and the potential for overmedicating yourself. But if you do have multiple symptoms and you want just one pill, your Smart Buy is Tylenol Cold Multi-Symptom Complete Formula Caplets. Just one tablet covers aches and fever, cough, runny nose, sneezing, and nasal congestion. It will cost you about 38 cents per dose, though, and if you experience side effects, it may be tough to say which ingredient is causing the problem.

If you don't need the all-inclusive multisymptom products, another Smart Buy is either Chlor-Trimeton Allergy D 4-hour tablets or Sudafed's Maximum Strength Dose Cold & Allergy Tablets. These alternatives will cost you about 21 cents and 25 cents, respectively. They don't include acetaminophen for pain and fever or dextromethorphan for cough suppression, and they're about 45 percent cheaper than products that contain these drugs. Talk with your pharmacist to see which may be better for you.

STOP THE COUGHING: ANTITUSSIVES AND EXPECTORANTS

Many things can cause a cough. To choose an over-the-counter cough product, though, you need only answer these three questions:

1. Do you have postnasal drip (drainage from your nose running down the back of your throat)?
2. Do you feel a tickle in your throat?
3. Do you feel like you have to cough something up?

The over-the-counter product that will work most effectively to reduce your cough depends on your answers to these questions.

COUGHS DUE TO POSTNASAL DRIP

Postnasal drip is a common symptom of sinus congestion that can result from allergies and colds. When the fluid from your nose drips down the back of your throat, it irritates your throat tissues. If you're taking an antihistamine to relieve other cold or allergy symptoms, this should also help your cough. Diphenhydramine, the well-known antihistamine in the name-brand product Benadryl, is particularly effective as a suppressant for coughs caused by postnasal drip. Drying up the nasal drip with an antihistamine such as diphenhydramine often eliminates the tickle, and thus the cough. And if you also need to treat that sore throat and get help with sleep, diphenhydramine can help.

COUGHS DUE TO A TICKLE IN YOUR THROAT

A tickle in your throat might result from breathing unusually dry air and is a common problem in the winter months when people are indoors with the heat running. An antitussive (which literally means "stop coughing") is a medication that stops a cough caused by a tickle in your throat. The most common over-the-counter antitussive is the active ingredient dextromethorphan, which works by suppressing the cough center in the brain. One familiar name-brand dextromethorphan product is Robitussin DM, and many store-brand and generic formulations exist, as well. The generic products are typically much cheaper, although you can score big savings by watching for store sales and manufacturer promotions.

Although dextromethorphan is a very effective cough suppressant, you must take it every 4 hours to keep your cough under control. If this isn't a problem for you, then stay with the regular dextromethorphan products. Often you can identify store brands and generic versions by looking for some variation of the word "tussin" and the letters "DM" on the label.

If you just can't break away every 4 hours to down another dose of cough syrup, consider the long-acting product Delsym, which contains a sustained-release formulation of dextromethorphan that lasts as long as 12 hours. There's a price for this convenience, of course. Delsym can cost 4 to 6 times as much as standard dextromethorphan preparations, and it isn't available in generic versions.

> ### ▶ Drink *Water*, Not Coffee and Colas
>
> When the label says, "Take with plenty of water," that means a *full 8 ounces of* water—not a sip, and not a soda or cup of coffee. This is important, because the drying-out effect of many cold and allergy products affects your entire body. If you're not drinking enough fluids, you easily can become dehydrated. Getting enough fluids also helps loosen congestion and mucous so you can get it out of your nose, throat, and chest, increasing the effectiveness of the guaifenesin. Caffeinated beverages aren't good substitutes. Caffeine-containing drinks actually act as diuretics—that is, they draw fluids from the body—and so have the opposite effect of what you want. ◀

DEEP COUGHS

If you have a deep-down cough, one that makes you feel like you need to cough something up, then the product you need is an expectorant. Expectorants thin and loosen mucous and secretions, making it easier for your body's normal cough mechanism to clear these substances from your bronchial tubes and throat. It's important to drink plenty of water when you take an expectorant, to help further liquefy the mucous and replace fluids your body loses as a result of the expectorant's actions. The only expectorant available in over-the-counter products is the ingredient guaifenesin. Many name-brand and generic cough and cold products contain this ingredient.

▶ A Cough with a Purpose

A "productive" cough, as the terminology implies, serves a purpose: It brings up whatever is causing

congestion in your airways and chest. Most of the time you don't want to stop a productive cough,

because doing so will allow congestion to accumulate, which provides a breeding ground for bacteria.

If your cough is productive, don't use a cough suppressant, such as dextromethorphan. ◀

Secretions due to allergies, colds, and other viral infections usually are clear or whitish in color. If you're bringing up mucous that's green or yellow, you need to see your doctor. This is a sign of a bacterial infection, which will likely require antibiotics. Antibiotics are no help for colds, viruses, and allergies, however.

$ SMART BUY
Cough Products

For a dry cough, the best choice is a store-brand version of Robitussin DM (look for a name like "Tussin DM"), at just over $5 for 12 ounces, or about 15 cents a dose (which provides 4 hours of relief). If this helps, but you still need something stronger, try Delsym. Although this product costs more (about $7 for 3 ounces, or 78 cents a dose), it provides relief for 12 hours—three times as long as name-brand and generic versions of regular dextromethorphan products.

Cough Preparations

PRODUCT	STRENGTH PER DOSE	ACTIVE INGREDIENT	USUAL DOSAGE	TYPICAL QUANTITY	TYPICAL PRICE	COST PER DOSE
Benylin Adult Formula Cough Suppressant, Raspberry Flavor Syrup SF	5mg	Dextromethorphan	Take 2 tsp. every 6–8 hrs.	4oz	$3.99	33¢
Buckley's Mixture, SF	12.5mg	Dextromethorphan	Take 1 tsp. every 4 hrs.	8oz	$7.99	25¢
Delsym Extended-Release Suspension 12 Hour Cough Relief, Orange Flavored Liquid	30mg dextromethorphan Hbr	Dextromethorphan polistirex	Take 2 tsp. every 12 hrs.	3oz	$7.99	89¢
Diabetic Tussin DM, Cough Suppressant/ Expectorant SF	100mg, 10mg	Guaifenesin, dextromethorphan	Take 2 tsp. every 4 hrs.	4oz	$5.99	50¢
Robitussin Cough & Congestion Liquid Formula	100mg, 10mg	Guaifenesin, dextromethorphan	Take 2 tsp. every 4 hrs.	4oz	$5.99	50¢
Robitussin Sugar Free Cough Formula, Children and Adult Syrup SF	100mg 10mg	Guaifenesin, dextromethorphan	Take 2 tsp. every 4 hrs.	4oz	$5.99	50¢
Robitussin DM Cough Suppressant, Expectorant Syrup	100mg, 10mg	Guaifenesin, dextromethorphan	Take 2 tsp. every 4 hrs.	12oz	$9.99	28¢
Robitussin plain	100mg	Guaifenesin	Take 2-4 tsp. every 4 hrs.	8oz	$7.50	31¢
Tussin DM Cough Suppressant (Generic version of Robitussin DM)	100mg 10mg	Guaifenesin, dextromethorphan	Take 2 tsp. every 4 hrs.	12oz	$6.49	18¢
Tussin Expectorant (Generic equivalent of Robitussin plain) (Rite Aid, Walgreens, Wal-Mart)	100mg	Guaifenesin	Take 2-4 tsp. every 4 hrs.	8oz	$5.99	25¢
Vicks 44D Cough Relief and Decongestant, Cherry	30mg, 60mg	Dextromethorphan, pseudoephedrine	Take 3 tsp. every 6 hrs.	8oz	$7.49	47¢
Vicks 44E Cough Relief and Expectorant	200mg, 20mg	Dextromethorphan guaifenesin	Take 3 tsp. every 4 hrs.	8oz	$7.99	50¢

For a "tight-chested" cough in which you feel you need to get something up and out, use an expectorant-only product containing guaifenesin. You can lower your per-dose cost to about 15 cents a dose by buying a generic version of plain Robitussin (usually on a nearby shelf, and including "tussin" as all or part of its name), about $5.25 for 12 ounces. Just be sure you don't see the letters "DM" or the words "cough suppressant" anywhere on the label. And if you're not sure what kind of cough you have or which cough product you need, ask your pharmacist.

▶ Hidden Sugar in Cough Suppressants

If you have diabetes or monitor the sugars in your diet for other reasons, read labels carefully when you purchase cough suppressants. Most contain significant amounts of sugar sweeteners to help mask the otherwise nasty tastes (sorry!) of the active ingredients. This can affect glucose levels. Products such as Diabetic Tussin, which contain no sugar, alcohol, fructose, sorbitol, or dyes, are excellent alternatives.

COUGH DROPS AND THROAT LOZENGES

If cough syrups are such a hassle to take, what with the measuring and the stickiness and all, why not just use cough drops, instead? Well, in many respects the term "cough drop" is misleading. Most cough drops contain no cough suppressant. Instead, they increase the flow of saliva as you suck on them, which lubricates your throat and helps soothe the irritation causing you to cough. If you have a tickle in your throat or need an expectorant to help you move secretions from your lungs, cough drops won't help much.

The active ingredient in most cough drops is menthol, which works by softening the mucous membranes to relieve irritation. (It also "feels" therapeutic, which helps you stop thinking so much about your cough.) The strength is fairly consistent across brands, 5mg to 10mg. Some cough drops also include eucalyptus oil and camphor. Those that say they include honey or lemon, which are naturally soothing, are often referring to flavor rather than ingredients (read the label carefully). If you choose to use cough drops to comfort a scratchy throat, choose a product that tastes good. But if your cough turns into a real nagging hack, don't linger with cough drops. Switch to a dextromethorphan preparation that will give you stronger relief.

Closely related to cough drops, at least on the store shelf, are lozenges and sprays designed to end your discomfort and your cough by numbing your sore throat. The active ingredient in such products is usually benzocaine, a topical anesthetic. Don't use these products for longer than two or three days! If your throat hurts badly enough that you want to numb it, you could have a bacterial infection, such as strep throat. Bacterial infections usually require prescription antibiotics—and that means a visit to the

Cough Drops and Throat Lozenges

PRODUCT	ACTIVE INGREDIENT	USUAL DOSAGE	TYPICAL QUANTITY	TYPICAL PRICE	COST PER DOSE
Cepacol Maximum Strength Sore Throat Lozenges, Cherry	Benzocaine 10mg, menthol 3.6mg	Dissolve 1 every 2 hrs. as needed.	18	$4.49	25¢
Cepacol Maximum Strength Sore Throat Spray	Dyclonine hydrochloride 0.1%	Spray throat 4 times, up to 4 such doses per 24 hrs.	4oz	$3.99	$1/oz.
Maximum Strength Halls-Plus Honey-Lemon Cough Drops	10mg menthol	Dissolve 1 lozenge every hour if needed.	25	$1.99	8¢
N'ICE Sugar Free Cough Suppressant/ Oral Anesthetic Drops, Citrus Flavor	5mg menthol	1 lozenge every 2 hrs, but no more than 10/24 hrs.	24	$2.99	12¢
Ricola Honey-Lemon Echinacea Throat Drops	Menthol 2.7mg	Dissolve 1 drop in mouth every 2 hrs. as needed.	24	$2.49	10¢
Robitussin Cough Drops (cherry and menthol eucalyptus)	7.4mg menthol, eucalyptus oil	Dissolve 1 lozenge every hour if needed.	25	$2.49	10¢
Robitussin Cough Drops (honey-lemon)	10mg menthol, eucalyptus oil	Dissolve 1 lozenge every hour if needed.	25	$2.79	11¢
Robitussin Honey Cough Drops	5mg menthol	Use as needed.	20	$2.49	12¢
Sucrets Sore Throat Wild Cherry Lozenge	Dyclonine hydrochloride 2.0mg	Dissolve 1 every 2 hrs as needed.	18	$3.49	19¢
Vicks Cherry Cough Drops	1.7mg menthol	Dissolve 1 lozenge every 2 hrs.	20	$1.29	6¢
Vicks Chloraseptic Sore Throat Lozenges Cherry	Benzocaine 6mg, menthol 10mg	Dissolve 1 every 2 hrs. as needed.	18	$4.49	25¢
Vicks Menthol Cough Drops	3.3mg menthol	Dissolve 1 lozenge every 2 hrs.	20	$1.29	6¢

doctor. Usually these products are fairly similar in price. When selecting one, go with products that have the most active ingredients.

 SMART BUY
Cough Drops and Throat Lozenges

For that little tickle in your throat, Hall's Maximum Strength cough drops contain the most menthol for a hard-to-beat price of about 7 cents a drop. If you have a sore throat, Vicks Chloraseptic currently is the strongest and most effective product, at about 20 cents a dose. Also try one of our favorite home remedies, the "Pharmacist's Special Sore Throat Formula" (which follows), or a simple salt-water gargle (1 teaspoon of salt in a warm glass of water; gargle as often as necessary). This gives great relief, you can do it as often as you like, it has no side effects, and costs next to nothing.

> ### ▶ Why a Salt-Water Gargle Helps
>
> What is it about a salt-water gargle that helps a sore throat feel better? In technical terms, it initiates an osmotic effect. In simple terms, the salt concentration in your gargle solution is higher than the salt concentration in your tissues. So the salt solution draws fluid out of the tissues, reducing swelling. And with reduced swelling comes lessened pain.

The aluminum/magnesium suspension coats and soothes the throat, and the diphenhydramine has a minor local anesthetic action that numbs the throat to some degree. If you do swallow the mixture, it won't hurt you—although the diphenhydramine will make you sleepy (which is why we recommend spitting it out). This mixture will cost you around 10 cents a dose, compared to about 24 cents a dose for Chloraseptic Throat Lozenges, a savings of 58 percent.

GUM WITH ASPIRIN

The product Aspergum basically is aspirin in a chewing gum marketed to help relieve sore throats. Is it a worthwhile product? Well, you will get aspirin into your system, which can help relieve pain in general. But there's no immediate or direct pain relief to the throat itself, it offers no topical anesthesia, and it's expensive. Although this product might give you relief, regular aspirin is just as effective and won't hurt your pocketbook nearly as much. We don't recommend it.

► The Pharmacist's Special Sore Throat Formula

Sore throats make people miserable. You can't talk, drink, eat, or even swallow without discomfort.

For an especially bothersome sore throat (after your doctor has ruled out a bacterial infection), try this mixture pharmacists recommend to patients receiving throat radiation for cancer treatments:

1. Mix equal amounts of generic aluminum and magnesium hydroxide suspension (brand name Maalox) and generic diphenhydramine elixir (brand name Benadryl).

2. Place the mixture in a bottle and shake well.

3. Gargle with 1 to 2 teaspoons of the mixture for 20 to 30 seconds every 3 or 4 hours, and spit it out.

VITAMIN C (ASCORBIC ACID)

Vitamin C is a popular remedy for colds and sore throats. There have been countless studies on the effects of vitamin C to treat such symptoms, but there still is no conclusive evidence supporting its use. You won't do yourself any harm by taking vitamin C, though, and it doesn't interact with other cold products. For sore throats and colds, try taking from 1 to 5 grams per dose up to 15 grams a day, which may shorten the length of time you have symptoms. However, if you're taking prescription medication, ask your pharmacist about the interactions that may take place with large amounts of vitamin C. Large doses of vitamin C also can cause some stomach upset and diarrhea.

Numerous brands and formulas of vitamin C exist on the market; no conclusive evidence exists that one (such as vitamin C with rose hips or acerola) absorbs any better than another. To keep your costs down, take the 500mg strength and purchase it in 1,000-count bottles. You should be able to find some for about $20 per bottle. Chewables are OK, but they're more expensive and you'll need to make sure you rinse your mouth well afterward to make sure the ascorbic acid of vitamin C doesn't eat away at the enamel on your teeth.

PAIN AND FEVER RELIEVERS

Often, pain and fever accompany colds, flus, and other viral infections. The drugs to relieve these symptoms, called analgesics, are the most widely used over-the-counter drugs. They're so widely used, in fact, that we've given them their own chapter—next!

$ SMART OPTIONS FOR SAVINGS
Cold, Flu, Cough, and Allergy Preparations

Nearly always, your best bet is to go with the least expensive product for cold, flu, cough, and allergy products. To keep things simple, we identified our picks at the end of each product section. But we know that when you have a cold or the flu, you want quick relief and easy choices. So here's a summary of our Smart Buys.

1. Oral decongestants: Buy a generic product that contains pseudoephedrine. Look for something like "pseudotabs" or "decongestant" tablets with pseudoephedrine.

2. Topical nasal decongestants: Buy generic original formula oxymetazoline (generic version of Afrin). Look for "12-Hour Nasal Spray." Don't let all the extras seduce you; they add nothing except cost.

3. Antihistamines: Buy a generic product that contains clemestine (a generic version of Tavist), such as Da-Hist (generic Tavist), if it's available. If it's not, buy a generic product containing bromphenerimine, such as Di Brom or Bromphen (generic versions of Dimetapp), or Chlor-Trimeton, such as Aller-Chlor or Chortabs.

4. Combination and "nighttime" products: Don't buy these. You pay more for less, and often end up treating symptoms you don't have.

5. Dry coughs: Buy a generic version of Robitussin DM (such as Tussin DM) containing dextromethorphan.

6. Productive coughs: Buy a generic version of plain Robitussin (such as Tussin), an expectorant containing guaifensesin (make sure the product does not include dextromethorphan).

7. Sore throats: Gargle with salt water or our Pharmacist's Special Sore Throat Formula (page 337). If this isn't possible or practical, go with Hall's Maximum Strength cough drops (if a cough is irritating your throat) or Vicks Chloraseptic spray.

Because viral infections (colds and flu) and allergies tend to roll around year after year (we even consider them "seasons!"), it often pays to buy in bulk so you have a supply on hand of the products you typically need. And because your needs usually aren't time-sensitive, especially if you plan ahead, it's worthwhile to investigate alternative sources for cold, flu, cough, and allergy products: These are great "buy ahead" products. If you live within driving distance of Canada, consider a day trip to compare products and prices. And no matter where you live, mail-order and Internet pharmacies can provide great savings. Just remember to check product expiration dates at the start of each "season" to make sure the drugs you're taking are still fresh and at optimum potency. And check our Web site at www.smartbuysdrugwise.com for the latest information about saving money on drugs!

Chapter 18

Over-the-Counter Pain Relief

M edications for pain relief, called analgesics, are some of the most widely used over-the-counter drugs. Helpful to relieve pain, swelling, and high tempera- tures, these miracle drugs have had a huge impact on our lives. Millions of people still follow the age-old advice, "Take two aspirin and call me in the morning." In fact, that analgesic is so popular that we consume 10 tons of it every year!

But aspirin might not be the right pain-reliever for you. The two other types of over-the-counter analgesics are acetaminophen and nonsteroidal anti-inflammatory drugs (NSAIDs, such as ibuprophen). The best product for you depends on your symp- toms and your medical history. Although choosing the right product is the first step toward saving money when you buy drugs, it's also the most important step when it comes to safeguarding your health.

Analgesics and Kidney Damage

All analgesics carry a risk for liver and kidney damage with overuse or overdose. If you drink alco- hol—even modest amounts—while you're taking over-the-counter analgesics, you compound your risk. Alcohol takes considerable resources from your liver, leaving it less capable of handling other challenges. Over-the-counter analgesics do the same. Confronted with alcohol and analgesics in combination, your liver might become unable to function.

ASPIRIN

From the beginning of time, people have used plant extracts containing forms of salicylic acid to relieve headaches, toothaches, and fevers. In 1899, scientists developed acetylsalicylic acid from salicylic acid, creating a consistent chemical compound that we know today as aspirin. Aspirin works to relieve pain by reducing inflammation and swelling. In the century since its development, aspirin in various forms has become the most widely used drug in the world. Although most people take aspirin to relieve aches and pains, aspirin's anticlotting (anticoagulant) properties led to another discovery in 1988: An aspirin a day can keep heart attacks away. Today, millions of people who take aspirin regularly do so on the advice of their cardiologists.

You might think that more than a hundred years of use means that aspirin is an extremely safe drug. For most people, this is true. But for some people, taking aspirin can have catastrophic health consequences. Those allergic to aspirin can have reactions ranging from mild rashes to hives to anaphylactic shock—a life-threatening condition in which the breathing passages swell shut and body systems begin to shut down. Because allergic reactions can jump from mild to life-threatening without warning, always contact your doctor or go to a hospital emergency department if you experience a reaction after taking aspirin. And if you know you're allergic to aspirin, never take any products containing it (including combination products for colds and flu, or arthritis preparations).

▶ Reye's Syndrome and Aspirin

A rare but potentially fatal condition called Reye's syndrome has been linked to aspirin use in children and teenagers who have influenza (the flu) or chickenpox. Because of this, the Centers for Disease Control, the U.S. Food and Drug Administration, the American Academy of Pediatrics' Committee on Infectious Diseases, and the U.S. Surgeon General's Office all advise parents not to give aspirin to anyone under age 18 who has the flu or chickenpox.

Aspirin also becomes a very dangerous drug if you take too much of it. Salicylates, the pain-relieving chemicals in aspirin, are very toxic in high doses. The greatest risk most people face is taking multiple products that contain aspirin (such as a pain reliever and a cold remedy). Always read product labels so you know what's in the products you're taking! And if you're taking an aspirin a day as a mild anticoagulant to reduce your risk for heart attack, remember to consider this when you take other aspirin products.

Aspirin can irritate your stomach, even to the point of causing bleeding. If you have an ulcer, don't take aspirin or products containing aspirin unless your doctor knows about your ulcer and tells you to take aspirin anyway. Some aspirin products have a coating that keeps the tablets from dissolving until they enter your small intestine. This is because aspirin (and some NSAIDs) depletes the mucous lining of the stomach; this lining protects the stomach from the hydrochloric acid that's normally there. This isn't a problem in the small intestine because very little if any hydrochloric acid is present there to cause damage. These enteric-coated ("enteric" means "intestinal") aspirin products cost more than regular aspirin, but they're the best choices for people with ulcers, a history of ulcers, or stomach sensitivity. Always swallow enteric-coated aspirin products whole; never chew, cut, or crush them as this destroys the protective coating.

Aspirin, like all drugs, can interfere with the actions of other medications. What makes aspirin a more significant risk in this regard is that many people who take it think of it as so commonplace that they don't consider themselves as "taking any other drugs or medications" when the doctor or pharmacist asks. Aspirin and aspirin products can interfere with the activity of (or cause adverse reactions to) the following medications:

+ Other salicylates, such as magnesium salicylate or choline salicylate, common ingredients in products such as Magan, Doan's Pills, Bayer Select Backache Pain Formula, Mobidin, Arthropan, Trilisate, and Trocosal.
+ PeptoBismol, because it contains bismuth subsalicylate, which becomes salicylate in the body.
+ Nonsteroidal anti-inflammatory drugs (NSAIDs), such as ibuprofen, ketoprofen, and naproxen. These drugs are marketed under many names, so be sure to read the label of any pain-relief product.
+ Prescription pain medications. Read the patient-information sheet carefully and study the warnings. If you have any questions, ask your pharmacist.
+ Prescription blood thinners (anticoagulants), such as Coumadin (warfarin), Plavix (clopidogrel), heparin, Lovenox (exoaprin), Dicumerol, Miradon (anisindione), and Fragmin (dalteparin) or other injected medications you might receive in a clinic or hospital. Aspirin and aspirin products will increase the effect of these medications, and can even cause life-threatening situations.

If you're using any of these drugs, check with your doctor or pharmacist before you take any over-the-counter products that contain aspirin or salicylates.

When it comes to buying aspirin, no differences exist among generic, name-brand, and store-brand products. Simply put, the cheaper the better. Using plain aspirin rather than highly advertised products will save you money. Some aspirin products are "buffered" to help them dissolve faster; that is, other chemicals have been added to neutralize aspirin's acidity. When these tablets reach the stomach, they dissolve slightly more quickly (a few minutes quicker than nonbuffered products, and about a half-hour faster than enteric-coated aspirin tablets). The idea is that the faster the tablets dissolve, the more quickly you'll get relief. Unlike Ascriptin, which contains an antacid but isn't buffered, Bufferin and other buffered products don't contain enough antacid to prevent potential stomach damage. Instead, speed is their advertised forte.

Although buffered aspirin does dissolve faster than regular aspirin, no conclusive evidence exists that this causes the drug's action to begin any faster. And although buffered aspirin might reduce stomach irritation, it's less effective at doing so than enteric-coated aspirin, which doesn't dissolve in your stomach at all, but rather, in your small intestine. And generic enteric-coated aspirin products are nearly as inexpensive as generic regular aspirin, so you save no money by buying regular aspirin. If you're taking an aspirin a day to prevent heart disease, as recommended by your doctor, you should probably be taking an enteric-coated product with a strength equivalent to baby aspirin (81mg).

As with most drugs, buying aspirin in larger quantities saves you money. Some pharmacies will allow you to purchase wholesale bottles containing 500 or 1,000 aspirin tablets, which drops the per-dose cost significantly. Shopping at warehouse stores such as Sam's Club or Costco is another way to find larger quantity products at good prices.

▶ Do You Need Child-Resistant Packaging?

Bulk- or wholesale-quantity over-the-counter drugs often come in bottles that don't have child-resistant caps. If you have children in your home, this poses a great risk for accidental poisoning. It's well worth the extra money to buy the largest quantity available *with* child-resistant packaging.

Aspirin Products

PRODUCT	STRENGTH	ACTIVE INGREDIENT	USUAL DOSAGE	TYPICAL QUANTITY	TYPICAL PRICE	COST PER DOSE
Anacin Pain Reliever Tablets	400mg, 32	Aspirin, caffeine	Take 1-2 tablets every 6 hrs., no more than 8 in 24 hrs.	300	$12.99	4.3¢
Aspircaf (generic version of Anacin) Tablets	400mg, 32	Aspirin, caffeine	Take 1-2 tablets every 6 hrs., no more than 8 in 24 hrs.	100	$3.99	4¢
Aspirin Tri-Buffered Tablets (generic version of Bufferin)	325mg	Aspirin	Take 1-2 tablets every 4 hrs., no more than 12 in 24 hrs.	250	$4.99	2¢
Bayer Aspirin Tablets	325mg	Aspirin	Take 1-2 tablets every 4 hrs., no more than 12 in 24 hrs.	100	$6.49	6.3¢
Bufferin Coated Aspirin Tablets	325mg	Aspirin	Take 1-2 tablets every 4 hrs., no more than 48 in 24 hrs.	130	$7.30	5.6¢
Ecotrin Low Strength Aspirin Tablets	81mg	Aspirin	Take 1-8 tablets every 4 hrs., no more than 48 in 24 hrs.	120	$6.99	5.8¢
Ecotrin Maximum Strength Coated Tablets	500mg	Aspirin	Take 1-2 tablets every 6 hrs., no more than 8 in 24 hrs.	150	$12.99	8.7¢
Ecotrin Regular Strength Coated Tablets	325mg	Aspirin	Take 1-2 tablets every 4 hrs., no more than 12 in 24 hrs.	250	$12.99	5.2¢
Excedrin Extra Strength Pain Reliever Tablets	500mg, 65mg	Aspirin, caffeine	Take 1-2 tablets every 6 hrs., no more than 8 in 24 hrs.	100	$8.99	9¢
Excedrin Migraine Coated Pain Reliever Tablets	250/250/65	Aspirin/acetaminophen /caffeine	Take 1-2 tablets every 6 hrs., no more than 8 in 24 hrs.	275	$13.99	5.1¢
Extraprin Migraine Pain Reliever Tablets	250/250/65	Aspirin/acetaminophen /caffeine	Take 1-2 tablets every 6 hrs., no more than 8 in 24 hrs.	250	$6.99	2.8¢
Genacote or Target or Wal-Mart brand Enteric-coated Maximum Strength (generic version of Ecotrin Maximum Strength Coated) Tablets	500mg	Aspirin	Take 1-2 tablets every 6 hrs., no more than 8 in 24 hrs.	150	$5.99	4¢
Genacote, or Target or Wal-Mart brand Enteric-coated Aspirin (generic version of Ecotrin Regular Strength) Tablets	325mg	Aspirin	Take 1-2 tablets every 4 hrs., no more than 12 in 24 hrs.	250	$5.99	2.4¢
Low Dose enteric-coated Aspirin (generic version of Ecotrin Low Strength) Tablets	81mg	Aspirin	Take 1-8 tablets every 4 hrs., no more than 48 in 24 hrs.	120	$3.99	3.3¢

PRODUCT	STRENGTH	ACTIVE INGREDIENT	USUAL DOSAGE	TYPICAL QUANTITY	TYPICAL PRICE	COST PER DOSE
Regular Aspirin (Target, Walgreens or Wal–Mart Brands) (generic version of Bayer Aspirin) Tablets	325mg	Aspirin	Take 1-2 tablets every 4 hrs., no more than 12 in 24 hrs.	500	$4.99	1¢

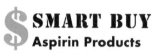

SMART BUY
Aspirin Products

Saving money with these products is simple: When you see a name-brand product, look away! Products such as Ecotrin, Bayer, and Excedrin should flash dollar signs. Buy generic, and buy the largest quantity available. A bottle of 500 aspirin tablets (325mg) from your local Walgreens, Target, or Wal-Mart costs around $5—a penny a tablet; name-brand Bayer Aspirin in a bottle of 100 tablets costs about $6.49: You save $1.49 right off the bat, and save more than $26 on an equivalent amount of the name-brand product, for a savings of 85 percent.

Go generic, buy bulk.

If your doctor wants you on the low-dose 81mg tablets, save yourself some money by skipping the popular but pricey name-brand product Ecotrin. Look for a label like "Low-Dose (or Low-Strength) Enteric-Coated Aspirin (81mg)." You can pick up 120-count bottles at a Wal-Mart or Target store for $4 to $5, a savings of at least $2 a bottle—29 percent—over Ecotrin. If you can find it in a larger quantity, you can save even more. If you have a sensitive stomach or history of ulcers and other gastrointestinal problems and have headache or arthritis pain, you may need the higher dosage 325mg enteric-coated aspirin. Again, visit your local Target, Walgreens or Wal-Mart and look for a generic version. It should cost you only around $6 for 250 tablets—about half the price of the name-brand product.

ACETAMINOPHEN

Although we think of acetaminophen—especially in its best-known name-brand form, Tylenol—as a relatively modern drug, doctors actually used it as long ago as the 1890s. It didn't become popular as an alternative to aspirin, however, until after the FDA approved its general use in 1955. Other acetaminophen-containing product lines include Excedrin, Midol, Anacin, and Pamprin. In fact, in the U.S. acetaminophen products are available in more than five dozen forms!

Unlike aspirin, which acts on the source of pain by reducing the inflammation that causes it, acetaminophen appears to act on the brain's pain threshold centers. Scientists believe it raises this threshold (the point at which you feel pain). They believe it reduces fever in much the same way, by acting on the heat regulatory centers and causing them to "direct" your blood vessels to dilate and your skin to sweat—actions that help cool your body. Thus, acetaminophen has no anti-inflammatory properties. Although it can help relieve the pain of conditions such as arthritis, it can't reduce the swelling that causes the pain.

Acetaminophen generally doesn't cause stomach irritation or upset, and doesn't appear to be linked to Reye's syndrome in children and teens who have the flu or chickenpox. However, if you drink alcohol moderately to heavily or have any kind of liver disease or disorder (such as one of the many forms of hepatitis), acetaminophen can cause life-threatening liver damage even at recommended doses. Your liver does most of the work of breaking drugs down into the forms your body will use. It also filters out the potentially harmful byproducts of this process (metabolism).

▶ Acetaminophen Bad for Pets

Never give acetaminophen to your pets. Just one-half of a regular-strength tablet of acetaminophen is enough to kill a cat or small dog and enough to cause irreversible liver damage in larger dogs. If you feel the need to medicate your pets, check with your veterinarian for drugs that are safe for use in animals.

Between 3 percent and 5 percent of acetaminophen's metabolic waste is a highly toxic byproduct. A healthy liver can produce a chemical that neutralizes this toxin. But if you take an overdose of acetaminophen or have even mild liver damage, the poison overwhelms your liver before it can do so. Acetaminophen poisoning is a leading cause of liver damage and failure, life-threatening medical conditions for which a liver transplant is often the only treatment.

And it doesn't take much acetaminophen, even with a healthy liver, to create an overdose situation. Indeed, just 8 extra-strength tablets taken in a 24-hour period can put enough acetaminophen in your system to put you at the threshold of toxicity. Never exceed the recommended dose or take acetaminophen for longer than the recommended period of time.

Acetaminophen and Liver Damage

Prolonged use of acetaminophen can cause liver damage. If you drink more than three alcoholic beverages daily or if you already have liver or kidney disease, do not take acetaminophen products without consulting your doctor. The point at which acetaminophen begins to cause liver damage in healthy adults is 4g in 24 hours (much lower for children). That's 8 tablets of the extra-strength (500mg, tablet) form. Never take more than this amount in 24 hours!

As with aspirin, no real differences exist among the many different name-brand and generic acetaminophen products. Of course, this is comparing like products—extra strength to extra strength, combination to combination. The most important thing is to buy the product strength that's appropriate for the dose you should take. Once you find the right product strength for you, buy the least expensive brand, which is usually a generic product. Acetaminophen products are available in many strengths and forms, including tablets, caplets (specially coated to make them easier to take), suppositories, and liquid preparations. It's particularly important to measure the correct dose with liquid products; read the label carefully.

Beware advertising claims! A manufacturer might add the term "arthritis strength" to its acetaminophen product line (Tylenol Arthritis Strength, for example), implying that this product has something special in it to relieve arthritis pain. Arthritis-strength products contain the pain reliever acetaminophen, but contain nothing to reduce inflammation, which is the source of most arthritis pain. So while this product might indeed give you relief from your arthritis pain, its only special feature is its higher potency—650mg compared to the regular strength of 325mg and the extra strength of 500mg. Unless you're willing to pay extra for the convenience of taking pills less frequently, we just don't think using arthritis-strength products makes sense. If you take acetaminophen regularly, it will cost you $50 a year more to take Tylenol Arthritis Strength than to take a generic extra-strength acetaminophen product. Whatever acetaminophen product and strength you buy, however, always read the label to make sure you take the correct dose.

Acetaminophen Products

PRODUCT	STRENGTH	ACTIVE INGREDIENT	USUAL DOSAGE	TYPICAL QUANTITY	TYPICAL PRICE	COST PER DOSE
Anacin Aspirin-Free Extra Strength Tablets	500mg	Acetaminophen	Take 1-2 tablets every 6 hrs., no more than 8 in 24 hrs.	100	$9.50	10¢
Excedrin Extra-Strength Tablets	250mg, 250mg, 65mg	Acetaminophen, aspirin, caffeine	Take 2 tablets every 6 hrs., no more than 8 in 24 hrs.	100	$9.79	20¢
Excedrin Migraine Caplets	250mg, 250mg, 65mg	Acetaminophen, aspirin, caffeine	Take 2 tablets every 6 hrs., no more than 8 in 24 hrs.	175	$12.99	15¢
Excedrin PM Aspirin-Free Pain Reliever/ Sleep Aid Tablets	500mg, 38mg	Acetaminophen, diphenhydramine citrate	Take 2 tablets at bedtime.	275	$15.99	12¢
Extra-Strength Non-Aspirin PM or No-Aspirin (generic version of Tylenol PM Extra-Strength Pain Reliever/Sleep Aid) Caplets	500mb	Acetaminophen, diphenhydramine	Take 2 tablets at bedtime.	100	$8.99	18¢
Genapap, "No-Aspirin," Acetaminophen or "Non-aspirin" extra-strength non-aspirin tablets	500mg	Acetaminophen	Take 1-2 tablets every 6 hrs., no more than 8 in 24 hrs.	500	$14.99	3¢
Genapap, "No-Aspirin," Acetaminophen or "Non-aspirin" (generic version of Tylenol Regular Strength) Tablets	325mg	Acetaminophen	Take 1-4 tablets every 4 hrs., no more than 12 in 24 hrs.	100	$4.99	5¢
Genapap, "No-Aspirin," Acetaminophen or "Non-aspirin" (generic version of Tylenol Regular Strength) Tablets	325mg	Acetaminophen	Take 1-4 tablets every 4 hrs., no more than 12 in 24 hrs.	500	$13.99	3¢
Midol Maximum Strength Menstrual Formula Caplets	500mg, 60mg, 15mg	Acetaminophen, caffeine, pyrilamine maleate	Take 2 caplets every 4 hrs., no more than 8 in 24 hrs.	24	$6.99	58¢

PRODUCT	STRENGTH	ACTIVE INGREDIENT	USUAL DOSAGE	TYPICAL QUANTITY	TYPICAL PRICE	COST PER DOSE
Pamprin Maximum Strength Menstrual Formula Caplets	250mg, 250mg 25mg	Acetaminophen / magnesium salicylate, pamabrom	Take 2 caplets every 4-6 hrs., no more than 8 in 24 hrs.	32	$6.99	44¢
Premsyn PMS Maximum Strength Menstrual Formula Caplets	500mg, 15mg, 25mg	Acetaminophen, pyrilamine maleate, pamabrom	Take 2 caplets every 4-6 hrs., no more than 8 in 24 hrs.	40	$7.49	38¢
Tylenol Arthritis Strength Tablets	650mg	Acetaminophen	Take 1-2 tablets every 8 hrs., no more than 6 in 24 hrs.	150	$13.99	9¢
Tylenol Extra Strength Tablets	500mg	Acetaminophen	Take 1-2 tablets every 6 hrs., no more than 8 in 24 hrs.	100	$9.99	10¢
Tylenol PM Extra-Strength Pain Reliever/ Sleep Aid Caplets	500mg, 25mg	Acetaminophen, diphenhydramine	Take 2 caplets at bedtime.	100	$10.99	22¢
Tylenol Regular Strength Tablets	325mg	Acetaminophen	Take 1-4 tablets every 4 hrs., no more than 12 in 24 hrs.	100	$8.99	9¢

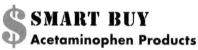

SMART BUY
Acetaminophen Products

Again, your Smart Buy is a generic product in a large quantity. These products, typically labeled "Non-Aspirin Pain Reliever" or "No-Aspirin," are made by seemingly endless numbers of manufacturers and sold through local discount stores, such as Target, Walgreens, Shopko, and Wal-Mart. Almost every household has a need for large quantities here, so purchase this product in 200-count bottles, at least. If you typically take 2 tablets each dose of the 325mg strength, you're probably better off bumping up to the extra-strength 500mg tablets and buying them in 500-count bottles. You should be able to find them at Walgreens or Wal-Mart for around $15 per bottle (about 3 cents a dose). Buying a generic product anywhere will save you lots of money. Because acetaminophen is a common ingredient in many multi-ingredient cold products, be sure you're getting only acetaminophen.

NONSTEROIDAL ANTI-INFLAMMATORY AGENTS (NSAIDs)

One of the fastest growing groups of over-the-counter drugs in recent years has been the NSAID (pronounced "EN-sed") family. Until a few years ago, the only NSAID available without a prescription was ibuprofen. Commonly found in Advil, Motrin-IB, and Nuprin, ibuprofen became very popular among people who needed relief from headaches, pain, arthritis, fever, and menstrual cramps. NSAIDs generally provide stronger pain relief than aspirin and acetaminophen. Although other NSAIDs now have joined it in over-the-counter status, ibuprofen remains the leading seller in this category.

Other NSAIDS include naproxen sodium, as in the name-brand product Aleve (the Walgreens brand is called Wal-proxen), and ketoprofen, as in the name-brand product Orudis KT. Orudis (ketoprofen) is slightly stronger than ibuprofen but weaker than naproxen; it must be taken less often than ibuprofen but more often than naproxen. As a rule, we prefer naproxen sodium over the other two because it lasts longer. But some people seem to do better with one of the others. Some trial-and-error may be necessary before some people find what works best for them.

> ### Allergy and Other Risks

All drugs carry the risk of allergy, overdose, and health problems resulting from overuse. And risks can be compounded with over-the-counter analgesics because these drugs show up in so many combinations and for so many uses. Your doctor or pharmacist might recommend aspirin, for example, as a mild anticoagulant (to reduce your risk for heart attack), to relieve headaches, to reduce arthritis inflammation, to lower fever, and to relieve minor aches and pains. If you have several of these complaints, you could end up taking several products, each of which targets a specific symptom, but which all contain the same active ingredient.

NSAIDs, like aspirin, have a mild anticoagulant (blood-thinning) effect. Your doctor might request that you suspend taking an NSAID for a short time if you're having scheduled surgery. Taking an NSAID in combination with aspirin or prescription blood-thinners (anticoagulants) can cause serious bleeding problems. And taking moderate to large doses of any NSAID regularly over an extended period can cause liver and kidney damage. Always follow the package directions, unless your doctor instructs you to do otherwise.

NSAIDs are often very effective for treating the pain and swelling of chronic arthritis, and can be taken safely for long periods as long as your doctor is monitoring your care. If your doctor recommends that you take an NSAID regularly, he or she often will want you to come in for a checkup and to have blood tests done to be sure your body is having no problems with the drug. Symptoms such as ringing in your ears, swollen ankles and hands (fluid retention), bloody or tarry stools, or mouth ulcers can indicate you're taking too much of the drug; stop taking it immediately and contact your doctor.

As with other kinds of analgesics, drinking moderate to heavy amounts of alcohol when you're taking an NSAID can set the stage for potentially life-threatening liver damage or failure. Alcohol and NSAIDs each put extra strain on your liver; in combination, the result quickly can become devastating.

When comparing NSAID products, and especially if you're switching to a different product because the one you're taking isn't giving you the relief you need, read the labels carefully. Many name-brand, store-brand, and generic products that sound like different drugs are really just the same drug in a different package. And be cautious when taking a combination product for a cold or the flu (see Chapter 17) with an NSAID for pain. Many combination flu-and-cold-symptom products contain an NSAID or acetaminophen.

Nonsteroidal Anti-Inflammatory Drugs (NSAIDs)

PRODUCT	STRENGTH	ACTIVE INGREDIENT	USUAL DOSAGE	TYPICAL QUANTITY	TYPICAL PRICE	COST PER DOSE
Advil	200mg	Ibuprofen	Take 1-2 tabs every 6 hrs., not more than 6 in 24 hrs.	100	$8.49	9¢
Advil Advanced Medicine for Pain, Coated Gel Caplets	200mg	Ibuprofen	Take 1-2 tabs every 6 hrs., not more than 6 in 24 hrs.	125	$8.49	7¢
Advil Migraine Solu-bilized Ibuprofen Liquid Filled Capsules	200mg	Ibuprofen	Take no more than directed. Adults: take 1 capsule. If migraine does not respond to 1 capsule, take 1 more capsule. Use the smallest effective dose.	80	$8.49	11¢
Aleve Arthritis Caplets	220mg	Naproxen sodium	Take 1 caplet every 8-12 hrs. For the first dose you may take 2 caplets within the first hr. Take no more than 2 caplets in any 8-12-hr. period, or 3 caplets in 24 hrs. Use the smallest effective dose.	100	$8.99	9¢

PRODUCT	STRENGTH	ACTIVE INGREDIENT	USUAL DOSAGE	TYPICAL QUANTITY	TYPICAL PRICE	COST PER DOSE
Aleve Arthritis Caplets	220mg	Naproxen sodium	Take 1 caplet every 8-12 hrs. For the first dose you may take 2 caplets within the first hour. Take no more than 2 caplets in any 8-12-hr. period, or 3 caplets in 24 hrs. Use the smallest effective dose.	200	$13.49	6.8¢
Ibuprofen, Genpril, Ibu-200, Wal-profen, Menadol (generic versions of Advil, Motrin IB) Tablets	200mg	Ibuprofen	Take 1-2 tabs every 6 hrs., not more than 6 in 24 hrs.	300	$12.99	4¢
Ibuprofen, Genpril, Ibu-200, Wal-profen, Menadol (generic versions of Advil, Motrin IB) Tablets	200mg	Ibuprofen	Take 1-2 tabs every 6 hrs., not more than 6 in 24 hrs.	500	$14.99	3¢
Motrin IB Ibuprofen Pain Reliever/Fever Reducer Gelcaps	200mg	Ibuprofen	Take 1-2 tabs every 6 hrs., not more than 6 in 24 hrs.	100	$7.99	8¢
Motrin IB Ibuprofen Pain Reliever/Fever Reducer Tablets	200mg	Ibuprofen	Take 1-2 tabs every 6 hrs., not more than 6 in 24 hrs.	100	$7.99	8¢
Naproxen Sodium, Wal-Proxen, (generic version of Aleve)	220mg	Naproxen sodium	Take 1 caplet every 8-12 hrs. For the first dose you may take 2 caplets within the first hour. Take no more than 2 caplets in any 8-12-hr. period, or 3 caplets in 24 hrs. Use the smallest effective dose.	200	$12.99	7¢
Orudis KT Tablets	12.5mg	Ketoprofen	Take 1 tablet every 4-6 hrs. while symptoms occur. If pain or fever does not improve, take 1 more tablet, but take no more than 2 tablets in any 4-6-hr. period, or 6 tablets in 24 hrs.	100	$10.49	11¢

$ SMART BUY
Nonsteroidal Anti-Inflammatory Drugs (NSAIDs)

The Smart Buy overall for an NSAID is a generic version of Aleve (naproxen sodium), such as the Walgreens brand Wal-proxen. A bottle of 200 tablets might cost about $12, or 6 cents a dose. Even though you can buy ibuprofen for about 3 cents a dose, you may have to take it as often as every 6 hours, and you may have to take 2 tablets per dose. This boosts your potential daily cost to 24 cents a day. One tablet of Wal-proxen (or any naproxen sodium product) may last 8 to 12 hours. Even if you don't take 3 tablets in

24 hours, your cost is about 20 cents a day, or a savings of as much as 17 percent, and you'll be getting a longer acting product, as well. Because Orudis KT isn't available yet in a generic version and you could need to take up to 6 tablets a day, it comes in at a very pricey 60 cents a day or more.

TOPICAL ANALGESICS

Topical analgesic products are those you rub into aching muscles to get relief. Many of these products, such as Icy Hot and Ben-Gay, work by generating warmth, which relaxes sore muscles to ease muscle tension and aching. Other products contain salicylates (the pain-relieving ingredients found in aspirin) that are supposed to soak into the tissues to provide pain relief. Some people find relief with topical analgesics; others do better taking oral products such as aspirin, ibuprophen, or other NSAID-type analgesics.

People who have arthritis and stiff muscles often get relief from the products that produce warmth (just as they might from a heating pad), technically called "counterirritants." Most of these products contain camphor, menthol, methyl salicylate, and phenol, which account for their familiar "locker room" smell. Some products also contain thymol, clove oil, and even turpentine. There is some debate about how counterirritants work. The accepted theory is that they stimulate nerve endings in the skin, "overloading" or confusing the nerve network that carries pain signals to the brain. Most counterirritants are also rubefacients; that is, they increase blood flow to the skin surface, which warms the skin.

Products such as Sportscreme (triethanolamine salicylate) and Aspercreme (trolamine salicylate) are related to aspirin, as you can tell from the salicylate both products contain. In fact, if you're allergic to aspirin or aspirin-type products, don't use these. Because these products aren't counterirritants, they provide no warmth. Controversy exists as to their effectiveness, because the skin is a very effective barrier to foreign substances. Some studies do show salicylate levels present in the tissues, indicating that the pain-relieving substance does make its way into the body. But research remains inconclusive when it comes to assessing just how well such products relieve pain. Although some salicylates probably make it through the skin, their concentration is unlikely to be high enough to have much effect.

Some products use capsaicin (the active ingredient in hot peppers) to generate heat. These odorless counterirritants include the name-brand products Zostrix and Capsaicin. The active ingredient in these creams also blocks the accumulation of a chemical called substance P, believed to play a role in transmitting pain signals to the brain. Although these products can be very effective in relieving localized pain, they can cause enough of a burning sensation to irritate your skin (especially if you happen to get any cream in an open cut or scrape). They're also more expensive than their menthol- and camphor-containing counterparts.

Read labels carefully and compare the percentages of active ingredients among products—even products with the same brand name. You'll find, for example, that Icy Hot Crème in a tube has different percentages than Icy Hot Ointment in a jar. And some products work better for some people than others. Finding what works best for you is often a matter of personal preference, as well as trial and error.

The form a product comes in also influences personal preference. Creams usually absorb well without leaving a film, and some contain emollients to moisten and soothe the skin. Ointments are petrolatum-based (Vaseline-like) and "trap" the ingredients into the skin. Ointments also offer a water-resistant barrier. Lotions typically are more liquid than creams or ointments, so they spread better over larger surfaces. Balms are really anything that relieves pain, and usually have some aromatic properties. The form a product comes in usually doesn't affect its cost.

Topical Analgesics

PRODUCT	STRENGTH	ACTIVE INGREDIENT	USUAL DOSAGE	TYPICAL QUANTITY	TYPICAL PRICE	COST PER OUNCE
Absorbine Jr. Linement	1.27%	Menthol	Apply 3-4 times a day.	4oz	$6.99	$1.75
Arthricare Ultra Arthritis Pain Relieving Rub	0.075%, 2%	Capsaicin, menthol	Apply 3-4 times a day.	1.5oz	$10.59	$7.06
Arthritis Hot Pain Relief Crème	15%, 10%	Methysalicylate, menthol	Apply 3-4 times a day.	3oz	$4.99	$1.67
Aspercreme Analgesic Crème Rub	10%	Trolamine salicylate	Apply 3-4 times a day.	3oz	$6.99	$2.33
Ben-Gay Penetrating Pain Relief Cream	15%, 10%	Methysalicylate, menthol	Apply 3-4 times a day.	6oz	$9.99	$1.67
Ben-Gay Ultra Strength Cream	30%, 10%, 4%	Methysalicylate, menthol, camphor	Apply 3-4 times a day.	6oz	$10.99	$1.83
Ben-Gay Unscented Pain Relieving Gel	2.5%	Menthol	Apply 3-4 times a day.	4oz	$7.99	$2
Capsagesic-HP Cream	0.075%	Capsaicin	Apply 3-4 times a day.	2 oz	$10.99	$5.50
Capzasin HP Arthritis Pain Relief Creme	0.075%	Capsaicin	Apply 3-4 times a day.	1.5oz	$12.99	$8.66
Capzasin P Arthritis Pain Relief Creme	0.025%	Capsaicin	Apply 3-4 times a day.	1.5oz	$10.49	$6.99

PRODUCT	STRENGTH	ACTIVE INGREDIENT	USUAL DOSAGE	TYPICAL QUANTITY	TYPICAL PRICE	COST PER OUNCE
Flexall Ultra Plus Gel	10%, 16%, 3.1%	Methysalicylate, menthol, camphor	Apply 3-4 times a day.	2oz	$6.49	$3.25
Icy Hot Balm	29%, 7.6%	Methysalicylate, menthol	Apply 3-4 times a day.	3.5oz	$6.99	$2
Icy Hot Cream	30%, 10%	Methysalicylate, menthol	Apply 3-4 times a day.	1.25oz	$3.69	$2.95
Joint-Ritis Arthritis Pain Reliever Ointment	16%	Menthol (also contains chondroitin, listed as inactive ingredient)	Apply 3-4 times a day.	2oz	$18.49	$9.25
$ Mineral Ice Gel	2%	Menthol	Apply 3-4 times a day.	8oz	$10.79	$1.35
Stop Pain Extra Strength Spray	8%	Menthol	Apply 3-4 times a day.	4oz	$10.59	$2.65
Thera-Patch	0.09%	Capsaicin	Apply 3-4 times a day.	7 patches	$7.89	$1.13 per patch
Tiger Balm Ultra Rub	Unlisted strengths	Camphor, menthol	Apply 3-4 times a day.	0.63oz	$6.99	$11.10
$ Walgreens Ultra-Strength Rub (generic version of Ben Gay Ultra Strength Cream)	30%, 10%, 4%	Methysalicylate, menthol, camphor	Apply 3-4 times a day.	4oz	$5.99	$1.50
Zostrix	0.025%	Capsaicin	Apply 3-4 times a day.	2oz	$15.99	$8
Zostrix HP	0.075%	Capsaicin	Apply 3-4 times a day.	2oz	$20.99	$10.50

$ SMART BUY
Topical Analgesics

Most people will find the more concentrated products their Smart Buys. These include the generic version of Ben-Gay's Ultra Strength Cream (such as Walgreens Ultra-Strength Rub), which costs about $6 for 4 ounces. Another Smart Buy is Mineral Ice in the larger 8-ounce jar, which lowers your cost per ounce to $1.35. Capsagesic-HP rub, which contains capsaicin (extracted from red chili peppers), is more expensive than most other topical analgesics, but still cheaper than the original name-brand product containing capsaicin, Zostrix-HP. The "HP" stands for "high potency," which is a strength of 0.075 percent (compared to regular strength 0.025 percent). You'll need a much smaller amount than with the lower strength. Capsagesic-HP rub will save you about $5, or about 48 percent over the name-brand Zostrix-HP.

$ SMART OPTIONS FOR SAVINGS
Over-the-Counter Pain-Relief Products

Pain-relief products are big sellers in the over-the-counter market, and there are dozens of products to choose from. But the Smart Buys can be yours just by following a few basic guidelines:

1. Always, always, always buy generic, and buy the largest quantity available. Talk to your pharmacist to see if you can order 500- or 1,000-count bottles to get a really great deal.

2. Watch for sales and coupon specials, especially during cold and flu season. Because there are so many uses for pain relievers, and your entire household can take these products, you can take advantage of great buys to stock up.

3. Consider buying generic pain-relief products in large quantities through mail-order and Internet pharmacies. You'll probably find the greatest savings through Internet drug stores located in Canada; just be cautious (read Chapter 4 first). And be sure to check the label's expiration date when the product arrives, so you know it's at peak potency.

4. If you live near Canada or travel there regularly, consider buying your generic pain-relief products there.

5. Check our Web site at www.smartbuysdrugwise.com for the latest information about more ways to save money on these drugs.

Chapter 19

Over-the-Counter Gastrointestinal Remedies

Gastrointestinal discomforts are among the leading reasons people visit their doctors, so it's not surprising that remedies to treat heartburn, upset stomach, and diarrhea are such popular drugstore purchases. Occasional intestinal upset is normal. Frequently the culprit is simply overdoing it—eating and drinking too much. Fried foods, baked goods, spicy foods, and beverages containing caffeine can irritate the sensitive tissues of your digestive tract, causing a burning sensation in your esophagus and stomach, as well as intestinal bloating and gas. If you feel the need to take products to relieve such symptoms, cut back on foods that can cause them.

If your discomfort continues longer than two weeks, keeps coming back, is intense enough to keep you from your usual activities, or if you have any bleeding, your problem could be serious; see your doctor. Unless your doctor tells you otherwise, don't exceed the recommended times and dosages of over-the-counter products that affect gastrointestinal discomfort.

The major products in this category include:

1. Antacids, which relieve indigestion
2. H2 blockers, which reduce the amount of acid the stomach produces
3. Antiemetic products, which relieve nausea and vomiting
4. Antidiarrheals, which relieve diarrhea
5. Laxative products, which relieve constipation
6. Gas-reducing products

ANTACIDS

Your stomach secretes 1 to 2 liters of hydrochloric acid and other fluids every day. This mixture, strong enough to remove Abraham Lincoln's face from a penny, starts the digestive process. Not surprisingly, a little hydrochloric acid goes a long way, and sometimes your stomach generates too much of it. Antacids neutralize stomach acid to relieve heartburn, indigestion, gastroesophageal reflux disorder (GERD), and sour stomach. Several antacid formulas simply combine mineral salts. These products work by interacting chemically with stomach acid to neutralize it. Less acid in your stomach means less irritation.

Three types of neutralizing antacids are used the most:

1. Aluminum hydroxide products
2. Calcium carbonate products
3. Magnesium oxide and magnesium hydroxide

They're relatively equal in effectiveness, but can have vastly different side effects.

ALUMINUM HYDROXIDE ANTACIDS

Aluminum hydroxide works well to relieve heartburn, but it's more likely than other formulations to cause constipation. These products are good choices if you have heartburn and diarrhea, but avoid them if your only problem is heartburn. Only one name-brand aluminum hydroxide product is available—Alternagel—and it has no generic alternatives. Other medications containing aluminum are combination products. (See the section "Aluminum–Magnesium Combination Products," later in this chapter.) Some people believe that aluminum can cause health problems, particularly in connection with Alzheimer's disease. No conclusive evidence exists to connect aluminum toxicity to Alzheimer's, however, or to any other toxicity in an individual with normally functioning kidneys. If you have kidney problems or disease, talk with your doctor before you use any over-the-counter products.

Aluminum Hydroxide Antacids

PRODUCT	STRENGTH PER DOSE	ACTIVE INGREDIENT	USUAL DOSAGE	TYPICAL QUANTITY	TYPICAL PRICE	COST PER OUNCE
AlternaGel Antacid Liquid	600mg	Aluminum hydroxide	Take 1-2 teaspoons between meals and at bedtime or as doctor directs.	12oz	$7.99	67¢

CALCIUM CARBONATE

Calcium carbonate is the main ingredient in antacids such as Tums and various generic products. It does a good job of relieving acid indigestion and is a good source of calcium. We hear much discussion about one form of calcium being better than another, but calcium is calcium. What does differ is that the various "salt" forms of calcium affect the rate at which each product dissolves. But it doesn't affect how much calcium you absorb at the end of the day.

Calcium Carbonate Products

PRODUCT	STRENGTH PER DOSE	ACTIVE INGREDIENT	USUAL DOSAGE	TYPICAL QUANTITY	TYPICAL PRICE	COST PER DOSE
Alka-Mints Antacid & Calcium Supplement	850mg	Calcium carbonate	Chew 1-2 tablets every 2 hrs. as needed (no more than 9 tabs in 24 hrs.;no longer than 2 weeks at maximum dose).	75	$2.69	36¢
Amitone Antacid, Tablets	420mg	Calcium carbonate	Chew 1-2 tablets as needed (no more than 18 tabs in 24 hrs.; no longer than 2 weeks at maximum dose).	90	$7.99	8.9¢
"Antacid Extra-Strength" (generic version of Tums Supplement) Tablets	750mg	Calcium carbonate	Chew 2-4 tablets as needed to treat symptoms (no more than 8 tablets in 24 hours).	110	$3.99	3.6¢
Antacid Tablets (generic version of Tums) Antacid/Calcium Supplement Chew Tabs	500mg	Calcium carbonate	Chew 2-4 tablets as needed (no more than 15 tabs in 24 hrs.; no longer than 2 weeks at maximum dose).	150	$3.99	2.7¢
Maalox Quick Dissolve Chewable Antacid Tablets, Assorted	600mg	Calcium carbonate	Chew 2-4 tablets as needed (no more than 13 tabs in 24 hrs.; no longer than 2 weeks at maximum dose).	85	$6.79	8¢
Maalox Antacid/ Calcium Supplement, Chewable Tablets, Regular Strength Lemon	600mg	Calcium carbonate	Chew 2-4 tablets as needed (no more than 13 pieces in 24 hrs.; no longer than 2 weeks at maximum dose).	85	$6.79	8¢
Surpass Antacid Chewing Gum Extra Strength, 450mg, Wintergreen	450mg	Calcium carbonate	Chew 1-2 pieces as needed (no more than 17 pieces in 24 hrs.; no longer than 2 weeks at maximum dose).	45	$5.99	13.3¢
Surpass Antacid Chewing Gum, 300mg, Wintergreen	300mg	Calcium carbonate	Chew 1-2 pieces as needed (no more than 26 pieces in 24 hrs.; no longer than 2 weeks at maximum dose).	60	$5.89	9.8¢
Titralac Extra Strength Antacid Tablets	750mg	Calcium carbonate	Chew 1-2 tablets every 3-4 hrs. as needed (no more than 8 tablets in 24 hrs).	100	$7.29	7.3¢

PRODUCT	STRENGTH PER DOSE	ACTIVE INGREDIENT	USUAL DOSAGE	TYPICAL QUANTITY	TYPICAL PRICE	COST PER DOSE
Titralac Instant Relief Antacid, Tablets	420mg	Calcium carbonate	Chew 2 tablets every 2-3 hrs. as needed(no more than 18 tabs in 24 hrs.; no longer than 2 weeks at maximum dose).	100	$5.99	6¢
Tums Calcium for Life Bone Health Calcium Supplement, 500mg	500mg	Calcium carbonate	Chew 2-4 tablets as needed (no more than 15 tabs in 24 hrs.; no longer than 2 weeks at maximum dose).	90	$6.89	7.7¢
Tums E-X Extra Strength Antacid /Calcium Supplement, Tablets	750mg	Calcium carbonate	Chew 2-4 tablets as needed to treat symptoms (no more than 8 tablets in 24 hrs.).	200	$8.39	4.2¢
Tums Extra Strength Fruit with Calcium tablets	750mg	Calcium carbonate	Chew 2-4 tablets as needed to treat symptoms (no more than 8 tablets in 24 hrs.).	48	$3.49	7.3¢
Tums Ultra Maximum Antacid/Calcium Supplement	1,000mg	Calcium carbonate	Chew 2-4 tablets as needed to treat symptoms (no more than 6 tablets in 24 hrs.).	36	$3.39	9.4¢
Tums Ultra Maximum Strength Antacid/Calcium Supplement, Mint Tablets	1,000mg	Calcium carbonate	Chew 2-4 tablets as needed to treat symptoms (no more than 6 tablets in 24 hrs.).	72	$4.99	7¢
Tums Ultra Maximum Strength Antacid/Calcium Supplement, Spearmint	1,000mg	Calcium carbonate	Chew 2-4 tablets as needed to treat symptoms (no more than 6 tablets in 24 hrs.).	160	$8.99	5.6¢
Tums Antacid/Calcium Supplement Tablets	500mg	Calcium carbonate	Chew 2-4 tablets as needed (no more than 15 tabs in 24 hrs.; no longer than 2 weeks at maximum dose).	150	$4.99	3.3¢

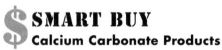

$ SMART BUY
Calcium Carbonate Products

If you're thinking that the first two Tums products in the foregoing table are the same strength, you're right. They're just labeled for different uses. More important is to notice that the antacid version is $2 less for 60 more tablets! Regardless of why you're taking a calcium supplement, whether as an antacid or as a calcium supplement, you probably need 1,000mg to 1,500mg a day. The Smart Buy is a generically equivalent product, such as "Antacid EX Tablets" or "Chewable Calcium Extra-Strength Tabs," in a bottle of 110 tablets of the 750mg strength, for about $4. A woman needing calcium supplementation probably will take 2 tablets a day, or 730 tablets a year, which is 7 bottles for an annual cost of about $28. This compares to an annual expense of about $35 for regular-strength name-brand Tums (500mg), a savings of 20 percent.

MAGNESIUM OXIDE AND MAGNESIUM HYDROXIDE PRODUCTS

Magnesium oxide and magnesium hydroxide are effective antacids and gentle laxatives. Doctors sometimes recommend magnesium to prevent leg cramps. Refer to the manufacturer's label for dosage, because it will vary depending on why you're taking the product.

Magnesium Oxide and Magnesium Hydroxide Products

PRODUCT	STRENGTH PER DOSE	ACTIVE INGREDIENT	USUAL DOSAGE	TYPICAL QUANTITY	TYPICAL PRICE	COST PER DOSE
Mag-Ox Tablets	400mg	Magnesium oxide	See label; depends on use.	100	$15.59	15.6¢
Phillips Milk of Magnesia Original	400mg/ teaspoon	Magnesium hydroxide	See label; depends on use.	26oz	$7.99	5.1¢
Phillips Milk of Magnesia Tablets	311mg	Magnesium hydroxide	See label; depends on use.	200	$7.99	4¢
Phillips Milk of Magnesia Original	400mg/ teaspoon	Magnesium hydroxide	See label; depends on use.	12oz	$4.79	6.6¢
Walgreens Magnesium Oxide Tablets	250mg	Magnesium oxide	See label; depends on use.	100	$3.49	3.5¢
Walgreens, Target, Wal-Mart Milk Of Magnesia Laxative & Antacid I	400mg/ teaspoon	Magnesium hydroxide	See label; depends on use.	26oz	$5.99	3.8¢
Your Life Magnesium Oxide Tablets	250mg	Magnesium oxide	See label; depends on use.	100	$4.89	4.9¢

$ SMART BUY
Magnesium Products

Name-brand products in this category cost significantly more and deliver nothing over their generic or store-brand equivalents. Whichever form of magnesium you buy, oxide or hydroxide, we recommend that you purchase a generic alternative. You'll find Smart Buys in stores such as Walgreens, Target, and Wal-Mart. Their economy-size (26 ounces or so) bottles of their "milk of magnesia" cost around $5—about half what you'd pay for the name-brand product Philips Milk of Magnesia. Be sure to visit our Web site at www.smartbuysdrugwise.com for updates on prescriptions and over-the-counter drugs.

ALUMINUM-MAGNESIUM COMBINATION PRODUCTS

Aluminum-magnesium products are among the most popular antacids on the market. Two familiar brands are Maalox and Mylanta. Maalox sound-alikes will have names like "Alu-Mag," "Alu-Drox," and "Alu-Hydrox." In combining aluminum and magnesium, the potential problems of each—constipation and laxative, respectively—cancel each other out. These products are available in liquid form.

Aluminum–Magnesium Products

PRODUCT	STRENGTH PER DOSE	ACTIVE INGREDIENT	USUAL DOSAGE	TYPICAL QUANTITY	TYPICAL PRICE	PRICE PER 5 ML DOSE
Alu-Mag, M-Antacid (generic version of Maalox)(Walgreens, Rite Aid)	225mg 200mg/ teaspoon	Aluminum, magnesium hydroxide	Take 2-4 teaspoons 4 times a day.	26oz	$4.49	2.9¢
Maalox Extra Strength Suspension	500mg 450mg 40mg/ teaspoon	Aluminum, magnesium hydroxide, simethicone	Take 2-4 teaspoons 4 times a day.	26oz	$9.99	6.4¢
Maalox Liquid Antacid	225mg 200mg /teaspoon	Aluminum, magnesium hydroxide	Take 2-4 teaspoons 4 times a day.	12oz	$4.79	13.3¢
Maalox TC Suspension	600mg 300mg/ teaspoon	Aluminum, magnesium hydroxide	Take 1-2 teaspoons 4 times a day.	12oz	$8.99	12.5¢
Mylanta Original Liquid	200mg 200mg 20mg/ teaspoon	Aluminum magnesium, hydroxide simethicone	Take 2-4 teaspoons between meals and at bedtime.	12oz	$4.69	6.5¢
Mylanta Original Maximum Strength Liquid	400mg 400mg 40mg/ teaspoon	Aluminum, magnesium hydroxide, simethicone	Take 2-4 teaspoons between meals and at bedtime.	12oz	$6.99	9.7¢
Wal-Mart or Walgreens Liquid Antacid (Generic version of Mylanta Liquid)	200mg 200mg 20mg/ teaspoon	Aluminum, magnesium hydroxide, simethicone	Take 2-4 teaspoonfuls between meals, and at bedtime.	26oz	$6.79	4.4¢

$ SMART BUY
Antacids

Among calcium carbonate products, your Smart Buy is a generic version of Tums EX (look for Chewable Calcium Antacid Extra-Strength 750mg Tablet) product in a 110-count bottle. If you shop at Walgreens or Wal-Mart, you shouldn't have to pay more than $4 or $5.

If you're buying a magnesium hydroxide product, you can buy the least expensive generic when you shop discount stores such as Walgreens. You'll get the best value if you purchase the large 26-ounce bottle for about $5, a savings of around $2 (about 29 percent) over the same size of the original brand Philips.

For aluminum-magnesium combination products, be sure to compare the amounts of active ingredients per dose. Again, buying big and generic will save you money. A generic for Maalox Original Strength is probably your best buy. Discount stores such as Walgreens carry a 26-ounce bottle of Antacid M Liquid for about $5, giving you twice as much for the price as the name-brand products, a 50 percent savings.

H$_2$ BLOCKERS

In the late 1970s, the first of a new class of drugs came onto the market. Called H$_2$ blockers, these drugs actually limit the amount of acid your stomach makes. Tagamet (cimetidine) was among the earliest H$_2$ blockers, and it remains among the most popular now that these drugs are available over the counter. Other familiar name-brands include Pepcid (generic name famotidine), Axid (generic name nizatidine), and Zantac (generic name ranitidine). H$_2$ blockers offer 6 to 12 hours of relief and are rapidly becoming the treatment of choice for gastroesophageal reflux disorder (GERD), and ulcers. They also provide rapid and effective relief for heartburn and acid indigestion.

Not much difference exists among the H$_2$ blockers in terms of effectiveness. Tagamet has several important drawbacks, however, and isn't the best choice for most people. For one thing, Axid, Pepcid, and Zantac and their generic or store-brand counterparts will give much longer relief per dose than Tagamet and its generic equivalents, reducing your cost and the number of times a day you have to take a dose. And Tagamet sometimes causes mental confusion in older people and can interact with a wide range of other prescription and over-the-counter drugs. Taking antacids along with Tagamet may interfere with its absorption, rendering it less effective. So you may end up taking more Tagamet and spending more money again. Caffeine may interfere with Tagamet metabolism by increasing its levels (and possible side effects) in your body. Because Tagamet interacts with numerous prescription medications, ask your pharmacist or read the warning labels carefully before you take it. Taking Tagamet while consuming alcohol will slow alcohol metabolism, so it will remain longer in your system.

Pepcid Complete has added calcium carbonate and magnesium hydroxide to the original product, which contains famotidine, to provide immediate relief until the famotidine takes effect. As you might expect, you pay more for this combination. If you often have an acid problem around mealtime and you can plan your efforts to subdue it, buy the generic version of Pepcid AC to save money and take a dose 15 to 60 minutes before eating. Then take a chewable antacid such as Tums to take the place of the added antacids in Pepcid Complete if you need the additional relief.

When it comes to H_2 blockers, generic isn't necessarily cheaper. Manufacturers often put these products on sale or offer extra tablets at no additional cost, making it possible to buy name-brand Pepcid for less than you'd pay for ranitidine, the generic

H2 Blockers

PRODUCT	STRENGTH PER DOSE	ACTIVE INGREDIENT	USUAL DOSAGE	TYPICAL QUANTITY	TYPICAL PRICE	COST PER DOSE
Axid AR Tablets	75mg	Nizatidine	Chew 1 tablet up to twice a day.	50	$14.99	30¢
Pepcid AC Chewable Tablets	10mg	Famotidine	Chew 1 tablet up to twice a day.	90	$23.99	27¢
Pepcid AC Tablets	10mg	Famotidine	Chew 1 tablet up to twice a day.	90	$23.99	27¢
Pepcid Complete Chewable Tablets	10mg 800mg 165mg	Famotidine, calcium carbonate, magnesium hydroxide	Chew 1 tablet up to twice a day.	50	$18.99	38¢
$ Rite Aid Generic Pepcid AC (famotidine)	10mg	Famotidine	Chew 1 tablet up to twice a day.	90	$16.99	19¢
$ Rite Aid Ranitidine 75mg Tablets Non-Prescription Strength	75mg	Ranitidine	Chew 1 tablet up to twice a day.	80	$15.99	20¢
Tagamet HB 200mg Tablet	200mg	Cimetidine	Chew 1 tablet up to twice a day.	70	$18.99	27¢
$ Walgreens Wal-zan 75 Acid Reducer	75mg	Ranitidine	Chew 1 tablet up to twice a day.	60	$12.99	22¢
Walgreens, Wal-Mart Cimetidine 200 mg Tablets	200mg	Cimetidine	Chew 1 tablet up to twice a day.	70	$14.99	21¢
Zantac 75mg Tablets	75mg	Ranitidine	Chew 1 tablet up to twice a day.	80	$22.99	29¢

form of Zantac. So watch your newspaper advertisements and each store's shelf tags for the bonus packs. Axid tends to be more expensive than other H_2 blockers at this point, but watch for a generic formula containing the active ingredient nizatidine to hit the market before long.

If you don't have insurance coverage for prescription drugs, buying over-the-counter often is significantly cheaper than purchasing a prescription-strength H_2 blocker. When Don came into the pharmacy to refill his wife's prescription for Pepcid 20mg, we noticed that he didn't have insurance. Don's wife had been taking the medication for some time, and he'd always just paid for the prescription, at a cost of $128 for 60 tablets, a one-month supply—$2.13 a day. We showed Don that he could buy a bottle of 90 tablets of the over-the-counter strength of generic Pepcid AC (famotidine) for $24. The over-the-counter strength is 10mg, so Don's wife would have to take 2 tablets to get her 20mg dose. This minor inconvenience of taking an extra tablet dropped her per dose cost to about $1.08 a day, for a 49 percent savings. Switching from a prescription name-brand product to a generic over-the-counter product saved Don $29 a month—a whopping $380 a year!

$ SMART BUY
H2 Blockers

Your Smart Buy is probably famotidine, the generic equivalent of Pepcid AC, for about 19 cents a dose. Check stores such as Walgreens, Wal-Mart, and Rite Aid for local specials. Name-brand manufacturers often offer promotional specials in which you get some "free" product, but overall you'll still do better buying generic. There's a lot of competition in this area, so watch prices and packaging, focusing on occasional bonus packs from time to time.

You can buy a generic such as Walgreens Wal-Zan 75 Acid Reducer (a generic version of Zantac-75) in a quantity of 60 (a one-month supply) for about $13, while 90 tablets of name-brand Zantac-75 will cost you around $23. This works out to 43 cents a day for Wal-Zan 75, compared to 51 cents a day for Zantac-75, a savings of about $30 annually, or 19 percent.

ANTIEMETIC PRODUCTS

Nausea and vomiting are unpleasant and unfortunately common accompaniments to a wide variety of gastrointestinal upsets and infections. For any vomiting that continues longer than two days, contact your regular healthcare provider or seek medical attention. For mild problems, though, a phosphorated carbohydrate solution might do the trick. Products containing this blend of sugars and phosphoric acid usually are effective and inexpensive. They help reduce nausea and vomiting by working directly on the stomach to reduce the smooth muscle wall contractions. Because of the sugar (fructose) these products contain, people with diabetes or HFI (high fructose intolerance) and pregnant women should not use them.

Antiemetic Products

PRODUCT	STRENGTH PER DOSE	ACTIVE INGREDIENT	USUAL DOSAGE	TYPICAL QUANTITY	TYPICAL PRICE	PRICE PER ML
"Nausea Relief" or "Anti-Nausea Liquid" Wal-Mart or Walgreens (generic version of Emetrol)	1.87g, 1.87g, 21.5mg	Glucose, levulose (fructose), phosphoric acid	Take 15–30ml undiluted, for no more than 1 hr. or 5 doses, or as doctor directs.	4oz	$4.99	21¢
$ Coca-Cola soft drink	N/A (trade secret	N/A (trade secret)	Sip small amounts of room-temperature soft drink.	12oz	$5.49 for 12 cans or 46¢ a can	64¢
$ Cola syrup	N/A	High fructose corn syrup, sucrose, water, caramel color, phosphoric acid	Pour 1–2 teaspoonfuls 5–10 ml) over crushed (ice and slip slowly. May repeat in 1–2 hrs.	4oz	$3.49	15¢
Emetrol Anti-Emetics for Nausea	1.87g 1.87g 21.5mg/ teaspoon	Dextrose, levulose (fructose), phosphoric acid	Take 15–30ml undiluted, for no more than 1 hr. or 5 doses or as doctor directs.	4oz	7.49	31¢
Store-brand cola soft drink (generic version of Coca-Cola)	N/A (trade secret)	N/A (trade secret)	Sip small amounts of room-temperature soft drink.	12oz	$2.99 for 12 cans or 25¢ a can	35¢

$ SMART BUY
Antiemetic Products

These products differ little in terms of effectiveness, but if you want to save money, cola syrup is the remedy of choice. Before you drive to the drugstore, though, try a home-remedy version of the same product. One inexpensive and readily available alternative is to take a room-temperature cola drink (such as regular Coca-Cola with sugar) and pour the cola back and forth between two glasses until the fizz is gone. Take small sips (1 to 2 teaspoons with brief intervals) until your stomach settles down. With a little shopping at your local grocery store, you should be able to get a store-brand cola for about 25 cents a can.

ANTIDIARRHEALS

When it comes to purchasing a product to treat diarrhea, do your homework first. You don't want to have to compare products and prices if you might have to run to the bathroom! As with vomiting, seek medical attention if you have diarrhea that continues for longer than two days, or for diarrhea that's bloody or accompanied by a fever.

Among the several kinds of antidiarrheal products, the most familiar is probably the pink liquid, Pepto-Bismol. Be aware that while using Pepto-Bismol, your stools may be dark in appearance. This is normal and doesn't indicate a problem. Pepto-Bismol's active ingredient is bismuth subsalicylate. This is related to the active ingredient in aspirin, so don't use Pepto-Bismol if you have an aspirin allergy. The bismuth component may have direct antimicrobial activity on various gastrointestinal bacteria and viruses; that is, it may help fight infections. The salicylate component possesses some antisecretory action, which also helps reduce diarrhea and possibly inflammation.

Another liquid product marketed as a treatment for diarrhea is Kaopectate. It also works as an absorbent and protectant. Kaopectate has replaced its old primary ingredients kaolin and pectin with the single active ingredient attapulgite. These medications aren't absorbed into your system; instead, they may relieve diarrhea by causing constipation.

Imodium, available in liquid and tablet forms, works by reducing the motility (movement) of the gastrointestinal tract. It also increases the thickness and density of stool and diminishes the loss of electrolytes and fluids.

In addition to using medicine to halt diarrhea, it's very important that you replace the fluid your body loses and follow a proper diet. For the first 24 hours, eat gelatin and drink plenty of caffeine-free clear liquids, such as ginger ale, decaffeinated cola, decaffeinated tea, and broth. Sports drinks aren't a good choice because they're high in sugars that could cause more digestive problems and potentially more diarrhea. For 24 hours, eat bland foods, such as cooked cereals, bread, crackers, and applesauce to help settle your system. Fruits, vegetables, fried or spicy foods, bran, candy, caffeine, and alcoholic beverages are likely to make your symptoms worse, so avoid them until everything returns to normal. As always, if you're pregnant, don't take these or any medications without consulting your physician first.

Sometimes convenience becomes the deciding factor in your purchasing decision. Many people who travel to other countries like to take an antidiarrheal product with them; products available in tablet form, such as Imodium or its generic counterparts, generally are the most convenient option for this.

Pepto-Bismol and Reye's Syndrome

Pepto-Bismol, that familiar pink liquid, carries an unexpected (and dangerous) risk when given to children—Reye's syndrome. Although Pepto-Bismol doesn't contain aspirin, a main ingredient is bismuth subsalicylate—a member of the same chemical family as aspirin (salicylates).

Never give Pepto-Bismol (or generic forms) to anyone under age 18!

Antidiarrheals

PRODUCT	STRENGTH PER DOSE	ACTIVE INGREDIENT	USUAL DOSAGE	TYPICAL QUANTITY	TYPICAL PRICE	PRICE PER DOSE
Bismuth Liquid, Smooth	262mg	Bismuth subsalicylate Antacid or Bis-Mate	Take 2 tablespoons every 1/2 to 1 hr. as needed, to a maximum of 8 doses in 24 hrs.	16oz	$4.99	25¢ per 2 tablespoons
Imodium A-D Anti-Diarrheal Caplets	2mg	Loperamide hcl	Take 2 caplets after the first loose bowel movement and 1 caplet after each following loose bowel movement, but no more than 4 caplets a day for no longer than 2 days.	24	$8.99	37.5¢ per tablet
Kaopectate Advanced Formula Regular Flavored Liquid	750mg	Attapulgite	Take 2 tablespoons at first sign of diarrhea, then after each loose bowel movement, no longer than 2 days.	12oz	$7.49	62.5¢ per 2 tablespoons
Pepto-Bismol Maximum Strength Liquid	525mg	Bismuth subsalicylate	Take 2 tablespoons every 1/2 to 1 hr. as needed, to a maximum of 4 doses in 24 hrs.	2oz	$6.99	58¢ per 2 tablespoons
Pepto-Bismol Maximum Strength Liquid	525mg	Bismuth subsalicylate	Take 2 tablespoons every 1/2 to 1 hour as needed, to a maximum of 4 doses in 24 hrs.	12oz	$4.99	41.6¢ per 2 tablespoons

PRODUCT	STRENGTH PER DOSE	ACTIVE INGREDIENT	USUAL DOSAGE	TYPICAL QUANTITY	TYPICAL PRICE	PRICE PER DOSE
Pepto-Bismol Original	262mg	Bismuth subsalicylate	Take 2 tablespoons every 1/2 to 1 hr. as needed, to a maximum of 8 doses in 24-hrs.	16oz	5.99	37.4¢ per 2 tablespoons
Pepto-Bismol Original Chewable Tablets	262mg	Bismuth subsalicylate	Chew 2 tablets (or dissolve in mouth) every 1/2 to 1 hr. as needed, to maximum of 8 doses in 24 hrs.	48	$6.79	28.3¢ per 2 tablespoons
Wal-Mart, Walgreens, Target Anti-Diarrheal Caplets	2mg	Loperamide hcl	Take 2 caplets after the first loose bowel movement and 1 caplet after each following loose bowel movement, but no more than 4 caplets a day for no longer than 2 days.	18	$4.99	27.7¢ per caplet

$ SMART BUY
Antidiarrheals

Your Smart Buy again is a generic version of Imodium called loperamide. It comes in 2mg strength only. Tablets typically cost less than liquids and travel more easily, too. Purchasing a generic generally saves you about $1 for a package of 18 tablets/caplets—about 20 percent over the name-brand product. Buying in large quantities usually isn't an option here, because you'll use these drugs for only 24 to 48 hours, unless your doctor instructs you otherwise and closely supervises your condition. Take these products only at the recommended dosages and for the recommended time period. Taking them longer can create the opposite problem—constipation.

▶ Managing Traveler's Diarrhea

If you're traveling outside the U.S., "traveler's diarrhea" is likely to be a serious concern. Prevention is the most effective treatment. In many locations, it's safest to use bottled water for drinking and brushing your teeth. Order drinks, even soft drinks, without ice; even ice cubes can be contaminated.

If you must drink from, or use, local water sources, consider boiling the water for 10 minutes or adding iodine tablets 30 minutes prior to consumption to kill bacteria. Your travel agent may have a more extensive list of precautions regarding the countries where you'll be traveling.

LAXATIVE PRODUCTS

The best treatment for constipation is prevention. Make sure you're getting plenty of fiber, fluids, and exercise. If constipation strikes despite these efforts, start with bulk-forming laxatives. These are mostly natural vegetable products that gently nudge your body back to its normal rhythms and regular bowel movements. It often helps to add a stool softener. Bulk-forming laxatives include products such as Metamucil and Cit-rucel. Stool softeners include products such as Colace and Surfak. Stool softeners work by bringing more water into the stool. If you're on a salt-restricted diet because of high blood pressure or other health problems, use Surfak. Colace contains docusate sodium, which will cause you to retain fluids and can lead to an increase in blood pressure. These products typically take a few days to work. It's important to drink plenty of fluids with each dose of these products and extra fluids throughout the day.

Mabel came to the pharmacy asking whether the pharmacist could recommend a less expensive laxative than the one she was using. She handed over an empty bottle of Senokot-S tablets, explaining that she'd been taking the product since having surgery, and, although it worked fine for her, it was quite expensive. She was right about the expense—this product retails for about $33 for 60 capsules, compared to half that or less for generic versions. But she was way off track for a different reason: She should-n't have been taking a stimulant laxative on a regular basis. Such laxatives will make the colon "lazy" to the point that, with continued daily use, it will rely on laxatives to stim-ulate bowel movements. We sometimes call this "laxative addiction."

Mabel's doctor had recommended Senokot-S because the pain pills Mabel was tak-ing after her surgery caused constipation (a common side effect of prescription pain medications). But now that Mabel wasn't taking pain medication very often, she really didn't need to take a stimulant laxative. Once Mabel understood the sequence of events and the consequences of taking stimulant laxatives long-term, she agreed to the fol-lowing regimen to restore her bowel to normal function.

First, we started with a bulk laxative—a sugar-free, generic version of Metamucil. At $9 for a 23.3-ounce bottle, this gave her 114 doses, costing about 8 cents a day. Sec-ond, we found a generic stool softener for $10, or about 10 to 20 cents a day, depend-ing on how many doses she needs to take. So we lowered her expense to as little as 28 cents a day, compared to the 55 cents a day she had been spending, a 49 percent sav-ings. Mabel was happy not only because we'd reduced her monthly costs, but also because she'd received valuable information regarding laxatives.

BULK-FORMING LAXATIVES

As you might expect, these products add bulk to the stool. Different products do this in different ways. The Metamucil, Perdiem, and Konsyl brands use psyllium seed husk to add bulk. Psyllium seeds also may be helpful in relieving irritable bowel syndrome (IBS). The name-brand product Citrucel contains methylcellulose, which holds water in the stool to facilitate bulk-forming peristalsis. You may also prefer Citrucel's smoother texture over some of the psyllium products. Another active ingredient, calcium polycarbophil, found in name-brand products such as Fibercon, works on the same bulk-laxative principle, but it's available in tablet form so you don't have to mix it with water. This product also contains 244mg of calcium per tablet, an added benefit.

Simple bulk-forming products are the safest kinds of laxatives. Remember these key points when using them:

1. A bulk laxative can take as little as 12 to 24 hours or as long as three days to work.
2. People who have swallowing difficulties probably should avoid the wafer forms, which are very dry.
3. When taking a powdered bulk laxative, always mix it with the amount of water the manufacturer recommends.
4. Bulk-forming laxatives may interfere with the absorption of other medications. To avoid this, space your laxative dose 30 to 60 minutes from any other medication you take.
5. Most of these products contain sugar, which can affect blood sugar levels in people who have diabetes (especially those who use insulin). Look for the sugar-free alternatives to most of these products.

Bulk-Forming Laxatives

PRODUCT	STRENGTH PER DOSE	ACTIVE INGREDIENT	USUAL DOSAGE	TYPICAL QUANTITY	TYPICAL PRICE	COST PER DOSE
Citrucel Convenience Packets Orange	2g	Methylcellulose	Take 1 pkt. in 8oz liquid 3 times a day.	20 pkts	$8.99	45¢
Citrucel Orange	2g	Methylcellulose	Take 1 level scoop (19g) in 8oz of liquid 3 times a day.	30oz	$15.99	36¢
Citrucel Sugar-Free Orange	2g	Methylcellulose	Take 1 level scoop (10.2g) in 8oz of liquid 3 times a day.	16.9oz	$15.89	33¢
Citrucel Sugar-Free Orange	2g	Methylcellulose	Take 1 level scoop (10.2g) in 8oz of liquid 3 times a day.	8.6oz	$8.99	37¢
Fibercon Tablets	625mg	Calcium polycarbophil	Take 2 tablets once a day, up to 4 times a day.	36	$6.99	39¢

PRODUCT	STRENGTH PER DOSE	ACTIVE INGREDIENT	USUAL DOSAGE	TYPICAL QUANTITY	TYPICAL PRICE	COST PER DOSE
Fibercon Tablets	625mg	Calcium polycarbophil	Take 2 tablets once a day, up to 4 times a day.	140	$15.99	23¢
Fiber-Lax Tablets (generic version of Fibercon)	625mg	Calcium polycarbophil	Take 2 tablets once a day, up to 4 times a day.	90	$9.99	22¢
Konsyl 75 Dose 450Gm	6g pysllium mucilloid	Pysllium seed	Take 1 rounded teaspoon in 8oz liquid 3 times a day.	75g	$18.99	25¢
Metamucil 114 Dose Original Texture Orange	3.4g of pysllium husk	Pysllium seed	Take 1 rounded teaspoon in 8oz liquid 3 times a day.	44.2oz	$12.49	11¢
Metamucil 114 Dose Smooth Texture Sugar-Free Orange	3.4g of pysllium husk	Pysllium seed	Take 1 rounded teaspoon in 8oz liquid 3 times a day.	23oz	$12.49	11¢
Metamucil 114 Doses Original Texture Regular	3.4g of pysllium husk	Pysllium seed	Take 1 rounded teaspoon in 8oz liquid 3 times a day.	29oz	$12.49	11¢
Metamucil 180 Dose Smooth Texture Sugar-Free Orange	3.4g of pysllium husk	Pysllium seed	Take 1 rounded teaspoon in 8oz liquid 3 times a day.	36.8oz	$17.99	10¢
Metamucil Fiber Wafers Apple Crisp	3.4g of pysllium husk	Pysllium seed	Eat 2 wafers with 8oz of your favorite hot or cold beverage up to 3 times a day.	24 wafers	$5.99	25¢
Metamucil Smooth Texture Sugar-Free Orange Single Serve Packets	3.4g of pysllium husk	Pysllium seed	Take 1 packet in 8oz of liquid 3 times a day.	30 pkts	$10.39	35¢
Natural Fiber Laxative Smooth Texture Sugar-Free Orange Wal-Mart, Walgreens (generic version of Metamucil)	3g	Pysllium seed	Take 1 rounded teaspoon in 8oz liquid 3 times a day.	23.3oz	$9.99	10¢
Natural Fiber Laxative Wal-Mart, Walgreens (generic version of Metamucil)	3g	Pysllium seed	Take 1 rounded teaspoon in 8oz liquid 3 times a day.	30oz	$9.99	9¢
Orange Fiber Therapy, Soluble Fiber Therapy (generic version of Citrucel)	2g	Methylcellulose	Take 1 level scoop in 8oz of liquid 3 times a day.	16oz	$6.89	15¢
Orange Soluble Fiber Laxative(Walgreen, Wal-Mart) (generic version of Citrucel Sugar-Free Orange)	2g	Methylcellulose	Take 1 level scoop in 8oz of liquid 3 times a day.	16.9oz	$10.99	23¢
Perdiem Fiber Therapy	6g pysllium	Pysllium seed	Take 1 rounded teaspoon in 8oz of liquid 1-2 times a day.	250g	$15.29	28¢

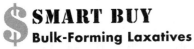

SMART BUY
Bulk-Forming Laxatives

Your Smart Buy is a generic form of Metamucil powder, such as Natural Vegetable Laxative or Natural Psyllium Husk Fiber Laxative. Just buy the regular formulation with sugar, if sugar isn't a problem in your diet. If you have diabetes or other concerns about sugar, then pay a little more for the sugar-free, orange-flavored product. Two doses of the Metamucil brand will cost you about 22 cents a day, or about $80 per year if you buy the 29-ounce size. Buy a generic version you can find in discount chain stores such as Walgreen, Wal-Mart, Shopko, or Target, and you'll cut your cost about 20 percent—you'll spend just 18cents a day, or about $64 a year.

> ### ▶ Compare Doses, Not Package Volume
>
> Watch the pricing on Metamucil and its generic versions! Do *not* compare how many ounces you're buying. Instead, compare how many *doses* the package contains: Read the label. For example, one Metamucil product listed in the foregoing table is 29 ounces; another is 44.2 ounces. You might think the greater amount would be the better buy, but if you look at the label, you get the same number of doses for the same price, so actually they're equally good buys. And although Metamucil Crisps might sound like a convenient product, note that you must consume 2 wafers per dose up to 3 times a day, or about 42 cents per dose, compared to about 10 cents a dose with the 180-dose options.

STOOL SOFTENERS

Stool softeners can be easy, effective alternatives to bulk laxatives and their associated problems. They don't interfere with other medications and require no mixing; nor do they contain sugar, like some bulk laxatives do. The only potential problem occurs if you must follow a salt-restricted diet because of other health problems. The active ingredient in most, but not all, stool softeners is docusate sodium, which adds significant sodium to your daily intake. If you're on a low-sodium diet, look for products containing docusate calcium instead.

Stool Softeners

PRODUCT	STRENGTH PER DOSE	ACTIVE INGREDIENT	USUAL DOSAGE	TYPICAL QUANTITY	TYPICAL PRICE	PRICE PER DOSE
Colace-100 Capsules	100mg	Docusate sodium	Take 2 capsules a day.	60	$24.99	41.6¢
Colace-50 Capsules	50mg	Docusate sodium	Take 2 capsules a day.	60	$20.99	35¢
Easy-Lax (Walgreens) Stool Softener Softgels (generic version of Surfak)	240mg	Docusate calcium	Take 1 capsule a day until bowel movements are normal or as doctor directs.	60	$9.99	16.6¢
Ex-Lax Stool Softener Caplets	100mg	Docusate sodium	Take 2 capsules a day.	40	$5.19	13¢
Peri-Colace Capsules	100mg 30mg	Docusate sodium, casanthranol	Take 1 capsule a day.	60	$26.99	45¢
Rite Aid Stool softener Capsules (generic version of Colace)	250mg	Docusate sodium	Take 1 capsule a day.	100	$9.99	10¢
Stool Softener Plus or Stool Softener Plus Stimulant Capsules (generic version of Peri-Colace Capsules)	100mg 30mg	Docusate sodium, casanthranol	Take 1 capsule a day.	100	$8.99	9¢
Surfak 240mg Capsules	240mg	Docusate calcium	Take 1 capsule a day until bowel movements are normal or as directed by a doctor.	100	$20.89	20.9¢
Wal-Mart or Walgreens Stool Softener Capsules	100mg	Docusate sodium	Take 2 capsules a day.	100	$6.49	6.5¢

$ SMART BUY
Stool Softeners

No surprises here: Buy bulk and buy generic. Taking name-brand Colace 100mg will cost you 80 cents a day if you take the recommended 2 capsules daily. If you purchase a generic 250mg capsule of docusate sodium (such as Stool Softener Laxative Capsules), you'll probably need only one capsule daily, because this product is twice the strength of regular Colace. This lowers your cost to about a dime a day, or about $36.50 annually, compared to a whopping $255 a year for the Colace brand! This nets you a savings of over $200 annually, or 86 percent.

▶ **Surfak for Salt-Restricted Diet**

If you're following a salt-restricted diet, look for a product called Surfak. It contains docusate calcium instead of docusate sodium, which is a salt.

STIMULANT LAXATIVES

For constipation that doesn't respond to these products, or when you want faster relief, the next category of products is the stimulant laxative. These drugs work by mildly irritating bowel tissue, causing the bowels to contract. This nearly always results in a bowel movement, although significant cramping can accompany the process. Be sure to read the manufacturer's warnings on the label before using any of these products. Common stimulant laxatives include Ex-Lax (senna), Dulcolax (bisacodyl), and Senokot (senna).

▶ **High Price for Fast Relief**

While you might think faster is better when it comes to relief from constipation, be warned that faster relief comes at a price. The faster a laxative works, the more intense the side effects of pain and cramping are likely to be. Stimulant laxatives can even cause diarrhea.

Although stimulant laxatives aren't "addictive" drugs in the classic sense, your colon (bowels) can become dependent on them with long-term use. You could find yourself unable to have a bowel movement without taking them. Healthcare professionals generally recommend that you limit the use of stimulant laxatives to no longer than 3 or 4 days. If your constipation continues beyond this time, see your regular healthcare provider to check for underlying health problems.

Some products combine a stool softener with a stimulant laxative, such as Correctol, Doxidan, and Feen-A-Mint. These products are fine to use for 3 or 4 days, although they're generally more expensive than the individual products. Usually you're better off taking a stool softener by itself if you need relief for longer than that to reduce the risk of taking a stimulant laxative for too long. ("Bowel addiction" isn't a concern with stool softeners.)

Stimulant Laxatives

PRODUCT	STRENGTH PER DOSE	ACTIVE INGREDIENT	USUAL DOSAGE	TYPICAL QUANTITY	TYPICAL PRICE	COST PER DOSE
Correctol Tablets	5mg	Bisacodyl	Take 1-3 tablets once a day.	90	$11.99	13.3¢
Doxidan Laxative Plus Stool Softener Liqui-gels	30/ 100mg	Casanthranol, docusate sodium	Take 1 or 2 capsules once a day.	30	$8.49	28¢
Dulcolax Suppositories	10mg	Bisacodyl	Insert 1 a day.	8	$11.89	$1.49 ea
Dulcolax Tablets	5mg	Bisacodyl	Take 1-3 tablets once a day.	25	$7.99	32¢
Ex-Lax Chocolate Laxative Tablets	15mg	Sennosides	Take 2 tablets 1-2 times a day.	18	$4.39	49¢
Ex-Lax Chocolate Laxative Tablets	15mg	Sennosides	Take 2 tablets 1-2 times a day.	48	$9.59	40¢
Ex-Lax Pills	15mg	Sennosides	Take 2 tablets 1-2 times a day.	30	$6.89	23¢
Ex-Lax Pills Maximum Relief Pills	25mg	Sennosides	Take 2 tablets 1-2 times a day.	24	$6.99	58¢
Peri-Colace Capsules	30/ 100mg	Casanthranol, docusate sodium	Take 1 or 2 capsules once a day.	60	$26.99	45¢
Senna Natural Laxative Tablets (generic version of Senokot Tablets)	8.6mg	Sennosides	Take 2 tablets 1-2 times a day.	100	$8.99	18¢
Senna-C Plus Tablets (generic version of Senokot-S tablets)	8.6mg/ 50mg	Sennosides, docusate sodium	Take 2 tablets 1-2 times a day.	60	$9.49	32¢
Senokot Tablets	8.6mg	Sennosides	Take 2 tablets 1-2 times a day.	100	$24.99	50¢
Senokot-S tablets	8.6mg/ 50mg	Sennosides, docusate sodium	Take 2 tablets 1-2 times a day.	60	$32.69	$1.09
Stool Softener Plus or Stool Softener Plus Stimulant Capsules (generic version of Peri-Colace Capsules)	100mg, 30mg	Docusate sodium, casanthranol	Take 1 capsule a day.	100	$8.99	9¢

PRODUCT	STRENGTH PER DOSE	ACTIVE INGREDIENT	USUAL DOSAGE	TYPICAL QUANTITY	TYPICAL PRICE	COST PER DOSE
Walgreens Women's Laxative (generic version of Correctol Tablets)	5mg	Bisacodyl	Take 1-3 tablets once a day.	90	$8.99	10¢
Walgreens, Wal-Mart Bisacodyl Laxative Tablets (generic version of Dulcolax)	5mg	Bisacodyl	Take 1-3 tablets once a day.	100	$9.99	10
Walgreens, Wal-Mart Regular Strength Laxative Pills (generic version of Ex-Lax Laxative Pills)	15mg	Sennosides	Take 2 tablets 1–2 times a day.	60	$5.99	10¢
Wal-Mart, Walgreens Bisacodyl Laxative Suppositories (generic version of Dulcolax Suppositories)	10mg	Bisacodyl	Insert 1 a day.	8	$6.99	88¢
Wal-Mart, Walgreens or Target Chocolate Laxative Tablets (generic version of Ex-Lax Chocolate Tabs)	15mg	Sennosides	Take 2 tablets 1-2 times a day.	18	$2.99	33¢

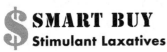

$ SMART BUY
Stimulant Laxatives

If you feel you need a stimulant laxative, first try a generic version of the name-brand product Peri-Colace (docusate sodium and casanthranol), which is a stimulant laxative and a stool softener. Stool softeners are underused, probably because results may take 12 to 72 hours, and many people don't want to wait that long. But they're more effective (with fewer side effects) over the long term. When purchasing this product for a chronic constipation problem, once your doctor has evaluated your overall health to rule out anything serious, buy larger quantities (60- or 100-count bottles) and go with a generic. Many discount stores stock their own generic brands (typically labeled "Stool Softener Plus" or "Stool Softener Plus Stimulant Laxative") for about $9 for 100 doses. Again, the savings potential is enormous: Peri-Colace can set you back around $160 a year (taking one capsule daily); the generic version will cost you less than $35 a year, a savings of 78 percent. You can probably think of many better ways to spend $125!

To really save money, though, maintain an adequate fluid intake, exercise, and consume plenty of fiber in your day-to-day routine. If lifestyle changes aren't enough, try a laxative for the short-term. Just remember three key points:

1. Start with just a stool softener or bulk-forming laxative.
2. Avoid stimulant laxatives unless absolutely necessary.
3. If stimulant laxatives haven't worked within a few days, stop taking them and see your doctor.

GAS-REDUCING PRODUCTS

Gas may take the form of flatulence, belching and burping, or abdominal fullness. Common causes include too much fiber in the diet, eating foods that don't digest easily, swallowing too much air while eating and drinking, taking antibiotics, consuming foods your body can't tolerate (lactose intolerance), and a condition called irritable bowel syndrome (IBS).

An effective and inexpensive remedy for abdominal fullness from excessive gas is simethicone. Simethicone doesn't act as an antacidinstead it lowers the surface tension of fluids in your stomach, which breaks up the gas bubbles. It's the active ingredient in name-brands products such as Gas-X, Mylanta Gas, and Phazyme. These products have generic forms that are usually cheaper. Buying in quantities of 100 can add further to your savings. Many antacid products also contain simethicone, because discomfort due to gas often accompanies indigestion.

Imodium A-D, an aid for diarrhea, has added simethicone to the original product to reduce some of the discomfort that accompanies diarrhea. Titralac, an antacid, also has added simethicone for antigas treatment. These combination products may be helpful, but often it's less expensive to purchase products independently. This improves your chances of being able to buy them in large quantities and generic forms, adding to your savings. Usually plain simethicone in 100-count bottles is your best buy. If your pharmacy doesn't stock this quantity, ask the pharmacist to order it for you.

$ SMART BUY
Gas-Reducing Products

Purchasing the generic versions Gas-X or Mylanta Gas in the higher dose maximum strength of 80mg in large quantities is your Smart Buy among these products. Look for names such as "Gas Relief" tablets or "Anti-Gas" tablets. These will cost you about 7 cents a dose, compared to 20 to 25 cents a dose for the name-brand products Mylanta Gas and Gas-X. Over a year, you might spend as much as $365 for a name-brand product, compared to about $100 annually for a generic version—a savings of about 73 percent. If you can't find 100-count bottles, talk with your pharmacist to see whether they

Gas-Reducing Products

PRODUCT	STRENGTH PER DOSE	ACTIVE INGREDIENT	USUAL DOSAGE	TYPICAL QUANTITY	TYPICAL PRICE	COST PER DOSE
Gas-X Extra Strength Peppermint Tablets	125mg	Simethicone	Chew 1-2 tablets after meals and at bedtime (no more than 4 in 24 hrs).	48	$9.99	20.8¢
Gas-X Peppermint Tablets	80mg	Simethicone	Chew 1-2 tablets after meals and at bedtime (no more than 6 in 24 hrs).	36	$7.49	20.8¢
Gas-X Softgels Maximum Strength Capsules	166mg	Simethicone	Swallow 1-2 softgels after meals and at bedtime (no more than 3 gels in 24 hrs).	50	$11.49	23¢
Mylanta Gas Softgels Maximum Strength	125mg	Simethicone	Chew 1-2 tablets after meals and at bedtime (no more than 4 in 24 hrs).	24	$6.89	28.8¢
Phazyme 180 mg Softgels	180mg	Simethicone	Swallow 1-2 softgels after meals and at bedtime (no more than 2 gels in 24 hrs).	36	$9.99	27.8¢
Shopko, Walgreens, Wal-Mart (generic version of Maximum Strength Gas Relief Tablets)	125mg	Simethicone	Chew 1-2 tablets after meals and at bedtime (no more than 4 in 24 hrs).	60	$6.99	11.6¢
Target, Wal-Mart, Walgreens (generic version of Gas Relief) Tablets	80mg	Simethicone	Chew 1-2 tablets after meals and at bedtime (no more than 6 in 24 hrs).	100	$6.99	7¢
Walgreens, Wal-Mart Ultra Strength (generic version of Anti-Gas) Softgels	180mg	Simethicone	Swallow 1-2 softgels after meals and at bedtime (no more than 2 gels in 24 hrs).	60	$9.49	15.8¢
Wal-Mart, Walgreens Maximum Strength (generic version of Mylanta Gas) Softgels	125mg	Simethicone	Chew 1-2 tablets after meals and at bedtime (no more than 4 in 24 hrs).	60	$9.49	15.8¢

might be in stock behind the counter or can be ordered from the wholesaler. (Most pharmacies receive deliveries from their wholesalers 5 or 6 times a week, so you won't have to wait longer than a day or two for a special order.)

$ SMART OPTIONS FOR SAVINGS
Over-the-Counter Gastrointestinal Remedies

Our leading recommendation among these products should be familiar to you by now: Buy generic! Although occasionally you might find a great deal on a name-brand product (when the store has the product on sale and you have a manufacturer's coupon and the moon is full), store brands and "no-name" brands nearly always provide the greatest savings. Because these are products you can stock up on, watch for sales and coupons, and check out virtual pharmacies.

To keep your digestive system functioning at its healthy best, eat nutritious foods (including plenty of fruits, vegetables, and whole grains for fiber), drink plenty of water, and include physical activity in your daily routine. Prevention is always the best medicine for most gastrointestinal problems and discomforts.

Over-the-Counter Treatments
for Eyes, Ears, Mouth, and Skin

You'll find a lot of over-the-counter products available for symptoms involving the eyes, ears, and mouth. But often the conditions causing these symptoms need the attention of a healthcare professional for proper diagnosis and treatment. The same is true for some skin conditions. As a general precaution, then, always see your doctor before seeking over-the-counter remedies for such symptoms, unless you've had the same problem before and know what relieves them successfully.

EYE-CARE PRODUCTS

How would your life change if you lost the sight in one or both eyes? Most people who have good vision can't even begin to imagine what it would be like. What might be a small scratch on another part of your body can quickly become a vision-threatening infection when it involves an eye. Many eye problems (although not all) cause enough pain to send you to the doctor right away. Only a medical professional (a physician or optometrist) can tell whether an eye problem is serious; it's never worth the risk to guess on your own.

See your doctor right away if any of the following circumstances is true for you:

+ Something has hit you in the eye.
+ Light hurts your eyes.
+ The insides of your eyelids are red and inflamed, or itch, or hurt.
+ There's a colored discharge from your eye, or you wake up with a crusty discharge on your eyelids.
+ You notice a sudden change in your vision, especially if it seems that you lose vision in a certain area (such as the image of a black curtain dropping down from the top of your field of vision, which can be the sign of a detached retina).

Untreated injuries and infections can result in loss of vision—partial or complete, temporary or permanent—and in some cases even the loss of an eye. Some eye infections, such as pinkeye (conjunctivitis), are highly contagious.

> ### Remove Your Contacts!
>
> Never wear contact lenses if you have an infection in your eye or eyelid, or if you suspect you may have an eye injury. Putting a contact lens into an infected or injured eye almost certainly will make the problem worse.

Because of the dangers of treating eye problems without medical guidance, only a few kinds of over-the-counter products are available for the eyes, including these:

1 Decongestants to reduce redness
2 Antihistamines for itchy and watery eyes due to allergies
3 Moisteners or artificial tears for short-term relief from dryness, such as that caused by being outdoors, working in a dry environment, or diminished tearing that often results as a function of aging
4 Lubricants for long-term moistening
5 Irrigating solutions to rinse the eyes

EYE DECONGESTANTS

Decongestant eye products remove the redness caused by engorged blood vessels in the eye. These products work by vasoconstriction, or shrinking the blood vessels. Most of the time, this intervention is probably unnecessary. The redness will go away whenever what is causing it goes away. Restricting blood flow is almost never a good thing to do. It can slow the healing process and can be hard on the eyes. But if it's your wedding day and you absolutely must get the redness out of your eyes, choose a generic product. Generic or store-brand products will be just as effective and are often much less expensive. You'll find the selection is limited, however. Making ophthalmic preparations sterile is costly and your savings may be less significant than with other over-the-counter products.

Eye Decongestants

PRODUCT	STRENGTH PER DOSE	ACTIVE INGREDIENT	USUAL DOSAGE	TYPICAL QUANTITY	TYPICAL PRICE	COST PER OUNCE
Bausch & Lomb All Clear AR Maximum Redness Relief Lubricant Eye Drops	0.5%, 0.03%	Hydroxypropyl methylcellulose, naphazoline hydrochloride	Put 1-2 drops in the affected eye up to 4 times a day.	15ml	$4.99	$9.98
Bausch & Lomb All Clear Eye Drop Regular	0.2%, 0.012%	Polyethylene glycol 300,naphazoline hydrochloride	Put 1-2 drops in the affected eye up to 4 times a day.	15ml	$5.49	$10.98
Clear Eyes ACR Eye Drops	0.012%, 0.25%	Naphazoline hydrochloride, zinc sulfate	Put 1-2 drops in the affected eye up to 4 times a day.	30ml	$7.79	$7.79
Clear Eyes Eye Drops	0.012%	Naphazoline hydrochloride	Put 1-2 drops in the affected eye up to 4 times a day.	15ml	$4.89	$9.78
Clear Eyes Eye Drops	0.012%	Naphazoline hydrochloride	Put 1-2 drops in the affected eye up to 4 times a day.	30ml	$6.49	$6.49
Murine Plus Tears Plus Redness Reliever Eye Drops	0.05%, 0.5%	Tetrahydrozoline hydrochloride, polyvinyl alcohol	Put 1-2 drops in the affected eye up to 4 times a day.	15ml	$4.59	$9.18
Vasoclear Eye Drops	0.02%, 0.25%	Naphazoline hydrochloride (0.02%)	Put 1-2 drops in the affected eye up to 4 times a day. polyvinyl alcohol (0.25%).	15ml	$11.59	$23.18
Visine A.C. Astringent Redness Reliever Eye Drops	0.05%, 0.25%	Tetrahydrozoline hydrochloride, zinc sulfate	Put 1-2 drops in the affected eye up to 4 times a day.	30ml	$6.99	$6.99
Visine Advanced Redness Reliever Eye Drops	0.05%	Tetrahydrozoline hydrochloride	Put 1-2 drops in the affected eye up to 4 times a day.	30ml	$6.99	$6.99
Wal-Mart, Walgreens, Target Eye Relief Drops	0.05%	Tetrahydrozoline hydrochloride	Put 1-2 drops in the affected eye up to 4 times a day.	15ml	$2.99	$5.98

$ SMART BUY
Eye Decongestants

As a rule, we don't recommend using these products; see a physician first. But if you absolutely must get the redness out of your eyes, check out the discount stores for a generic version of Visine (with a name like "Eye Relief Drops"). You'll save about $1 over name-brand counterparts.

ALLERGY EYE PRODUCTS

If your eyes are itchy and watery due to pollen allergies or the family cat, and you use Visine or a generic counterpart, you'll probably notice that it doesn't work. That's because the decongestant-only Visine-type products won't reduce the allergy response. You need an antihistamine to do this. If your allergy symptoms are limited to just your eyes, an antihistamine eye drop is a better choice. It will provide immediate relief and you won't experience the drowsiness that comes with using oral antihistamines.

Knowing which antihistamine eye product to buy can be a challenge, because the product's name doesn't always describe what it does accurately. Some vasoconstrictor products have tried to join the allergy-relief category by marketing products you'd think contain antihistamines—but they don't. For example, Visine A.C. Allergy Relief Drops contains no antihistamine. Its active ingredient is tetrahydrozoline, a decongestant, and it includes some zinc to remove proteins and mucous from the outer surface of the eyeball. Although this might take the redness out of your itchy, watery eyes, it won't relieve the itching and tearing. Read the ingredients list very carefully when choosing an antihistamine eye product. Ophthlamic antihistamine products will contain ingredients such as pheniramine maleate or antazoline.

$ SMART BUY
Allergy Eye Products

Few name-brand products are available in this special-use category. Don't be surprised to find name-brand products such as Visine-A or Opcon-A priced close to their generic versions. You may save $1 or so, but for a quick product selection that's easy to find, your Smart Buy is Visine-A, at about $7 for one-half ounce.

ARTIFICIAL TEARS/EYE LUBRICANTS

Artificial tears/eye lubricants are drops that relieve dry eyes and come in two forms, drops and ointments. Typically you'd use the drop form during the day, because these

Allergy Eye Products

PRODUCT	STRENGTH PER DOSE	ACTIVE INGREDIENT	USUAL DOSAGE	TYPICAL QUANTITY	TYPICAL PRICE	COST PER 0.5 OUNCE
Bausch & Lomb Opcon-A Eye Drops	0.315, 0.2675%	Pheniramine maleate, naphazoline hydrochloride	Put 1-2 drops in the affected eye up to 4 times a day.	15ml	$6.99	$6.99
Naphcon A Eye Drops	0.3%, 0.025%	Pheniramine maleate, naphazoline hydrochloride	Put 1-2 drops in the affected eye up to 4 times a day.	15ml	$8.99	$8.99
Vasocon A Allergy Relief Eye Drops	0.5%, 0.05%	Antazoline phosphate, naphazoline hydrochloride	Put 1-2 drops in the affected eye up to 4 times a day.	15ml	$8.99	$8.99
Visine-A Eye Allergy Relief, Antihistamine/ Decongestant, Drops	0.3%, 0.25%	Pheniramine maleate, naphazoline hydrochloride	Put 1-2 drops in the affected eye up to 4 times a day.	15ml	$6.99	$6.99
Wal-Mart, Walgreens, or Rite Aid Allergy Relief Eye Drops (generic version of Naphcon-A, Opcon A & Visine-A)	0.315, 0.2675%	Pheniramine maleate, naphazoline hydrochloride	Put 1-2 drops in the affected eye up to 4 times a day.	15ml	$7.29	$7.29

products produce less blurred vision for less time than ointment-based products. If you have a chronic problem with dry eyes, your doctor or optometrist may recommend you use the ointment during the night while sleeping. The advantage of using ointment is that it will lubricate your eyes during most of your non-waking hours.

Because artificial tears products use several different vehicles to moisturize the eye, it often takes experimentation to find the product that works best. Most people find that products containing polyvinyl alcohols, such as Hypo Tears and Murine, work well with little blurred vision. Sometimes these products fail to relieve symptoms, however. Then you'll need to find a product that has either a stronger percentage of polyvinyl alcohol or a different active ingredient. The stronger the active ingredient, the thicker the product; for many people, this means more blurred vision, at least after first applying the drops. Thicker but longer lasting lubricating ingredients are carboxymethylcellulose sodium and hydroxypropyl methylcellulose.

How Many Drops?

Comparing the cost per dose among ophthalmic products is something of a guessing game. Calculate roughly 15 drops for each milliliter (ml) of the product you buy. Since the average over-the-counter eye product comes in 15ml size, you can figure about 15 drops per milliliter times the 15ml size, or 225 drops. This depends on the product's viscosity (how thick the liquid is), so consider it a "guesstimate," not an exact figure.

Some doctors and optometrists may recommend that you use a product that has no preservatives, because some people have allergic responses to them. Although preservative-free products are available over-the-counter, they're manufactured in a unit-dose, or single-use, form only, so they're expensive. Because these products contain no preservatives, they easily become contaminated, so after applying the product once to your eye, you must throw away what's left. Using the same package more than once can spread the contamination to your eye, causing irritation and even infection. Unit-dose products generally cost more money than multiple-use products, because you're paying for the packaging. Many of the artificial tears products, with and without preservatives, are available both as name-brands and as generic or store-brand products.

$ SMART BUY
Artificial Tears and Eye Lubricants

For mildly to moderately dry eyes, look for a product that contains polyvinyl alcohol as its active ingredient. Use the drops rather than the ointment. These products will cause fewer problems with blurred vision and tend to cost less. Surprisingly, one of the Smart Buys is Murine Lubricant Eye Drops in the 30ml size, for about $7. You'll save around $1.50, or 30 percent, compared to the 15ml (half-ounce) size of even some generic equivalents, at about $5. Many generic versions are priced very close, so they don't afford much savings. Remember that single-use packaging is much more expensive. Because

Artificial Tears/Eye Lubricants

PRODUCT	STRENGTH PER DOSE	ACTIVE INGREDIENT	USUAL DOSAGE	TYPICAL QUANTITY	TYPICAL PRICE	COST PER 0.5 OUNCE
Akwa Tears Solution	1.4%	Polyvinyl alcohol	Put 1–2 drops in affected eye as needed.	15ml	$4.99	$4.99
Bausch & Lomb Moisture Eyes Drops	1%, 0.3%	Propylene glycol, glycerin	Put 1–2 drops in affected eye as needed.	15ml	$8.99	$8.99
Bausch & Lomb Moisture Eyes Drops	1%, 0.3%	Propylene glycol, glycerin	Put 1–2 drops in affected eye as needed.	30ml	$12.99	$6.50
Bion Tears Lubricant Eye Drops 0.4ml PF	0.1%, 0.3%	Dextran 70, hydroxypropyl methylcellulose 2910	Put 1–2 drops in affected eye as needed.	28 unit dose (discard after 1 use)	$10.89	$14.58
Celluvisc Lubricant Eye Drops 0.4ml Containers PF	1.0%	Carboxymethy-cellulose sodium	Put 1–2 drops in affected eye as needed.	30 unit dose (discard after 1 use)	$10.59	$13.24
GenTeal Lubricant Eye Drops	0.3%	Hydroxypropyl methylcellulose	Put 1–2 drops in affected eye as needed.	15ml	$9.99	$9.99
Hypo Tears Lubricant Eye Drops	1.0%, 1.0%	Polyvinyl alcohol / polyethylene glycol 400	Put 1–2 drops in affected eye as needed.	30ml	$10.49	$5.25
Murine Tears Lubricant Eye Drops	0.5%	Polyvinyl alcohol	Put 1–2 drops in affected eye as needed.	30ml	$6.99	$3.50
Refresh Lubricant Eye Drops 0.4ml PF	1.4%	Polyvinyl alcohol	Put 1–2 drops in affected eye as needed.	50 unit dose (discard after 1 use)	$13.99	$10.50
Refresh Plus Lubricant Eye Drops 0.4ml PF	0.5%	Carboxylmethyl-cellulose sodium	Put 1–2 drops in affected eye as needed.	50 unit dose (discard after 1 use)	$13.29	$9.97
Refresh Tears Lubricant Eye Drops (2 pack)	0.5%	Carboxylmethyl-cellulose sodium	Put 1–2 drops in affected eye as needed.	2 X 30ml	$19.99	$5
Tears Naturale Lubricant Eye Drops	0.1%, 0.3%	Dextran 70, hydroxypropyl methylcellulose	Put 1–2 drops in affected eye as needed.	30ml	$11.49	$5.75
Visine Tears Lubricant Eye Drops	1.0%, 0.2%, 0.2%	Polyethylene glycol 400, glycerin, hydroxypropyl methylcellulose	Put 1–2 drops in affected eye as needed.	30ml	$8.59	$4.30
Walgreens or Wal-Mart Artificial Tears Drops (generic version of HypoTears, Akwa Tears)	1.4%	Polyvinyl alcohol	Put 1–2 drops in affected eye as needed.	15ml	$4.99	$4.99

these products contain no preservatives, be sure to discard what's left after each use. If you save it to use later, it could become contaminated, and then so might your eyes.

EYE-IRRIGATING SOLUTIONS

Irrigating solutions are used to relieve eye irritation from loose foreign matter (such as dust), chlorine, and air pollutants. These products may contain several ingredients, ranging from simple sodium chloride (saline solution) to boric acid. Even if the solution contains an antibacterial agent (such as boric acid), it won't cure or prevent an eye infection. These products are intended only to remove debris from your eyes, not for extended use.

▶ Using an Eyecup

Some eye irrigating solutions come with an *eyecup*—a small container you fill with irrigating solution, and then place over your eye to bathe it. Although eyecups are useful in certain situations, most routine eye irrigation is better done *without* an eyecup. Once the eyecup touches your eye, it becomes contaminated. Unless you sterilize it before each use—impractical and sometimes impossible—you risk introducing or extending an infection.

Because irrigation solutions aren't used to treat eye infections, there's no particular advantage to buying a product that contains boric acid or any other antibacterial agent. Compare ingredients and prices, and buy generic or store brand when possible. Price is really the only consideration here, because product selection is limited.

Some general recommendations:

1. Always wash your hands before doing anything with your eyes.
2. Examine your eye before using an irrigating solution or any other eye product.
3. Remove contact lenses if you wear them.
4. If you can't find the foreign object causing the irritation, gently pull the upper

eyelid over the lower one; using an irrigating solution may dislodge loose debris.

5. If a foreign object is stuck in your eye, do not attempt to remove it. This could cause permanent or serious damage to your eye. Cover your eye with a cup or glass and seek professional help immediately.

6. For chemical exposure, rinse your eyes with fresh, cool water for 15 minutes, and then seek medical attention.

Eye Irrigating Solutions

PRODUCT	STRENGTH PER DOSE	ACTIVE INGREDIENT	USUAL DOSAGE	TYPICAL QUANTITY	TYPICAL PRICE	COST PER OUNCE
Bausch & Lomb Eye Wash	N/A	Boric acid, purified water, sodium borate, sodium chloride	Irrigate eye as needed.	4oz	$6.39	$1.60
Collyrium Eye Wash	N/A	Boric acid, sodium borate, water	Irrigate eye as needed.	4oz	$6.89	$1.72
Rite Aid, Walgreens Sterile Buffered Eye Wash (generic version of B & L Eye Wash)	N/A	Boric acid, sodium borate, water	Irrigate eye as needed.	4oz	$4.99	$1.25

$ SMART BUY
Eye Irrigating Solutions

Look for simple saline (salt water) solutions. Many people believe they must have boric acid in case there's an infection. Boric acid is an old-time remedy that's never been proven to work, and is more expensive than plain saline. A number of chain stores sell their own brands labeled "Eye Wash." You shouldn't have to pay more than $4 or $5 for 4 ounces.

EAR PRODUCTS

Ear products you'll find over the counter are used either to remove earwax or for drying fluid in the ear. Wax-removal products use a mild type of peroxide that softens the wax, allowing it to be flushed from the ear with water squirted from a bulb syringe. Be careful when flushing with these syringes. Too much pressure can damage the eardrum. Swimmers with a history of ear infections often use specialized products that contain alcohol and glycerin to dry the excess water from their ears. (The alcohol's job is to dry the excess water; the glycerin prevents irritation to the ear canal from the alcohol. You want the alcohol to remove the excess water from the ear canal, but not from the ear canal's surrounding tissues.) These products can be very helpful to prevent infection when used immediately after swimming.

Ear Products

PRODUCT	STRENGTH PER DOSE	ACTIVE INGREDIENT	USUAL DOSAGE	TYPICAL QUANTITY	TYPICAL PRICE	COST PER OUNCE
Auro-Dri	95%	Isopropyl alcohol and propylene glycol	Use 4-5 drops after swimming or bathing.	1oz	$3.99	$3.99
Auro Ear Drops	6.5%	Carbamide peroxide	Use 5-10 drops twice a day for up to 4 days.	0.75oz	$4.99	$6.65
Debrox Earwax Removal Aid	6.5%	Carbamide peroxide	Use 5-10 drops twice a day for up to 4 days.	1oz	$9.99	$9.99
Murine Ear Drops	6.5%	Carbamide peroxide	Use 5-10 drops twice a day for up to 4 days.	0.5oz	$4.69	$9.38
Murine Ear System (includes ear bulb syringe)	6.5%	Carbamide peroxide	Use 5-10 drops twice a day for up to 4 days.	0.5oz	$8.99	$17.98
Swim-Ear Ear Drying Aid	95%	Isopropyl alcohol, glycerin	Use 4-5 drops after swimming or bathing.	1oz	$3.29	$3.29
Wal-Mart, Walgreens "Ear Wax Removal" Drops (generic version of Debrox, Murine, or Auro Ear Wax Removal)	6.5%	Carbamide peroxide	Use 5-10 drops twice a day for up to 4 days.	0.5oz	$4.99	$9.98

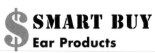

SMART BUY
Ear Products

Your Smart Buy among earwax removal products is a generic version of Debrox or Murine brand products, often simply labeled "Ear Wax Removal Drops." You'll spend about as much as you would for Murine, but you'll get 50 percent more product. The better value on your first purchase, however, may be the Murine Ear Wax Removal Kit, which includes a bulb syringe in the box, for about $9. The syringe is critical for rinsing out the loosened wax after 3 or 4 days of using the drops, and will save you a trip to the doctor for rinsing. Among the ear-drying products (to prevent "swimmer's ear"), look for Swim Ear to save about 60 cents a bottle over similar products, a 15 percent savings.

How to Use an Ear Syringe

Fill the ear bulb syringe with lukewarm water, and turn the affected ear downward toward a sink or basin. As you *gently* squeeze the syringe, aim the stream at an angle to avoid directly hitting the eardrum and prevent pain or damage.

ORAL ANTIBACTERIAL AND ANESTHETIC PRODUCTS

ANTIBACTERIAL PRODUCTS FOR THE MOUTH

Mouthwash products are designed to get rid of germs in your mouth. The jury is still out as to whether they actually do so. As far as the American Dental Association is concerned, medicinal mouthwashes don't achieve much. If you really feel you need a mouthwash, use a flavor that appeals to you or your significant other. Generic and store-brand products are available that contain the same active ingredients as popular brands such as Scope; the only difference is taste. Go with the cheaper generic or store brands.

$ SMART BUY
Antibacterial Products for the Mouth

Buying a large quantity of generic product wins you big savings once again. Look on the store shelf next to a major brand such as Scope and you should find a generic "antibacterial" mouthwash. Buying a 50-ounce bottle can lower your cost to about 9 cents an ounce. That will save you about $2 a bottle, or around 31 percent, over the name-brand equivalent.

Antibacterial Products for the Mouth

PRODUCT	STRENGTH PER DOSE	ACTIVE INGREDIENT	USUAL DOSAGE	TYPICAL QUANTITY	TYPICAL PRICE	COST PER OUNCE
Cepacol Antiseptic Mouthwash and Gargle, Gold	0.05%	Cetylpyridinium chloride	Rinse or gargle before/ after brushing.	32oz (946ml)	$4.99	16¢
Cepacol Antiseptic Mouthwash and Gargle, Mint	0.05%	Cetylpyridinium chloride	Rinse or gargle before/ after brushing.	24oz (710ml)	$4.99	21¢
Lavoris Mouthwash, Cinnamon	See next column.	SD alcohol 38-B, citric acid, clove oil, glycerin polysorbate 80, poloxamer 407, saccharin, sodium hydroxide, sorbitol, zinc chloride, water, zinc oxide	Rinse or gargle before/ after brushing.	32oz (946ml)	$3.99	13¢
Listerine Antiseptic Mouthwash	See next column.	Thymol 0.064%, eucalyptol 0.092% methyl salicylate 0.060%, menthol 0.042%	Rinse with 4 teaspoonfuls for about 30 seconds twice a day.	33.9oz (1,000ml)	$5.49	16¢
Listerine Antiseptic Mouthwash Tartar Control, Wintermint	See next column.	Thymol 0.064%, eucalyptol 0.092%, methyl salicylate 0.060%, menthol 0.042%	Rinse with 4 teaspoonfuls twice a day for about 30 seconds.	32.5oz (1,000ml)	$5.49	17¢
Listerine Antiseptic Mouthwash, Cool Mint	See next column.	Eucalyptol (0.092%), methyl salicylate 0.060%), menthol (0.042%), thymol (0.064%),	Rinse with 4 teaspoonfuls for about 30 seconds twice a day.	50.7fl oz (1,500ml)	$7.99	16¢
Plax Anti-Plaque Dental Rinse	See next column.	Water, sorbitol solution, alcohol (8.7%),tetrasodium pyrophosphate,	Rinse with 1 tablespoon about 30 seconds before brushing.	24oz	$5.99	25¢
Scope Mouthwash, Original Mint	See next column.	Water, alcohol (15 wt%), glycerin, flavor, polysorbate 80, sodium saccharin, sodium benzoate, cetylpyridinium Cl, domiphen bromide, benzoic acid, FD&C blue #1, FD&C yellow #5	Rinse or gargle for 30 seconds with approximately 2/3 capful twice a day.	33fl oz (1,000ml)	$4.49	14¢

PRODUCT	STRENGTH PER DOSE	ACTIVE INGREDIENT	USUAL DOSAGE	TYPICAL QUANTITY	TYPICAL PRICE	COST PER OUNCE
Scope Mouthwash, Original Mint	See next column.	Water, alcohol (15 wt%), glycerin, flavor, polysorbate 80, sodium saccharin, sodium benzoate, cetylpyridinium Cl, domiphen bromide, benzoic acid, FD&C blue #1, FD&C yellow #5	Rinse or gargle for 30 seconds with approximately 2/3 capful twice a day.	50fl oz (1,500ml)	$6.49	13¢
Target, Wal-Mart, Walgreens, Original Mint Original Mint (generic version of Scope Mouthwash)	See next column.	Water, alcohol (15 wt%), glycerin, flavor, polysorbate 80, sodium saccharin, sodium benzoate, cetylpyridinium Cl, domiphen bromide, benzoic acid, FD&C blue #1, FD&C yellow #5	Rinse or gargle for 30 seconds with approximately 2/3 capful twice a day.	50fl oz (1,500ml)	$4.49	9¢
Targon Smokers' Mouthwash, Original	See next column.	Water, alcohol (16.0 %), glycerin, sodium lauryl sulfate, sodium benzoate, flavor, saccharin, PEG-40 hydrogenated castor oil	Rinse with 20m (2/3 ounce) for 30 seconds in the morning and evening before brushing. Spit out the wash after rinsing.	24fl oz (709ml)	$5.79	24¢
Wal-Mart, Target, Walgreens "Anti-Plaque" Pre-Rinse (Generic version of Plax)	See next column.	Water, sorbitol solution, alcohol (8.7%), tetrasodium pyrophosphate,	Rinse 1 tablespoon about 30 seconds before brushing.	24oz	$3.99	17¢
Wal-Mart, Target, Walgreens Antiseptic Mouthwash (generic version of Listerine)	See next column.	Thymol 0.064%, eucalyptol 0.092%, methyl salicylate	Rinse with 4 teaspoonfuls for about 30 seconds twice a day.	33.8oz	$3.99	12¢

PRODUCTS TO RELIEVE TOOTHACHE

Most people experience a toothache at some point in their lives. Often, it results from an infection. Although you must see your dentist promptly for proper treatment of whatever is causing your toothache, there are two ways to alleviate the pain until you can: Apply an oral topical anesthetic to numb the area that hurts, or take an over-the-counter pain medication, such as ibuprofen or naproxen sodium, as you would for any other ache or pain. Most people get the highest level of relief by combining these methods.

Most topical dental products contain benzocaine, either by itself or combined with menthol or phenol. These ingredients provide pain relief. Another product that's both effective and cheap is clove oil, which you can buy in pharmacies, health food stores, and many grocery stores. Clove oil contains a natural local anesthetic called eugenol. (One folk remedy for toothache is to place a whole clove over the painful tooth and bite down.) Although you can buy a Red Cross Toothache kit that contains a clove oil product, it's less expensive to buy pure clove oil.

Dental Pain Not Always from Your Teeth

Dental pain can occur due to earaches, sinus problems, or even heart attacks. If your toothache lasts longer than a day or two, consult your dentist, doctor, or pharmacist. A condition even more serious than an infection may be causing the problem.

While clove oil is the cheapest remedy for relieving tooth pain, Orajel P.M. may give longer lasting relief, because its formulation keeps the benzocaine in place for a longer period of time. When it comes to toothache, price isn't always an issue! For sore areas on the inside of the lip, gums, or tongue, benzocaine products work well, although their relief is temporary. (They'll go to work 20 to 30 minutes faster than oral pain-relievers, such as aspirin or NSAIDs.) If the pain continues or becomes worse, see your doctor or dentist.

$ SMART BUY
Products to Relieve Toothache

For the money, you can't beat pure clove oil. You'll need to apply it a little more frequently than any of the benzocaine gels, but it's effective and cheap. But be sure to apply it to the tooth and not the surrounding tissue, as it may irritate the area. For a long-acting product, your Smart Buy is Orajel Maximum Strength Gel. Although this product is expensive ($7 or $8), it will keep that pain away for a long time.

How to Use Clove Oil for Toothache

To use clove oil, first rinse the tooth with water. Then moisten a small plug of cotton with the clove oil and put it on the affected tooth. Be careful not to get clove oil on your gums or mouth tissue; it can be quite irritating. You should feel relief almost immediately, and can apply clove oil up to 4 times a day. Be sure to follow up with your dentist to get treatment for the cause of your pain.

Products to Relieve Toothache

PRODUCT	STRENGTH PER DOSE	ACTIVE INGREDIENT	USUAL DOSAGE	TYPICAL QUANTITY	TYPICAL PRICE	COST PER 0.5 OUNCE
Anbesol Gel Maximum Strength	20%	Benzocaine	Apply to the affected area up to 4 times a day.	0.25oz	$7.49	$14.98
Clove oil	100%	Eugenol	Apply to affected area up to 4 times a day.	4ml	$2.47	$9.26
Orajel Oral Pain Reliever Maximum Strength Liquid	20%	Benzocaine	Apply a small amount of Orajel topically with cotton swab or clean finger tip into cavity and around gum surrounding the teeth.	0.45oz	$7.49	$8.32
Orajel P.M. Nighttime	20%	Benzocaine Formula	Apply a small amount of Orajel topically with cotton swab or clean finger tip into cavity and around gum surrounding the teeth.	0.18oz	$7.49	$20.80
Red Cross Toothache Drops	85%	Eugenol (clove oil)	Use tweezers to moisten pellet, remove excess, and place in cavity (no more than 4 times a day).	0.33oz	$5.79	$8.79
Temparin Dental First Aid Kit (for toothaches and cavity filling)	85%	Eugenol (clove oil)	Rinse the affected tooth with water to remove any food particles. Pat dry with cotton swab. Saturate tip of cotton applicator with liquid in vial and apply to tooth. Avoid touching surrounding gum tissues, cheek, or tongue with wet applicator tip.	1 kit	$6.99	

COLD SORE PRODUCTS

Cold sores—those ugly, painful sores that form on the lips and around the mouth—have various causes, including high fever; exposure to the sun, which may trigger Type 1 herpes simplex virus (HSV-1) infections; stress; even too much acid in your diet, as from eating too much fruit. Numerous products are available to provide relief from the pain and itching of cold sores. Most contain either benzocaine or combinations of phenol, camphor, and allantoin. These ingredients provide symptomatic relief by numbing and keeping the area from drying and cracking to cause further pain.

One product that appears to head off cold sores before they develop is Herpecin-L, which contains the sunscreens octyl methoxycinnamate (7.5 percent), oxybenzone (6 percent), and octyl salicylate (5 percent), and a silicone oil used as a protectant, dimethicone (1 percent). The sunscreens in this product may prevent sun-triggered HSV-1 recurrence.

A new and promising over-the-counter product for preventing HSV-1 outbreaks is Abreva, which contains 10 percent docosanol. Abreva must be applied immediately when you feel the first telltale tingle on your lip, and then 5 times daily over a day or two. Once the blister forms, however, the best you can do is treat the discomfort. For this, choose a product that contains a topical painkiller, such as benzocaine. Orajel Mouth-Aid contains the most benzocaine among these products. More generic products are beginning to appear on the market, but they aren't yet widespread. As in treating many other types of minor pain, you can take ibuprofen, naproxen sodium, or acetaminophen in addition to a using a topical product.

If you get cold sores often due to stress, the amino acid L-lysine 500mg (sold as a nutritional supplement) taken once daily might help as a preventive measure. If you get them from eating too many high-acid foods (such as tomatoes), try drinking a solution of one teaspoonful of baking soda mixed in a full glass of water. This concoction works to neutralize acid systemically.

Cold Sore Products

PRODUCT	STRENGTH PER DOSE	ACTIVE INGREDIENT	USUAL DOSAGE	TYPICAL QUANTITY	TYPICAL PRICE	COST PER 0.5 OUNCE
Abreva Cold Sore/ Fever Blister Treatment	(10%)	Docosanol	Apply every hour at first sign of cold sore/ fever blister.	0.07oz (2g)	$15	$112.50
Campho-phenique Maximum Strength Cold Sore Gel	N/A	Camphorated phenol, colloidal silicon dioxide, eucalyptus oil, glycerin, light mineral oil	Apply 1-3 times a day at first sign of cold sore/ fever blister.	0.23oz (6.5g)	$3.60	$8.30
Carmex Cold Sore Reliever and Lip Moisturizer, Jar	N/A	Alum, phenol, petrol-atum, lanolium, cocoa butter, wax base	Apply every hour at first sign of cold sore/ fever blister.	0.25oz (7.5g)	$1.20	$2.40
Herpecin-L Lip Balm Stick, SPF 36	7.5%, 6.0%, 5.0%, 1.0%	Octyl methoxy-cinnamate, oxyben-zone, octyl salicylate, dimethicone	Apply every hour at first sign of cold sore/ fever blister.	0.1oz (2.8g)	$4.70	$25.18
Orajel Mouth Aid Cold & Canker Sore Medicine, Gel	20%	Benzocaine up to 4 times a day.	Apply to the affected area (5.3g)	0.18oz	$4	$11.32
Zilactin Canker Sore, Cold Sore, Fever Blister Reliever	10%	Benzyl alcohol	Apply to the affected area every 4-6 hrs.	0.25oz (7g)	$7.70	$16.50

$ SMART BUY
Cold Sore Products

Mail-order and Internet pharmacies such as drugstore.com or cvspharmacy.com often offer the best prices on these products. Price isn't always the main concern when it comes to products to relieve cold sores, however. You might prefer to pay more to get faster relief. For quick results, your Smart Buy is Abreva, purchased at a local drugstore such as Walgreens. This is the only true antiviral product for cold sores available at present. If you want to spend less and are willing to take a chance of not catching the cold sore in time, try Carmex or Herpecin-L.

And visit www.smartbuysdrugwise.com for regular updates on prescription and over-the-counter drugs.

SKIN-CARE PRODUCTS

Your skin is your body's largest organ. It literally holds you together, protecting your other organ systems from the potential hazards of living in the world. It's amazing that most of the problems that afflict the skin are relatively minor and respond so well to the over-the-counter products available to treat them.

SKIN MOISTURIZING PRODUCTS

From time to time, many people need a skin moisturizer. Harsh weather, wind, sunburn—many things can dry out the skin. When it comes to products proclaiming to provide relief, results can vary considerably from person to person. When there's no infection present, just about any product is adequate. For conditions that don't improve in about a week, consult your doctor.

> ### ► Drink More Water!
>
> A surprising number of people who have simple dry skin simply don't drink enough water. The dehydration that results causes their skin to become dry, even cracked. Be sure to drink 8 full glasses of water each day. Once the body concentration of water falls below 10 percent, skin will exhibit dryness. Using a humidifier can help, too.

Good-quality lotions such as Curel, Lubriderm, and Nivea provide as much moisturizing as most people with dry skin need. For products that are less costly, yet just as effective, consider Cornhusker's Lotion, Bag Balm, and Udder Cream. These products typically work just as well for minor skin dryness, but they're priced considerably lower. The differences among them are mostly cosmetic. Cornhusker's Lotion and Udder Cream absorb into the skin better, without the greasy, petrolatum residue Bag Balm leaves. However, Bag Balm also contains a mild antiseptic (hydroxyquinoline) and a moisturizer (lanolin). Bag Balm gets rave reviews from people whose hands suffer from constant work-related exposure; they find it's the only product that heals the fissures they often develop, especially on their palms. Bag Balm's antiseptic properties may prevent infection, but it's not the same as an antibiotic, so don't expect it to cure an infection that's already present.

> ## Bag Balm for Soft Hands
>
> If you have really rough, chapped hands, a great treatment is to soak your hands in warm water for 5 to 10 minutes right before you go to bed, pat them dry with a towel, apply a liberal amount of Bag Balm, and then wear a pair of cotton gloves overnight. You'll be surprised how soft your skin becomes after just one night's treatment.

Here are some other useful and inexpensive treatments for dry skin:

1. Reduce bathing time to decrease body moisture loss, and bathe in warm (not hot) water.
2. Bathe less often, if possible.
3. Decrease the use of soap.
4. Drink plenty of fluids.
5. Use bath oils and moisturizers to lessen fluid loss.
6. If you live in a dry region, use a humidifier.

One inexpensive alternative to products such as Eucerin cream is to buy a one-pound container of plain hydrogenated vegetable oil (such as Crisco) at the grocery store. This will feel greasier when you apply it, but it has the same moisturizing qualities. (Just don't buy butter flavor!)

Skin Moisturizing Products

PRODUCT	STRENGTH PER DOSE	ACTIVE INGREDIENT	USUAL DOSAGE	TYPICAL QUANTITY	TYPICAL PRICE	COST PER OUNCE
Aquaphor Ointment Original	N/A	Petrolatum, mineral oil, ceresin, lanolin alcohol	Apply to the affected area(s) as needed.	16oz	$17.99	$1.13
Aveeno Moisturizing Lotion	1.25%, 1.0%	Dimethicone, colloidal oatmeal	Apply to the affected area(s) as needed.	12oz	$7.79	65¢
Bag Balm	See next column.	8-Hydroxyquinoline sulfate 0.3%; base: petrolatum, lanolin	Apply to the affected area(s) as needed.	10oz	$7.99	80¢
Carmol-20 Cream	See next column.	Carbomer 940, hypoallergenic fragrance, isopropyl myristate, isopropyl palmitate, propylene glycol, purified water, sodium laureth sulfate, stearic acid, trolamine, urea (carbamide), xanthan gum	Apply 1–2 times a day Moisturizes rough, dry skin, especially on hands, elbows, and heels.	3oz	$7.09	$2.36
Cetaphil Moisture Lotion	See next column.	Purified water, glycerin, hydrogenated poly-isobutene, cetearyl alcohol (And) ceteareth-20, maca-damia nut oil, dime-thicone, tocopheryl acetate, stearoxytri-methylsilane (and) stearyl alcohol, pan-thenol, farnesol, benzyl alcohol, phen-oxyethanol, acrylates/C10-30 alkyl acrylate crosspolymer, sodium hydroxide, citric acid	Apply to affected area(s) as needed.	16oz	$9.99	62¢
Corn Husker's Lotion		Water, glycerin, SD alcohol 40, sodium calcium alginate, oleyl sarcosine, methyl-paraben, guar gum, triethanolamine, calcium sulfate, fragrance, calcium chloride, fumaric acid, boric acid	Apply to affected area(s) as needed.	7oz	$3.69	53¢

PRODUCT	STRENGTH PER DOSE	ACTIVE INGREDIENT	USUAL DOSAGE	TYPICAL QUANTITY	TYPICAL PRICE	COST PER OUNCE
Curel Lotion Age Defying	See next column.	Water, glycerin, distearyldimonium chloride, petrolatum, lactic acid, isopropyl palmitate, cetyl alcohol, sodium lactate, dimethicone, PEG-150/decyl/SMDI co-polymer, methylparaben, propylparaben	Apply to affected area(s) as needed.	18oz	$9.49	.53¢
Curel Lotion Original	See next column.	Deionized water, glycerin, distearyl-dimonium chloride, petrolatum, isopropyl palmitate, 1-hex-adecanol, dimethicone, sodium chloride, fragrance, methyl-paraben, propylparaben	Apply to affected area(s) as needed.	6oz	$3.53	59¢
Eucerin Crème Original	See next column.	Water, petrolatum, mineral oil, ceresin, lanolin alcohol, methyl-chloroisothiazolinone, methylisothiazolinone	Apply to affected area(s) as needed.	16oz	$14.59	91¢
Keri Original Formula Scented Lotion	See next column.	Water, mineral oil, propylene glycol, PEG-40 stearate, glyceryl stearate/PEG-100 stearate, PEG-4 dilaurate, laureth-4, lanolin oil, methylparaben, carbomer, propyl-paraben, fragrance, triethanolamine, dioctyl sodium sulfo-succinate, quaternium-15	Apply to affected area(s) as needed.	15oz	$7.99	53¢
Lubriderm Lotion Fragrance Free	See next column.	Water, mineral oil, petrolatum, lanolin, sorbitol solution, stearic acid, lanolin alcohol, cetyl alcohol, glyceryl stearate/PEG-100 stearate, triethanolamine, dimethicone, pro-pylene glycol, tri (PPG-3 myristyl ether) citrate, disodium EDTA, methylparaben, ethyl-paraben, propylparaben xanthan gum, butyl-paraben, methyldibromo glutaronitrile	Apply to affected area(s) as needed.	16oz	$8.79	55¢

PRODUCT	STRENGTH PER DOSE	ACTIVE INGREDIENT	USUAL DOSAGE	TYPICAL QUANTITY	TYPICAL PRICE	COST PER OUNCE
Moisturel Cream	See next column.	Dimethicone 1%, petrolatum 30%, carbomer-934, cetyl alcohol, diazolidinyl urea, glycerin, laureth-23, magnesium aluminum silicate, methylchloroisothiazolinone, methylisothiazolinone, PG dioctanoate, PVP, hexadecene copolymer, sodium hydroxide, steareth-2, water	Apply to affected area(s) as needed.	16oz	$17.49	$1.09
Neutrogena Body Moisturizer	See next column.	Purified water, glycerin, emulsifying wax NF, octyl isononanoate, dimethicone, propylene glycol isoceteth-3 acetate, cyclomethicone, stearic acid aloe extract, matricaria extract, tocopheryl acetate, dimethicone copolyol, acrylates/C10-30 alkyl acrylate crosspolymer, cetearyl alcohol, sodium cetearyl sulfate, sodium sulfate, hydrogenated lanolin, glyceryl aurate, tetrasodium EDTA, triethanolamine, BHT, propylene glycol, methylparaben, ethylparaben, propylparaben, diazolidinyl urea, benzalkonium chloride, fragrance	Apply to affected area(s) as needed.	15.2oz	$8.99	59¢
Nivea Body Original Lotion	See next column.	Triple-purified water, mineral oil, glycerin, isopropyl palmitate, glyceryl stearate SE, cetearyl alcohol, tocopheryl acetate (vitamin E), lanolin alcohol, isopropyl myristate, simethicone, fragrance, carbomer, hydroxypropyl methylcellulose, sodium hydroxide, methylchloroisothiazolinone, methylisothiazolinone	Apply to affected area(s) as needed.	12oz	$7.39	62¢

PRODUCT	STRENGTH PER DOSE	ACTIVE INGREDIENT	USUAL DOSAGE	TYPICAL QUANTITY	TYPICAL PRICE	COST PER OUNCE
Suave Skin Lotion Vitamin E & Lanolin	See next column.	Water, stearic acid, glycerin, mineral oil, tea, petrolatum, aloe barbadensis gel, tocopheryl acetate (vitamin E acetate), lanolin oil, glyceryl stearate, fragrance, dimethicone, magnesium aluminum silicate, carbomer, methylparaben, tetrasodium, DMDM Hydantoin	Apply to affected area(s) as needed.	18oz	$3.99	22¢
Udder Cream	See next column.	Allantoin, dimethicone, lanolin oil, propylene glycol in emollient base	Apply to affected area(s) as needed.	10oz	$5.99	60¢
Vaseline Brand Advanced Healing Intensive Care Lotion	See next column.	Dimethicone, water, petrolatum, glycerin, stearic acid, glycol stearate, glyceryl stearate, TEA, sunflower (helianthus annuus) seed oil, soybean sterol, lecithin, tocopheryl acetate (vitamin E acetate), cetyl alcohol, PEG-40 stearate, magnesium aluminum silicate, carbomer, stearamide AMP, ethylene brassylate, methylparaben, DMDM hydantoin, iodopropynyl butylcarbamate, disodium EDTA, titanium dioxide	Apply to affected area(s) as needed.	24.5oz	$5.50	23¢
Walgreens, Wal-Mart (generic version of Lubriderm Lotion)	See next column.	Water, mineral oil, petrolatum, lanolin, sorbitol solution, stearic acid, lanolin alcohol, cetyl alcohol, glyceryl stearate/PEG-100 stearate, triethanolamine, dimethicone, propylene glycol, tri (PPG-3 myristyl ether) citrate, disodium EDTA, methylparaben, ethylparaben, propylparaben, xanthan gum, butylparaben, methyldibromo glutaronitrile	Apply to affected area(s) as needed.	16oz	$6.99	44¢
Wal-Mart, Walgreens Hydrating Ointment (generic equivalent of Aquaphor)	N/A	Petrolatum, mineral oil, ceresin, lanolin alcohol	Apply to affected area(s) as needed.	14oz	$12.99	93¢

$ SMART BUY
Skin Moisturizers

For mildly dry skin, your Smart Buys are Suave's Lotion with Vitamin E and Lanolin, or Vaseline Brand Advanced Healing Intensive Care Lotion. These are both good moisturizers that usually will do the job, and they cost less than other name-brand products such as Nivea, Lubriderm, and Keri-lotion moisturizers. Your cost per ounce for these is about 25 cents, compared to about 45 cents for a generic version of Lubriderm.

BURN CARE PRODUCTS

One minute you're cooking dinner and the next your fingers are on fire—literally. Who hasn't burned themselves while cooking in the kitchen or at the barbecue grill? The most important and effective action you can take to minimize a burn's severity is to apply cold to the area immediately. Put the burned part in cold water, or apply a cold compress (such as a cold, wet washcloth) for about 20 minutes. Don't use ice! It's too cold and can damage your skin further. After 20 minutes, inspect your burn to determine its severity. A first-degree burn causes pain, redness, and swelling; this is the least serious kind of burn. A second-degree burn causes pain, redness, swelling, and blistering. A third-degree burn is the most serious, and includes obvious damage to the tissues beneath the skin. Ironically, a third-degree burn might hurt less than a first-degree burn, but this is not a good thing: It means there's been damage to the nerves.

1. A third-degree burn requires emergency medical attention. Go to the hospital emergency department.
2. A second-degree burn requires prompt medical attention. Call your doctor right away, or seek care at an urgent care clinic.
3. A first-degree burn requires medical attention if it covers a large area (bigger than the back of your hand), involves your face, or doesn't respond to home treatment.

The only level of burn you should attempt to treat with over-the-counter products is a minor first-degree burn. Some people find that a pattern of 20 minutes on/20 minutes off cold compresses or water provides relief that's just as effective as any medication. Other people prefer the relief of anesthetic-containing products that numb the burned area, such as Americaine, Dermoplast, or Solarcaine sprays. Although there are burn products available in cream forms, the sprays provide faster and less intrusive relief at about the same cost.

Another excellent product is Water-Jel Burn Jel. It contains lidocaine to numb the pain and a gel that draws the heat out of the burn to limit further damage. If your pharmacy doesn't stock Water-Jel Burn Jel, ask the pharmacist to order it for you. It's an excellent addition to any first-aid kit. Gauze pads permeated with Water-Jel are available over the counter. This is a unique product; there are no generic equivalents.

Burn Care Products

PRODUCT	STRENGTH PER DOSE	ACTIVE INGREDIENT	USUAL DOSAGE	TYPICAL QUANTITY	TYPICAL PRICE	COST PER OUNCE
Bactine Squeeze Bottle	2.5%	Lidocaine	Apply as directed up to 3 times a day.	4oz	$6.89	$1.72
Foille Ointment	5%	Benzocaine	Apply as directed up to 4 times a day.	1oz	$4.59	$4.59
Solarcaine Aloe Extra Burn Relief Gel	0.5%	Lidocaine	Apply as directed up to 4 times a day.	8oz (226g)	$8.49	$1.06
Solarcaine Aloe Extra Burn Relief Spray	0.5%	Lidocaine	Spray as directed up to 4 times a day.	4.5oz (127g)	$8.49	$1.89
Target, Rite Aid, Walgreens Aloe Vera Gel with Lidocaine	0.5%	Lidocaine	Apply as directed up to 4 times a day.	16oz	$5.49	34¢
Water-Jel Burn Jel	2%	Lidocaine	Apply as directed 3-4 times a day.	4oz	$9.99	$2.50

$ SMART BUY
Burn Care Products

For burns, use Water-Jel. This very effective product is well worth the price. If the cost is too steep for you, try a store-brand aloe-vera-with-lidocaine product (generic version of Solarcaine Gel). A 16-ounce bottle shouldn't cost you more than $6 or $7.

TOPICAL ANTIFUNGAL PRODUCTS

Many kinds of fungal (yeast) infections plague mankind. Athlete's foot, jock itch, and toenail fungus are among the most common. Basically the same fungus causes all of these afflictions; only the location on the body varies.

Although Tinactin (tolnaftate) was the first antifungal product available in over-the-counter form, it's no longer the most effective, because its active ingredient covers a narrow range of fungal agents. Other products, such as Micatin (active ingredient miconazole) and Lotrimin (active ingredient clotrimazole), provide a broader spectrum of antifungal action. Generic forms of these products are also available, and are just as effective as their name-brand counterparts at a lower cost. If Micatin or Lotrimin is ineffective, seek professional help. If your doctor says you simply have athlete's foot, and the other products seem to be losing the battle, try one of the new products previously available by prescription and now available over the counter—Lamisil AT or Nizoral. They're a lot more expensive, but they cover a broader spectrum and probably will be more effective for you.

Applying the cream form of an antifungal product between the toes and on the feet twice daily for 10 to 14 days is quite effective. If you have a severe fungal infection, you might also use a miconazole spray or powder in your socks or shoes once a day until your infection is under control. Although antifungal products can control and ultimately eliminate fungal infections, the most effective treatment is prevention. Adopt these basic lifestyle habits that make it difficult for fungi to thrive:

1. Make sure your shoes fit correctly and are made of materials that "breathe." Leather is a better choice than vinyl or other manmade materials. This reduces the amount of moisture that remains in your shoes.
2. Wear cotton, not nylon, socks, and change your socks at least twice daily to help keep your feet dry. Cotton helps to move moisture away from your feet.
3. Make sure your feet are dry before you put on your socks and shoes. If athlete's foot is a chronic problem for you, consider using a hairdryer to get your feet absolutely dry. The less moisture you have on your foot, the harder you make it for the fungi to multiply.

Some people have serious foot perspiration problems. If you're one of them, ask your local pharmacist to make an aluminum chloride solution for you. This is the most effective drying agent, but it doesn't come in an over-the-counter product you can just buy off the shelf. Another aluminum chloride product, Drysol, is available by prescription; your doctor can give you a prescription for this if you or your pharmacist prefers to go that route. Applying aluminum chloride to the bottoms of your feet will limit the amount that they sweat, which will reduce the moisture available to promote fungi.

One of the most difficult fungal infections to treat is one that involves the toenails. It's very hard to penetrate the nail bed with a concentration of any drug sufficient to totally wipe out the infection. You might be among the fortunate few who have some success when treating these infections with over-the-counter topical preparations, but most people succeed only in controlling the infection briefly before the fungus returns.

The most effective over-the-counter product for treating toenail fungal infections is tea tree oil. This substance possesses both antifungal and antiseptic (bacteria-killing) properties. Tea tree oil smells like Pine-Sol cleaner. It's applied to the infected toenail 2 to 4 times a day; treatment takes 6 to 12 months. Even though tea tree oil is expensive (about $9 an ounce), it goes a long way, because you apply just a few drops a day. A 6-month treatment typically requires one or two bottles. And although tea tree oil may seem somewhat expensive per bottle, it's more cost-effective in the long run than other over-the-counter products that probably will never completely cure the problem.

Topical Antifungal Products

PRODUCT	STRENGTH PER DOSE	ACTIVE INGREDIENT	USUAL DOSAGE	TYPICAL QUANTITY	TYPICAL PRICE	COST PER OUNCE
Absorbine Jr. Topical Analgesic Rub	1.27%	Menthol	Apply up to 4 times a day.	4oz	$7.99	$2
Cruex Cream	1%	Clotrimazole	Apply twice a day.	0.5oz	$8.79	$17.58
Desenex Antifungal Liquid Powder	2%	Miconazole	Spray twice a day.	3.5oz	$6.99	$2
Desenex Antifungal	2%	Miconazole	Spray twice a day.	3oz Spray	$6.99	$2.33
Fungi-cure Antifungal	10%	Undecylenic acid	Apply twice a day.	1oz Liquid	$12.99	$12.99
Fungi-nail Liquid	1%, 2%, 2%	Resorcinol, salicylic acid, chloroxylenol	Apply twice a day.	30ml	$13.99	$13.99
Lamisil AT Cream	1%	Terbenafine	Apply twice a day.	12g	$10.99	$27.47
Lamisil AT Cream	1%	Terbenafine	Apply twice a day.	24g	$16.99	$21.23
Lamisil AT Full Prescription Strength Anitfungal Spray	1%	Terbenafine	Apply twice a day.	1oz	$11.99	$11.99
Lotrimin AF Antifungal Liquid Spray	1%	Clotrimazole	Apply twice a day.	4oz	$7.99	$2
Lotrimin AF Cream	1%	Clotrimazole	Apply twice a day.	0.42oz	$9.99	$23.79
Micatin Cream	2%	Miconazole	Apply twice a day.	0.5oz	$7.49	$14.98
Rite Aid, Walgreens (generic version of Miconazole Cream)	2%	Miconazole	Apply twice a day.	0.5ounce	$6.59	$13.18
Target, Wal-Mart Tolnaftate Cream (generic version of Tinactin)	1%	Tolnaftate	Apply twice a day.	1oz	$8.99	$8.99

PRODUCT	STRENGTH PER DOSE	ACTIVE INGREDIENT	USUAL DOSAGE	TYPICAL QUANTITY	TYPICAL PRICE	COST PER OUNCE
Tea Tree Oil	100%	Tea tree oil	Apply 2–4 times a day.	30ml	$9.99	$9.99
Tinactin Cream	1%	Tolnaftate	Apply twice a day.	0.5oz	$7.49	$14.98
Walgreens, Wal-Mart Clotrimazole Cream (generic version of Lotrim AF)	1%	Clotrimazole	Apply twice a day.	1oz	$8.99	$8.99

SMART BUY
Topical Antifungal Products

Your Smart Buy in a cream formula is a generic version of Lotrimin AF cream, such as Wal-Mart's or Walgreen's; the label typically says "Anti-Fungal Cream" or just the generic name Clotrimazole (the active ingredient). This will give you twice the cream for the same money you'd spend for Lotrimin AF. Clotrimazole covers more types of fungi than products such as the older versions of Desenex and Tinactin.

If you prefer a spray powder, your Smart Buy is Desenex. It's stronger than the other products and tends to cost less. And to treat a nail fungus, the only over-the-counter product we recommend is tea tree oil. It's less expensive than Fungi-Nail and does a better job.

TOPICAL FIRST-AID PRODUCTS

The first thing you should know about over-the-counter first-aid topical products is that they're useful only for minor infections. For example, topical antibiotics are poor choices for treating serious burns, because they don't help prevent the kinds of infections that typically occur with them. Most antibiotic preparations are ointments that cover the burn and prevent it from getting the air exposure it needs to heal.

Burns aside, a generic version of Neosporin is the best over-the-counter product for treating most minor infections. Because it contains three different antibiotics, it will kill more bacteria than a single-antibiotic product. The only drawback to using it is that many people are allergic to neomycin, one of the antibiotics in Neosporin. If you're one of them, you might experience itching, redness, and even hives after using it. Polysporin contains the other two antibiotics in Neosporin (polymyxin B sulfate and bacitracin zinc), but no neomycin. It may not be quite as effective as Neosporin, however, and it's also more difficult to find in generic form. Some of these products come in a "plus" version that includes the topical anesthetic pramoxine to help reduce pain and itching. These products will cost about $1 a tube more than regular versions, and don't usually provide enough relief to make the extra expense worthwhile.

Some people remember treating their childhood scrapes and cuts with iodine, mercurochrome, or merthiolate, and still want to buy these products. While these medications may have been good at one time, topical antibiotics, such as Neosporin, which kill many more kinds of bacteria, are far better choices. And these old remedies are poisonous if ingested. For cleaning a wound or scrape, hydrogen peroxide is an old-time favorite that remains highly effective and is very inexpensive. If you decide to use it, be sure to follow with an antibiotic ointment such as Neosporin.

Topical First-Aid Products

PRODUCT	STRENGTH PER DOSE	ACTIVE INGREDIENT	USUAL DOSAGE	TYPICAL QUANTITY	TYPICAL PRICE	COST PER OUNCE
Bacitracin Ointment		Bacitracin	Apply up to 4 times a day.	1oz	$3.99	$3.99
Neosporin +Plus Pain Relief Antibiotic Ointment	5,000 units 3.5mg 400 units 10mg	Polymyxin B, neomycin, bacitracin, pramoxine	Apply 4 times a day.	1oz	$8.59	$8.59
Neosporin First Aid Antibiotic ointment	5,000 units 3.5mg 400 units	Polymyxin B, neomycin, bacitracin	Apply 4 times a day.	0.5oz	$5.49	$10.98
Polysporin ointment	10,000 units	Polymyxin B, bacitracin 500 units	Apply 4 times a day.	1oz	$6.99	$6.99
Rite Aid, Wal-Mart, or Walgreens Hydrogen Peroxide	3%	Hydrogen peroxide	Apply as directed.	16oz	99¢	6¢
Rite Aid, Wal-Mart, or Walgreens Hydrogen Peroxide	3%	Hydrogen peroxide	Apply as directed.	32oz	$1.79	6¢
Spectrocin ointment	0.25% and 0.025%	Neomycin and gramicidin	Apply 4 times a day.	1oz	$5.89	$5.89
Target, Rite Aid, Walgreens (generic versions) of Polysporin ointment	10,000 units 500 units	Polymyxin B, bacitracin	Apply 4 times a day.	1oz	$5.99	$5.99
Walgreens, Wal-Mart Triple Antibiotic Ointment (generic version of Neosporin)	5,000 units 3.5mg 400 units	Polymyxin B, neomycin, bacitracin	Apply 4 times a day.	2oz	$5.99	$3

PRODUCT	STRENGTH PER DOSE	ACTIVE INGREDIENT	USUAL DOSAGE	TYPICAL QUANTITY	TYPICAL PRICE	COST PER OUNCE
Walgreens, Wal-Mart Triple Antibiotic Ointment (generic version of Neosporin)	5,000 units 3.5mg 400 units	Polymyxin B, neomycin, bacitracin	Apply 4 times a day.	1oz	$3.99	$3.99
Walgreens, Wal-Mart Triple Antibiotic Plus Ointment (generic version of Neosporin Plus Pain Relief)	5,000 units 3.5mg 400 units 10mg	Polymyxin B, neomycin, bacitracin, pramoxine	Apply 4 times a day.	1oz	$4.99	$4.99

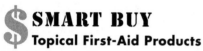

$ SMART BUY
Topical First-Aid Products

The Smart Buy here is a generic triple antibiotic ointment (a generic version of Neosporin Ointment). A common generic labeling is "Triple Antibiotic Ointment" or "First Aid Ointment." You can find these products even on many supermarket shelves. If you're allergic to neomycin, one of the three antibiotics in Neosporin Ointment, go with a generic version of Polysporin Ointment that contains the other two antibiotics only, bacitracin and polymyxin B. Don't be surprised to find this product is more expensive than triple antibiotic ointment, even though it contains just two antibiotics.

SUNSCREEN PRODUCTS

Outdoor activities are more popular than ever, and that almost always means exposure to the sun—and sunburn. Sunburn is unpleasant enough, but a more serious problem is the potential for skin cancer. Sunburn can damage the skin significantly, setting the stage for cancer's most common (and most preventable) form. Using sunscreen can help prevent or reduce sunburn and consequently reduce the risk of cancerous skin conditions. Sunscreen also dramatically reduces the skin damage that causes the appearance of premature aging. With hundreds of sunscreen products available, your choices are almost overwhelming. The most important factor to consider when selecting a sunscreen product is that it provides protection against both UV-A and UV-B radiation. UV-A radiation is believed to cause more cancerous, precancerous, and premature aging conditions than UV-B.

> ## ▶ Cheap But Not Easy
>
> Hydrogen peroxide is unquestionably the cheapest product available to treat topical infections, but it fails to get a Smart Buy nod because it's also the least convenient product to use. You can't carry it with you, and you need some sort of vehicle to apply it to your wound. The best use for hydrogen peroxide is to cleanse your wound, following with an antibiotic ointment, 3 or 4 times daily until the wound has healed. ◀

Sunscreen products are rated or classified by SPF (sun protection factor) level. The SPF numbers on the packaging can range from as low as 2 to as high as 60. These numbers refer to the product's ability to screen or block the sun's burning rays. However, SPF protection doesn't actually increase in proportion to the SPF number. A product with an SPF of 15 will absorb 93 percent of sunburn rays. When you go to a product with an SPF of 30, you increase sunburn-ray absorption by only an additional 4 percent, for a total of 97 percent. Even a suntan lotion with an SPF of 2 will absorb 50 percent of sunburn rays.

As you can see, any suntan or sunscreen product will give you some protection. As a rule of thumb, however, go with a product that has an SPF of 30. If you're very fair-skinned, you can go higher to give yourself maximum protection. However, a higher SPF doesn't mean you can apply the sunscreen less frequently. All sunscreens recommend you apply the product every few hours, depending on your activities. Waterproof products tend to stay on longer, especially if you're in the water or perspire heavily, but they still need to be reapplied.

And everyone should use sunscreen, regardless of natural skin color or tendency to tan. Anyone can get skin cancer.

Most sunscreens contain para-aminobenzoic acid, commonly known as PABA, first developed in the late 1970s. Today's PABA formulations are far more sophisticated and effective than earlier ones. One early problem with PABA was that it left stains on clothing. You can relax now: This doesn't happen with the new formulas. However, many people are allergic to PABA. Other sunscreen formulas use benzophenones (oxybenzone), cinnamates (octylmethyl cinnamate and cinoxate), and salicylates instead of PABA, and these are just as effective.

Apply Sunscreen *Before* Sun Exposure

Always remember that you need to apply sunscreen 30 minutes prior to your sun exposure. And don't forget your lips! Many lip balms are available with sun-blocking ingredients.

Another ingredient that works quite well is the sunblock micronized titanium dioxide, which came onto the market in the late 1990s. It works by reflecting the sun's rays away from the skin. This product is a godsend for people who spend long periods in the sun, like Roger, who enjoys mountain-climbing. Roger got pretty good protection from conventional waterproof sunscreens—except on his nose. He tended to perspire a lot and consequently wound up sunburning his nose to the point of blisters. Then he tried a product with titanium dioxide, and that was the end of his sunburn.

When it comes to sunscreen products, name-brand products are much more expensive than store-brand products! Find the SPF you need, consider buying the waterproof versions, and avoid PABA if you're allergic to it. Sometimes buying larger sizes can save you money. When applying sunscreen, be sure to shake liquid forms well to ensure an even distribution of active ingredients. Most creams and gels remain well-mixed. Spray-type sunscreens have lower SPF factors, and so provide less protection. For this reason, we don't recommend them.

Sunscreen Products

PRODUCT	ACTIVE INGREDIENT	TYPICAL QUANTITY	TYPICAL PRICE	COST PER OUNCE
Bain de Soleil Orange Gelee Sunscreen, SPF 15	Octocrylene, octyl methoxycinnamate, octyl salicylate, oxybenzone	3.12oz (88g)	$9	$2.89
Banana Boat Sport Spray Gel, SPF 25	Homosalate (4.8%), octyl methoxycinnamate (7.5%), octyl salicylate (5.0%), oxybenzone (4.0%), sunscreen	6oz (180 ml)	$7	$1.17
Bull Frog The Quik Gel Sunblock, 36 SPF	Octocrylene (10%), octyl methoxycinnamate (7.5%), oxybenzone (6%), octyl salicylate (5%)	4oz	$8	$2
Coppertone All Day Sunblock Lotion, SPF 15	Ethylhexyl P-methoxycinnamate, oxybenzone	4oz	$7	$1.75
Coppertone Gel UVA/UVB Sunblock, SPF 30	Avobenzone (parsol 1789), octocrylene, octyl salicylate, oxybenzone	6fl oz (177 ml)	$9	$1.50
Coppertone Oil Free Sunblock Lotion, SPF 45	Ethylhexyl P-methoxycinnamate, oxybenzone, 2-ethylhexyl salicylate, homosalate	8 floz (237 ml)	$9	$1.13
Hawaiian-Style Dark Tanning Oil SPF 2 (sound-alikes for Hawaiian Tropic Tanning Oil)	Octyl methoxycinnamate mineral oil; sorbitan oleate; fragrance; coconut oil; oils of plumeria, manako mango, kuawa guava, mikana papaya, lilikoi passion fruit, taro & kukui; cocoa butter; amyl acetate; aloe extract; lanolin; eucalyptus oil	8oz	$5	63¢
Neutrogena Healthy Defense Oil-Free UVA/UVB Block SPF 30+	Homosalate (17%), octyl methoxycinnamate (7.5%), oxybenzone (6%), octyl salicylate (5%), (118 ml) avobenzone (2%)	4oz	$9	$2.25
Neutrogena Sensitive Skin UVA/UVB Block, SPF 30	9.1% Titanium dioxide (inert physical blocker)	4oz (118 ml)	$8	$2
No-Ad SPF 30 Sunblock Lotion PABA-free		16oz	$6.99	44¢
PreSun Sensitive Sunblock, SPF 28 Cream	Titanium dioxide (16% w/w)	3.5oz (100ml)	$9	$2.57
Walgreens SPF 15 Sunblock Lotion	Octyl methoxycinnamate, oxybenzone, water, stearic acid, sorbitol, sorbitan oleate, glyceryl stearate Se, hydrogenated vegetable oil, isopropyl myristate, trie-thanolamine, PVP/eicosene copolymer, benzyl alcohol, imidazolidinyl urea, methylparaben, dimethicone, carbomer, fragrance, jojoba oil, propylparaben, tocopherol, vitamin E, aloe barbadensis gel, disodium EDTA	10oz	$6.99	70¢
Walgreens SPF 30 Sunblock Lotion	Ethylhexyl p-methoxycinnamate, oxybenzone, water, stearic acid, sorbitol, sorbitan oleate, glyceryl stearate Se, hydrogenated vegetable oil, PVP/eicosene copolymer, triethanolamine, benzyl alcohol, fragrance, dimethicone, methylparaben, imidazolidinyl urea, tocopheryl acetate, vitamin E acetate, propylparaben, aloe barbadensis gel, jojoba oil, disodium EDTA, polysorbate 20	10oz	$7.99	80¢

PRODUCT	ACTIVE INGREDIENT	TYPICAL QUANTITY	TYPICAL PRICE	COST PER OUNCE
Walgreens Waterproof SPF 8 Sunblock Lotion	Octyl methoxcinnamate, oxybenzone, water, sorbitan sesquioleate, sorbitol, glyceryl stearate Se, stearic acid, isopropyl myristate, triethanolamine, aloe barbadensis gel, PVP/eicosene copolymer, benzyl alcohol, methyl-paraben, dimethicone, carbomer, fragrance, jojoba oil, propylparaben, tocopheryl acetate, vitamin E acetate, disodium EDTA	10oz	$6.99	70¢
Zia Natural Skincare Solar Intelligence SPF 30 Gel, Body	Benzopehenone-3 3%, octyl methoxycinnamate 7%, octyl salicylate 2%	4oz	$15	$3.75

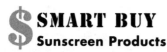

SMART BUY
Sunscreen Products

Your Smart Buy for sunscreen products is a store brand, hands down. Look for water-proof, PABA-free products with an SPF of at least 30. The "No Ad" product line (whose manufacturer does advertise) is an excellent buy you can find in stores such as Rite Aid, Long's Drugs, and even supermarkets.

WART-REMOVAL PRODUCTS

Warts are skin growths caused by a virus. The typical wart is a rough round or oval raised lump on the skin; it might be lighter or darker than the surrounding normal skin, skin-colored, or even (rarely) black. Typically, most warts can be removed by using top-ical over-the-counter medications containing either salicylic acid or lactic acid. If you don't have good results after 12 weeks of treatment using these medications, seek med-ical attention.

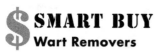

SMART BUY
Wart Removers

The Smart Buy for wart removers is a generic version of Compound W, typically sold as a store-brand "Wart Remover Liquid." You should have to pay no more than $6 for a half-ounce bottle—about a 40 percent savings over the name-brand equivalent.

Wart-Removal Products

PRODUCT	STRENGTH PER DOSE	ACTIVE INGREDIENT	USUAL DOSAGE	TYPICAL QUANTITY	TYPICAL PRICE	COST PER OUNCE
Compound W Plantar Wart Remover Gel	17%	Salicylic acid	Apply 1-2 times a day up to 12 weeks.	0.25oz	$9.99	$39.96
Compound W Plantar Wart Remover Pads	40%	Salicylic acid	Apply 1 pad every 48 hours up to 12 weeks.	20	$9.99	50¢ per pad
Compound W Wart Remover Liquid	17%	Salicylic acid	Apply 1-2 times a day up to 12 weeks.	0.31oz	$9.49	$30.61
Compound W Wart Remover Pads	40%	Salicylic acid	Apply 1 pad every 48 hours up to 12 weeks.	14	$9.99	71¢ per patch
Occlusal-HP Wart Remover	17%	Salicylic acid	Apply 1-2 times a day up to 12 weeks.	10ml	$17.99	$53.97
Wal-Mart, Walgreens "Plantar Wart-Remover" (generic version of Compound W Plantar Wart Remover) Pads	40%	Salicylic acid	Apply 1 pad every 48 hours up to 12 weeks.	24	$6.99	29¢ per pad
Wal-Mart, Walgreens, Rite Aid, "Wart Remover" Liquid	17%	Salicylic acid	Apply 1-2 times a day up to 12 weeks.	0.5oz	$5.49	$10.98

Protect Your Skin When Treating Warts

Wart removers use salicylic acid to "eat away" the wart. To prevent the acid from also eating away the unaffected skin near the wart, try this: Before applying the wart-remover liquid, put a light film of petroleum jelly (such as Vaseline) on the skin around the wart (but not on the wart). Then when you apply the salicylic acid, it will come in contact only with the wart itself.

ACNE PRODUCTS

Acne develops when the skin pores become plugged with facial oils and other debris, resulting in an outbreak of lesions. Benzoyl peroxide, resorcinol, salicylic acid, and sulfur are common active ingredients in topical over-the-counter medications used to treat acne. Each works a little differently, but benzoyl peroxide is the best at killing "P. acnes" (Propionibacterium acnes), the most common bacteria associated with acne, and it may reduce oil production.

The first step in fighting acne is to keep your face clean. Many antiperspirant-type soaps can actually clog the pores and make acne worse. Change to a good-quality facial soap, such as Neutrogena facial acne bar; you'll probably see a significant improvement. Another product that may facilitate cleansing is called Buf Puf. Don't scrub too hard, though; this can irritate your skin and possibly spread bacteria. Dermatologists often recommend Dove soap because it doesn't clog pores or aggravate acne. It's an inexpensive skin-cleansing solution, at just over $1 a bar. Cetaphil is another good choice, although at $6 for 8 ounces, it's pricier. Look for less expensive store brands. A generic form of Cetaphil is a gentle (and inexpensive) option for removing eye makeup, as well as cleansing your skin.

► Use Cosmetics that Keep Your Pores Clear

If you use facial cosmetics, look for products labeled "noncomedogenic." Regular cosmetics (as well as deodorant bar soaps) are often comedogenic, which means they plug the pores in your skin. This sets the stage for the form of acne most common in women, acne cosmetica. Noncomedogenic cosmetics don't clog pores.

If simple face-washing doesn't solve your problem, it's time to add benzoyl peroxide to your arsenal. Start with a product containing a 5 percent concentration; many people find that the higher strength irritates and excessively dries their skin. If you use a benzoyl peroxide product for a month without good results, then try a 10 percent formula. If this, too, fails to clear your skin, or if it causes irritation and dryness, it's time

to see your doctor. Buying another over-the-counter product probably will be a waste
of money.

Acne Products

PRODUCT	STRENGTH PER DOSE	ACTIVE INGREDIENT	USUAL DOSAGE	TYPICAL QUANTITY	TYPICAL PRICE	COST PER OUNCE
Biore Blemish Double Agent, Salicylic Acid Acne Treatment	2%	Salicylic acid	Apply in morning and rinse in evening.	0.75oz (21g)	$7.49	$9.99
Biore Blemish Fighting Cleanser, Salicylic Acid Acne Treatment	(0.5%)	Salicylic acid	Lather up small amt. with water, massage on face & rinse thoroughly.	5 floz (147 ml)	$6.49	$1.30
Cetaphil Daily Face Cleanser	See next column.	Water, cetyl alcohol, propylene glycol, sodium lauryl sulfate, stearyl alcohol	Massage into wet skin 1-2 times a day and rinse.	8oz	$6.99	88¢
Clean & Clear Persa-Gel 10, Maximum Strength	(10%)	Benzoyl peroxide	Apply 2-3 times a day.	1oz (28g)	$5.49	$5.49
Clearasil Acne Fighting Cream, Maximum Strength, Vanishing	(10%)	Benzoyl peroxide	Apply 2-3 times a day.	0.65oz (18g)	$5.49	$8.45
Neutrogena Oil-Free Acne Wash Foam Cleanser	2%	Salicylilc acid	Wash up to twice a day.	5.1oz	$6.99	$1.40
Oxy Balance Maximum Acne Treatment, Vanishing Cream	10%	Benzoyl peroxide	Apply 2–3 times a day.	1oz (28g)	$5.69	$5.69
Stridex Maximum Strength Acne Medication Pads with Salicylic Acid	(2.0%)	Salicylic acid	Use 1-3 times a day.	55 pads	$4.49	8¢ per pad
Target, Wal-Mart, Walgreens Oil-Free Acne Wash (generic version of Neutrogena Oil-Free Acne Wash)	2%	Salicylilc acid	Wash up to twice a day.	8oz	$5.49	69¢
Walgreens, Wal-Mart Daily Facial Cleanser (generic version of Cetaphil Daily Face Cleanser)	See next column	Water, cetyl alcohol, propylene glycol, sodium lauryl sulfate, stearyl alcohol	Massage into wet skin and rinse 1-2 times a day.	16oz	$7.99	50¢

PRODUCT	STRENGTH PER DOSE	ACTIVE INGREDIENT	USUAL DOSAGE	TYPICAL QUANTITY	TYPICAL PRICE	COST PER OUNCE
Walgreens, Wal-Mart, Rite Aid Acne Medication (generic version of of Oxy Balance Acne Cream)	10%	Benzoyl peroxide	Apply 2-3 times a day.	1oz (28g)	$3.99	$3.99
Wal-Mart, Walgreens Maximum Strength Acne Gel (generic version of of Persa-Gel 10, Maximum Strength)	10%	Benzoyl peroxide	Apply 2-3 times a day.	1oz (28g)	$4.99	$4.99

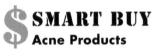

SMART BUY
Acne Products

Your Smart Buys among products to treat acne are generic or store-brand products. One good, gentle facial cleanser is a generic version of Cetaphil Facial Cleanser from a Wal-Mart or Walgreens, usually labeled simply "Daily Face Cleaner" or "Gentle Face Cleanser." You can get 16 ounces of such a product for about $1 more than you'll pay for 8 ounces of a name-brand product. (The generic version of Cetaphil is a great makeup remover, too.) Choose a generic benzoyl peroxide product to save about 30 percent over name-brand products such as Oxy Acne Products and Clearasil. Look for plain-sounding names like "Medicated Acne Cream" or "Acne Treatment," and you'll pay around $4 for an ounce.

SMART OPTIONS FOR SAVINGS
Over-the-Counter Treatments for Eyes, Ears, Mouth, and Skin

Again, generic versions offer the best savings. Usually, larger sizes cost less per dose or per use than smaller sizes. Mail-order and Internet pharmacies might offer better prices than your local stores, although it pays to watch for store sales and manufacturer coupons. Membership warehouse stores such as Costco and Sam's Club sell larger sizes or several packages bundled together for bargain prices.

Chapter 21

Other Over-the-Counter Products

M any over-the-counter products have specific uses that don't fit into broad categories. In this chapter we discuss those products.

PRODUCTS FOR DIABETES

Diabetes mellitus afflicts as many as 16 million Americans (about 5 million undiagnosed), over half of whom use insulin injections to treat the condition. Diabetes occurs when damage to the pancreas causes it to stop producing insulin, the hormone that makes it possible for the body to use glucose (a form of sugar your cells require as the energy that enables them to function). When insulin production stops suddenly and completely, it's called type 1 diabetes. When insulin production slows gradually, it's called type 2 diabetes. All people with type 1 diabetes must take insulin; about half of those who have type 2 diabetes eventually will require insulin injections.

INSULIN

Although insulin is the standard treatment for diabetes today, and it permits people with diabetes to live fairly normal lives, it was discovered only in the late 1930s. Before that time, a diagnosis of diabetes was a death sentence. Without insulin to metabolize glucose, the body can't survive. Countless types and brands of insulin are available today, as well as many combinations of vials, prefilled syringes, and cartridges. But only two major American companies manufacture insulin—Lilly and Novo Nordisk.

Insulin is available without a prescription (with the exception of Lilly's Humalog and Novolin's Novolog, a fast-acting insulin that requires a prescription), and must be kept refrigerated. Unopened, it's good for about six months; it stays good for about 30 days once it's been opened. Insulin is one product that pharmacies sell without much of a profit margin; that is, they charge only a small amount over what it costs them to buy the drug. One manufacturer's products might be cheaper than another in different parts of the country, and often chain stores can sell insulin at lower prices because they buy in quantities large enough to pay lower prices themselves. Because insulin must remain refrigerated, it's not a good idea to buy it from mail-order suppliers.

Multiuse vials of insulin usually cost less than pre-filled cartridges or syringes, but they aren't always the best buy. Pre-filled syringes and cartridges offer more accurate dosages, reducing the insulin that might be wasted when preparing injections: Insulin syringes are very small. Sometimes it's hard to read the numbers and see the measurement lines on the syringe's barrel. Add less-than-steady hands to the mix, and it can be tricky indeed to draw up the correct amount of insulin. This can waste insulin and deliver the wrong dose—which can land you in the hospital emergency room.

Two 10ml vials of Novolin R insulin, for example, typically last about a month and cost $42 to $46; you'll also need to spend about $25 a month on syringes. NovoPen pre-filled syringes containing the same one-month supply of insulin cost about $84, or $20 more. If your hands are steady and your vision is good, go with the multiuse vials for economy. But if your vision makes seeing the syringe markings a challenge or your hands can be a little shaky, the NovoPen might be a more cost-effective (as well as medically prudent) option, because it ensures that you'll receive the correct dose without waste. Devices such as the NovoPen are also a good choice for people who, because their diabetes is not well controlled, must take varying amounts of insulin.

Insulin

PRODUCT	USUAL DOSAGE	TYPICAL QUANTITY	TYPICAL PRICE	COST PER MILLILITER
Humalog Insulin	Variable	10ml	$46.99	$4.70
Humalog Insulin	Variable	5 x 1.5ml cartridge	$48.99	$6.53
Humalog MIX 75/25	Variable	10ml vial	$24.99	$2.50
Humalog MIX 75/25	Variable	5 x 3ml PFS	$92.99	$6.20
Humalog Pen	Variable	5 x 1.5ml cartridge	$91.99	$12.27
Humulin 70/30	Variable	10ml vial	$24.99	$2.50
Humulin 70/30	Variable	5 x 3ml PFS	$74.99	$5
Humulin L	Variable	10ml vial	$24.99	$2.50

PRODUCT	USUAL DOSAGE	TYPICAL QUANTITY	TYPICAL PRICE	COST PER MILLILITER
Humulin N	Variable	10ml vial	$24.99	$2.50
Humulin R	Variable	10ml vial	$24.99	$2.50
Humulin U	Variable	10ml vial	$24.99	$2.50
Humulin 50/50	Variable	10ml vial	$24.99	$2.50
Lantus Insulin	Variable	10ml vial	$46.99	$4.70
Novolin 70/30	Variable	10ml vial	$22.99	$2.30
Novolin 70/30	Variable	5 x 1.5ml cartridge	$44.99	$3
Novolin 70/30	Variable	5 x 3ml cartridge	$73.99	$4.93
Novolin L	Variable	10ml vial	$22.99	$2.30
Novolin N	Variable	10ml	$22.99	$2.30
Novolin N	Variable	5 x 1.5ml cartridge	$44.99	$3
Novolin N	Variable	5 x 3ml cartridge	$73.99	$4.93
Novolin R	Variable	10ml vial	$22.99	$2.30
Novolin R	Variable	5 x 1.5ml cartridge	$44.99	$6
Novolin R	Variable	5 x 3ml cartridge	$73.99	$4.93
Novolog	Variable	10ml vial	$46.99	$4.70
Novolog	Variable	5 x 3ml PFS	$88.99	$5.93

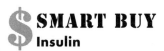

SMART BUY
Insulin

When it comes to insulin, your Smart Buy is the multidose vial, as long as you can read the numbers on the syringe and hold the vial easily and steadily to draw up an accurate dose. Beyond this, insulin prices are all about the same. (Talk to your doctor before changing manufacturers. Changing on your own is never advisable.)

INSULIN SYRINGES/NEEDLES

There isn't a huge difference among the various brands of needles and syringes for use with insulin. Look for ultrafine 29-gauge syringes. These are slightly smaller in diameter (same length), thus somewhat less painful to use, than the older 28-gauge options. Becton-Dickenson (BD) needles are triple-beveled for easier skin penetration.

Insulin Syringes/Needles

PRODUCT	TYPICAL QUANTITY	TYPICAL PRICE	COST PER SYRINGE
Becton-Dickenson Micro-fine 28 Ga. 0.3cc, 0.5cc, & 1cc (Short & Regular Length Needle) Insulin Syringe	100	$25.99	26¢
Becton-Dickenson Ultra-Fine 29 Ga. 0.3cc, 0.5cc & 1cc (Short & Regular Length Needle) Insulin Syringe	100	$24.99	25¢
Becton-Dickenson Ultra-Fine II 30 Ga. 0.3cc, 0.5cc & 1cc (Short & Regular Length Needle) Insulin Syringe	100	$26.99	27¢
Monoject 28 Ga. 0.5cc & 1cc Insulin Syringe	100	$17.99	18¢
Monoject 29 Ga. 0.5cc & 1cc Insulin Syringe	100	$18.99	19¢
Precision Sure-Dose 29 Ga. 0.3cc, 0.5cc & 1cc Insulin Syringe	100	$20.99	21¢
Terumo 27Ga. 1cc Insulin Syringe	100	$14.99	15¢
Terumo 28Ga. 1cc Insulin Syringe	100	$16.99	17¢

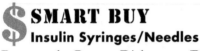

$ SMART BUY
Insulin Syringes/Needles

Because the Becton-Dickenson (BD) brand is usually the most expensive, ask what other brands your pharmacy carries and try those first. Either Monoject or Terumo brand may be your Smart Buy. These can save you as much as 12 cents a syringe, a savings of up to 44 percent.

BLOOD GLUCOSE MONITORS

Blood glucose monitors, or glucometers, read blood sugar levels for people with diabetes. Many brands and types of blood glucose monitors are available, and no one is best for everybody. All provide the same basic functions; the more expensive models typically offer more sophisticated computerized features, such as data storage or the ability to link to a computer. Many manufacturers offer rebates that can bring the cost of a glucometer down to nearly nothing.

Consider the following factors when buying a blood glucose monitor:

1. Do you take insulin or oral medication to control your diabetes? Blood sugar levels for people taking oral medication tend to stay more consistent, and so a basic model will meet your needs.

2. How easy is it for you to operate the machine and handle the test strips? Your pharmacy should have display models you can test.

3. How easy is it for you to obtain a large enough blood sample to get an accurate blood glucose reading? Some machines require a smaller sample.

As tempting as the rebates might appear, base your selection on your needs. Although cost is always a consideration, don't let it be your only guide. After all, your health is at stake. Ask a certified diabetes educator or a pharmacist knowledgeable about blood glucose monitoring for suggestions and recommendations.

Blood Glucose Monitors

PRODUCT	TYPICAL PRICE	COST OF 50 STRIPS	COST PER STRIP (50 COUNT)	COST OF 100 STRIPS	COST PER STRIP (100 COUNT)
Accu-Chek Advantage	$65 Monitor Kit	$45 (curve)	90¢ (comfort	$80 (curve)	80¢ (comfort
Accu-Chek Compact Monitor Kit	$75	$45 (3 drums = 51 tests)	88¢	N/A	N/A
Accu-Chek Complete Monitor Kit (comfort curve)	$110	$45	90¢	$80	80¢
FreeStyle Glucose Monitor System	$75	$40	80¢	$75	75¢
Glucometer DEX Diabetes Care System	$70	$42	84¢	$74	74¢
Glucometer Elite Diabetes Care System	$50	$44	88¢	$72	72¢
Lifescan One Touch Basic Diabetes Monitor System	$55	$41	82¢	$75	75¢
Lifescan One Touch Fast Take Diabetes Monitor System	$75	$40	80¢	$75	75¢
Lifescan One Touch InDuo Blood Glucose & Insulin Dosing System (uses One Touch Ultra Strips)	$100	$43	86¢	$80	80¢

PRODUCT	TYPICAL PRICE	COST OF 50 STRIPS	COST PER STRIP (50 COUNT)	COST OF 100 STRIPS	COST PER STRIP (100 COUNT)
Lifescan One Touch Profile Diabetes Monitor System (uses One Touch Basic Strips)	$100	$41	82¢	$75	75¢
Lifescan One Touch Sure Step Diabetes Monitor System	$65	$40	80¢	$75	75¢
Lifescan One Touch Ultra Diabetes Monitor System	$65	$43	86¢	$80	80¢
Medisense Precision QID Blood Glucose Monitor Management System	$50	$41	82¢	$77	77¢
Medisense Precision Xtra Advanced Diabetes Management System	$77	$43	86¢	$76	76¢

$ SMART BUY
Blood Glucose Monitors

Choose the blood glucose monitor that best suits your needs. With all the rebates available, price isn't really an issue. The important economical consideration when it comes to saving money is the price of the test strips each machine uses. The glucometer will last you a few years, but you'll have to buy test strips each month. Compare prices on test strips before you buy your glucometer, so you can factor in their cost. To save money on strips, buy boxes that contain at least a hundred.

Recently a popular consumer magazine tested and rated 11 blood glucose monitors. The product rated as both accurate and easiest to use, and consistent was Lifescan's One Touch Ultra Glucose Monitor. Consistency from test to test is almost as critical as a monitor's accuracy. Although it's a bit more expensive than the other monitors, the Ultra's reliability makes this blood glucose monitor the Smart Buy. This monitor's strips may cost a little more, but factor in how critical accuracy is to this disease state. If money really is the all-deciding factor for you, then the Glucometer Elite will save you up to 8 cents a strip over higher-priced brands—about 10 percent. This might not sound like a lot, but if you're using two strips a day at 8 cents a strip, you'll save about $58 in a year.

LANCETS

Lancets pierce your fingertip to get blood for checking your blood glucose, or blood sugar, level. More people complain about the discomfort of this than of giving themselves insulin injections! Some meters come with lancet devices that require a specific, proprietary lancet. This means you have to buy that particular type and brand of lancet, which is a definite disadvantage. Look for lancet devices that accept other brands. The Penlet lancet device that comes with One Touch brand glucose monitors can use many other brands of lancet and adjusts for the depth of penetration (how far the lancet goes into the skin).

Lancets

PRODUCT	TYPICAL QUANTITY	TYPICAL PRICE	COST PER LANCET
Accu-Chek Soft Touch Lancets	100	$11.99	12¢
Accu-Chek Soft Touch Lancets	200	$13.99	7¢
Accu-Chek Softclix Lancets	100	$13.99	14¢
Accu-Chek Softclix Lancets	200	$19.99	10¢
Becton-Dickenson Ultra-Fine II Lancets	200	$13.99	7¢
Microlet Lancets	100	$10.49	11¢
One Touch Fine Point Lancets	100	$11.49	12¢
One Touch Ultra Soft Lancets	100	$11.99	12¢
One Touch Ultra Soft Lancets	100	$12.99	13¢
Value Plus Thin Lancets	100	$5.99	6¢

$ SMART BUY
Lancets

For comfort and low price, it's hard to beat Becton-Dickenson's Ultra-Fine II Lancets. You can expect to pay $12 to $14 for 200 lancets, $1 or $2 more than 100-count of name-brand lancets, such as Accu-Chek Soft Touch. But if you really want the least expensive, have your friendly pharmacist shop his wholesaler for off-brands. We were able to find a box of a hundred thin lancets manufactured by Inverness for $5.99. If you're using Accu-Chek's Softclix brand of lancets, you're paying as much as 14 cents each. If you purchase off-brands, such as those by Inverness, you'll pay about 6 cents each—a savings of about 57 percent.

PRODUCTS THAT RELIEVE MENSTRUAL DISCOMFORT

Monthly premenstrual and menstrual discomforts are a fact of life for many women. Symptoms range from cramps, backache, and headache to bloating, swelling, and tension. Many over-the-counter products claim to relieve these symptoms, but their effectiveness varies. Many of these compounds contain acetaminophen or ibuprofen for pain relief; some, such as Midol 200 and Pamprin IB, contain only ibuprofen. Others combine a pain reliever with a diuretic, such as ammonium chloride or pamabrom, to relieve bloating and swelling.

Some menstrual relief products also contain the antihistamine pyrilamine maleate because of its ability to relax certain muscles; this helps reduce cramping. Although this might make you feel better, it can cause drowsiness—a side effect that can create complications if you need to be alert. Many women take such products only at night. And some products contain caffeine, which can intensify the pain relief effect and acts as a diuretic to help with bloating and swelling. These have the side effect of keeping you awake. It's usually best to take products containing caffeine only during the day, and not within 4 to 6 hours of bedtime.

If you experience swelling and bloating, try drinking extra coffee or cola drinks containing caffeine during the day. For many women, this provides enough of a diuretic effect to relieve the discomfort. This is a more economical choice than buying caffeine-containing combination products! If you usually drink coffee or caffeinated soft drinks, remember that taking a menstrual relief product that contains caffeine will boost your daily caffeine intake. If you feel shaky, switch to noncaffeinated beverages while taking the medication.

Many women get relief with relatively few side effects just from taking ibuprofen or naproxen. Because cramping causes most of the discomfort, we suggest starting with a generic form of Alleve (naproxen sodium). Naproxen sodium seems to reduce cramping more than ibuprofen and you'll get 8 to 12 hours of relief, compared to 4 to 6 hours with ibuprofen. In addition to their pain-relief qualities, these drugs are believed to have an effect on prostaglandin levels that can affect cramping. These products are most effective when you begin taking them 2 to 3 days before you expect your period to start, and then continue taking them during your period. If your symptoms are severe, you can start taking the product 5 to 7 days ahead of your period. If you miss the advance time and your pain is severe, you can take an initial dose of 2 tablets, and then return to the recommended dose of one tablet every 8 to 12 hours.

Products to Relieve Menstrual Discomfort

PRODUCT	STRENGTH	ACTIVE INGREDIENT	TYPICAL DIRECTIONS	TYPICAL QUANTITY	TYPICAL PRICE	COST PER TABLET/CAPSULE
Aleve Arthritis Caplets, Caplets	220mg	Naproxen sodium	Take 1 caplet every 8 to 12 hrs.	100	$8.99	9¢
Diurex PMS Formula Caplets	1,000mg, 50mg, 30mg	Acetaminophen, pamabrom, pyrilamine	Take 2 caplets every 6 hrs.	12	$4.99	42¢
Ibuprofen, Genpril, Ibu-200, Wal-profen, Menadol(generic versions of Advil, Motrin IB) Tablets	200mg	Ibuprofen	Take 1-2 tabs every 6 hrs. (not more than 6 in 24 hrs.).	300	$12.99	4¢
Ibuprofen, Genpril, Ibu-200, Wal-profen, Menadol(generic versions of Advil, Motrin IB) Tablets	200mg	Ibuprofen	Take 1-2 tabs every 6 hrs. (not more than 6 in 24 hrs.).	500	$14.99	3¢
Midol Maximum Strength Pain & Menstrual Relief Caplets	500mg, 60mg, 15mg	Acetaminophen, caffeine, pyrilamine	Take 2 gelcaps every 4 hrs.	16	$5.49	34¢
Midol Maximum Strength Pain/Cramp Formula Tablets	200mg	Ibuprofen	Take 1 tablet every 4—6 hrs.	24	$6.99	29¢
Midol Pain Relief Teen Formula Caplets	500mg, 25mg	Acetaminophen, pamabrom	Take 2 caplets every 4 hrs.	24	$6.99	29¢
Midol PMS Relief Aspirin-Free Gelcaps	500mg, 60mg, 15mg	Acetaminophen, caffeine, pyrilamine	Take 2 gelcaps every 4 hrs.	24	$6.99	29¢
Midol Maximum Strength Pain & Multi-Symptom Menstrual Relief Caplets	500mg, 25mg, 15mg	Acetaminophen, pamabrom, pyrilamine	Take 2 caplets every 4 hrs.	40	$9.59	24¢
Motrin IB Ibuprofen Pain Reliever/Fever Reducer Gelcaps	200mg	Ibuprofen	Take 1-2 tabs every 6 hrs. (no more than 6 in 24 hrs.).	100	$7.99	8¢

PRODUCT	STRENGTH	ACTIVE INGREDIENT	TYPICAL DIRECTIONS	TYPICAL QUANTITY	TYPICAL PRICE	COST PER TABLET/CAPSULE
Naproxen Sodium, Wal-Proxen, (Walgreens Generic version of Aleve)	220mg	Naproxen sodium	Take 1 caplet every 8 to 12 hrs.	200	$12.99	7¢
Pamprin Maximum Cramp Relief Caplets	250mg, 250mg, 25mg	Acetaminophen, magnesium salicylate, pamabrom	Take 2 caplets every 4-6 hrs.	32	$6.99	22¢
Pamprin Multi-Symptom Menstrual Relief Caplets	500mg, 25mg, 15mg	Acetaminophen, pamabrom, pyrilamine	Take 2 caplets every 4-6 hrs.	40	$7.49	19¢
Premsyn PMS Caplets	500mg, 25mg, 15mg	Acetaminophen, pamabrom, pyrilamine	Take 2 caplets every 4-6 hrs.	40	$7.99	20¢
Tylenol Women's Multi-Symptom Menstrual Relief Caplets	500mg, 25mg	Acetaminophen, pamabrom	Take 2 caplets every. 4-6 hrs.	40	$7.99	20¢
Walgreens Women's Multi-Symptom Menstrual Relief Caplets	500mg, 25mg	Acetaminophen, pamabrom	Take 2 caplets every 4-6 hrs.	24	$3.99	17¢

 # SMART BUY
Products to Relieve Menstrual Discomfort

Your Smart Buy here is a 500-count bottle of ibuprofen 200mg tablets (generic version of Motrin IB & Advil), for $15 to $20: Ask your pharmacist to order in this larger, cost-cutting size from the wholesaler, because most stores don't stock them. This will cut your per-tablet cost to 3 or 4 cents, a savings of about 50 cents over the name-brand Motrin IB in 100-count bottles. If you have some water retention, save money by simply drinking a caffeinated beverage. (The diuretic in menstrual products is caffeine.)

VAGINAL PRODUCTS

Yeast infections are among the most common vaginal problems women experience, and not surprisingly, numerous over-the-counter products are available to treat them. Doctors prescribed brands such as Monistat (miconazole), Gyne-Lotrimin (clotrimazole), Vagistat-1 (tioconazole), and Mycelex-G (butoconazole nitrate) for many years before these products became available for self-treatment of these common infections. Now you can choose from a wide variety of generic, store-brand, and name-brand products. Those with the same active ingredient are unlikely to differ much. What does seem to matter are the product's form and the length of time you use the medication.

Vaginal yeast products come in three forms—cream, vaginal tablet, and vaginal suppository. Which one is better for you is a largely matter of personal preference. Many gynecologists believe that because they dissolve slowly and consistently, vaginal tablets or suppositories do a better job of keeping the antifungal agent inside the vagina where it needs to stay. Creams, although they provide immediate relief from itching and burning, tend to drain out more quickly. But because it might take a day or two for the treatment to affect the symptoms, many tablet and suppository products also include a small tube of cream to relieve external itching.

You may be tempted to go with a one-day product, but these work best for mild infections. Yeast infections, which are actually fungal, can be stubborn to treat. Even the 3-day products often are not enough to eliminate the infection. Cost differences are rarely more than $1 or $2; it's usually worth your while to go with the 7-day product to ensure you get rid of the infection. Product strengths are the same no matter the length of treatment.

Name-brand and generic products with the same active ingredient differ little, and nearly all vaginal yeast products contain the maximum percentage of active ingredient. The only consideration might be the thickness of the various creams—again, a personal determination. The thicker the cream, the longer it stays in place. Because length of treatment determines cost, we don't provide a cost per course of therapy in the table.

Vaginal Products

PRODUCT	STRENGTH PER DOSE	ACTIVE INGREDIENT	USUAL DOSAGE	TYPICAL QUANTITY	TYPICAL PRICE
Gyne-Lotrimin Vaginal Inserts	200mg	Clotrimazole	Insert 1 vaginally at bedtime for 3 nights.	3 inserts	$12.99
Monistat-1 Vaginal Ointment	1%	Tioconazole	Insert one time at bedtime.	1 prefilled applicator	$16.99
Monistat-3 Vaginal Cream	4%	Miconazole	Insert 1 applicator at bedtime for 3 nights.	3 prefilled applicators	$15.99
Monistat-3 Vaginal Insert	200mg	Miconazole	Insert 1 at bedtime for 3 nights.	3 inserts	$15.99
Monistat-7 Vaginal Cream	2%	Miconazole	Insert 1 applicator at bedtime for 7 nights.	7 disposable applicators	$14.99
Monistat-7 Vaginal suppositories	100mg	Miconazole	Insert 1 suppository at bedtime for 7 nights.	7 suppositories	$14.99

PRODUCT	STRENGTH PER DOSE	ACTIVE INGREDIENT	USUAL DOSAGE	TYPICAL QUANTITY	TYPICAL PRICE
Mycelex-3 Vaginal Cream	2%	Butoconazole	Insert 1 applicator at bedtime for 3 nights.	3 prefilled applicators	$12.99
Vagistat-1 Vaginal	1% Ointment	Tioconazole	Insert 1 time at bedtime.	1 applicator	$14.49
Walgreens Clotrimazole Vaginal Cream	2%	Clotrimazole	Insert 1 applicator at bedtime for 3 nights.	3 disposable applicators	$10.99
Walgreens Clotrimazole Vaginal Cream	1%	Clotrimazole	Insert 1 applicator at bedtime for 7 nights.	1.5oz w/applicator	$8.99
Walgreens Miconazole-7 Vaginal Cream (generic version of Monistat-7)	2%	Miconazole	Insert 1 applicator at bedtime for 7 nights.	7 disposable applicators	$8.99

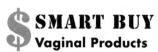

SMART BUY
Vaginal Products

Smart Buys among the vaginal products are generic versions of Monistat-7 cream. The cream form allows more even coverage, which helps affect a complete cure. And you can apply the cream topically for external irritation. A generic version of Monistat-7 Vaginal cream, such as the Walgreens or Rite Aid store brand, will cost you $9 or $10, a savings of about 50 percent over the name brand, which will cost $4 or $5 more.

SLEEP AIDS

No doubt you've seen TV, newspaper, and magazine ads for sleep-aid products such as Compoz, Excedrin PM, Nytol, Sleepinal, Sominex, and Unisom. These products contain one of three active ingredients—diphenhydramine, doxylamine, and pyrilamine. Once again, diphenhydramine—best-known as the familiar antihistamine Benadryl—enters the picture. The other drugs are antihistamines, too. In fact, most sleep-aid products exploit the notorious side effect of most antihistamines, drowsiness.

So which sleep-aid product is the wisest purchase? As far as effectiveness, no one is better than the others. But when it comes to saving money, there's one big step you can take to save a lot: Walk away from the sleep-aid section, go straight to the cough-and-cold section, and buy a generic antihistamine such as diphenhydramine (plain old Benadryl). These drugs are significantly less expensive than sleep aids, and the savings add up quickly. If you use a sleep aid fairly regularly, consider buying a large quantity. A 1,000-count bottle of diphenhydramine sells for about $20, for example—just $2 per 100 tablets. You don't have to be an accountant to calculate the savings compared to an equivalent amount of Sominex (around $22 per 100 tablets)—90 percent!

Don't use Tylenol PM or Motrin PM as a continual remedy for insomnia. If you have chronic pain that might be causing the insomnia, see a doctor. If your sleeping problems have nothing to do with pain, then don't take combination products that include pain relievers. Instead, use just an antihistamine.

Sleep Aids

PRODUCT	STRENGTH PER DOSE	ACTIVE INGREDIENT	USUAL DOSAGE	TYPICAL QUANTITY	TYPICAL PRICE	COST PER DOSE
Alluna Sleep Tablets	200mg, 120mg	Valerian root extract, hops extract	Take 1-2 tablets before bedtime.	56	$17.99	32¢
Compoz Nighttime Sleep Aid, Caplets	50mg	Diphenhydramine hydrochloride	Take 1 capsule at bedtime.	24	$6.99	29¢
Diphenhydramine Capsules (URL, MAJOR, IVAX brands) (special order through your pharmacist)	25mg	Diphenhydramine hydrochloride	Take 1-2 capsules at bedtime.	1,000	$24.99	2¢
Excedrin PM Caplets, Aspirin Free Analgesic with Sleep Aid	38mg, 500mg	Diphenhydramine citrate, acetaminophen	Take 2 capsules at bedtime.	100	$10.49	24¢
Legatrin PM Caplets, Advanced Formula Pain Reliever with Sleep Aid	50mg, 500mg	Diphenhydramine hydrochloride, acetaminophen	Take 1 caplet at bedtime.	50	$11.99	22¢
Nytol Maximum Strength, Nighttime Sleep-Aid, SoftGels	50mg	Diphenhydramine hydrochloride	Take 1 capsule at bedtime.	32	$6.99	19¢
Simply Sleep Nighttime Sleep Aid Mini-Caplets	25mg	Diphenhydramine hydrochloride	Take 2 caplets at bedtime.	48	$8.99	31¢
Sleepinal Nighttime Sleep Aid Capsules	50mg	Diphenhydramine hydrochloride	Take 1 capsule at bedtime.	32	$9.99	15¢
Sominex Tablets, Nighttime Sleep-Aid	25mg	Diphenhydramine hydrochloride	Take 2 tablets at bedtime.	72	$7.99	11¢
Tylenol Extra Strength PM Caplets, Pain Reliever & Sleep Aid	25mg, 500mg	Diphenhydramine hydrochloride, acetaminophen	Take 2 caplets at bedtime.	150	$11.99	8¢
Unisom Maximum Strength, Night Time Sleep Aid SleepGels	50mg	Diphenhydramine hydrochloride	Take 1 softgel at bedtime.	32	$9.99	31¢

PRODUCT	STRENGTH PER DOSE	ACTIVE INGREDIENT	USUAL DOSAGE	TYPICAL QUANTITY	TYPICAL PRICE	COST PER DOSE
Unisom Night Time Sleep Aid Tablets	25mg	Doxylamine succinate	Take 1 tablet at bedtime.	48	$11.99	25¢
Walgreens Nighttime Sleep Aid Caplets	25mg	Diphenhydramine Hcl	Take 2 caplets at bedtime.	48	$6.99	8¢
Walgreens, Wal-Mart, Diphenhydramine Capsules (special order through your pharmacist)	25mg	Diphenhydramine hydrochloride	Take 1-2 capsules at bedtime.	100	$7.49	3¢
Walgreens, Wal-Mart, Diphenhydramine Capsules (special order through your pharmacist)	25mg	Diphenhydramine hydrochloride	Take 1-2 capsules at bedtime.	100	$7.49	3¢

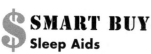

$ SMART BUY
Sleep Aids

When choosing a sleep-aid product, look in the cough-and-cold section. That's where you'll find Benadryl (active ingredient diphenhydramine) and its generic counterparts. It's significantly cheaper than traditional insomnia remedies, especially when you buy generic and in bulk packages. If you use a sleep aid regularly, your Smart Buy will be a 1,000-count bottle of diphenhydramine, which your pharmacist can order for you. At $20 to $30 per thousand, your cost per capsule drops to less than 3 cents. When you compare this to a Tylenol PM, you'll find you save about 60 percent. Avoid the "night-time pain reliever" combinations. Most are simply acetaminophen (Tylenol) and diphenhydramine (Benadryl). Not only are these products more expensive, you'll end up taking acetaminophen you probably don't need.

STIMULANTS

Sometimes you need to stay awake when your body wants nothing more than to fall asleep, or you want to maintain a high level of alertness when you might otherwise feel inclined to get a bit drowsy. Perhaps you need to drive a long distance, or you have to cram for a big test. The product to reach for is an over-the-counter stimulant. These products contain the caffeine equivalent of 2 to 4 cups of coffee. Indeed, drinking coffee is usually a more cost-effective alternative, but it might not be practical, depending on your circumstances or your tastes. One of the most familiar name brands among over-the-counter stimulants is No-Doz.

The first factor to consider when buying stimulant products is that upset stomach is a common side effect. If you have a touchy stomach already, look for products containing citrated caffeine. The citric acid component will reduce the level of upset. The next factor to consider is product strength. Some products contain twice the caffeine of others. If you find that 100mg does the job for you, then you can save money by taking half a tablet of a product that's 200mg strength.

It's not a good idea to take stimulants for an extended period or on a regular basis. Even though the body seems to adjust to the many effects of caffeine (as our love affair with coffee demonstrates), caffeine is known to interact with numerous prescription and other over-the-counter medications. It also can affect maladies such as thyroid disease and heart disease. Read the label precautions and warnings, and talk with your doctor before using the product if you have any conditions or take any of the medications listed there.

Stimulants

PRODUCT	STRENGTH PER DOSE	ACTIVE INGREDIENT	USUAL DOSAGE	TYPICAL QUANTITY	TYPICAL PRICE	COST PER DOSE
No-Doz Maximum Strength Caplets	200mg	Caffeine	Take 1-2 caplets every 3-4 hrs. as needed.	36	$5.99	17¢
No-Doz Maximum Strength Caplets	200mg	Caffeine	Take 1-2 caplets every 3-4 hrs. as needed.	60	$8.99	15¢
Ultra Pep-Back Stimulant Caplets	200mg	Eleveine	Take 1-2 caplets every 3-4 hrs. as needed.	18	$4.89	27¢
Vivarin Caplets	200mg	Caffeine	Take 1 caplet every 3-4 hrs. as needed.	24	$5.79	24¢
Vivarin Tablets Maximum Strength	200mg	Caffeine	Take 1 tablet every 3-4 hrs. as needed.	80	$14.29	18¢
Walgreens Maximum Strength Awake Caplets	200mg	Caffeine	Take 1 caplet every 3-4 hrs. as needed.	36	$4.89	14¢

Let's compare these over-the-counter stimulant products with commonplace beverages and food products that contain caffeine. Per dose, these products might not be the most economical choices, but they offer the unique benefit of pleasure! If you routinely consume these items, use caution when adding any additional stimulants. And be sure to check the ingredients of any herbal products you take, especially those that promote increased energy or weight loss.

Foods and Drinks that Contain Caffeine

PRODUCT	STRENGTH PER DOSE	ACTIVE INGREDIENT	USUAL DOSAGE	TYPICAL QUANTITY	TYPICAL PRICE	COST PER DOSE
Brewed coffee	137mg	Caffeine	1 cup	8oz	$1	$1
Carbonated colas	37mg	Caffeine	1 can or bottle	12oz	$1	$1
Dark chocolate	30mg, 180mg	Caffeine, theobromide	1 candy bar (plain)	1.5oz	75¢	75¢
Espresso	212mg	Caffeine	1 shot	3.3oz	$1	$1
High caffeine colas	100mg	Caffeine	1 can or bottle	12oz	$1	$1
Milk chocolate	12mg, 74mg	Caffeine, theobromide	1 candy bar (plain)	1.5oz	75¢	75¢
Red Bull energy drink	130mg	Caffeine	1 can	250ml (about 8oz)	$2	$2

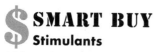

SMART BUY
Stimulants

Although you might enjoy foods and drinks containing caffeine more than swallowing tablets and caplets, as you can see, they're not Smart Buys. For the best savings, buy a generic product, such as Walgreens' Awake tablets containing caffeine; choose the 200mg strength.

MOTION-SICKNESS (ANTIVERTIGO) PRODUCTS

Some people experience motion sickness when they travel by plane or boat; others feel nauseated just from watching the rides at a carnival. If you read the labels on the products marketed to treat the dizziness, nausea, and vomiting of motion sickness, you'll see a familiar friend—the antihistamine. In addition to their other actions, antihistamines slow nerve conduction to the nausea center of the brain. This reduces the sensations of motion sickness. Of course, you'll pay a price for this relief, in the form of another familiar friend—drowsiness. Most motion-sickness products aren't appropriate if you're driving or operating machinery (such as a boat), or if you need to remain alert.

The antihistamines Meclizine (brand name Dramamine II Less Drowsy) and dimen-hydrinate (brand name Dramamine or Bonine) do an excellent job of reducing the symptoms of motion sickness without putting you to sleep. If you take these products frequently, look for large quantities (or ask your pharmacist to order them for you). A new product is the acupressure band, marketed under names such as Travel-Eze. The band activates an acupressure point on the wrist that affects the nausea center. You can use the band again and again, because it contains no drug and has no side effects.

In addition to taking a motion-sickness product, you can take other steps to reduce the motion sickness you feel. If you're riding in a car or bus, sit near the front, where you can see out the front window. Look toward distant objects ahead, not at the road or at roadside objects. If you're flying, request a seat in the middle of the plane to experience the least effect from the plane's regular movement and turbulence.

Motion-Sickness (Antivertigo) Products

PRODUCT	STRENGTH PER DOSE	ACTIVE INGREDIENT	USUAL DOSAGE	TYPICAL QUANTITY	TYPICAL PRICE	COST PER DOSE
Bonine Tablets	25mg	Meclizine hydrochloride	Take 1-2 daily as directed.	8	$4.99	63¢
Dramamine II Tablets Less Drowsy Formula Tablets	25mg	Meclizine hydrochloride	Take 1-2 daily as directed.	8	$5.29	66¢
Dramamine Original Formula Tablets	50mg	Dimenhydrinate hydrochloride	Take 1-2 tablets every 4-6 hrs.	12	$5.49	46¢
Dramamine Original Formula Tablets	50mg	Dimenhydrinate hydrochloride	Take 1-2 tablets every 4-6 hrs.	36	$11.99	33¢
Marezine Motion Sickness Prevention Tablets	50mg	Cyclizine	Take 1 tablet every 4-6 hrs.	12	$4.99	42¢
Meclizine HCl, USP 25mg, Antiemetic, Tablets	25mg	Meclizine hydrochloride	Take 1-2 daily as directed.	100	$5.99	6¢
Nauzene Chewable Tablet for Nausea	920mg	Sodium citrate dihydrate	Chew 2-4 tablets every 15 minutes	40	$6.99	17¢
Relief Band for Motion Sickness Relief	N/A	Drug-free (works by acupressure)	Apply as directed.	1	$99.99	Virtually unlimited (reusable)
Sea-Band Wrist Bands for Travel Sickness	N/A	Drug-free (works by acupressure)	Apply as directed.	1 pair	$10.99	Virtually unlimited (reusable)

PRODUCT	STRENGTH PER DOSE	ACTIVE INGREDIENT	USUAL DOSAGE	TYPICAL QUANTITY	TYPICAL PRICE	COST PER DOSE
Travel-Eze Wrist Bands for the Traveler	N/A	Drug-free (works by acupressure)	Apply as directed.	1 pair	$8.99	Virtually unlimited (reusable)
Wal-Dram For Adults & Children Tablets (Walgreens)	50mg	Dimenhydrinate hydrochloride	Take 1-2 tablets every 4-6 hrs.	24	$5.99	25¢
Wal-Dram II Tablets (Walgreens)	25mg	Meclizine hydrochloride	Take 1-2 daily as directed.	16	$4.99	31¢

$ SMART BUY
Motion-Sickness (Antivertigo) Products

Smart Buys here are the acupressure-type wristbands, such as the Travel-Eze brand. Many people find them very effective, and because they're reusable, they're very cost-effective.

If you've tried the wristband without success, then talk to your pharmacist about purchasing larger quantities of a generic version of Dramamine II tablets (25mg strength). You'll have to ask for this, and your pharmacist might need to order it for you. But it will be worthwhile, because it will cost you only about $6 for 100 tablets.

DIET AIDS

With health officials estimating that nearly 60 percent of Americans are overweight, it's little wonder that the diet aid business generates nearly $30 billion a year in revenues. Despite the perception of myriad choices, however, your options again are much fewer than you'd think. Basically, there are just two ways to lose weight with standard over-the-counter products. Both aim to reduce the amount of food you eat. Although we discuss weight-loss products in this section, we don't recommend them. Some of these products, especially those that contain ephedra, can be dangerous to your health.

Some products affect the appetite by working on the brain's "appetite center." This is a part of the brain that responds to adrenaline or drugs like adrenaline by sending a message telling the thought center that the stomach is full. You're not actually full, your brain just thinks so, so you feel less interested in eating.

Until 2000, most of these products contained phenylpropanolamine (PPA), a common decongestant. But after numerous reports of adverse health effects, including stroke, the FDA pulled all PPA-containing products from the market. The number of products on today's market that work this way is very limited. Many of these products were reissued with a different active ingredient, often the decongestant pseu-doephedrine. Many formerly popular over-the-counter diet aids didn't return in new formulas, however.

Some ephedra-containing over-the-counter products, such as Metab-O-Life, remain on the market. This drug is chemically similar to PPA and may cause the same kinds of health problems in certain people, especially those who have high blood pressure or glaucoma. Some weight-control products sold in health food stores also contain ephedra (sometimes identified as "ma huong" on the label). Because you have no way to know for sure whether you're susceptible to the potentially dangerous side effects of these products, avoid them.

The second over-the-counter weight-management product you'll find in most phar-macies is the "canned diet." These are meal-replacement products, usually liquids with a milkshake-like consistency, that use controlled calories rather than drugs to help with weight loss. Most provide balanced nutritional content, including appropriate vitamins, minerals, and percentages of carbohydrate, protein, and fat, but they don't contain the complex nutritional benefits of fresh whole foods and shouldn't be considered ade-quate substitutes. Some of these products have a low salt content, which causes your body to lose water. This is why you seem to lose large amounts of weight quickly and then find your weight loss slows. You can only lose so much water! These products are intended for limited use. Again, we don't recommend these products. They're not cost-effective, and studies show that 90 percent or more of dieters are back to their original weight or more two years after they started dieting if they've used over-the-counter or prescription diet aids. This is because effective, long-term weight loss and maintenance requires lifestyle changes.

The most effective and economical way to lose weight is to reduce the number of calories you consume and increase your physical activity. Add more vegetables, fruits, and whole grains to your diet, and cut back on fats and carbohydrates (sugars and starches). Get at least 30 minutes of moderate exercise at least 4 days a week—every day is best. Some people benefit from commercial programs such as Weight Watchers or Jenny Craig, although these "diet aids" aren't cheap. These programs aren't worth the expense if you can eat right and exercise. And most such programs charge extra for the food the program requires you to buy and for consultations. The costs add up quickly, when you could accomplish the same result by eating smaller portions, eating a balanced diet, and being more physically active. (Even just walking for 30 minutes a day can make a huge difference in both weight and fitness.)

Because we don't recommend these products, we can't consider any of them Smart Buys.

PRODUCTS TO RELIEVE HEMORRHOID DISCOMFORT

Hemorrhoids are swollen veins around the anus that sometimes become inflamed or irritated. They can be inside the anus, where you can't see them, or outside. Although hemorrhoids can be quite uncomfortable, most of the time the problem is a simple one that will go away on its own. Some people find this an embarrassing topic. However, hemorrhoids are very common and have many causes. Common symptoms include itching, burning, pain, and sometimes bleeding. Bleeding can be a sign of a more serious problem. If you're having rectal bleeding, see your doctor!

Many types of products are on the market to relieve the discomfort of hemorrhoids. The one that will work best for you depends on your symptoms. External hemorrhoids generally respond well to creams and ointments. Ointments last longer, but they're greasy, which can be messy and annoying. Relieving the symptoms of internal hemorrhoids usually requires a product that can be inserted into the rectum, such as applicator-applied creams and ointments or suppositories.

Many hemorrhoidal products contain topical anesthetics, which relieve pain for 20 minutes to several hours. Some products contain topical steroids, such as hydrocortisone, that act to reduce the swelling and inflammation. A few products include vasoconstrictor drugs, such as ephedrine, epinephrine, or phenylephrine, to shrink swollen tissues. And still other products contain a combination of anesthetic and steroid, along with other ingredients to lubricate and soothe irritated tissues.

Products of similar name aren't necessarily the same. If your doctor or pharmacist recommends Preparation H, for example, clarify which Preparation H product you should use. Preparation H Hemorrhoidal Cream and Preparation H Hemorrhoidal Ointment each contain about 75 percent petrolatum (the substance most people know as Vaseline), along with about 3 percent shark liver oil (a "topical protectant" that prevents irritation of and water loss from the skin by forming a physical barrier), with other ingredients to soften and moisturize tissues. Preparation H Anti-Itch Formula also contains 1 percent hydrocortisone, which reduces swelling. You can obtain the same relief at a much lower cost by buying plain 1 percent hydrocortisone cream, however. It also feels cool and soothing, and it reduces swelling and inflammation. No studies prove that popular products containing shark liver oil (such as Preparation H) help "shrink" hemorrhoids. They may lubricate, but they don't shrink anything—except maybe your wallet!

You might not like the idea of using suppositories, but this method is very effective for treating internal hemorrhoids. Once inserted, a suppository dissolves quickly to release pain- and itch-relieving medication. Just remember to remove the outer wrapper before inserting the suppository. (A surprising number of people don't!) It's a good idea to consult your doctor before using suppositories, just to be sure the problem is really hemorrhoids. Anusol-HC and its generic counterparts provide effective relief for most people.

▶ Use Vasoconstrictors with Caution

Don't use hemorrhoidal preparations containing vasoconstrictors (such as ephedrine, epinephrine, or phenylephrine) if you have heart disease, thyroid problems, diabetes, or difficulty urinating. Vasoconstrictors can make these conditions worse. Vasoconstrictors also can cause trouble sleeping, nervousness, and loss of appetite or nausea.

A nondrug therapy that's both inexpensive and soothing is the simple sitz bath. You can purchase a sitz bath at your pharmacy for $8 to $10. The sitz bath localizes body contact with astringents and other products used in the bath to just the affected areas, so you don't dry out other parts of your body as you might by sitting in a bathtub. Another product you'll find among the hemorrhoidal products is Tuck's pads. These are used more for cleansing, but they may also help shrink external hemorrhoids. And, to save money, a generic version is available. Tuck's and similar products contain witch hazel, an astringent (substance that dries the skin). Other inexpensive steps you can take are to increase fluid intake, use stool softeners, and increase fiber in your diet. These methods will reduce constipation, and thus reduce straining during bowel movements, which ,in turn, reduces irritation to the hemorrhoids so they can heal.

Products that Relieve Hemorrhoid Discomfort

PRODUCT	STRENGTH PER DOSE	ACTIVE INGREDIENT	USUAL DOSAGE	TYPICAL QUANTITY	TYPICAL PRICE	COST PER OUNCE OR SUPPOSITORY
Americaine Hemorrhoidal Ointment w/Benzocaine	20%	Benzocaine	Apply as needed as directed.	1oz	$7.99	$7.99
Anusol Hemorrhoidal Ointment	1%, 12.5%	Pramoxine hydrochloride, zinc oxide, mineral oil	Apply as needed as directed up to 5 times a day.	1oz	$4.99	$9.99
Anusol HC-1% Ointment	1%	Hydrocortisone	Apply as directed 3-4 times a day.	0.7oz	$6.99	$4.99
Anusol Hemorrhoidal Suppositories	51%	Topical starch	Insert 1 up to 6 times a day.	12	$5.99	50¢ each
Cortaid 1% Cream Maximum Strength	1%	Hydrocortisone	Apply as directed 3-4 times a day.	0.5oz	$4.99	$9.98
Hemorid Maximum Strength Hemorrhoidal Creme with Aloe	30%, 20%, 1%, 0.25%	Petrolatum, mineral oil, pramoxine hydrochloride, phenylephrine hydrochloride	Apply as needed as directed.	1oz	$5.99	$5.99
Hydrocortisone 1% Cream (Wal-Mart, Target, Walgreens)	1%	Hydrocortisone	Apply as directed 3-4 times a day.	1oz	$3.49	$3.49
Hydrocortisone 1% Ointment (Wal-Mart, Target, Walgreens)	1%	Hydrocortisone	Apply as directed 3-4 times a day.	2oz	$4.49	$2.25
Nupercainal Hemorrhoidal & Anesthetic Ointment	1%	Dibucaine	Apply as needed as directed up to 4 times a day.	1oz	$7.99	$7.99
Preparation H Cream 3%, 0.25%	18%, 12%,	Petrolatum, glycerin, shark liver oil, phenyl-ephrine hydrochloride	Apply as needed as directed.	1.8oz	$8.99	$4.99
Preparation H Hemorrhoidal Cooling Gel	0.25%, 50%	Phenylephrine hydrochloride, witch hazel	Apply as needed as directed.	1.8oz	$10.99	$6.10
Preparation H Hemorrhoidal Suppositories	85.5%, 0.25%, 3.0%	Cocoa butter, phenylephrine hydrochloride, shark liver oil	Insert 1 up to 4 times a day.	24	$12.99	54¢ each
Tronolane Anesthetic Hemorrhoid Cream	1%	Pramoxine hydrochloride	Apply as needed. as directed.	2oz	$7.99	$4
Tucks Hemorrhoidal Pads with Witch Hazel	50%	Witch hazel	Apply as needed as directed up to 6 times a day.	40	$4.99	13¢ each

PRODUCT	STRENGTH PER DOSE	ACTIVE INGREDIENT	USUAL DOSAGE	TYPICAL QUANTITY	TYPICAL PRICE	COST PER OUNCE OR SUPPOSITORY
Tucks Hemorrhoidal Pads with Witch Hazel	50%	Witch hazel	Apply as needed as directed up to 6 times a day.	100	$6.99	7¢ each
Walgreens Hemorrhoidal Cream	18%, 12%, 3%, 0.25%	Petrolatum, glycerin, shark liver oil, phenylephrine hydrochloride	Apply as needed as directed.	1.8oz	$5.99	$3.32
Walgreens Hemorrhoidal Suppositories	79%, 3%	Cocoa butter, shark liver oil	Insert 1 up to 4 times a day.	48	$10.79	$2.25
Walgreens Pre-Moistened Hemorrhoidal Pads with Witch Hazel	50%	Witch hazel	Apply as needed as directed.	100	$5.79	6¢ each

 ## SMART BUY
Products to Relieve Hemorrhoid Discomfort

Of the many ingredients in these types of products, none work better than hydrocortisone. It effectively reduces inflammation, itching, and discomfort, both inside and out (or, more technically speaking, internally and externally). Walgreens sells 2 ounces of hydrocortisone 1 percent ointment for $4 or $5. Not only can you use this product for hemorrhoidal discomfort, but also for other minor skin rashes and irritations. If you don't like the greasy feel of the ointment base, try the cream. You should be able to purchase a one-ounce tube from any discount drug store, such as Wal-Mart or Target, for about $3.

HEAD LICE TREATMENTS

For parents of school-aged children, head lice are among the most fearsome creatures in the animal kingdom. Every school year, thousands of American children come home from school with notes from school nurses announcing outbreaks of infestations and advising parents about how to eliminate the creepy but harmless pests. Contrary to common belief, head lice can't jump or fly. Instead, they spread via head-to-head contact or shared personal items, such as combs or hats.

As easy as it is to acquire head lice, you'd think it would be simple to get rid of them. It's much harder to eliminate head lice than it is to get them, however. Head lice have a handy (for them) adaptive feature: They can suspend breathing for up to 8 hours.

This allows them to survive shampooing and even treatment with products that work only while they're on the hair. Getting rid of lice requires a multipronged attack (and might involve treating all family members). To eliminate head lice from your household, you must take the following steps.

First, treat the hair with Nix. This liquid, which contains permethrin 1 percent, is the most effective over-the-counter product available. Although prescription products are stronger, they're not necessarily more effective and usually have the potential for more side effects. Unlike products that come out in the rinse water, permethrin binds to the protein in hair shafts. This gives the drug 7 to 14 days of further activity. All other products are effective only for the length of time they're on the head (usually 5 to 10 minutes). For maximum effectiveness, apply Nix to clean, dry hair (shampoo with the cheapest non-conditioning shampoo you can find). This differs from the package directions, but many physicians now recommend that you wash your hair and then use a hair dryer to completely dry it. (Don't towel-dry, as package instructions direct.)

▶ Alternative Nix Method

In some resistant cases, doctors recommend you apply Nix to completely dry hair (following a wash with a non-conditioning shampoo), cover the head with a loose-fitting shower cap, leave it on overnight, and then thoroughly rinse the Nix from the hair 8 hours later. Although this will be safe and effective for most people, check with your family doctor before trying it (as you should before using any product in a way that varies from package directions).

Next, remove all the nits (eggs). The only effective way to do this is to purchase a metal comb manufactured for this purpose. (Don't use the ones supplied with the medication; they don't do the job.) Starting at the ends, comb the hair toward the scalp. You must literally strip the egg from the hair shaft, which can be a challenge, because they're very sticky. Over-the-counter products, such as Clear, are available to help remove the eggs; they loosen the eggs chemically so that a comb can remove them more easily.

These products are quite effective and well worth the money. Also try dipping the comb in a 1:1 solution of vinegar and water to loosen the eggs.

Don't use a conditioner on the hair for the 14 days of treatment. Conditioner coats the hair and any nits and eggs still there, shielding them from Nix's insecticide action.

Finally, wash clothing and bedding in hot soapy water and dry in a hot dryer. No further treatment is necessary; the heat of the dryer will kill any lice that manage to survive the washing machine. Some people feel the need to use commercial sprays on their furniture. This is OK, but it's not usually necessary. Vacuuming your furniture and carpeting will suffice. Lice are hard to kill while they're on a person, but they can't live without a host to supply blood. Getting stuck in a vacuum-cleaner bag means certain death.

Following these steps nearly always eliminates head lice. You might be tempted to try a special shampoo that's cheaper than Nix, but this can be false economy. If you fail to attack this problem aggressively and thoroughly right from the first, you'll confront it again and again.

Head Lice Treatments

PRODUCT	STRENGTH PER DOSE	ACTIVE INGREDIENT	USUAL DOSAGE	TYPICAL QUANTITY	TYPICAL PRICE	COST PER OUNCE
A 200 Maximum Lice Killing Shampoo	0.33%, 4%	Pyrethrum extract, piperonyl butoxide	Shampoo hair; apply shampoo; leave in 10 minutes, then rinse.	4oz	$13.99	$3.50
Lice Killing Shampoo Wal-Mart, Rite Aid, Wal-Mart (generic version of A200, Pronto, Rid)	0.33%, 4%	Pyrethrum extract, piperonyl butoxide	Shampoo hair; apply shampoo; leave in 10 minutes, then rinse.	4oz	$8.99	$2.25
Liceguard Robi Comb (electronic)	N/A	N/A	Follow package instructions.	1 unit	$31.99	$31.99
Nix Lice Treatment Rinse	1%	Permethrin	Shampoo hair, dry hair thoroughly; apply shampoo; leave in 10 minutes, then rinse.	4oz	$18.99	$4.75
Nix Lice Treatment Rinse	1%	Permethrin	Shampoo hair; dry thoroughly; apply shampoo; leave in 10 minutes, then rinse.	2oz	$12.99	$6.50
NPA LiceMeister (mechanical)	N/A	N/A	Follow package instructions.	1oz	$11.99	$11.99

PRODUCT	STRENGTH PER DOSE	ACTIVE INGREDIENT	USUAL DOSAGE	TYPICAL QUANTITY	TYPICAL PRICE	COST PER OUNCE
Permethrin Lice Treatment Rinse (generic version of Nix Lice Treatment) Rite Aid, Walgreens, Wal-Mart	1%	Permethrin	Shampoo hair, dry hair thoroughly; apply shampoo; leave in 10 minutes, then rinse.	4oz	$14.99	$3.75
Pronto Lice Killing Shampoo	0.33%, 4%	Pyrethrum extract, piperonyl butoxide	Shampoo hair; apply shampoo; leave in 10 minutes, then rinse.	2oz	$10.99	$5.50
Rid Maximum Strength Lice Killing Shampoo	0.33%, 4%	Pyrethrum extract, piperonyl butoxide	Shampoo hair; apply shampoo; leave in 10 minutes, then rinse.	4oz	$12.99	$3.25
Rid Maximum Strength Lice Killing Shampoo	0.33%, 4%	Pyrethrum extract, piperonyl butoxide	Shampoo hair; apply shampoo; leave in 10 minutes, then rinse.	8oz	$18.99	$2.37

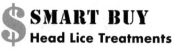

$ SMART BUY
Head Lice Treatments

The Smart Buy here is a generic version of Nix (such as "Permethrin Lice Treatment Rinse"). Such a product gives 7 to 14 days' residual activity, helping to prevent reinfestation from any missed nits that hatch after shampooing. Try your local Rite Aid, Wal-Mart, or Walgreens store to find this effective treatment at about a 20-percent savings over the name brand.

SMOKING-CESSATION PRODUCTS

Cigarette smoking is an addictive habit that has no health benefits and considerable health risks. If you smoke, stop.

If only it were that easy! It's not, of course. In fact, it's one of the most difficult things to do. Many health experts say nicotine, a chemical in tobacco, is as addictive as heroin. Breaking free of its grip often takes more than willpower—although your mental readiness to give up smoking is key to your success.

Smoking-cessation products contain nicotine in gum, topical-patch, and inhalant forms. This helps you to satisfy your body's craving for nicotine as you taper off slowly. Which form works best? Statistics show that the gum is 50 to 60 percent effective and the patches approximately 80 percent effective. Patches are so effective, many health experts recommend them above anything else. Some people resist buying the patches because of the cost. But how much do you spend for cigarettes? In most cases, you'll spend no more than you spend already, because you won't be buying cigarettes. And in 8 to 12 weeks, the usual course of treatment, you won't be spending anything!

> ## ▶ A Warning to Moms-to-Be
>
> If you're pregnant, don't use stop-smoking products unless directed to by your physician. Miscarriages
>
> have occurred among women who used these products during pregnancy. ◀

There are two systems of nicotine-patch therapy. Nicoderm CQ incorporates three strengths—21mg, 14mg, and 7mg—in a three-step program. The Nicotrol Transdermal System's 6-week program uses one strength of 15mg in a patch you wear for 16 hours at a time.

To make your experience with the patch the best it can be, apply it to a clean, dry area on your upper arm, chest, or back. Choose an area that's not very oily, has little or no hair, and is free of scars, cuts, burns, or other skin irritations. Press the patch firmly in place with the palm of your hand and hold the pressure for about 10 seconds. Make sure there's good contact with your skin, especially around the edges of the patch. When you remove the patch, fold it in half, sticky sides together, before you discard it. (If you leave the surface of the patch exposed, the small amount of nicotine that remains can be poisonous to young children and pets.)

Generic versions of Nicoderm CQ are available now, such as Nicotine Transdermal Patches (found at Walgreens or Rite Aid). These work just as well as the name brand at providing nicotine. However, we do hear from people who use the patches that some prefer the adhesive of the Nicoderm product to that of the generic. As far as we know, there are no differences in effectiveness, so this might be just a matter of personal preference. If you prefer the Nicoderm adhesive, you'll probably have more success with the treatment if you continue using Nicoderm. But if the generic's adhesive works for you, this is a good way to save some money.

The other smoking-cessation option is nicotine chewing gum (brand name Nicorette). If you smoke more than 25 cigarettes a day, use the 4mg strength; otherwise, use the 2mg strength. Typically, you'll chew one piece every hour or two for the first 6 weeks, reduce to one piece every 2 to 4 hours for the next 3 weeks, and finally one piece every 4 to 8 hours for the last 3 weeks, for a total of 12 weeks. If you have a strong craving after 12 weeks, talk to your doctor.

Smoking-Cessation Products: Patches

PRODUCT	STRENGTH PER DOSE	ACTIVE INGREDIENT	USUAL DOSAGE	TYPICAL QUANTITY	TYPICAL PRICE	COST PER PATCH
Nicoderm CQ Smoking Cessation Aid	21mg	Nicotine	Apply 1 patch daily per package schedule.	7	$29.99	$4.28
Nicoderm CQ Smoking Cessation Aid	21mg	Nicotine	Apply 1 patch daily per package schedule.	14	$49.99	$3.57
Nicoderm CQ Smoking Cessation Aid	14mg	Nicotine	Apply 1 patch daily per package schedule.	7	$29.99	$4.28
Nicoderm CQ Smoking Cessation Aid	14mg	Nicotine	Apply 1 patch daily per package schedule.	14	$49.99	$3.57
Nicoderm CQ Smoking Cessation Aid	7mg	Nicotine	Apply 1 patch daily per package schedule.	7	$29.99	$4.28
Nicoderm CQ Smoking Cessation Aid	7mg	Nicotine	Apply 1 patch daily per package schedule.	14	$49.99	$3.57
$ Nicotine Transdermal System (generic version of Nicoderm CQ)	22mg	Nicotine	Apply 1 patch daily per package schedule.	14	$36.99	$2.64
$ Nicotine Transdermal System (generic version of Nicoderm CQ)	14mg	Nicotine	Apply 1 patch daily per package schedule.	14	$36.99	$2.64
$ Nicotine Transdermal System (generic version of Nicoderm CQ)	7mg	Nicotine	Apply 1 patch daily per package schedule.	7	$23.99	$3.43
Nicotrol Transdermal System	15mg	Nicotine	Apply 1 patch daily for 6-week period.	7	$29.99	$4.28

Smoking-Cessation Products: Gums

PRODUCT	STRENGTH PER DOSE	ACTIVE INGREDIENT	USUAL DOSAGE	TYPICAL QUANTITY	TYPICAL PRICE	COST PER PIECE
Nicorette 2mg Gum (orange & mint flavors)	2mg	Nicotine	Use per package schedule.	48	$29.99	62¢
Nicorette 2mg Gum (orange & mint flavors)	2mg	Nicotine	Use per package schedule.	108	$52.99	49¢
Nicorette 2mg Gum (orange & mint flavors)	2mg	Nicotine	Use per package schedule.	168	$66.99	40¢
Nicorette 4mg Gum (orange & mint flavors)	4mg	Nicotine	Use per package schedule.	48	$32.99	69¢
Nicorette 4mg Gum (orange & mint flavors)	4mg	Nicotine	Use per package schedule.	108	$55.99	52¢
Nicorette 4mg Gum (orange & mint flavors)	4mg	Nicotine	Use per package schedule.	168	$77.99	46¢
Nicotine Polacrilex 2mg Gum or Nicotine Gum Stop Smoking Aid	2mg	Nicotine	Use per package schedule.	108	$38.99	36¢
Nicotine Polacrilex 4mg Gum or Nicotine Gum Stop Smoking Aid	4mg	Nicotine	Use per package schedule.	108	$44.99	42¢

$ SMART BUY
Smoking-Cessation Products

Choose the nicotine patches. Success rates are higher with patches than with the inhaled prescription products (such as Nicotrol Nasal Spray) or chewing gum products. Look to save money with generic versions, but be aware that some products stick to your skin better than others. People tell us Nicoderm CQ seems to stick better than other brands.

If you smoke a pack a day (20 cigarettes), completing the smoking-cessation schedule using the 2mg strength of a nicotine gum will cost you about $350. Completing the schedule using a generic nicotine patch, such as Rite Aid or Walgreens Nicotine Transdermal Patch (a generic version of Nicoderm CQ), will cost about $195. (This compares to $380 for cigarettes for a comparable period of time!) So the generic equivalent Nicoderm Patch will save you about 44 percent over the nicotine gum—and about 49 percent over smoking.

PRODUCTS FOR OSTEOARTHRITIS

Nearly 20 million people in the U.S. live with osteoarthritis, an often painful and some-times debilitating condition in which the joints become stiff and inflamed. Not sur-prisingly, prescription and over-the-counter drugs to treat osteoarthritis generate billions of dollars in sales each year. For a long time, the most effective products for treating osteoarthritis were the nonsteroidal anti-inflammatory drugs (NSAIDs). But although NSAIDs are quite effective, they can cause problems. Stomach-related prob-lems, including ulcers, are among the leading reasons people stop taking these drugs. In recent years, new products that have shown some success (without the stomach-related side effects) have come to market in the U.S. The active ingredients glucosamine, chon-droitin, and MSM (methyl sulfonyl methane) are manufactured both as single-compo-nent products and in various combinations.

Glucosamine is a natural building block of healthy cartilage and may help repair and maintain cartilage and stimulate growth of cartilage cells. Chondroitin may help to maintain the natural lubricating fluid in joints and cartilage. MSM is a natural source of dietary sulfur. Sulfur is responsible for maintaining the elasticity and flexibility of the connective tissue that makes up joints.

GLUCOSAMINE

Glucosamine technically is an amino sugar the body manufactures naturally. It's essen-tial in the production of cartilage, the "shock absorber" material that cushions the joints to prevent bone from grinding on bone. For many years, European physicians (and American veterinarians) have used glucosamine to treat and prevent osteoarthri-tis.

Glucosamine comes in three forms—glucosamine sulfate, glucosamine hydrochlo-ride, and N-acetyl-glucosamine. No one really knows for sure whether one "salt" form is better than another. In nature, glucosamine is found in abundance in shellfish. Some manufacturers combine different forms in one tablet. Dosage is usually 500mg taken 3 times daily. Unlike with NSAIDs, you'll need to be patient: It can take a month or longer before you notice improvement.

The University of Maryland School of Pharmacy in Baltimore has evaluated several manufacturers of glucosamine. Their findings showed differences between the strengths stated on the packaging and what was actually in the tablets. A popular con-sumer advocate survey of glucosamine products found some brands to be less than acceptable, because actual amounts of the ingredients were about 50 percent less than the amounts stated on the manufacturer's label. Another study showed that glucosamine alone was as effective as combination products. Refer to the following tables; then read our Smart Buy comments on glucosamine products that follow.

> ### Chondroitin–Heparin Caution
>
> Chondroitin has a chemical structure similar to that of heparin, an anticoagulant (blood thinner). If you're already taking any prescription anticoagulant, check with your doctor before taking chondroitin or combination products containing it.

CHONDROITIN

Chondroitin is a naturally produced component of shark cartilage that might be helpful, either in combination with glucosamine or by itself, in offering some protection to cartilage. You can get chondroitin from your diet by eating "gristle"—cartilage left in meat products—although most people don't find this idea very appealing. The usual dose of the supplement is 400mg taken 3 times daily. Most products combine glucosamine and chondroitin in a single tablet that provides 500mg of glucosamine and 400mg of chondroitin.

MSM (METHYL SULFONYL METHANE)

MSM is another substance that's often combined with glucosamine or added to glucosamine/chondroitin combination products. You might remember a topical product sold seemingly everywhere, from pharmacies to gas stations, in the 1970s: DMSO (dimethyl sulfoxide), originally used by veterinarians, became a fad treatment for many ailments (although it never received approval for such uses); arthritis relief seemed to be the most common use. But the product's side effects of garlic-like breath and body odor, as well as some damage to the liver, eventually led to DSMO's removal from the marketplace.

In the body, however, metabolism converts DMSO into MSM. When DMSO was no longer available, people began taking MSM, instead. It appears that MSM might offer the positive effects of DSMO without the harmful side effects. Many arthritis sufferers claim taking MSM has improved their conditions, although no conclusive studies exist that demonstrate any effectiveness in treating the numerous ailments people use it to treat. We don't recommend taking MSM, unless it's included in combination with glucosamine and chondroitin at a better price than glucosamine and chondroitin alone.

SAMe (S-Adenosylmethionine)

Originally SAMe was used to treat depression. By accident, doctors and patients discovered that it had an additional property: It seemed to help arthritis sufferers. So over the years, it also has been used to treat arthritis. The use of SAMe for this purpose is controversial. As is the case with MSM, no studies have been performed to show its effectiveness. Despite this, some people are willing to pay nearly $200 a month for this product.

You probably shouldn't become one of them. The evidence is too sketchy to justify the very high cost. Most people can find more effective and less expensive options. Aside from the controversy surrounding its use, SAMe also might interact with other antidepressants, as well as with drugs prescribed to treat Parkinson's disease. If you want to take SAMe for arthritis symptoms and you already take medication for depression or Parkinson's, talk with your physician first.

Glucosamine/Chondroitin Products for Joint Pain

PRODUCT	STRENGTH PER DOSE	ACTIVE INGREDIENT	USUAL DOSAGE	TYPICAL QUANTITY	TYPICAL PRICE	DAILY COST (AT 1500 MG)
ARTHx DS Glucosamine Chondroitin Capsules	500mg, 400mg	Glucosamine, chondroitin	Take 1 capsule 3 times a day.	180	$52.99	88¢
Cosamin DS Joint Health Supplement, Double Strength Capsules	500mg, 400mg	Glucosamine hydrochloride, sodium chondroitin sulfate	Take 1 tablet 3 times a day.	210	$87.99	$1.26
CVS Glucosamine Chondroitin Double Strength Caplets	500mg, 400mg	Glucosamine, chondroitin	Take 1 caplet 3 times a day.	180	$39.99	67¢
Flexagen Glucosamine, Chondroitin & Vitamin C, Caplets	500mg, 400mg, 20mg	Glucosamine hydrochloride, chondroitin sulfate, vitamin C	Take 1 caplet up to 3 times a day.	100	$29.99	90¢

PRODUCT	STRENGTH PER DOSE	ACTIVE INGREDIENT	USUAL DOSAGE	TYPICAL QUANTITY	TYPICAL PRICE	DAILY COST (AT 1500 MG)
Move Free Tablets	500mg, 400mg	Glucosamine, chondroitin	Take 1 tablet 3 times a day.	120	$31.99	80¢
Nature's Way Flexmax Glucosamine Chondroitin	375mg, 300mg	Glucosamine, chondroitin	Take 2 tablets twice a day.	240	$63.99	$1.07
Sundown Osteo Bi-Flex Glucosamine Chondroitin Tablets	250mg, 200mg	Glucosamine, chondroitin	Take 2 tablets 3 times a day.	120	$28.99	$1.45
Sundown Osteo Bi-Flex Glucosamine & Chondroitin Double Strength Chews, Cherry	500mg, 400mg	Glucosamine hydrochloride, chondroitin sulfate	Take 1 tablet 3 times a day.	60	$26.99	$1.35
Sundown Osteo Bi-Flex Caplets Triple Strength	750mg, 600mg chondroitin sulfate	Glucosamine hydrochloride,	Take 1 tablet 2 times a day.	80	$31.99	80¢
Walgreens Glucosamine Chondroitin Double-Strength Capsules	500mg, 400mg	Glucosamine sulfate, chondroitin sulfate	Take 1 capsule 3 times a day.	120	$31.99	80¢

Glucosamine + MSM Products

PRODUCT	STRENGTH PER DOSE	ACTIVE INGREDIENT	USUAL DOSAGE	TYPICAL QUANTITY	TYPICAL PRICE	DAILY COST (AT 1500 MG)
Flex-A-Min Glucosamine Chondroitin MSM Tablets	500mg, 400mg, 167mg	Glucosamine hydrochloride, sodium chondroitin sulfate, methylsulfonylmethane (MSM)	Take 1 tablet 3 times a day.	180	$41.99	70¢
Move Free Plus MSM Tablets	375mg, 300mg, 375mg	Glucosamine, chondroitin, methylsulfonylmethane (MSM)	Take 2 tablets twice a day.	120	$33.99	$1.13
Natrol Glucosamine + MSM Double-Strength Tablets	500mg, 500mg	Glucosamine, methylsulfonylmethane (MSM)	Take 1 tablet 3 times a day.	60	$18.59	93¢
Nature Made TripleFlex, Maximum Strength Glucosamine Chondroitin plus MSM, Tablets	500mg, 400mg, 125mg	Glucosamine hydrochloride, chondroitin sulfate, methylsulfonylmethane (MSM)	Take 1 tablet 3 times a day.	50	$16.49	99¢
Osteo Bi-Flex + MSM Caplets	375mg, 250mg	Glucosamine, methylsulfonylmethane (MSM)	Take 2 tablets twice a day.	120	$31.99	$1.07

PRODUCT	STRENGTH PER DOSE	ACTIVE INGREDIENT	USUAL DOSAGE	TYPICAL QUANTITY	TYPICAL PRICE	DAILY COST (AT 1500 MG)
Sundown Osteo Bi-Flex Plus MSM Caplets	375mg, 300mg, 250mg	Glucosamine, chondroitin methylsulfonylmethane (MSM)	Take 2 caplets twice a day.	120	$34.99	$1.17
Walgreens Glucosamine + MSM Tablets	500mg, 500mg	Glucosamine, methyl-sulfonylmethane (MSM)	Take 1 tablet 3 times a day.	180	$21.99	37¢

Glucosamine + SAMe Products

PRODUCT	STRENGTH PER DOSE	ACTIVE INGREDIENT	USUAL DOSAGE	TYPICAL QUANTITY	TYPICAL PRICE	DAILY COST
Move Free Plus SAMe Tablets	500mg, 133mg	Glucosamine, SAMe	Take 1 tablet 3 times a day.	30	$22.99	$2.30
Natrol SAMe Joint Formula Caplets	200mg, 250mg, 200mg	Glucosamine methyl-sulfonylmethane (MSM), SAMe	Take 2 caplets a day.	20	$25.99	$9.75
Nature Made Joint Action Tablets	500mg, 200mg	Glucosamine, SAMe	Take 1 tablet 3 times a day.	50	$41.99	$2.52

$ SMART BUY
Products for Osteoarthritis

The best buy to date is either Walgreen's Finest Natural Glucosamine Sulfate 500mg capsules, at 42 cents, or a Basic Nutrition brand from Rite Aid, for about 40 cents a day for a 1,500mg dose. Remember to take this supplement regularly and be patient. It may take two or even three months before you notice results.

> ## ▶ Glucosamine's Effectiveness
>
> A study conducted in 2002 suggests that glucosamine alone is as effective as glucosamine in combination with chondroitin. Further research is needed to explore this preliminary finding. Check our Web site at www.smartbuysdrugwise.com for updates! ◀

PRODUCTS TO RELIEVE URINARY IRRITATION

The burning that accompanies a urinary tract infection commands your immediate attention. Doctors have long prescribed phenazopyridine, in 100mg or 200mg doses, to relieve this sometimes intense discomfort. Now versions of this drug are available over the counter; all contain 95 milligrams of phenazopyridine (except for UTI Relief 32, which contains 97.2mg). You'll find this medication under the brand names Azo-Gesic, Azo-Standard, Uristat, UTI Relief 32, and Prodium. Azo-Gesic is technically a generic; it's just that some companies (in this case Major Pharmaceuticals) like to use a pseudo-"brand name." Walgreens also markets a version called Urinary Relief Tablets. Phenazopyridine has mild antiseptic properties, and so might be effective at killing bacteria in very mild infections.

Another product for urinary tract discomfort is Cystex, which contains the active ingredients methenamine mandelate and sodium salicylate. It was a good product in its time, but since the prescription name-brand Pyridium (generic name phenazopyridine) became available in an over-the-counter version, it and its generic counterparts are the better choice, because they provide a higher degree of urinary tract pain relief.

Pyridium is used for its urinary analgesic properties. It acts to numb the nerve endings in the urethra, which eliminates the burning that occurs when urinating. The usual dose for an adult is 1 to 2 tablets, 3 times daily. If your symptoms aren't better in two days, or if they become worse, seek medical attention promptly. Also be aware that using this medication may change the color of your urine from a faint yellow to an intense red: Don't be alarmed!

Products to Relieve Urinary Irritation

PRODUCT	STRENGTH PER DOSE	ACTIVE INGREDIENT	USUAL DOSAGE	TYPICAL QUANTITY	TYPICAL PRICE	COST PER DOSE
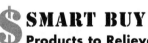 Azo-Gesic	95mg	Phenazopyridine Hcl	Take 2 tablets up to 3 times daily (not for more than 2 days).	30	$5.99	40¢
Azo-Standard Tablets	95mg	Phenazopyridine Hcl	Take 2 tablets up to 3 times daily (not for more than 2 days).	30	$8.99	60¢
Consumers Choice Systems UTI Relief 32, Urinary Tract Pain Relief Tablets	97.2mg	Phenazopyridine Hcl	Take 2 tablets up to 3 times daily (not for more than 2 days).	32	$7.49	47¢
Cystex Tablets	162mg, 162.5mg	Methenamine mandelate, sodium salicylate	Take 2 tablets up to 3 times daily (not for more than 2 days).	40	$9.99	50¢
Prodium Tablets	95mg	Phenazopyridine Hcl	Take 2 tablets up to 3 times daily (not for more than 2 days).	24	$8.39	70¢
Uristat Urinary Pain Relief Tablets	95mg	Phenazopyridine Hcl	Take 2 tablets up to 3 times daily (not for more than 2 days).	24	$8.99	75¢
Walgreens Urinary Pain Relief	95mg	Phenazopyridine Hcl	Take 2 tablets up to 3 times daily (not for more than 2 days).	32	$6.99	44¢

$ SMART BUY
Products to Relieve Urinary Irritation

The Smart Buy here is Azo-Gesic, made by Major Pharmaceuticals. (You may have to ask your pharmacist to special order it.) You can get 30 tablets for about $6. The Azo-Gesic will save you about 30 percent over its name-brand counterpart, Azo-Standard. Just remember not to use this product for longer than two days, because phenazopyridine does such a good job of stopping the burning upon urination that, if you do have an infection, you won't be able to tell.

$ SMART OPTIONS FOR SAVINGS
Other Over-the-Counter Products

For most of the products covered in this chapter, buying generic and in the largest quantity possible are your Smart Options for Savings. The exception is insulin, because it has a short potency period. Buy insulin only as you need it, and follow all handling and storage recommendations.

Keep the following points in mind when you shop for the kinds of over-the-counter products featured in this chapter:

1. Mail-order and Internet ("virtual") pharmacies often offer the lowest prices on many of these products. It's worth comparing prices before you buy; be sure to factor in shipping costs and the length of time it will take for your order to arrive. (The savings, too, may be "virtual.") Two factors that can offset online pharmacy savings—poor planning and needing your insulin before it's mailed. If you do order insulin by mail, make certain the pharmacy packages it properly: Most insulins must be kept cold, but not frozen.

2. Unless you know you're getting exactly the same product you'd get in the U.S., we don't recommend buying these products outside the country.

3. Look for coupons and manufacturer's rebates, especially on blood glucose monitors and other items of equipment.

Consider the cost of related items before you make a purchasing decision for items such as blood glucose monitors and lancet devices. Choose products that will accept various brands of test strips and lancets, so you won't be trapped into buying expensive proprietary ones.

Chapter 22

Over-the-Counter Drugs for Children

Children's bodies function quite differently from those of adults. Because of their size and metabolism, children easily can overdose on medications such as cough/cold products. Never give a child an adult dose of any over-the-counter drug unless the child's physician specifically tells you to do so! And always use caution in giving a child any drug, even preparations made especially for children. Read the product's label carefully and thoroughly, so you know what side effects can occur. If you're unsure whether the drug is appropriate for your child's condition and health background, what dose to give, or what relief to expect the product to provide for your child, check with your child's doctor or your pharmacist before administering it.

Many children's medications come in liquid form, which can make giving the correct dose a challenge. The product's label will tell you how much of the drug to give, based on the child's age and weight. If a child weighs more or less than the label indicates for a child of the same age, use the dose that corresponds with the child's weight. It's very important to measure children's doses accurately. And sometimes it can be a surprising challenge. When the directions say "1 teaspoon," does that mean to use the same spoon you use for eating cereal? Only if you have no other means for measuring 1 teaspoon. Kitchen spoons vary considerably in terms of how much fluid they hold.

Even the measuring devices that come with many children's products (usually small cups with dose markings) can be difficult to use. The markings are often embossed in the plastic material the cup is made from—and making those raised lines, numbers, and letters tiny enough to fit on the cup is an amazing tribute to modern manufacturing methods! Unfortunately, it's also a reminder of the human eye's limitations. Struggling to read what number goes with which line can make the administering of medication feel more like a cruel vision test! Be sure to place the measuring cups that come with children's drug products on a flat surface (such as a countertop or table) and bend down to look at the markings at eye level. Pour the liquid into the cup to the line that represents the correct dose for your child. Holding the cup in your hand makes it too easy to tip the cup, so an amount that looks just right is either too little or too much.

Don't use the measuring cup from one product to measure any other drug! Product measuring cups (and other devices such as droppers and special spoons) are specific to the product and aren't interchangeable. Some cups are marked for "1 dose;" others mark teaspoons (tsp.) or milliliters (ml). Tragically, each year emergency rooms across the country treat drug overdoses in hundreds of children who receive the wrong measurement of drug.

The most accurate measuring device to use is an oral syringe, which you can get from your pharmacist. (You can't attach a needle to an oral syringe, so it can't be used for injections.) Most oral syringes have measurement markings on the barrel that show both teaspoons and milliliters. Please note that your measuring device may show cubic centimeters (ccs); for all basic measuring purposes, cc (cubic centimeters) is synonymous with ml (milliliters). Your pharmacist can show you how to use an oral syringe, or you can follow these easy steps:

1. Make sure the plunger is pushed all the way into the barrel.
2. Place the tip of the syringe into the liquid drug.
3. Slowly pull back the plunger until it reaches the line indicating the appropriate dose for the child.
4. Remove the syringe from the drug and wipe off excess liquid. Double-check the amount; it doesn't matter how you hold the syringe, because the fluid level won't change. Make sure you have no air bubbles inside the syringe, or your measurement will be inaccurate.
5. Put the tip of the syringe in the child's mouth and gently depress the plunger to release the medication, making sure you direct the stream to the side so as not to hit the uvula (the flap of tissue hanging down in the back of the throat). Otherwise you may end up wearing what you're trying to administer.
6. Encourage the child to swallow several times, to get it all down. Unless the label says otherwise, you can give the child a drink of water or juice to make this easier.
7. Pull the plunger completely out of the barrel and rinse both parts under running water. Reinsert the plunger and push water through the tip. Again, remove the plunger so that both parts can dry.

> ### ► Throw Away Those Syringe Tips!
>
> An oral medication syringe often comes with a small cap over the tip. Always remove and discard this cap immediately! A baby or young child could easily choke on or swallow the cap. The cap is like a safety seal; it's there only to make it clear that the syringe has never been used. The pharmacist might remove the cap before giving the syringe to you, as a precaution. ◄

Most products for children are sweetened and flavored, so kids take them pretty easily. If your child resists, try putting the syringe back farther in the mouth, toward the back of the tongue. (Be careful; if you go too far, you'll activate your child's gag reflex!) Squirting out the medicine will cause your child to swallow instinctively. Don't worry if some of the drug dribbles out of your child's mouth, and don't give more medicine unless you're certain your child spit out all of what you tried to give. If you have problems or questions, call your pharmacist or pediatrician.

CHILDREN'S COUGH, COLD, FLU, AND ALLERGY PRODUCTS

Children's products to ease the symptoms of viruses and allergies are similar to their adult counterparts. As with the adult products, the many name-brands are just various combinations and strengths of the same drugs. Much of the information in Chapter 17, "Over-the-Counter Cough, Cold, Flu, and Allergy Preparations," applies to children's products for the same symptoms.

Unless the child's doctor instructs you otherwise, use these products only when the child shows symptoms. The label may say "every 4 hours," but don't give the product by the clock; administer it only when the child displays the symptoms you're medicating for. Don't overmedicate the child. Many children's flu products show dosages for adults, too, so you (the adult) can take them as well (although, again, we recommend you avoid combination products).

> ### Read Labels Carefully
>
> Take care when you pick a name-brand product (which we usually discourage, because the generic versions are less expensive and just as effective) to make sure you get what you think you're getting. For example, if you choose Tylenol for a child's fever, be sure you buy just Tylenol and not Tylenol Cold Plus Cough Liquid (just one of the many combination products under the Tylenol brand). The latter contains not only Tylenol (acetaminophen), but also an antihistamine, a decongestant, and a cough suppressant. Not only are you likely to spend more than you planned or need to, you're also likely to overmedicate the child.

CHILDREN'S OVER-THE-COUNTER ANTIHISTAMINE PRODUCTS

Antihistamines dry up a runny nose, watery eyes, sneezing, and allergic reactions such as rashes, itching, and hives. Examples include the name-brand products Benadryl (active ingredient diphenhydramine) and Chlor-trimeton (active ingredient chlorpheniramine). The popular product Dimetapp combines the antihistamine brompheniramine and the decongestant pseudoephedrine.

$ SMART BUY
Children's Over-the-Counter Antihistamine Products

The best choice for your money among children's over-the-counter antihistamines is a generic chlorpheniramine product. A number of comparably priced store-brand and generic products are available. Soundalike names might be something like "Chlortabs" or "Aller-Chlor." If a product has "chlor" in its name, it's probably an allergy product. Your pharmacist probably can order you a 100-count bottle for around $6, which is about 80 percent less per dose that what you'd spend for the name-brand Chlor-Trimeton in 24-count packages.

Antihistamine Products

PRODUCT	STRENGTH PER DOSE (5ML = 1TSP)	ACTIVE INGREDIENT	USUAL DOSAGE	TYPICAL QUANTITY	TYPICAL PRICE	COST PER DOSE
Aller-Chlor or Chlortabs 4-hr Tablets (generic version of Chlor-Trimeton)	4mg	Chlorpheniramine	Children ages 6–11, 2mg (1/2 tablet) every 4–6 hrs., not more than 6 tablets in 24 hrs.	100	$5.99	3¢ per 1/2 tab
Benadryl Liquid	12.5mg/5ml	Diphenhydramine	Children ages 6–11, 1–2 tsp. every 4–6 hrs.; 12 years and older, 2–4 tsp. every 4–6 hrs.	236ml	$8.99	19¢ per tsp.
Benahist or Diphenhist Allergy Liquid (generic version of Benadryl)	12.5mg/5ml	Diphenhydramine	Children ages 6–11, 1–2 tsp. every 4–6 hrs.; 12 years and older, 2–4 tsp. every 4–6 hrs.	236ml	$6.99	15¢ per tsp.
Chlor-trimeton Allergy Relief 4-hour Tablets	4mg	Chlorpheniramine	Children ages 6–11, 2mg (1/2 tablet) every 4–6 hours, not more than 6 tablets in 24 hrs.	24	$6.99	15¢ per tab
DiBromm or Bromphen (generic version of Dimetapp Liquid)	1mg/5ml, 15mg/5ml	Brompheniramine, pseudoephedrine	Children ages 2–5, 1 tsp. every 4 hrs.; ages 6–11, 2 tsp. every 4 hrs.; 12 & older, 4 tsp. every 4 hrs.	118ml	$3.99	17¢ per tsp.
Dimetapp Children's Cold & Allergy Liquid	1mg/5ml, 15mg/5ml	Brompheniramine, pseudoephedrine	Children ages 2–5, 1 tsp. every 4 hrs.; ages 6-11, 2 tsp. every 4 hrs.; 12 & older, 4 tsp. every 4 hrs.	236ml	$8.99	19¢ per tsp.
Triaminic Allergy Runny Nose & Congestion Orange Softchew Tablets	1mg, 15mg	Chlorpheniramine, pseudoephedrine	Children ages 6–11, 2 tablets every 4–6 hrs., not more than 4 doses in 24 hrs.	18	$4.99	55¢ per 2 tabs

If your child needs a stronger antihistamine because chlorpheniramine doesn't handle your child's symptoms, try a generic version of diphenhydramine, which is a little stronger. These single-ingredient products offer more uses: They'll relieve your child's runny nose due to cough or allergy, and they're also effective for treating allergic responses or the itching that accompanies childhood diseases such as chickenpox. You might see generic soundalike names like "Benahist," "Histadryl," or "Diphen"-something.

CHILDREN'S OVER-THE-COUNTER DECONGESTANT PRODUCTS

Decongestants help clear stuffed nasal passages so your child can breathe better, and may then relieve pressure in the Eustachian tubes in the ears. Examples include the name-brand product Sudafed (active ingredient pseudoephedrine) and Dimetapp (which also contains an antihistamine). Some Dimetapp generic version soundalikes might be "Bromatap," "Genetap," or "DiBromm."

Decongestants

PRODUCT	STRENGTH PER DOSE (5ML =1TSP)	ACTIVE INGREDIENT	USUAL DOSAGE	TYPICAL QUANTITY	TYPICAL PRICE	COST PER DOSE
DiBromm, Bromaline, Bromanate or Bromphen Liquid (Generic Dimetapp Liquid)	1mg/5ml, 15mg/5ml	Brompheniramine, pseudoephedrine	Children ages 2-5, 1 tsp. every 4 hrs.; 6-11, 2 tsp every 4 hrs; over 12, 4 tsp. every 4 hrs.	118ml	$3.99	17¢ per tsp.
DiBromm, Bromaline or Bromphen Liquid (Generic Dimetapp Liquid)	1mg/5ml, 15mg/5ml	Brompheniramine, pseudoephedrine	Children ages 2-5, 1 tsp. every 4 hrs; 6-11, 2 tsp. every 4 hrs.; over 12, 4 tsp. every 4 hrs.	16oz.	$11.99	13¢ per tsp.
Dimetapp Children's Cold & Allergy Liquid	1mg, 15mg	Brompheniramine, pseudoephedrine	Children ages 2-5, 1 tsp. every 4 hrs.; 6-11, 2 tsp. every 4 hrs; over 12, 4 tsp. every 4 hrs.	236ml	$8.99	19¢ per tsp.
Dimetapp Children's Decongestant Pediatric Drops	7.5mg/0.8ml	Pseudoephedrine	Children ages 2-3, 2 droppers (1.6ml) every 4-6 hrs., not more than 4 doses in 24 hrs.	15ml	$4.99	53¢ per 1.6ml
Little Noses, Decongestant Nose Drops, Gentle 1/8% Formula, Infants & Children (For Nasal Use Only)	1/8%	Phenylephrine	Children ages 2-5, 2-3 drops in each nostril every 4 hrs. USE NO LONGER THAN 3 DAYS.	15ml	$3.49	About 4¢ per dose
Pediacare Decongestant Drops for Infants	15mg/0.8ml	Pseudoephedrine	Children ages 2-3, 2 droppers (1.6ml) every 4-6 hrs., not more than 4 doses in 24 hrs.	15ml	$4.99	53¢ per 1.6ml
Sudafed Children's Non-Drowsy Nasal Decongestant Liquid	15mg/5ml	Pseudoephedrine	Children ages 2-5, 1 tsp.; 6-11, 2 tsp.; over 12, 4 tsp.	118ml	$4.99	21¢ per tsp.
Sudafed	30mg	Pseudoephedrine	Take 1-2 tabs every 4-6 hrs., not more than 8 in 24 hrs.	48	$8.49	18¢ per tab

PRODUCT	STRENGTH PER DOSE (5ML =1TSP)	ACTIVE INGREDIENT	USUAL DOSAGE	TYPICAL QUANTITY	TYPICAL PRICE	COST PER DOSE
Susphrine, Pseudogest, or Pseudotabs, (generic for Sudafed Tablets)	30mg	Pseudoephedrine	Children ages 6-12, 1 tab every 4-6 hrs., not more than 4 in 24 hrs. Children younger than 6 use liquid.	100	$5.99	6¢ per tab
Triaminic Allergy Runny Nose & Congestion Orange Softchew Tablets	1mg, 15mg	Chlorpheniramine, pseudoephedrine	Children ages 6-11, 2 tablets every 4-6 hrs., not more than 4 doses in 24 hrs.	18	$4.99	55¢ per 2 tabs
Triaminic Chest Congestion Liquid	15mg/5ml, 50mg/5ml	Pseudoephedrine, guaifenesin	Children ages 2-5, 1 tsp.; 6-11, 2 tsp., every 4-6 hrs., not more than 4 doses in 24 hrs.	120ml	$5.79	24¢ per tsp.

$ SMART BUY
Children's Decongestant Products

Most oral decongestants for children contain pseudoephedrine. Soundalike generic forms of Sudafed might be "Pseudogest," "Pseudotabs," or "Genaphed." If your child is 6 years of age or older, then the generic equivalent in tablet form will cost you about 6 cents a dose, compared to about 18 cents a dose—a 65 percent savings.

If your child is younger than 6 years, we recommend a generic equivalent of Dimetapp liquid. You'll probably find names similar to "DiBromm," "Bromanate," "Bromaline," or "Bromphen Liquid" (something with "brom" in the name). Most pharmacies carry 4-ounce sizes, but ask your pharmacist to order in 8-, 12-, or even 16-ounce sizes. Bromaline Liquid in a 16-ounce size costs about $12. This is a savings of about 24 percent over the smaller size of generic, and a 32 percent savings over the 8-ounce size of the name brand.

The Convenience of Dimetapp

Many parents like the convenience of Dimetapp (and its generic counterparts) for treating a child's cold symptoms. Although we generally don't recommend combination products, there are times when such convenience has its value. Just be sure to buy a generic product that offers the best savings. And keep in mind that Dimetapp has its limits. If later you should need to give your child an antihistamine for an allergic reaction, you'll have to buy one. The brompheniramine in Dimetapp isn't as strong as an antihistamine such as diphenhydramine (Benadryl). And your child won't need a decongestant to combat the symptoms of an allergic reaction.

CHILDREN'S OVER-THE-COUNTER FEVER RELIEVERS

Fever-reducers do just that, and also relieve pain. Examples include Tylenol (acetaminophen) and Motrin (ibuprofen). Although aspirin is an effective drug for reducing fever and relieving pain in adults, don't give aspirin to children under age 16 unless your child's doctor specifically instructs you to do so. Aspirin can cause serious complications in children. (More on this later in this chapter.)

$ SMART BUY
Children's Over-the-Counter Fever Relievers

Generally, infant drop products offer the best value and are the easiest product to give to children under age 2. Always read label directions carefully and thoroughly to be sure you give your child the correct dose! Older children (ages 5 to 11) can take, and typically enjoy taking, chewable tablets. Buy generic or store-brand products for the most significant savings; Smart Buy products you find in your community might be regional store brands. This is where shopping around can add up to significant savings. Because of the risk for a rare but serious complication, Reye's syndrome, do not administer aspirin or other salicylate-containing products (such as Pepto-Bismol) if your child has (or could have) a viral infection such as influenza, a cold, or chickenpox. Instead, use a generic equivalent of Tylenol (acetaminophen), such as Genapap, Myapap, Ty-Pap, or

Children's Pain/Fever Reducer. The 4-ounce generic will save you somewhere in the neighborhood of 37 percent over the name-brand in the same size.

Children's Over-the-Counter Fever and Pain Relievers

PRODUCT	STRENGTH PER DOSE (5ML = 1TSP)	ACTIVE INGREDIENT	USUAL DOSAGE	TYPICAL QUANTITY	TYPICAL PRICE	COST PER DOSE
Advil Children's Fever & Pain Reducer Drops	100mg/2.5ml	Ibuprofen	Children ages 2-3 (24-35 lb.), 2.5ml (1/2 tsp.) every 6-8 hrs., not more than 4 doses in 24 hrs.	15ml	$5.49	92¢ per 1/2 tsp.
Ibuprofen (generic version of Motrin) Children's Oral Suspension	100mg/5ml	Ibuprofen	Children ages 2-3 (24-35 lb.), 1 tsp.; 4-5 (36-47 lb.), 1.5 tsp.; 6-8 (48-59 lb.), 2 tsp.; 9-10 (60-71 lb.), 2.5 tsp.; 11 (72-95 lb.), 3 tsp., every 6-8 hrs., not more than 4 doses in 24 hrs.	120ml	$5.49	23¢ per tsp.
Motrin Children's, Ibuprofen Oral Suspension, Fever Reducer/Pain Reliever	100mg/5ml	Ibuprofen	Children ages 2-3 (24-35 lb.), 1 tsp.; 4-5 (36-47 lb.), 1-1/2 tsp.; 6-8 (48-59 lb.), 2 tsp.; 9-10 (60-71 lb.), 2.5 tsp.; 11 (72-95 lb.), 3 tsp. every 6-8 hrs., not more than 4 doses in 24 hrs.	120ml	$6.49	27¢ per tsp.
Motrin Children's Chewable Tablets (Fever & Pain Reducer)	50mg	Ibuprofen	Ages 4-5 (36-47 lb.), 3 tabs; 6-8 (48-59 lb.), 4 tabs; 9-10 (60-71 lb.), 5 tabs; over 11 (72-95 lb.), 6 tabs every 6-8 hours, not more than 4 doses in 24 hrs. Under 4 years of age (and under 36 lb.) consult a physician.	24	$4.29	54¢ per 3 tabs
Myapap, Genapap, Pain/Fever Reducer Generic formula, Acetaminophen Infant Concentrated Drops	80mg, 0.8ml	Acetaminophen	Children ages 2-3, (24-35 lb.)1.6ml (2 droppers) every 4 hrs., not more than 5 doses in 24 hrs.	30ml	$7.29	39¢ per 1.6ml
Myapap, Genapap, Pain/Fever Reducer or Acetaminophen Suspension (Generic Tylenol Suspension)	160mg/5ml	Acetaminophen	Children ages 2-3 (24-35 lb.), 5ml; 4-5 (36-47 lb.), 7.5ml; 6-8 (48-59 lb.), 10ml; 9-10 (60-71 lb.), 12.5ml; over 11 (72-95 lb.), 15ml, every 4 hrs., not more than 5 doses in 24 hrs.	120ml	$3.99	17¢ per tsp.

PRODUCT	STRENGTH PER DOSE (5ML = 1TSP)	ACTIVE INGREDIENT	USUAL DOSAGE	TYPICAL QUANTITY	TYPICAL PRICE	COST PER DOSE
Tylenol Children's Fever & Pain Reducer Chewable Tablets	80mg	Acetaminophen	Children ages 2-3 (24-35 lb.), 2 tabs; 4-5 (36-47 lb.), 3 tabs; 6-8 (48-59 lb.), 4 tabs; 9-10 (60-71 lb.), 5 tabs; over 11 (72-95 lb.), 6 tabs, every 4 hrs., not more than 5 doses in 24 hrs.	60	$5.49	18¢
Tylenol Children's Fever & Pain Reducer Suspension	160mg/5ml	Acetaminophen	Children ages 2-3 (24-35 lb.), 5ml; 4-5 (36-47 lb.), 7.5ml; 6-8 (48-59 lb.), 10ml; 9-10 (60-71 lb.), 12.5ml; over 11 (72-95 lb.), 15ml, every 4 hrs., not more than 5 doses in 24 hrs.	120ml	$6.49	27¢ per tsp.
Tylenol Infants Concentrated Pain & Fever Reducer Drops	80mg, 0.8ml	Acetaminophen	Children ages 2-3 (24-35 lb.), 1.6ml (2 droppers) every 4 hrs., not more than 5 doses in 24 hrs.	30ml	$8.49	45¢ per 1.6ml

CHILDREN'S OVER-THE-COUNTER COUGH SUPPRESSANTS

Cough suppressants stop a cough. Use a cough suppressant when your child has a "throat tickle" kind of cough, not for a "chest rattle" kind of cough (which needs an expectorant). Robitussin DM (dextromethorphan) is commonly recommended, and most generic and store brands advertise themselves as "same active ingredients as Robitussin DM."

 SMART BUY
Children's Over-the-Counter Cough Suppressants

In general, use pediatric drops for children age 2 and under. These products are more concentrated than regular liquids, so you don't have to give as much. Buy generic or store brand products whenever possible. And because we prefer single-ingredient products over combinations, we suggest a generic version of Robitussin DM for your best cost-per-dose savings. Soundalikes usually will have "Tussin" somewhere in the product name. Because we recommend a generic version of Robitussin DM, look for Tussin-DM or something similar on the label. The generic equivalent of Robitussin DM will save you about 2 cents per teaspoon, or about 14 percent over the name brand.

Children's Over-the-Counter Cough Suppressants

PRODUCT	STRENGTH PER DOSE (5ML =1TSP)	ACTIVE INGREDIENT	USUAL DOSAGE	TYPICAL QUANTITY	TYPICAL PRICE	COST PER DOSE
Delsym Extended-Release 12 hour Cough Relief	30mg*/5ml dextrome-thorphan hbr	Dextromethorphan polistirex	Children ages 2-5, 2.5ml; 6-11, 5ml; over 12, 10ml, every 12 hours, not more than 2 doses in 24 hrs.	89ml	$7.99	45¢ per tsp.
Dimetapp Children's Cold & Cough Elixir	1mg, 15mg, 5mg all per 5ml	Brompheniramine, pseudoephedrine, dextromethorphan	Children ages 2-5, 1 tsp. every 4 hrs.; 6-11, 2 tsp. every 4 hrs.;12 & older, 4 tsp. every 4 hrs.	237ml	$9.99	21¢ per tsp.
Dimetapp Children's Decongestant Plus Infant Cough Drops	7.5mg/0.8ml, 2.5mg/0.8ml	Pseudoephedrine, dextromethorphan	Children ages 2-3, 2 droppers (1.6ml) every 4-6 hrs., not more than 2 doses in 24 hrs.	15ml	$5.99	64¢ per 1.6ml
Motrin Children's Cold Berry-Flavored Suspension	100mg/5ml, 15mg/5ml	Ibuprofen, pseudoephedrine	Children ages 2-5, 1 tsp.; 6-11, 2 tsp., every 6-8 hrs., not more than 4 doses in 24 hrs. Do not give to children under age 2.	120ml	$6.49	27¢ per tsp.
Pediacare Decon-gestant & Cough Drops for Infants	7.5mg/0.8ml, 2.5mg/0.8ml	Pseudoephedrine, dextromethorphan	Children ages 2-3, 2 droppers (1.6ml) every 4-6 hrs., not more than 4 doses in 24 hours.	15ml	$5.99	64¢ per tsp.
Pediacare Long Lasting Cough Plus Cold Liquid	7.5mg/5ml, 15mg/5ml	Dextromethorphan, pseudoephedrine	Children ages 2-5, 5ml; 6-11, 10ml, every 6-8 hrs., not more than 4 doses in 24 hrs.	120ml	$5.99	25¢ per tsp.
Robitussin DM Cough Suppressant Expectorant Syrup	10mg, 100mg both per 5ml	Dextromethorphan, guaifenesin	Children ages 2-5, 1/2 tsp.; 6-11, 1 tsp.; over 12, 4 tsp., up to every 4 hrs., not more than 4 doses in 24 hrs.	355ml	$9.99	14¢ per tsp.
Robitussin DM Infant Drops; cough suppressant & expectorant	2.5mg/2.5ml, 100mg/2.5ml	Dextromethorphan, guaifenesin	Children ages 2-6, 2.5ml every 4 hrs., not more than 6 doses in 24 hrs.	30ml	$5.49	92¢ per tsp.
Robitussin Pediatric Cough Formula Liquid	7.5mg/5ml	Dextromethorphan	Children ages 2-5, 5ml; 6-11, 10ml; over 12, 20ml, every 6 hrs, not more than 4 doses in 24 hrs.	118ml	$5.79	25¢ per tsp.

PRODUCT	STRENGTH PER DOSE (5ML =1TSP)	ACTIVE INGREDIENT	USUAL DOSAGE	TYPICAL QUANTITY	TYPICAL PRICE	COST PER DOSE
Tussin DM, (generic version of Robitussin DM) Cough (Walgreens, Wal-Mart) Suppressant Expectorant Syrup	10mg, 100mg both per 5ml	Dextromethorphan, guaifenesin	Children ages 2-5, 1/2 tsp.; 6-11, 1 tsp.; over 12, 4 tsp., up to every 4 hrs., not more than 4 doses in 24 hrs.	355ml	$8.29	12¢ per tsp.
Triaminic AM non-drowsy Cough & Decongestant	15mg/5ml; 7.5mg/5ml	Pseudoephedrine, dextromethorphan	Children ages 2-5 (24-47 lb.), 1 tsp. every 6 hrs.; 6-11 (48-95 lb.), 2 tsp. every 6 hrs.; over 12 (96+ lb.), 4 tsp. every 6 hrs.	118ml	$6.29	27¢ per tsp.
Tylenol Plus Cold Plus Cough Suspension	180mg, 1mg, 15mg, 5mg all per 5ml	Acetaminophen, chlorpheniramine, pseudoephedrine, dextromethorphan	Children ages 6-11, 2 tsp. every 4-6 hrs., not more than 4 doses in 24 hrs.	120ml	$5.99	25¢ per tsp.

CHILDREN'S OVER-THE-COUNTER COUGH EXPECTORANTS

Expectorants help loosen mucous (phlegm) in both the head and chest, so your child can blow her nose and cough up what might be causing chest tightness. If your child has a loose, rattling cough, an expectorant will make the cough more effective in bringing up mucous, so the need to cough eases.

Children's Over-the-Counter Cough Expectorants

PRODUCT	STRENGTH PER DOSE (5ML =1TSP)	ACTIVE INGREDIENT	USUAL DOSAGE	TYPICAL QUANTITY	TYPICAL PRICE	COST PER DOSE
Robitussin Plain Expectorant Cough Syrup	100mg/5ml	Guaifenesin	Children ages 2-5, 2.5ml every 4 hrs.; 6-11, 5-10ml every 4 hrs.; over 12, 10-20ml every 4 hrs.	237ml	$5.99	13¢ per tsp.
Tussin Plain or Guaituss Plain, (generic version of Robitussin Plain) Expectorant Cough Syrup	100mg/5ml	Guaifenesin	Children ages 2-5, 2.5ml every 4 hrs.; 6-11, 5-10ml every 4 hrs.; over 12, 10-20ml every 4 hrs.	237ml	$4.99	11¢

$ SMART BUY
Children's Over-the-Counter Cough Expectorants

Buy a generic formula of guaifenesin only; you don't want to stop a productive cough, because doing so allows the mucous to collect and become home for nasty bacteria. Any cough product with a "DM" in the name contains dextromethorphan, a cough suppressant, which you only want if the cough isn't productive. The best expectorant will have the word "Tussin" or "Guiatuss" in it, but not a "DM." Nor should it have a "PE" or "CF." And remember to provide plenty of water during the day, or the expectorant won't loosen that phlegm. Again, the generic equivalent product will save you money. We know 2 cents a teaspoon isn't a lot, but it makes for a 15 percent savings over the name brand.

CHILDREN'S OVER-THE-COUNTER MULTI-SYMPTOM COMBINATION PRODUCTS FOR "COLD AND COUGH"

When you buy combination products, you're paying for the convenience of giving your child a single dose of medication. Now, we have nothing against convenience. It does concern us, however, that combination products often give children drugs they don't

Children's Over-the-Counter "Cold and Cough" Combination Products

PRODUCT	STRENGTH PER DOSE (5ML = 1TSP)	ACTIVE INGREDIENT	USUAL DOSAGE	TYPICAL QUANTITY	TYPICAL PRICE	COST PER DOSAGE
Bromtapp, Bromaline, Bromphen or Di Bromm Liquid (generic version of Dimetapp Liquid)	1mg/5ml; 15mg/5ml	Brompheniramine, pseudoephedrine	Children ages 2-5, 1 tsp. every 4 hrs.; 6-11, 2 tsp. every 4 hrs.; over 12, 4 tsp. every 4 hrs.	118ml	$4.99	21¢ per dose
DiBromm, Bromaline, Bromtapp or Bromphen Liquid (generic version of Dimetapp Liquid)	1mg/5ml; 15mg/5ml	Brompheniramine, pseudoephedrine	Children ages 2-5, 1 tsp. every 4 hrs.; 6-11, 2 tsp. every 4 hrs.; over 12, 4 tsp. every 4 hrs.	16oz.	$11.99	13¢ per tsp.
Dimetapp Children's Cold & Allergy Liquid	1mg, 15mg	Brompheniramine, pseudoephedrine	Children ages 2-5, 1 tsp. every 4 hrs.; 6-11, 2 tsp. every 4 hrs.; over 12, 4 tsp. every 4 hrs.	236ml	$9.99	21¢ per tsp.
Dimetapp Children's Cold & Cough Elixir	1mg, 15mg, 5mg all in 5ml	Brompheniramine, pseudoephedrine, dextromethorphan	Children ages 2-5, 1 tsp. every 4 hrs.; 6-11, 2 tsp. every 4 hrs.; over 12, 4 tsp. every 4 hrs.	237ml	$9.99	21¢ per tsp.

PRODUCT	STRENGTH PER DOSE (5ML = 1TSP)	ACTIVE INGREDIENT	USUAL DOSAGE	TYPICAL QUANTITY	TYPICAL PRICE	COST PER DOSE
Dimetapp Children's Decongestant Plus Infant Cough Drops	7.5mg/0.8ml, 2.5mg/0.8ml	Pseudoephedrine, dextromethorphan	Children ages 2-3, 2 droppers (1.6ml) every 4-6 hrs., not more than 4 doses in 24 hrs.	15ml	$5.99	64¢ per 1.6ml
Motrin Children's Cold Berry-Flavored Suspension	100mg, 5ml, 15mg, 5ml	Ibuprofen, pseudoephedrine	Children ages 2-5, 1 tsp.; 6-11, 2 tsp., every 6-8 hrs., not more than 4 doses in 24 hrs. Do not give to children under age 2.	120ml	$6.49	27¢ per tsp.
Pediacare Decongestant & Cough Drops for Infants	7.5mg/0.8ml, 2.5mg/0.8ml	Pseudoephedrine, dextromethorphan	Children ages 2-3, 2 droppers (1.6ml) every 4-6 hrs., not more than 4 doses in 24 hrs.	15ml	$5.99	64¢ per 1.6ml
Robitussin DM Infant Drops, cough suppressant & expectorant	2.5mg/2.5ml, 100mg/2.5ml	Dextromethorphan, guaifenesin	Children ages 2-6, 2.5ml every 4 hrs., not more than 6 doses in 24 hrs.	30ml	$5.49	46¢ per1/2 tsp.
Sudafed Children's Non-Drowsy Cold & Cough Liquid	5mg/5ml, 15mg/5ml	Dextromethorphan, pseudoephedrine	Children ages 2-5, 5ml; 6-11, 10ml; over 12, 20ml.	118ml	$5.99	25¢ per tsp.
Triaminic AM nondrowsy Cough & Decongestant	15mg/5ml 7.5mg/5ml	Pseudoephedrine, dextromethorphan	Children ages 2-5 (24-47 lb.), 1 tsp. every	118ml	$6.29	27¢ per tsp.

need in addition to the ones they do need. Most of the time, this probably doesn't cause any problems. But the more medications your child takes, the greater the risk for adverse reactions and other complications. We prefer going the more cautious route of giving a separate drug for each symptom, despite the potential inconvenience.

As with the adult products, we advise against buying most combination drugs. It's generally more cost-effective—and safer—to buy and use only the drugs actually needed to relieve your child's symptoms. If your child has a fever and a stuffy nose, but no cough, there's no reason to give a combination product that contains a cough suppressant.

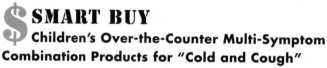

$ SMART BUY
Children's Over-the-Counter Multi-Symptom
Combination Products for "Cold and Cough"

As you know by now, we don't consider most combination products to be Smart Buys. If you want to use one because your child has multiple symptoms and resists taking medications, Tylenol Cold Plus Cough Suspension covers the bases. For big savings, go with a generic equivalent of Dimetapp Liquid. You'll find it under names like DiBromm, Bromonate, Bromphen or Bromaline Liquid. These generic equivalents do not stop a cough; nor do they contain a fever or pain reducer. But you probably have a generic equivalent of Tylenol for pain/fever at home already. Because you're most likely trying to treat the symptoms of a cold (runny nose and/or congestion), the generic equivalents of Dimetapp will treat both annoyances and reduce your cost per teaspoon from 50 cents a day for the Tylenol Cold Plus Cough Suspension to about 13 cents a day, for a savings of 74 percent! These types of multi-symptom products with the same ingredients are often marketed as "flu" preparations, particularly during peak "cold and flu season" (November through March in much of the United States). Manufacturers and drugstores offer coupons, sale prices, and other discounts at this time. Combining a manufacturer's coupon from the advertising supplement of the Sunday newspaper with a drugstore's sale price can save you quite a bit of money, even on a name-brand product.

Children's Over-the-Counter Multi-Symptom Combination Products for Flu

PRODUCT	STRENGTH PER DOSE (5ML =1TSP)	ACTIVE INGREDIENT	USUAL DOSAGE	TYPICAL QUANTITY	TYPICAL PRICE	COST PER DOSE
Dimetapp Nighttime Flu Syrup	160mg, 1mg, 5mg, 15mg all per 5ml	Acetaminophen brompheniramine maleate, dextro-methorphan, pseudo-ephedrine	Children ages 6-11, 2 tsp. every 4 hrs.	120ml	$6.59	60¢ per 2 tsp.
Dimetapp Syrup Non-Drowsy Flu Syrup	160mg, 15mg, 5mg all per 5ml	Acetaminophen, pseudoephedrine, dextromethorphan	Children ages 2-5, 1 tsp.; 6-11, 2 tsp., every 4 hrs., not more than 4 doses in 24 hrs.	120ml	$6.59	56¢ per 2 tsp
Robitussin Flu Liquid	160mg, 1mg, 5mg, 15mg all per 5ml	Acetaminophen chlorpheniramine, dextromethorphan, pseudoephedrine	Children ages 6-11, 2 tsp.; over 12, 4 tsp., every 4 hrs., not more than 4 doses in 24 hrs.	118ml	$5.89	50¢ per 2 tsp.
Tylenol Flu Children's Suspension Liquid	160mg, 1mg, 7.5mg, 15mg all per 5ml	Acetaminophen, chlorpheniramine, dextromethorphan, pseudoephedrine	Children ages 6-11, 10ml every 6 hrs., not more than 4 doses in 24 hrs. For children younger than age 6 or under 48 lb., consult a physician first.	120ml	$5.99	50¢ per 2 tsp.

$ SMART BUY
Children's Over-the-Counter
Multi-Symptom Combination Products for Flu

For both safety (your child's) and savings, buy individual products in generic forms, rather than combination products for flu symptoms, even though the symptoms are varied—cough, congestion, fever, aches, and pains. Although it might seem that you're buying (and spending) more up front, you'll actually get significantly lower per-dose costs by doing it this way. You also get better use of the products, and limit the amounts of drugs that your child takes. A child might need a pain reliever and decongestant for a cold, and two months later need just a pain reliever for the discomfort of teething. A child rarely will have all the symptoms the drugs in a combination product can relieve.

Calculating your savings can be a bit complicated because they'll vary depending on the products you actually use. Tylenol Cold Plus Cough Suspension costs about $5 for a 4-ounce bottle, or about 42 cents a dose (2 teaspoons every 4 hours). If your child just has a head cold (stuffy and runny nose, itchy eyes), a generic form of Dimetapp (combination of an antihistamine and decongestant such as Bromatap or DiBromm) will cost about 13 cents a dose. Need to add a cough suppressant? Generic Robitussin DM (such as Tussin DM or Guiatuss DM) is just 12 cents a dose. Adding a generic form of Tylenol for pain and/or fever will cost you about 23 cents per teaspoon.

We know you're doing the math: 13¢ + 12¢ + 23¢ = 48¢ per teaspoon, if you had to give all these generics at once. That's 6 cents more per dose than the Tylenol Cold Plus Cough Suspension. But here's where the value lies: When your child has just a runny nose next month, which was the smarter buy? Giving the Tylenol Cold Plus Cough Suspension at 42 cents a dose (and overmedicating your child) or generic equivalent Dimetapp Liquid, at 13 cents a dose? Generic Dimetapp, of course, at a savings of 73 percent! You're armed with as many medications as the multi-symptom product, but now you can save money each time a symptom comes up, and you won't overmedicate.

Notice how similar these "flu" combinations are to the cough/cold combinations. In fact, the Tylenol Cold Plus Cough Suspension is listed in both categories, and could be used in both situations, if you still want to give the multi-symptom product. But use only one of these products at a time. Watch how your child reacts to the medications. Besides looking for symptomatic relief, watch for unwanted side effects.

CHILDREN'S PAIN RELIEF PRODUCTS

Tylenol (acetaminophen)—the name-brand products as well as the generic forms—comes in different strengths. Know what you're buying and giving to your child! It's very easy for children to overdose on acetaminophen because their livers aren't fully developed yet and can't metabolize the drug completely. This means it takes longer for it to leave your child's body. With repeated regular doses, it takes very little time for a crisis to develop; how little depends on your child's physical development and age.

Tylenol (acetaminophen) for children and infants comes in three strengths and forms—a chewable 80mg tablet and two strengths of oral liquid (drops and suspension). The oral drops are intended only for infants and come in a concentration of 80mg per 0.8ml; the oral liquids and suspensions come in a concentration of 160mg per teaspoon (5 ml) and up. When your child has a fever, you want to relieve it now. It's uncomfortable for kids and scary for parents when children get fevers. Many parents rush right to the drugstore and grab the first Tylenol product they see. Frighteningly often, they grab the wrong one. Always double-check your choice. And if you have any uncertainty about which product to buy, ask the pharmacist.

> ▶ ## Use Weight to Determine Correct Dose
>
> Know your child's weight! This is far more important than your child's age when it comes to both determining the correct strength of product to buy and calculating the appropriate dose.

Children's Pain Relief Products

PRODUCT	STRENGTH PER DOSE (5ML = 1TSP)	ACTIVE INGREDIENT	USUAL DOSAGE	TYPICAL QUANTITY	TYPICAL PRICE	COST PER DOSE
Advil Children's Fever & Pain Reducer Drops	100mg/2.5ml	Ibuprofen	Children ages 2-3 (24-35 lb.), 2.5ml (1/2 tsp.) every 6-8 hrs., not more than 4 doses in 24 hrs.	15ml	$5.49	92¢ per 1/2 tsp.
Children's, Ibuprofen or Fever Reducer/Pain Oral Ibuprofen Suspension, Reliever	100mg/5ml	Ibuprofen	Children ages 2-3 (24-35 lb.), 1tsp.; 4-5 (36-47 lb.), 1-1/2 tsp.; 6-8 (48-59 lb.), 2 tsp.; 9-10 (60-71 lb.), 2-1/2 tsp.; 11 (72-95 lb.), 3 tsp. every 6-8 hrs., not more than 4 doses in 24 hrs.	120ml	$5.79	24¢ per tsp.

PRODUCT	STRENGTH PER DOSE (5ML =1TSP)	ACTIVE INGREDIENT	USUAL DOSAGE	TYPICAL QUANTITY	TYPICAL PRICE	COST PER DOSE
Motrin Children's Chewable Tablets (Fever & Pain Reducer)	50mg	Ibuprofen	Children ages 4-5 (36-47 lb.), 3 tabs; 6-8 (48-59 lb.), 4 tabs; 9-10 (60-71 lb.), 5 tabs; over 11 (72-95 lb.), 6 tabs, every 6-8 hrs., not more than 4 doses in 24 hrs.Under 4 years of age (and under 36 lb.) consult a physician first.	24	$4.29	54¢ per 3 tab dose
Motrin Children's, Ibuprofen Oral Suspension, Fever Reducer/Pain Reliever	100mg/5ml	Ibuprofen	Children ages 2-3 (24-35 lb.), 1 tsp.; 4-5 (36-4/ lb.), 1.5 tsp.; 6-8 (48-59 lb.), 2 tsp.; 9-10 (60-71 lb.), 2.5 tsp.; 11 (72-95 lb.), 3 tsp. every 6-8 hrs., not more than 4 doses in 24 hrs.	120ml	$6.49	27¢ per tsp.
Myapap, Genapap or "Pain/Fever Reducer" (generic version of Tylenol Suspension) Wal-Mart, Rite Aid, Walgreens	160mg/5ml	Acetaminophen	Children ages 2-3 (24-35 lb.), 5ml; 4-5 (36-47 lb.), 7.5ml; 6-8 (48-59 lb.), 10ml; 9-10 (60-71 lb.), 12.5ml; over 11 (72-95 lb.), 15ml, every 4 hrs., not more than 5 doses in 24 hrs.	120ml	$5.49	23¢ per tsp.
Myapap, Genapap, or "Pain & Fever" Reducer Drops(generic version of Tylenol) Wal-Mart, Rite Aid, Walgreens	80mg, 0.8ml	Acetaminophen	Children ages 2-3 (24-35 lb.), 1.6ml (2 droppers), every 4 hrs., not more than 5 doses in 24 hrs.	30ml	$7.29	39¢ per 1.6ml
Tylenol Children's Fever & Pain Reducer Chewable Tablets	80mg	Acetaminophen	Children ages 2-3 (24-35 lb.), 2 tabs; 4-5 (36-47 lb.), 3 tabs; 6-8 (48-59 lb.), 4 tabs; 9-10 (60-71 lb.), 5 tabs; over 11 (72-95 lb.), 6 tabs, every 4 hrs., not more than 5 doses in 24 hrs.	60	$5.49	18¢ per 2 tab dose
Tylenol Children's Fever & Pain Reducer Suspension	160mg/5ml	Acetaminophen	Children ages 2-3 (24-35 lb.), 5ml; 4-5 (36-47 lb.), 7.5ml; 6-8 (48-59 lb.), 10ml; 9-10 (60-71 lb.), 12.5ml; over 11 (72-95 lb.), 15ml, every 4 hrs., not more than 5 doses in 24 hrs.	120ml	$6.49	27¢ per tsp.
Tylenol Infants Concentrated Pain & Fever Reducer Drops Antacid, Tablets	80mg, 0.8ml	Acetaminophen	Children ages 2-3 (24-35 lb.), 1.6ml (2 droppers) every 4 hrs., not more than 5 doses in 24 hrs.	30ml	$8.49	45¢ per 1.6ml dose

$ SMART BUY
Children's Over-the-Counter Fever and Pain Relievers

For pain and fever, we recommend generic acetaminophen (Tylenol) liquid for children. Comparable store-brand or generic versions you may encounter could be "Genapap," "Fever/Pain Reducer," "Myapap," "Ty-Pap," or "Acetatabs." For infants (under age 2), concentrated drops are the more cost-effective and easier to administer. Give your child the dose that's appropriate for his or her weight.

CHILDREN'S GASTROINTESTINAL REMEDIES

Over-the-counter products for children generally target four areas of gastrointestinal upset—nausea (upset stomach), gas, diarrhea, and constipation.

CHILDREN'S PRODUCTS FOR UPSET STOMACH

Cola syrup is one of the more inexpensive and effective anti-nausea medications for both adults and children. Typically, 1 to 2 teaspoons over some chipped or crushed ice, sipped slowly, provides quick relief. Cola syrup does contain high amounts of sugars and is quite palatable for most children. An even less expensive option is to use a non-diet store-brand cola. Sipping small amounts can be a good substitute, especially in the middle of the night when the pharmacy is closed.

> ### ► Pepto-Bismol Caution
>
> Don't give Pepto-Bismol to your child if he or she is allergic to aspirin; might have chickenpox, cold, or influenza; or has a fever. Pepto-Bismol contains salicylates, the chemicals in aspirin. Aspirin has been linked to Reye's syndrome, a rare but serious and potentially fatal complication of certain viral infections (most notably chickenpox). Of the people who contract Reye's syndrome, 90 to 95 percent of them took some salicylate-type product prior to having a viral infection. About half of those who survive end up with some degree of permanent brain damage.

Children's Over-the-Counter Remedies for Upset Stomach (Nausea)

PRODUCT	STRENGTH PER DOSE (5ML =1TSP)	ACTIVE INGREDIENT	USUAL DOSAGE	TYPICAL QUANTITY	TYPICAL PRICE	COST PER DOSE
Coca Cola soft drink	N/A (trade secret)	N/A (trade secret)	Sip small amounts of room-temperature soft drink.	12oz	$5.49 for 12 cans or; 46¢ a can	0.64¢ per tsp.
Cola Syrup		High-fructose corn syrup, sucrose, water, caramel color, phosphoric acid, natural flavors, caffeine	Pour 1-2 tsp. over ice, sip slowly; may be repeated every 1-2 hrs., not more than 6 doses in 24 hrs.	4oz	$2.99	12¢ per tsp.
Emetrol Anti-Emetics for Nausea	1.87g, 1.87g, 21.5mg all per 5ml	Dextrose, levulose (fructose), phosphoric acid	Children ages 2-11, 5-10ml; over 12, 15-30ml; undiluted, not more than 1 hr. or 5 doses or as directed by physician.	118ml	$7.49	32¢ per tsp.
Gassy Gator Tummy Pops	9g, 1g	Sugars, calcium gylcinate chelate	Dissolve slowly in mouth (do not chew), not more than 8 pops in 24 hrs.	10	$3.49	35¢ each
Little Tummys Nausea Relief	1.87g, 1.87g 21.5mg	Dextrose, levulose (fructose), phosphoric acid, natural ginger extract	Children ages 2-11, 5-10ml; over 12, 15-30ml, about every 15 mins., undiluted, not more than 1 hr. or 5 doses, or as directed by physician.	150ml	$6.99	14¢ per tsp.
Maximum Strength Bismuth Liquid	525mg/15ml	Bismuth subsalicylate	Children ages 3-5, 5ml; 6-8, 10ml; 9-11, 15ml; over 12, 20ml, every 60 min. not more than 4 doses in 24 hrs.	360ml	$4.99	7¢ per tsp.
Mylanta Children's Upset Stomach Bubblegum Chew Tabs	400mg	Calcium carbonate	Children ages 2-4, 1 tab; 5-11, 2 tabs, not more than 3 times a day.	24	$4.99	21¢ per tab
"Nausea Relief" (generic version of Emetrol)		Dextrose, levulose (fructose), phosphoric acid	Children ages 2-11, 5-10ml; over 12, 15-30ml; undiluted, not more than 1 hr. or 5 doses or as directed by physician.	118ml	$6.49	28¢ per tsp.
Original Strength Bismuth Liquid	262mg/15ml	Bismuth subsalicylate	Children ages 3-5, 5ml; 6-8, 10ml; 9-11, 15ml; over 12, 20ml, every 30-60 min., not more than 8 doses in 24 hrs.	240ml	$3.39	7¢ per tsp.

PRODUCT	STRENGTH PER DOSE (5ML =1TSP)	ACTIVE INGREDIENT	USUAL DOSAGE	TYPICAL QUANTITY	TYPICAL PRICE	COST PER DOSE
Pepto-Bismol Maximum Strength Liquid	525mg/15ml	Bismuth subsalicylate	Children ages 3-5, 5ml; 6-8, 10ml; 9-11, 15ml; over 12, 20ml, every 60 min. not more than 4 doses in 24 hrs.	360ml	$6.69	9¢ per tsp.
Pepto-Bismol Original Liquid	262mg/15ml	Bismuth subsalicylate	Children ages 3-5, 5ml; 6-8, 10ml; 9-11, 15ml; over 12, 20ml, every 30-60 min., not more than 8 doses in 24 hrs.	480	$6.69	7¢ per tsp.
Store Brand Cola Soft Drink (generic version of Coca Cola)	N/A (trade secret)	N/A (trade secret)	Sip small amounts of room-temperature soft drink.	12oz	$2.99 for 12 cans or 25¢ a can	0.35¢ per tsp.
Titralac, Instant Relief Antacid, Tablets	420mg	Calcium carbonate	Take 2 tablets every 2-3 hrs. as needed, not more than 18 tabs in 24 hrs., not longer than 2 wks. at maximum dose.	100	$5.99	12¢ per 2 tabs

$ SMART BUY

Children's Over-the-Counter Remedies for Upset Stomach (Nausea)

If your child is vomiting, Emetrol is an effective product to help stop it; look for a generic product with a name that includes "Nausea Relief" or something similar. Another product with a formulation very close to Emetrol is Little Tummys Nausea Relief; this will save you about 13 percent over Emetrol. The soft-drink remedy we describe in Chapter 19 (sips of room-temperature, flat cola) works for children, too, and is, without question, the cheapest and safest option (although it might not be as effective once nausea has taken hold).

CHILDREN'S OVER-THE-COUNTER REMEDIES FOR GAS

Infants and children getting used to different foods (for example, when attending a new daycare or returning to school) often have problems with intestinal gas, which causes cramping and discomfort. The safest and most effective over-the-counter products to give to your child to relieve the discomfort of gas contain simethicone. Buy generic for considerable savings. Children, especially younger ones, generally do better with liquids.

Children's Over-the-Counter Remedies for Gas

PRODUCT	STRENGTH PER DOSE (5ML =1TSP)	ACTIVE INGREDIENT	USUAL DOSAGE	TYPICAL QUANTITY	TYPICAL PRICE	COST PER DOSE
Gerber Gas Drops	20mg/0.3ml	Simethicone	Children under age 2 (less than 24 lb.), 0.3ml; 2 & older (over 24 lb.), 0.6ml, as needed after meals and bedtime, not more than 12 doses in 24 hrs.	30ml	$13.79	28¢ per 0.6ml
Infant "Gas Relief" Drops, Walgreens, Rite Aid, Wal-Mart	20mg/0.3ml	Simethicone	Children under age 2 (less than 24 lb.), 0.3ml; 2 & older (over 24 lb.), 0.6ml, as needed after meals and bedtime, not more than 12 doses in 24 hrs.	30ml	$5.99	12¢ per 0.6ml
Little Tummy's Gas for Infants & Children	20mg/0.3ml	Simethicone	Children under age 2 (less than 24 lb.), 0.3ml; 2 & older (over 24 lb.), 0.6ml, as needed after meals and bedtime, not more than 12 doses in 24 hrs.	30ml	$6.49	13¢ per 0.6ml
Mylicon Infant Gas Relief Drops	20mg/0.3ml	Simethicone	Children under age 2 (less than 24 lb.), 0.3ml; 2 and older (over 24 lb.), 0.6ml, as needed after meals and bedtime, not more than 12 doses in 24 hrs.	30ml	$12.49	25¢ per 0.6ml

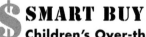

$ SMART BUY
Children's Over-the-Counter Remedies for Gas

To relieve the discomfort of intestinal gas, use a generic simethicone product. Liquid forms usually are easier for children to take. Your Smart Buy is a generic version of simethicone drops, which sells for about $5 for a 1-ounce bottle, compared to about $12 for the same amount of name-brand Mylanta Gas Drops. You'll most likely find the generic version of Infant's Gas Relief on the store shelf to the right of Mylicon Infant Gas Relief, which will save you about 52 percent over the name brand.

CHILDREN'S OVER-THE-COUNTER PRODUCTS FOR DIARRHEA

Diarrhea is a nuisance at best; at worst, it can indicate a medical problem your child's doctor should evaluate and treat. Diarrhea in children under age 2 is especially danger-ous; young children can become dehydrated quickly. Often it's best to contact your child's doctor before treating for diarrhea, particularly if your child is age 2 or younger.

Two kinds of products are available to treat diarrhea in children—Kaopectate (con-taining attapulgite) and Imodium (containing loperamide). Both come in various generic and store-brand versions that will be much less expensive than the name brand.

Do not give any antidiarrheal product to a child who has a temperature over 101 degrees, blood or mucous in the stool, or for longer than two days. If your child is age 2 or under, or your child's diarrhea persists longer than two days, contact your pedia-trician. It's also important for a child with diarrhea to drink plenty of liquids to help

Children's Over-the-Counter Remedies for Diarrhea

PRODUCT	STRENGTH PER DOSE (5ML =1TSP)	ACTIVE INGREDIENT	USUAL DOSAGE	TYPICAL QUANTITY	TYPICAL PRICE	COST PER DOSE
Anti-diarrheal Liquid, Wal-Mart, Walgreens (generic version of Imodium A-D Liquid)	1mg/5ml	Loperamide	Children ages 6-8 (48-59 lb.), 10ml to start, then 5ml after each loose bowel movement, up to 4 doses in 24 hrs., not longer than 2 days; ages 9-11 (60-95 lb.), 10ml to start, then 5ml after each loose bowel movement, up to 6 doses in 24 hrs, not longer than 2 days; over age 12, 20ml to start then 10ml after each loose bowel movement, up to 8 doses in 24 hrs., not longer than 2 days.	120ml	$5.99	25¢ per tsp.
Imodium A-D Anti-diarrheal Liquid	1mg/5ml	Loperamide	Children ages 6-8 (48-59 lb.), 10ml to start, then 5ml after each loose bowel movement, up to 4 doses in 24 hrs., not longer than 2 days; ages 9-11 (60-95 lb.), 10ml to start, then 5ml after each loose bowel movement, up to 6 doses in 24 hrs, not longer than 2 days; over age 12, 20ml to start then 10ml after each loose bowel movement, up to 8 doses in 24 hrs., not longer than 2 days.	120ml	$7.99	33¢ per tsp.

PRODUCT	STRENGTH PER DOSE (5ML =1TSP)	ACTIVE INGREDIENT	USUAL DOSAGE	TYPICAL QUANTITY	TYPICAL PRICE	COST PER DOSE
Kaopectate Children's Cherry Liquid	300mg/15ml	Attapulgite	Children ages 3-5, 7.5ml; ages 6-11, 15ml; over age 12, 30ml, not more than 7 doses in 24 hrs.	172ml	$6.79	20¢ per tsp.
Maximum Strength Bismuth Liquid	525mg/15ml	Bismuth subsalicylate	Children ages 3-5, 5ml; ages 6-8, 10ml; ages 9-11, 15ml; over age 12, 20ml, every 60 min., not more than 4 doses in 24 hrs.	360ml	$4.99	7¢ per tsp.
Original Strength Bismuth Liquid	262mg/15ml	Bismuth subsalicylate	Children ages 3-5, 5ml; ages 6-8, 10ml; ages 9-11, 15ml; over 12, 20ml, every 30-60 min., not more than 8 doses in 24 hrs.	240ml	$3.39	7¢ per tsp.
Pepto-Bismol Maximum Strength Liquid	525mg/15ml	Bismuth subsalicylate	Children ages 3-5, 5ml; ages 6-8, 10ml; ages 9-11, 15ml; over age 12, 20ml, every 60 min., not more than 4 doses in 24 hrs.	360ml	$6.69	9¢ per tsp.
Pepto-Bismol Original Liquid	262mg/15ml	Bismuth subsalicylate	Children ages 3-5, 5ml; ages 6-8, 10ml; ages 9-11, 15ml; over age 12, 20ml, every 30-60 min., not more than 8 doses in 24 hrs.	480	$6.69	7¢ per tsp.

replace the fluids lost through the diarrhea to prevent dehydration. Unless your child's doctor instructs you otherwise, give your child only water to drink.

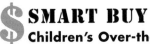 SMART BUY
Children's Over-the-Counter Remedies for Diarrhea

The Imodium A-D kinds of products generally are most effective and require the fewest doses to remedy the problem. Buying a generic version will save you around 8 cents a teaspoon, or about 24 percent. Look for a label that says something like "Anti-Diarrheal Liquid."

ELECTROLYTE REPLACEMENT PRODUCTS

Electrolyte replacement products help restore vital chemicals and fluid if your child has had diarrhea or vomiting, or becomes dehydrated. Products come in many generics and flavors, including freezer pops. Premixed electrolyte products (already liquid) are good for only 48 hours after you open them. After that, they begin to deteriorate. Write the date and time you opened the container on the label. Put the lid back on tightly and store it in the refrigerator. Try to get your child to drink 1 or 2 bottles of electrolyte liquid (or eat 1 or 2 electrolyte freezer pops) every 24 hours, until the child is back to his or her usual eating and drinking habits. Sports drinks aren't a good choice for electrolyte replacement; they contain large quantities of sugar, which can cause other digestive problems.

Children's Over-the-Counter Electrolyte Replacement Products

PRODUCT	STRENGTH PER DOSE	ACTIVE INGREDIENT	USUAL DOSAGE	TYPICAL QUANTITY	TYPICAL PRICE	COST PER DOSE
Infantlyte or Pediatric "Electrolyte" Oral Maintenance Solution	45mEq, 20mEq, 35mEq, 30mEq, 20g, 5g per 1,000ml of solution	Sodium, potassium chloride, citrate, dextrose, fructose, water	Children age 2 and older, offer solution every 3-4 hrs., 1,000-2,000ml per day while diarrhea continues.	1,000ml	$3.99	$3.99 per 1,000ml
Kaolectrolyte Electrolyte Replenisher	48mEq, 20mEq, 40mEq, 28mEq, 20g per 960ml of solution	Sodium, potassium chloride, citrate, dextrose, fructose, water	Children age 2 and older, offer solution every 3-4 hrs., 1,000-2,000ml per day while diarrhea continues.	32oz (in 4 pkts)	$4.99	$5.20 per 1,000ml
Pedialyte Flavored Liquid	$5.20 per 1,000ml 35mEq, 30mEq,20g, 5g per 1,000 ml of solution	Sodium, potassium chloride, citrate, dextrose, fructose, water	Children age 2 and older, offer solution every 3-4 hrs., 1,000-2,000ml per day while diarrhea continues.	1,000ml	$6.49	$6.49 per 1,000ml
Pedialyte Freezer Pops Assorted Flavors 20g, 5g per	45mEq, 20mEq, 35mEq, 30mEq, 1,000 ml of solution	Sodium, potassium, chloride, citrate, dextrose, fructose, water	Children age 2 and older, offer solution every 3-4 hrs.1,000-2,000ml per day while diarrhea continues.	16 pops, 1,000ml of solution	$6.49	$6.49 per 1,000ml
Revital Oral Electrolyte Jell Cups	45mEq 20mEq 35mEq 30mEq 25g per 1,000ml of gel	Sodium, potassium chloride, citrate, dextrose, fructose, water	Children age 1 and older, offer as often as desired.	20oz (4 5oz cups)	$5.99	$10 per 1,000ml

$ SMART BUY
Children's Over-the-Counter Electrolyte Replacement Products

A generic product is your Smart Buy in this category. Look for "-lyte" in the product's name. Stay with simple electrolyte solutions for best results. Don't substitute these types of products with sports drinks, which contain lots of sugars that may upset your child's stomach. The generic equivalent of Pedialyte will save you about 38 percent over the name-brand products. You want to get about 1,000ml of solution into your child over the course of a day.

If experience tells you that's unlikely to happen, consider using Kaolectrolyte individual packets. This product comes in 8-ounce containers (about 240ml) and helps reduce waste, saving your money. (In case you don't read labels, most electrolyte products require refrigeration. Note the date and time you open them; most should be destroyed 48 hours after opening.) If your child will drink only 8 ounces a day (about 240ml), you'll have to throw out a half-full container: Your cost just doubled. So even if you purchased a generic equivalent of Pedialyte for $3.99 per 1,000ml, your cost would increase to about $8 per 1,000ml. In this instance only, you'll be better off purchasing individual packets of Kaolectrolyte, at about $5 per 1,000ml.

CHILDREN'S OVER-THE-COUNTER PRODUCTS FOR CONSTIPATION

Constipation can be chronic or temporary. For an occasional bout, you may use either a stimulant laxative, such as Fletcher's Castoria, or a glycerine suppository. If constipation is a chronic problem, make sure your child drinks lots of liquids and eats foods high in fiber (such as raw fruits and vegetables and whole grains). Routinely using stimulant laxatives (such as Fletcher's Castoria or Senokot) or enemas will set up a dependence situation in which your child's colon won't function properly on its own, so use these products sparingly. For a child age 2 or under, check with the doctor before giving any products to treat constipation.

$ SMART BUY
Children's Over-the-Counter Products for Constipation

Fleet's Babylax glycerin suppositories are a Smart Buy, at about 70 cents a dose, although you should give no more than 1 dose unless your child's doctor instructs you otherwise. Children 6 years of age and older who have chronic constipation problems can take a generic version of Metamucil, a bulk-forming laxative that's gentle on the system. Look for labels that say "Natural Vegetable Laxative" or "Natural Fiber Laxative" to identify generic versions. Don't use Senokot and other stimulant laxatives unless your child's

Children's Over-the-Counter Remedies for Constipation

PRODUCT	STRENGTH PER DOSE (5ML=1TSP.)	ACTIVE INGREDIENT	USUAL DOSAGE	TYPICAL QUANTITY	TYPICAL PRICE	COST PER DOSE
Colace -50 Stool Softener	50mg	Docusate sodium	Children ages 6-11, 1-2 capsules a day; age 12 years and older, 1-4 capsules a day.	60	$17.99	30¢ each
Fleet's Babylax Glycerin Rectal Suppositories	Glycerin USP	Glycerin	Children ages 2-5, 1 suppository, or as directed by physician.	6 suppos-itories	$5.29	88¢ each
Fleet's Children's Enema per enema	9.5g, 3.5g	Monobasic sodium phosphate, dibasic sodium phosphate	Children ages 2-11, 1 enema, or as directed by physician.	66ml (1 enema)	$1.99	$1.99 each
Fleet's Glycerin Laxative Rectal Applicators	Glycerin USP	Glycerin	Children over age 6, 1 suppository or as directed by physician.	4 suppos-itories	$4.99	$1.25 each
Fletcher's Castoria	166.5mg/5ml	Senna concentrate	Children ages 2-5, 5-10ml; 6-15, 10-15ml, not more than twice a day.	75ml	; 6.49	43¢ per tsp.
Natural Fiber Laxative (generic version of Metamucil), 114 doses	3g/5ml	Psyllium seed	Children ages 6-11, 1/2 rounded tsp. in 8oz liquid 3 times a day.	30oz	$7.79	7¢ per dose
Senokot Children's Natural Laxative Liquid Syrup	8.8mg/5ml	Purified senna	Children ages 2-5, 2.5 to 3.75ml; 6-12, 5-7.5ml, not more than twice a day.	74ml	7.49	51¢ per tsp.

doctor instructs you to, and then only for a limited time. Consult your child's doctor before giving your child any laxative product on a regular basis.

Consult Your Doctor for Eye, Ear, Nose, and Mouth Problems

Don't use adult products for problems involving your child's eyes, ears, nose, or mouth unless your child's pediatrician specifically instructs you to. If your child has a problem, have the doctor give you an accurate diagnosis. Many eye, ear, nose, and mouth problems in children are infections you'll need prescription medications to treat.

CHILDREN'S OVER-THE-COUNTER PRODUCTS FOR DIAPER RASH

Many babies get diaper rash, an irritation of the skin in the diaper area. The best treatment, of course, is prevention: Keep your baby clean and dry. When diaper rash appears to be the problem, it's still a good idea to have the doctor make sure it's not something more serious (and always take your child to the doctor if the rash has open sores or is bleeding). If it's just diaper rash, you'll find a number of products available to ease your little one's discomfort.

Children's Over-the-Counter Products for Diaper Rash

PRODUCT	STRENGTH PER DOSE	ACTIVE INGREDIENT	USUAL DOSAGE	TYPICAL QUANTITY	TYPICAL PRICE	COST PER 30 GRAMS
A & D Original Diaper Rash Ointment	53.4%, 15.5%	Petrolatum, lanolin	Apply as often as necessary.	113g	$5.29	$1.40
A & D Original Diaper Rash Ointment	53.4%, 15.5%	Petrolatum, lanolin	Apply as often as necessary.	454g	$11.19	74¢
Boudreaux's Butt Paste, Diaper Rash Ointment	16%	Zinc oxide	Apply as often as necessary.	113g	$8.49	$2.25
Desitin Diaper Rash Ointment	40%	Zinc oxide	Apply as often as necessary.	454g	$13.99	93¢
Desitin Ultra Smooth Cream Formula Diaper Rash Ointment	10%	Zinc oxide	Apply as often as necessary.	57g	$3.99	$2.10
Gold Bond Medicated Baby Powder		Zinc oxide, talc	Apply as often as necessary.	283g	$8.29	88¢
Gold Bond Medicated Baby Powder, Cornstarch Plus		Cornstarch, zinc oxide, kaolin	Apply as often as necessary.	113g	$4.99	$1.32
Vitamin A & D Ointment	53.4%, 15.5%	Petrolatum, lanolin	Apply as often as necessary.	120g	$3.99	$1
Zinc Oxide Ointment	40%	Zinc oxide	Apply as often as necessary.	454g	$9.99	66¢

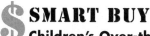 SMART BUY
Children's Over-the-Counter Products for Diaper Rash

The most inexpensive, and often the most effective, product here is a 1-pound jar of zinc oxide ointment. This has the same active ingredient as in Desitin Diaper Rash Ointment; purchasing the generic equivalent will save you 33 percent. However, with most skin-care products, a process of trial and error may be necessary before you find the right one. Start with the most cost-effective products first, such as a simple zinc oxide ointment or a vitamin A and D ointment. If those don't work for your child, try other products. (And see the sidebar for Pharmacist Rick's Diaper Rash Remedy!)

▶ Pharmacist Rick's Diaper Rash Remedy

Pharmacist Rick says, "When my son was an infant, he had horrible diaper rash. We tried everything under the sun, from over-the-counter products to all the prescription products the dermatologist suggested. We changed his diapers so often he was rarely wet, but he still had an inflamed rash. Finally the dermatologist said, 'I know this is going to sound weird, but go to the grocery store and look for a product called Saffola in the cooking section.' As it turns out, Saffola is a safflower cooking oil that's highest in polyunsaturated fats and termed a 'drying oil.' After just two days of treatment with Saffola, my son's rash was completely gone! Over the years, I've been somewhat reluctant to recommend this treatment, because it sounds, in the words of my son's dermatologist, weird. But when people do try it, they find that it works—and not just for diaper rash. It can be effective to treat the itching and scaling of eczema and psoriasis, too."

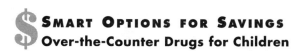 SMART OPTIONS FOR SAVINGS
Over-the-Counter Drugs for Children

Buying over-the-counter drugs for children is no different than buying them for yourself in terms of the ways you can find the Smart Buys and best savings. Overall, our

Smart Options for Savings on over-the-counter drugs for children include the following tips:

1. Check the prices of store brands and generic versions in your local area. These will vary depending on where you live. And watch for sales and store specials. Sometimes it's worthwhile to buy a product on sale, when you know it's something your child will need soon enough, such as a pain reliever.

2. Watch for manufacturer's coupons in magazines and advertising inserts. A savings great enough can make a name-brand product less expensive than a generic version.

3. If you're buying to stock up, rather than rushing to the store because your child is sick, check prices through mail-order and Internet pharmacies (including those in Canada; see Chapter 4, "Saving on Drugs Across the Border," for precautions).

4. If you live near the Canadian border or plan a trip to Canada, plan to pick up products you know you're likely to need. Make a list of what you need and what you'd pay for the products through your usual purchasing sources, so you'll know whether the Canadian price is a good deal. And remember to factor in the currency exchange rate!

5. When treating cold, flu, cough, and allergy symptoms, buy single-ingredient products so you can give just the medication your child needs for specific symptoms.

And remember to check our Web site at www.smartbuysdrugwise.com for the latest information about more ways to save money on these drugs.

4-Way Cold Tablets, 316
5-HT3 receptor antagonists, 265
29-gauge syringes, 423

A
A/T/S, 281
AARP (American Association of Retired Persons) pharmacy, 33–34, 36, 56
Abbott, patient assistance program, 52
abdominal contractions, 263
Abreva, 398–399
absorption into the skin, 290
acarbose, 173
Accolate, 201, 203
Accu-Chek, 428
Accutane, 281
ACE inhibitors, 137, 143
acetaminophen
    as over-the-counter analgesic, 341, 346–350
    conditions and symptoms relieved by, 122, 326, 398, 428
    for children, 466–467, 474–477
    in combination products, 325
    in narcotics, 246–247
    in sleep aids, 434
Acetatabs, 477
acetazolamide, 270
acetohexamide, 171
acetylcholine, 233
acetylsalicylic acid, 342
Aciphex, 260
acne, 280–283, 418–420

acteylcholine-blocking drugs, 229–230
Actifed, 298
Actonel, 169
Actos, 172
Acular, 274
acupressure-type wristbands, 438
acyclovir, 284–285
AD, 19
ADA (American Dental Association), 393
ADD (attention deficit disorder), 234–238
Adderall, 234–235
adult onset (type 2) diabetes, 171
advertising, 4–5, 9–10, 30, 310–311. See also marketing strategies by pharmaceutical companies
Advil, 244, 298, 307, 316, 350, 430
AeroBid, 198
Afrin, 298, 320, 322–323
aggression, 234
aging, effects of drugs on, 22–24
agranulocytosis, 223
akathisia, 222–223
Albalon, 276
albuterol, 195–197, 203
alcohol (beverage), 173, 264, 326–327, 347, 352
alcohol (medicine), 392
alendronate, 168–169
Aleve, 298

Ali, Muhammad, 239
Alka Seltzer, 316
Allegra, 204–206
Aller-Chlor, 462
Allerest, 316–317
allergic reactions, 111, 115, 351, 354
allergies, 20–21, 117, 204–207, 275
allergy eye products, 386–387
allergy preparations
    analgesics. See pain medications
    antihistamines. See antihistamines
    antitussives and expectorants, 330–334
    categories of, 315–316
    combination products, 325–330
    cough drops and throat lozenges, 334–336
    decongestants, 317–323, 325
    for children, 461–474
    gum with aspirin, 336–337
    vitamin C (ascorbic acid), 337–338
allopurinol, 181–182
almotriptan, 255
Alomide, 275
alpha-blockers, 137, 143–144
Alphagan, 270
alprazolam, 209–210
alprostadil, 189
Alrex, 274
Alternagel, 360
Alu-Drox, 364

Alu-Hydrox, 364

Alu-Mag, 364

aluminum, 184

aluminum hydroxide antacids, 360

aluminum-magnesium combination products, 364

aluminum/magnesium suspension, 336

Alupent, 195–196

Alzheimer's disease, 233–234, 360

AMA (American Medical Association), 147

amantadine, 230

Amaryl, 171

Ambien, 210, 213

Americaine, 406

American Academy of Pediatrics, Committee on Infectious Diseases, 342

American Association of Retired Persons (AARP) pharmacy, 33–34, 36, 56

American Dental Association (ADA), 393

American Diabetes Association, 171, 173

American Medical Association (AMA), 147

amitriptyline, 215, 250, 254, 265

ammonium chloride, 184, 428

amoxicillin, 90, 102, 105–106, 108

amphetamines, 234

ampicillin, 105–106, 260

Anacin, 346

Anafranil, 215

analgesics. See pain medications

anaphylactic shock, 342

Androderm, 168

androgens, 167–168

Android, 168

anemia, 226

anesthetic products, 393–397

angina, 126–130

angiotensin II receptor antagonists, 137, 143

animal bites, 102

anisindione, 343

Ansaid, 240

Antacid EX Tablets, 362

Antacid M Liquid, 365

antacids, 184, 259, 261, 359–365, 380

antazoline, 386

anthrax, 113

Anti-Diarrheal Liquid, 482

Anti-inflammatory drugs, 240–246, 265–268

antianxiety drugs, 209–213

antibacterial products, 393–397

antibiotic ointment, 412

antibiotics
choosing, 116–117
effects on viruses, 90
families of, 105–116
how long to take, 94
prescriptions for, 74
pricing of, 94–102, 107, 109–111, 113–114
resistance to, 89–90
side effects of, 21, 103–105, 150
See also infections

anticholinergic drugs, 230

anticoagulants (blood thinners), 119–122, 343

antidepressants, 213–222, 250–251, 264–265

antidiarrheals, 369–372

antiemetic products, 367–369

antifungal products, 407–410

antihistamines
dangers of, 299
for children, 462–463, 466
oral, 323–325, 386
pricing of, 303
side effects of, 75
symptoms and conditions

relieved by, 204–206, 258, 275, 302, 436–438
when to buy, 326

antipsychotic drugs, 222–226

antiseizure drugs, 226–229

antitussives, 330–334

antivertigo treatments, 436–438

antiviral drugs, 284

Anusol-HC, 441

anxiety, 209–213

apple juice, 264

aqueous humor, 269–270

Arava, 245–246

Aricept, 233–234

Armour Thyroid, 177

arrythmias, 122, 124–127, 130–136

Artane, 230, 232

arthritis, 240–246, 450–455

Arthritis Foundation, 316

arthritis strength products, 348–349

Arthropan, 343

artificial tears, 386–390

AS, 19

Asacol, 265–266

ascorbic acid (vitamin C), 184, 337–338

Ascriptin, 344

Aspercreme, 354

Aspergum, 336–337

aspirin, 20–21, 121–122, 181, 336–337, 342–346, 466

aspirin powder, 289

assistance services, 54–55

asthma, 143, 193–204

atenolol, 136, 143

athlete's foot, 286–287, 407

Ativan, 209–210, 213

atorvastatin, 150

atria, 122

Atrovent, 200, 203

attapulgite, 481

attention deficit disorder (ADD), 234–238

atypical antipsychotics, 222–223
AU, 19
Augmentin, 90, 102, 104
Avandia, 171
Avelox, 104, 110–111
Awake tablets, 436
Axert, 255
Axid, 258, 298, 365
Azmacort, 198
Azo-Gesic, 455–456
Azo-Standard, 455–456
Azopt, 270
Azulfidine, 265–266

B
baby aspirin, 344
Babylax glycerin suppositories, 484
bacitracin, 276, 412
bacitracin zinc, 410
baclofen, 251
bacteria, 89–92, 257, 276–277
bacterial infections, 283–286, 332, 335–336
Bactrim, 105, 114–115, 188
Bactroban, 284–285
Bag Balm, 400–401
balms, 355, 414
bananas, 144–145, 264
bat bites, 102
baths, 263, 401, 441
Baycol, 114, 150
Bayer, 346
Bayer Children's Cough Syrup, 316
Bayer Corporation Pharmaceutical Division, patient assistant program, 52
Bayer Select Backache Pain Formula, 343
Bayer Select Pain Relief, 316
BD (Becton-Dickenson), 423–424, 427–428
beans, 264

beclomethasone, 198
Beclovent, 198
Becton-Dickenson (BD), 423–424, 427–428
belladonna alkaloids, 263–264
Bellergal-S, 263
Ben-Gay, 354, 356
Benadryl
    as antihistamine, 323–325
    as cough suppressant, 330
    as sleep aid, 432, 434
    effects on the stomach, 258
    over-the-counter status, 298
Benahist, 463
Bentyl, 264, 267
Benzamycin, 281, 283
benzocaine, 335, 395–396
benzodiazepines, 209–210
benzonatate, 206
benzophenones, 413–414
benzoyl peroxide, 281, 418–420
benztropine, 230
beta agonists, 193, 195–197, 203–204
beta-blockers, 133–137
beta-receptors, 133–134
Betagan, 270, 273
betaxolol, 270
bethanechol, 187
Betoptic, 270
Biaxin, 102, 113
bicarbonate, 183–184
biguanides, 171–172
bile acid sequestrants, 148–149
biphasic oral contraceptives, 156, 159
bipolar disorder, 222
birth control pills. *See* oral contraceptives
bisacodyl, 377
bismuth subsalicylate, 369
bites, 102
blackened skin burns, 286
bladder, 184
bladder infections, 102, 187

bleeding, breakthrough, 156
blindness, 170
blistered burns, 286
blisters, 398, 414
blood cholesterol, 147–154
blood glucose monitors, 424–426
blood tests, 69
blood thinners (anticoagulants), 119–122, 343
blood vessels, 171
Boehringer-Ingelheim Pharmaceuticals, patient assistance program, 52
bone loss, 161–162, 168–170
bowel movements, 377, 441
bradykinesia, 222–223
brand loyalty, 310–311
breakthrough bleeding, 156
breast cancer, 163, 167
breast infections, 102
brick-and-mortar pharmacies, 29
brimonidine, 270
brinzolamide, 270
Bristol-Myers Squibb, patient assistance program, 52
broccoli, 264
Bromaline, 465
Bromanate, 465
Bromatap, 464, 474
bromocriptine, 230
Bromotap Elixir, 316
Bromphen Liquid, 465
brompheniramine, 323
bronchitis, 102
budesonide, 198–199
Buf Puf, 418
buffered aspirin, 344
Bufferin, 344
bulb syringes, 392–393
bulk-forming laxatives, 372–375
bulk purchases, over-the-counter drugs, 307–308, 344

bupropion, 217
burns, 286, 406–407
Buspar, 114, 209–210, 213
buspirone, 209
butoconazole nitrate, 430

C
cabbage, 264
caffeine
    amplification of side effects
        by, 201
    as diuretic, 331
    benefits of removing from
        diet, 264
    consuming with fluoro-
        quinolones, 111
    food and drinks containing,
        436
    in pain relievers, 428
    in stimulants, 435–436
calcium, 169–170, 183, 362, 373
calcium carbonate, 360–362,
    366
calcium channel blockers,
    130–133, 137
California, pharmaceutical
    assistance programs in, 57
camphor, 334
Canada, buying drugs in, 37–49
Canadameds.com, 44
Canadarx.com, 44
Canadianmedusa.com, 44
cancer, 163, 167–168
canned diet, 439
Capsagesic-HP rub, 356
capsaicin, 354–356
capsules, splitting, 79
Carafate, 76, 261
carbachol, 269–270
carbamazepine, 226–227
carbidopa, 230, 233
carbonated beverages, 264, 331,
    368–369, 428
carboxymethylcellulose
    sodium, 387

Cardizem CD, 130
Cardura, 143–144, 191
carisoprodol, 251
Carmex, 399
carteolol, 270
cartilage, 451
casanthranol, 379
cat bites, 102
Catapress, 234–235
cats, giving acetaminophen to,
    347
Caverject, 189
cavities, 216
CDC (Centers for Disease
    Control), 342
Ceclor, 108
Cedax, 104, 108
cefaclor, 108
cefadroxil, 108
cefdinir, 108
cefpodoxime, 108
cefprozil, 108
ceftibuten, 108
Ceftin, 102, 108
cefuroxime, 108
Cefzil, 108
Celebrex, 17, 240, 241, 244
celecoxib, 240
Celexa, 17, 216, 222
cellophane wrap, 290
Center for Drug Evaluation
    and Research, 17
Centers for Disease Control
    (CDC), 342
central nervous system condi-
    tions
    Alzheimer's disease, 233–234
    anxiety, 209–213
    depression, 213–222
    insomnia, 209–213
    Parkinson's disease, 222,
        229–233
    psychotic disorders, 222–226
    seizure disorders, 226–229
cephalexin, 108, 110

cephalosporins, 105–106,
    108–110
cephradine, 108
Cerebryx, prescription errors
    with, 17
Cetaphil, 418, 420
cetirizine, 204
Cheracol Plus Syrup, 316
Chewable Calcium Extra-
    Strength Tabs, 362
CHF (congestive heart failure),
    122–123, 183
chickenpox, 342
child-resistant packaging, 344
children
    applying steroids to, 290
    attention deficit disorder
        (ADD), treatments for,
        234–238
    diaper rashes, 286–287
    giving acetaminophen to, 347
    giving aspirin to, 342
    measuring dosages for,
        459–460
    over-the-counter products
        for
        cough, cold, flu, and
            allergy products,
            461–474
        diaper rashes, 486–487
        gastrointestinal remedies,
            477–485
        pain medications, 467–468,
            474–477
Children's Allerest Tablets, 317
Chlor-Trimeton, 323, 325, 330,
    462
Chloraseptic Throat Lozenges,
    336
chlordiazepoxide, 209, 264
chlorpheniramine, 323, 463
chlorpromazine, 222
chlorpropamide, 171
Chlortabs, 462
chlorzoxazone, 251

chocolate, 264

cholesterol, 147–154, 162, 172

cholestyramine, 149

cholestyramine powder, 264–264, 268

choline salicylate, 343

cholinesterase inhibitors, 233

chondroitin, 450–453

cigarette smoking, cessation products, 446–450

Cigna Tel–Drug, 34

Ciloxin, 276, 280

Ciloxin eye drops, 102

cimetidine, 201, 258–259

cinnamates, 414

cinoxate, 414

Cipro, 104–105, 110–111, 115, 188

Cipro HC ear drops, 102

ciprofloxacin, 110, 188, 276

citalopram, 216

Citrucel, 372–373

Claritin, 76, 204–206

clavulanic acid, 106

Clear, 444

Clearasil, 280, 420

clemestine, 323

Cleocin, 281

clidinium, 264

Climara, 163

clindamycin, 105, 281

Clinoril, 76, 240

clomipramine, 215

clonidine, 234

clopidogrel, 121, 343

clorazepate, 209

clotrimazole, 408, 410, 430

clove oil, 354, 396–397

cloxacillin, 105

clozapine, 223

Clozaril, 223

Co–Benemid, 182

co–pay, 84

coal tar, 288–289

Coca-Cola, 368–369

codeine, 21, 206, 246, 255

coffee, 331, 428

Cogentin, 230

Cognex, 233–234

cola, 260, 264, 331, 368–369, 428

cola syrup, 477

Colace, 372, 376

colchicine, 181

cold preparations
    analgesics. See pain medications
    antihistamines. See antihistamines
    antitussives and expectorants, 330–334
    categories of, 315–316
    combination products, 325–330
    cough drops and throat lozenges, 334–336
    decongestants, 317–323, 325
    for children, 461–474
    gum with aspirin, 336–337
    vitamin C (ascorbic acid), 337–338

cold sores, 284, 398–399

colds, 90–92

colitis, ulcerative, 265–268

colon, 377

combination products, 302–305, 325–330, 471–474

Combivent, 203

comedogenic cosmetics, 418

Committee on Infectious Diseases, American Academy of Pediatrics, 342

Compound W, 416

Compoz, 432

Comtrex, 316

Comtrex Liquid, 317

Comtrex Tablets and Caplets, 317

Conar-A Tablets, 317

Concerta, 234, 237–238

conditioner, 445

Congesprin Cold Tablets for Children, 317

congestion in eyes, 276–279

congestive heart failure (CHF), 122–123, 183

conjugated estrogens, 162

Connecticut Pharmaceutical Assistance Contract to the Elderly and Disabled (ConnPACE), 57

ConnPACE (Connecticut Pharmaceutical Assistance Contract to the Elderly and Disabled), 57

constipation, 247, 264–265, 372–380, 441, 484–486

Contac, 317

contact lenses, 277, 384

contractions, abdominal, 263

controlled substances, 74

cooking oil, 487

Cordarone, 122

Coreg, 81

Coricidin, 317

Cornhusker's Lotion, 400

corpus cavernosum, 189

Correctol, 377

Cortaid, 77, 298

Cortisporin, 97

cosmetics, 418

Cosopt, 270, 273

costs of prescription drugs. See pricing of over-the-counter drugs; pricing of prescription drugs

cough, 143, 196

cough drops, 334–336

cough preparations
    analgesics. See pain medications
    antihistamines. See antihistamines
    antitussives and expectorants, 330–334
    categories of, 315–316

combination products,
325–330
cough drops and throat
lozenges, 334–336
decongestants, 317–323, 325
for children, 461–474
gum with aspirin, 336–337
narcotics in, 206
vitamin C (ascorbic acid),
337–338
cough suppressants, 330–334,
468–470
Coumadin, 343
counterirritants, 354
coupons, 309–311
Covera, 122
COX-1 and -2 inhibitors, 241
Cozaar, 137
creams, 288, 293, 355, 431, 443
credit card transactions over
the Internet, 32–33
Crisco, 401
Crohn's disease, 265–268
cromolyn, 200, 275, 279
Crossborderpharmacy.com,
44–45
cultures, 117
Curel, 400
currency exchange, 41
cutting tablets, 78–84
CVS.com, 31, 34
cyanocobalamin, 260
cyclo-oxygenase (COX)
inhibitors, 241
cyclobenzaprine, 23, 251
cyclosporine, 114–115
Cylert, 234, 238
Cystex, 455
cystitis, 187
Cytotec, 261

D
dairy products, 112, 264
Dalmane, 210

dalteparin, 343
Darvocet, 246–247
Darvon, 246–247, 250
Daypro, 240, 244
Debrox, 392
decongestant eye products,
384–386
decongestants, 206, 214,
317–323, 325, 464–466
Delaware Prescription Drug
Assistance Program, 57
Delsym, 331
Demerol, 246, 246–247, 255
Denavir, 284–285
Depakene, 226
Depakote, 226
depression, 213–222
Dermoplast, 406
Desenex, 410
desipramine, 215, 251, 265
Desitin Diaper Rash Ointment,
487
Desyrel, 217
Detrol, 185, 187
Dexedrine, 234–235, 237
dextroamphetamine, 234
dextromethorphan, 326,
331–332, 468
Diabeta, 171
diabetes, 102, 170–176,
421–428
Diabinese, 22, 171
Diamox, 270
diaper rash, 286–287
diaper rashes, 486–487
diarrhea, 264–265, 369–371,
377, 480–482
diazepam, 209–210, 227
DiBromm, 464–465, 474
diclofenac, 241, 274
dicloxacillin, 96, 102, 105–106
Dicumerol, 343
dicyclomine, 23, 264
diet aids, 438–439

Diflucan, 76
diflunisal, 240
digitalis. See digoxin
digoxin, 17, 114, 122–124, 144
Dilantin, 226–227
Dilaudid, 246–247
diltiazem, 143
dimenhydrinate, 437
Dimetapp, 298, 317, 323,
464–466
Dimetapp Liquid, 473–474
dimethyl sulfoxide (DMSO),
451–452
Dipentum, 266, 268
Diphen, 463
diphenhydramine
as antihistamine, 323, 325
as cough suppressant, 330
as sore throat treatment, 336
buying in bulk, 307
in sleep aids, 432, 434
strength of, 466
dipivefrin, 270
dipyridamole, 121
"direct-to-consumer" advertising, 9–10
Discount Prescription Medication Program, 57
disease-modifying
antirheumatic drugs
(DMARDs), 240, 245
disopyramide, 114
Ditropan, 185, 187
diuretics, 123, 137, 144–147,
331, 428
divalproex, 226
Divalproex sodium. See
Depakote
DM, 331, 333–334
DMARDs (disease-modifying
antirheumatic drugs), 240,
245
DMSO (dimethyl sulfoxide),
451–452

Doan's Pills, 343

docosanol, 398

doctors

finding in Canada, 43, 46

measuring of drug's safety by, 69

pharmaceutical sales representatives' influence on, 5–6, 10–11

prescription mistakes by, 13–16, 18–19

questions to ask about before accepting prescriptions from, 11

Doctorsolve.com, 44–45

docusate calcium, 375, 377

docusate sodium, 375–376, 379

dog bites, 102

dogs, giving acetaminophen to, 347

Dolobid, 76, 240

Dolophine, 246–247

donepezil, 233

Donnatal, 22, 264

dopamine, 229–231

Doral, 210

dorzolamide, 270

dosages

antibiotics, 95–102, 107

measuring for children, 459–460, 475

Metamucil, 375

Dove soap, 418

doxazosin, 143–144, 191

doxepin, 23, 215, 251

Doxidan, 377

doxycycline, 102, 105, 112, 281

Dramamine, 437–438

drinks

sports, 483–484

warm, 263

Drixoral, 298

drug interactions

allergies and, 20–21

antiseizure drugs, 227

aspirin, 343

checking before trying new products, 299

erythromycin, 113–114

H2 blockers, 259

xanthine derivatives, 201

drug representatives, 5–6, 10–11

Drugstore.com, 31, 34

dry mouth, 216

dry skin, 287, 293–294, 400–406

Drysol, 408

Dulcolax, 377

DuoNeb, 203

Duragesic patches, 246–247

Duricef, 108

Dymelor, 171

Dynabac, 105

dyskinesia, 223

E

ear-care products, 391–393

ear drops, 102

ear infections, 102, 391–393, 485

earaches, 396

Eckerd.com, 29, 31, 33–34

Econopred, 274, 279

Ecotrin, 346

eczema, 280, 289

edema, 183

Effexor, 217

eggs, head lice, 444–445

Elavil, 215, 250, 254

Eldepryl, 230

Elder Prescription Insurance Coverage (EPIC), 59

Elderly Pharmaceutical Insurance Coverage (EPIC), 60

electrolyte replacement products, 483–484

electronic transactions over the Internet, 32–33

Eli Lilly and Company, patient assistance program, 52

Emetrol, 479

Enbrel, 245

endometrial cancer, 163

energy, improvement of, 167

enteric-coated aspirin, 344

ephedra, 439

EPIC (Elder Prescription Insurance Coverage), 59

EPIC (Elderly Pharmaceutical Insurance Coverage), 60

epilepsy, 226–229

erectile dysfunction, 188–190

erections, 217

ergotamine, 263

Ery-Tab, 281

erythromycin, 113–114, 150, 276, 281

Eskalith, 70

estazolam, 210

esterified estrogens, 163

Estinyl, 163

Estrace, 163, 166, 170

estradiol, 163, 166

Estratab, 163

estrogen, 156–157, 160–167, 169

estrogen receptor modulator, 168

estropipate, 163

etodolac, 240

eucalyptus oil, 334

Eucerin cream, 293–294, 401

eugenol, 396

Eustachian tubes, 464

Evista, 168

Ex-Lax, 377

Excedrin, 346

Excedrin PM, 298, 432

exchange rates, 41

exoaprin, 343

expectorants, 206, 330–334, 470–471

expiration dates, 78

Express Pharmacy Services, 33–34

eye-care products, 383–391
eye conditions
    congestion in, 276–279
    glaucoma, 269–274, 276
    infections of, 276–279, 384,
        485
    inflammation of, 274,
        276–279
eye decongestants, 384–386
eye drops, 102, 269–271,
    275–277, 279–280, 386–390
eye infections, 102
eye-irrigating solutions,
    390–391
eye lubricants, 386–390
eyecups, 390
eyes, contact between steroids
    and, 290

F
facial cosmetics, 418
famciclovir, 284
Familymeds.com, 35
famotidine, 258, 365–366
Famvir, 284
FDA. See U.S. Food and Drug
    Administration
Feen-A-Mint, 377
felbamate, 226
Felbatol, 226
Feldene, 76, 240–241
fenofibrate, 151
fentanyl, 246
fever, 122, 338, 347, 466–468
fexofenadine, 204
first-aid products, 410–412
first-degree burns, 286, 406
first generation cephalosporins,
    108
flavoxate, 185
Fleet's Babylax glycerin sup-
    positories, 484
Fletcher's Castoria, 484
Flexeril, 76, 251, 254
Flomax, 17, 191–192

Florida, pharmaceutical assis-
    tance programs in, 57
Flovent, 198–199
Floxin, 104–105, 110
flu
    giving aspirin to children suf-
        fering from, 342
    treatments for
        analgesics. See pain medica-
            tions
        antihistamines. See antihist-
            amines
        antitussives and expecto-
            rants, 330–334
        categories of, 315–316
        combination products,
            325–330
        cough drops and throat
            lozenges, 334–336
        decongestants, 317–323,
            325
        for children, 461–474
        gum with aspirin, 336–337
        vitamin C (ascorbic acid),
            337–338
fluid retention, 242
flunsolide, 198
fluorometholone, 274
fluoroquinolones, 105, 110–112
fluoxetine, 216, 221
fluoxymesterone, 167
flurazepam, 210
flurbiprofen, 240, 274, 279
fluticasone, 198–199
fluvastatin, 150
fluvoxamine, 216
FML, 274
Food and Drug Administra-
    tion. See U.S. Food and Drug
    Administration
foot infections, 102
foot perspiration, 408
Fosamax, 161, 168, 176
Fox, Michael J., 239
foxglove, 122

Fragmin, 343
freezer pops, 483
fructose, 264, 368
fungal infections, 104, 286–288,
    407–410

G
gabapentin, 226, 250
gallbladder disease, 163
Garamycin, 276, 279
gargles, salt-water, 336
gas, 479–480
gas-reducing products, 380–382
Gas-X, 380
gastric upset, 103–104
gastroesophageal reflux disor-
    der (GERD), 360, 365
gastrointestinal conditions
    excess stomach acid, 257–263
    intestinal problems, 263–268
    over-the-counter remedies
        antacids, 359–365, 380
        antidiarrheals, 369–372
        antiemetic products,
            367–369
        for children, 477–485
        gas-reducing products,
            380–382
        H2 blockers, 365–367
        laxatives, 373–380
gatifloxacin, 110
gemfibrozil, 149–151
Genaphed, 318, 465
Genepap, 466, 477
generations of antibiotics, 90
generic drugs, 19, 67–72, 85,
    305–307
Genetap, 464
genital herpes, 284
genitourinary conditions treat-
    ments
    male erectile dysfunction,
        188–190
    urinary acidifiers, 184
    urinary alkalinizers, 183

urinary tract infections,
187–188
urinary tract relaxers, 185–187
urinary tract stimulators, 187
urine flow through prostate,
191–192
gentamicin, 276, 279
GERD (gastroesophageal
reflux disorder), 360, 365
glaucoma, 185, 269–274, 276
Glaxo Wellcome, patient assistance program, 53
GLD Pharmaceuticals, 35
glimepiride, 171
glipizide, 171
Glucometer Elite, 426
glucometers, 424–426
Glucophage, 172, 176
glucosamine, 450–455
glucose, 170, 421
Glucotrol, 171
Glucovance, 173
glyburide, 171, 173, 176
glycerin, 392, 484
Golden Mountaineer Discount
Card, 62
gout, 181–182
gramicidin, 276
grape juice, 264
grapefruits, 130
gristle, 451
guaifenesin, 326, 331–332
guanfacine, 234
Guiatuss DM, 474
gum
aspirin, 336–337
nicotine, 77, 446–449
Gyne-Lotrimin, 298, 430

H
H2 blockers, 257–260, 262–263,
365–367
hair growth, 144
Halcion, 114, 210, 213

Haldol, 222
Hall's Maximum Strength
cough drops, 336
Halls Mentho-Lyptus Decongestant Liquid, 317
haloperidol, 222
Halotestin, 168
Haltran, 316
handwriting, quality of, 13–16,
18–19
hay fever, 204, 258
HDL, 149, 151, 162, 172
head lice, 443–446
headaches, 122, 254–256
Healthmeds.com, 44
heart, 171
heart attacks, 396
heart conditions
causes of, 435
congestive heart failure, 183
treatments for
angina, 126–130
blood thinners, 119–122
cardiovascular, 122–124
high blood pressure,
136–147
irregular heartbeats,
124–127, 130–136
lower blood cholesterol
and triglycerides,
147–154
other heart problems,
130–136
heartburn, 360
heating pads, 263, 354
Helicobacter pylori, 113
hemorrhoids, 440–443
heparin, 343, 451
hepatitis, 347
herbal (natural) products, 300
Herpecin-L, 398, 399
herpes, genital, 284
HFI (high fructose intolerance), 368

high blood pressure, 130, 134,
136–147, 325
high-fat foods, 264
high fructose intolerance
(HFI), 368
Histadryl, 463
histamine, 204
histamine H2 blockers,
257–260
histamines, 75
HMG-CoA reductase
inhibitors. *See* statins
HMO coverage for prescription drugs, 75–76
Hold Children's Formula
Lozenges, 317
honey, 334
HoosieRx, 58
hormone replacement therapy
(HRT), 161–168
hormones
androgens, 167–168
diabetes treatments, 170–176
gout treatments, 181–182
hormone replacement ther-
arpies (HRTs), 161–168
hypothyroidism treatments,
176–181
oral contraceptives, 155–160
horses, estrogen taken from,
162–163
hot baths, 263
HRT (hormone replacement
therapy), 161–168
HS, 19
HSV-1 (Type 1 herpes simplex
virus), 398
humidifiers, 401
hydrochloric acid, 343, 359–360
hydrochlorothiazide, 137
hydrocodone, 247, 250
hydrocortisone, 102, 440, 443
hydrogen peroxide, 411, 413
hydromorphone, 246

hydroxypropyl methylcellulose, 387
hydroxyquinoline, 400
hyoscyamine, 264
hyperactivity, 234
hypersensitivity, 103
hypertension. *See* high blood pressure
Hypo Tears, 387
hypoglycemia, 171
hypothyroidism, 176–181
Hytrin, 143–144, 191

I
ibuprofen
  conditions and symptoms relieved by, 240, 244, 302, 350–351, 395, 398, 428–430
  drug interactions, 343
  name-brand products containing, 315–316
  pricing of, 244, 353–354
  taking with blood thinners, 122
ice, 406
Icy Hot, 354–355
idiopathic, 288–289
illegal drug sales, 30–31, 46
Illinois, pharmaceutical assistance programs in, 57–58
Ilotycin, 276
Imdur, 127, 129
imipramine, 215, 251
Imitrex, 255
Imodium, 264, 267–268, 298, 370, 481
Imodium A-D, 380, 482
importing drugs into U.S., 41–42
impotence, 167, 188–190
index, narrow therapeutic (NTI), over-the-counter drugs, 305, 307

indexes
  narrow therapeutic (NTI), 19–20, 69
    antiseizure drugs, 227, 229
    drugs for treating heart conditions, 119–120, 124, 126, 153–154
    thyroid treatments, 177, 180
    xanthine derivatives, 200–201
  therapeutic, 69
Indiana, pharmaceutical assistance programs in, 58
indigestion, 360
Indocin, 240–241
indomethacin, 181, 240
infected wounds, treatments for, 100–101
infections
  acne, 280–283
  bacterial, 283–286
  bladder, 187
  body's resistance to, 89–90
  breast, 102
  causes of, 90–92
  ear, 102, 391–393
  eyes, 276–279, 384
  fungal, 104–105, 407–410
  in children, 485
  urinary tract, 186–188
  viral skin, 283–286
  yeast, 104–105, 430–432
  See also antibiotics
influenza. *See* flu
"informational" letters, 7–9
inhalant solutions, 194
insomnia, 209–213, 234, 432–434
insulin, 170, 421–423
insulin sensitizers, 171–172
insulin syringes, 422–424
insurance coverage
  over-the-counter drugs, 259

prescription drugs, 29, 74–76, 84–85, 263, 281
Intal, 200
intercourse, 189
Internet pharmacies, 27–36, 43–45
intestinal cramping, 263–268
intestinal inflammation and irritation, 265–268
intestinal upset, 103–104
intestines, 343
iodine, 411
Iowa Priority Prescription Savings Program, The, 58
ipratropium, 200, 203
iron, 260
irregular heartbeats, 122, 124–127, 130–136
irritable bowel syndrome (IBS), 263–265
Ismo, 127
isocarboxazid, 214
Isopto Carbachol, 269
Isopto Carpine, 269
isosorbide, 126–127
isotonic preparations, 290
itching, 288–292
itraconazole, 287

J
Jenny Craig, 439
jock itch, 286, 407

K
Kansas Senior Pharmacy Assistance Program, 58
Kaolectrolyte, 484
Kaopectate, 369, 481
Keflex, 108
Kenalog, 289–290
Keri-lotion, 293
ketoconazole, 286, 288
ketoprofen, 122, 241, 343, 351
ketorolac, 241, 274

Ketotifen, 275
Key Pharmaceuticals, patient
    assistance program, 53
kidney damage, 170, 242–243,
    341
kidney disease, 348
kidney infections, 102
kidneys, 144, 150–151
Kmart, 320
Konsyl, 373

L
labels, children's products, 462
Lac-Hydrin, 293
lactic acid, 293, 416
Lactobacillus acidophilus, 104
Lamictal, 226
lamotrigine, 226
lancets, 427–428
lanolin, 400
Lanoxin, 17, 122–123, 260
lansoprazole, 260
Lasix, 68, 73, 81
latanoprost, 269–270
laxative addiction, 372
laxatives, 373–380, 484–485
LDL, 149–151, 162
leflunomide, 245–246
leg cramps, 363
legumes, 264
lemon, 334
Lescol, 114, 150
leukotriene receptor antago-
    nists, 201
Levaquin, 104–105, 110
levobunolol, 270
levocabastine, 275
levodopa, 230, 233
levofloxacin, 110
levothyroxine, 177
Levoxyl, 177, 180
Levsin, 264, 267
Levsinex, 264
Librax, 264
Librium, 209

lice, 443–446
Lidex, 289
lidocaine, 406–407
Lifescan, 426
Lilly, 421
limbs, loss of, 170–171
Lioresal, 251
lip balms, 414
Lipitor, 21, 114, 150
Little Tummys Nausea Relief,
    479
liver, 150
liver damage, 242–243,
    347–348
Livostin, 275
lobbyists, 3
Lodine, 76, 240
lodoxamide, 275
Longs Drugs, 35
loop diuretics, 145
loperamide, 264, 268, 371, 481
Lopid, 149–151
Lopressor, 136
loratadine, 204
lorazepam, 209
loss leaders, 308
Lotemax, 274
loteprednol, 274
Lotrimin, 298, 408, 410
Lotronex, 265
lovastatin, 150
Lovenox, 343
Low Cost Drugs for the
    Elderly Program, 58
low-sodium diets, 375, 377
loxapine, 222
Loxitane, 222
lozenges, 334–336
Lubriderm, 400
Luvox, 216, 222

M
ma huong, 439
Maalox, 112, 364, 365
macrolides, 105, 113–114

Magan, 343
magnesium, 184
magnesium hydroxide, 363,
    365–366
magnesium oxide, 363
magnesium salicylate, 343
mail-order pharmacies, 27, 29,
    43–45
Maine, pharmaceutical assis-
    tance programs in, 58
Major Pharmaceuticals, 456
male erectile dysfunction,
    188–190
male hormones, 167–168
manic-depressive disorder, 222
manufacturer rebates, 311–312
MAOIs (monoamine oxidase
    inhibitors), 214–215
marketing strategies by phar-
    maceutical companies
    "direct-to-consumer" adver-
        tising, 9–10
    "patient information" cam-
        paigns, 7–9
    by sales representatives, 5–6,
        10–11
    creating markets for new
        drugs, 75
    distributing samples to doc-
        tors, 10–11
    drugs with similar-sounding
        names, 16–18
    rebate programs for bulk
        purchases, 6–7
    See also advertising
Marplan, 214
Maryland Pharmacy Assistance
    Program, 58
Massachusetts, pharmaceutical
    assistance programs in, 59
mast cell stabilizers, 193, 200
Maxair, 195, 196
Maxalt, 255–256
Maxaquin, side effects of,
    104–105

mcg, 19
MDIs. *See* metered-dose
    inhalers
meal-replacement products,
    439
measuring cups, 459–460
Meclizine, 437
medical care, when to seek,
    299–300
medical shorthand, 18–19
Medicare, 55
MediFlu, 316
medroxyprogesterone, 167
meglitinides, 171–172
Mellaril, 222
meloxicam, 240
membership programs, 85
membership stores, 308, 312
menopause, 162, 167
menstruation, 166, 428–430
menthol, 334, 395
meperidine, 246
Merck, 7–8, 53
Merck Medco, 33, 35
mercurochrome, 411
merthiolate, 411
mesalamine, 265, 266
Metab-O-Life, 439
metabolic waste, 347
Metamucil, 372, 373, 375, 484
metaproterenol, 195–196
Metaxalone, 251
metered–dose inhalers (MDIs),
    193–195, 198–199, 203
metformin, 172–173
methadone, 246
methazolamide, 270
methenamine, 184
methocarbamol, 251
methotrexate, 115, 245,
    245–246
methyl sulfonyl methane
    (MSM), 451–454
methylphenidate, 234, 237–238
methyltestosterone, 167

metipranolol, 270
metoprolol, 136
Mevacor, 114, 149–150
Mexico, buying drugs in, 49–50
mg, 19
Micatin, 298, 407–408
Michigan, pharmaceutical
    assistance programs in, 59
miconazole, 408, 430
Micronase, 171
Micronor, 156
Midol, 316, 346, 428
migraines, 254–256
milkshakes, 439
Mineral Ice, 356
Minimum Medical Program, 62
Minitran patches, 127, 129
Minnesota, pharmaceutical
    assistance programs in, 59
Minocin, 281, 283
minocycline, 105, 112, 281, 283
minoxidil, 144
Miradon, 343
Mirapex, 230
mirtazapine, 215
misoprostol, 261
Missouri SenioRx Program,
    59–60
mistakes in dispensing drugs
    drug interactions and aller-
        gies, 20–21
    drugs with similar-sounding
        names, 16–18
    medical shorthand misread,
        18–19
    poor handwriting, 13–16
    protecting yourself from, 24,
        26
    substituting drugs, 19–20
    transcription errors, 18
Mobic, 240
Mobidin, 343
moisture on the skin, limiting
    amount of, 287
moisturizing creams, 293

Monistat, 298, 430, 432
monoamine oxidase inhibitors
    (MAOIs), 214–215
Monoject, 424
Monoket, 127
mononitrate, 127
monophasic oral contracep-
    tives, 156–159
montelukast, 201
"morning-after" pills, 157
morphine, 246–247
motion-sickness (antivertigo)
    treatments, 436–438
Motrin, 240, 244, 307, 316, 466
Motrin IB, 298–299, 316, 350,
    430
Motrin PM, 433
mouth
    antibacterial and anesthetic
        products, 393–397
    antibiotics used to treat
        infections in, 98–99
    cold sore treatments,
        398–399
    dryness in, 216
    problems with in children,
        485
    toothache treatments,
        395–397
mouthwash, 393
moxifloxacin, 110
MS Contin, 247
MSIR, 247
MSM (methyl sulfonyl
    methane), 451–454
mucous, 332, 386, 470
multi-component products,
    302–305, 471–474
mupirocin, 284
Murine, 276, 387, 392
muscle damage, 150
muscle relaxers, 251–254
Muse, 189
Myapap, 466, 477
Mycelex-G, 430

Mycoplasma pneumonia, 112
Mycostatin, 286
Mylanta, 112, 364
Mylanta Gas, 380
Mylanta Gas Drops, 480
Mysoline, 226

N
N-acetyl-glucosamine, 450
NABP (National Association
    of Boards of Pharmacy), 31
nabumetone, 241
nail fungus, 286–287, 407–409
Naldecon, 317
naphazoline, 276
Naprosyn, 76, 240
naproxen, 122, 240, 343, 428
naproxen sodium, 351, 395, 398
narcotics, 74, 206, 246–250
Nardil, 214
narrow therapeutic index
    (NTI)
    antiseizure drugs, 227, 229
    definition of, 19–20
    drugs for treating heart con-
        ditions, 119–120, 124, 126,
        153–154
    generic drugs, 69–71
    over-the-counter drugs, 305,
        307
    thyroid treatments, 177, 180
    xanthine derivatives, 200–201
nasal decongestants, 320–323,
    325
nasal sprays, 317, 320–323
National Association of
    Boards of Pharmacy
    (NABP), 31
natural (herbal) products, 300
nausea, 367–369, 477–480
Navane, 223
nebulizers, 194
Necon, 135, 160
necon (Ortho-Novum), 68
needles, 423–424

Needymeds.com, 54
nefazodone, 217
neomycin, 102, 276, 410
Neosporin, 276
Neosporin Ointment, 298,
    410–412
Neptazane, 270
nerve pain, 227
nervous system. *See* central
    nervous system
Neurontin, 226, 250, 254
Neutrogena, 418
Neutrogena T-gel shampoo,
    288
Nevada, pharmaceutical assis-
    tance programs in, 60
New Hampshire Prescription
    Drug Discount Program, 60
New Jersey, pharmaceutical
    assistance programs in, 60
New York, pharmaceutical
    assistance programs in, 60
Nicoderm CQ, 298, 447, 449
Nicorette, 298, 447–448
nicotine, 446
nicotine cravings, 217
Nicotine Transdermal Patch,
    449
nifedipine, 143
"nighttime" preparations,
    326–327
nitric acid, 189
Nitro-Dur, 127, 129
nitroglycerin, 126–127, 189
Nitrolingual spray, 127
Nitrostat, 127
nits, 444–446
Nivea, 400
Nix, 444–446
nizatidine, 258, 365
Nizoral, 260, 286, 288, 408
No-Doz, 434
noncomedogenic cosmetics, 418
nonphenothiazines, 222–223
nonsteroidal anti-inflammatory

drugs (NSAIDs)
    as arthritis treatment,
        239–246, 450
    eye conditions, 266, 274,
        279–280
    as pain reliever, 254, 341,
        350–354
    taking with blood thinners,
        122
norepinephrine, 217, 234, 248
Norflex, 251
Norpace CR, 126
Norpramin, 215, 251
North Carolina, pharmaceuti-
    cal assistance programs in,
    61
nortriptyline, 215, 251
noses, 317–320, 485
Novo Nordisk, 421
Novolin, 421–422
NovoPen, 422
NSAIDs. *See* nonsteroidal anti-
    inflammatory drugs
NTI. *See* narrow therapeutic
    index
Nuprin, 298, 350
Nyquil, 316, 327
Nyquil Liqui-gels, 303
nystatin, 286
Nytol, 298, 432

O
obsessive-compulsive disorder
    (OCD), 216
OCD (obsessive-compulsive
    disorder), 216
octyl methoxycinnamate, 398
octyl salicylate, 398
octylmethyl cinnamate, 414
Ocufen, 274, 279
Ocuflox, 280
Ocupres, 270
OD, 19
Office of Postmarketing Drug
    Risk Assessment, 17

ofloxacin, 110
Ogen, 163
ointments, 288, 355, 387–388, 410–412, 440
olanzapine, 223
olopatadine, 275
olsalazine, 266
omeprazole, 260
Omnicef, 108
One Touch Ultra Glucose Monitor, 426–427
online pharmacies, 27–36, 43–45
Opcon-A, 386
ophthalmic steroids, 290
opiate derivatives, 246
OptiPranolol, 270
Orajel Mouth-Aid, 398
Orajel P.M., 396
oral antibacterial and anesthetic products, 393–397
oral antihistimes, 323–325, 386
oral contraceptives, 105, 114, 155–160, 172
oral decongestants, 317–320
oral prednisone, 198
oral syringes, 460–461
orange juice, 144
oranges, 130
Orap, 223
Orinase, 171
orphenadrine, 251
Ortho-Novum, 135, 156, 160
Orudis, 241, 351, 353
OS, 19
osteoarthritis, 450–455
osteoporosis, 161–162, 168–170
OU, 19
over-the-counter drugs
    arthritis, 244
    growth of, 297–299
    pricing of. See pricing of over-the-counter drugs
    saving money on

bulk purchases, 307–308
buying generic drugs, 305–307
choosing the correct drug type, 301–305
coupons and store sales, 309–311
manufacturer rebates, 311–312
shopping around for bargains, 308–309
when to seek medical attention for symptoms, 299–300
See also specific drug names
ovulation, 172
oxaprozin, 240, 244
oxazepam, 209
Oxy Acne Products, 420
oxybenzone, 398, 413–414
oxybutynin, 185
Oxycontin, 247, 250
oxymetazoline, 320

P
PAAD (Pharmaceutical Assistance for the Aged and Disabled), 60
PABA (para-aminobenzoic acid), 413–414, 416
PACE (Pharmaceutical Assistance Elderly), 61
P.acnes (Propionibacterium acnes), 418
pain medications
    nonsteroidal anti-inflammatory drugs (NSAIDs). See nonsteroidal anti-inflammatory drugs
    over-the-counter
        acetaminophen, 122, 246–247, 325–326, 341, 346–350
        aspirin, 20–21, 121–122, 181, 336–337, 342–346

for children, 467–468, 474–477
        kidney damage from, 341
        topical analgesics, 354–356
prescriptions
    arthritis treatments, 240–246
    migraine treatments, 254–256
    muscle relaxers, 251–254
    narcotics, 74, 206, 239, 246–250
    non-narcotics, 239
    specialized pain relief, 250–251
pamabrom, 428
Pamelor, 215, 251
Pamprin, 298, 346, 428
pantoprazole, 260
para-aminobenzoic acid (PABA), 413–414, 416
Parafon, 251
Parke-Davis, patient assistance program, 53
Parkinson's disease, 222, 229–233
Parlodel, 230
Parnate, 214
paroxetine, 216
Patanol, 275
patches, 163–164, 246, 447, 449
patents, 4–5, 40–41, 67, 72
patient assistance programs, 51–64
"patient information" campaigns, 7–9
Paxil, 216, 222
PCN, 19
Pedialyte, 484
pemoline, 234
penicillin, 19, 105–108
penicillin G, 106
penicillin V, 99, 101, 106
penicillin VK, 102
penicillinase, 106

penis, 189, 217
Penlet, 427
Pennsylvania, pharmaceutical
   assistance programs in, 61
Pentasa, 266
pentoxifylline, 120–121
Pepcid, 258–259, 263, 365–367
Pepcid AC, 298
Pepto-Bismol, 343, 369–370,
   466, 477
Percocet, 247
Perdiem, 373
pergolide, 230
Peri-Colace, 379
periods, 166, 428–430
Permax, 230
permethrin, 444
peroxide
   benzoyl, 418–420
   hydrogen, 411, 413
perphenazine, 222
perspiration, 408
Persantine, 121
petrolatum, 440
petroleum jelly, 417
pets, giving acetaminophen to,
   347
Pharmaceutical Assistance
   Elderly (PACE), 61
Pharmaceutical Assistance for
   the Aged and Disabled
   (PAAD), 60
Pharmaceutical Assistance Program, 57–58
pharmaceutical companies
   executives' annual salary
      range, 3
   marketing strategies of
      "direct-to-consumer"
         advertising, 9–10
      "patient information"
         campaigns, 7–9
      by sales representatives,
         5–6, 10–11
      creating markets for new

drugs, 75
distributing samples to
   doctors, 10–11
rebate programs for bulk
   purchases, 6–7
See also advertising
patient assistance programs,
   51–54
Pharmaceutical Research and
   Manufacturers of America
   (PhRMA), 3–4
pharmacies
   in Canada, 42–46
   on the Internet, 27–36,
      43–45
Pharmacist Rick's Diaper Rash
   Remedy, 487
Pharmacist's Special Sore
   Throat Formula, 337
Phazyme, 380
phenazopyridine, 455
phenelzine, 214
pheniramine maleate, 386
phenobarbital, 226–227,
   263–264
phenol, 395
phenothiazines, 222
phenylephrine, 320
phenylpropanolamine (PPA),
   316–317, 438–439
phenytoin, 115, 226–227
Philips, 365
phosphorated carbohydrate
   solution, 367–368
photosensitivity, 105
PhRMA (Pharmaceutical
   Research and Manufacturers
   of America), 3–4
Phrma.org, 54
pilocarpine, 269–270
pimozide, 223
pioglitazone, 172
pirbuterol, 195
piroxicam, 240
Plavix, 121, 343

Pletal, 120
pneumonia, 102, 112
poison oak, 289
poisons, 122–123
Poly-Histine Expectorant
   Syrup, 317
polymyxin B, 102, 276, 410,
   412
polyneuropathy, 151
Polysporin Ointment, 412
Polysporin, 276
Polytrim, 276
polyvinyl alcohols, 387–388
pores, 418
Postal Prescription Services, 35
postnasal drip, 330
potassium, 123, 144–145
potassium acid phosphate, 184
potassium citrate, 183
potassium-sparing diuretics,
   145
PPA (phenylpropanolamine),
   316–317, 438–439
pramipexole, 230
pramoxine, 410–411
Pravachol, 114, 150
pravastatin, 150
PrecisionRX, 35
Precose, 173
Pred Forte, 274, 279
prednisolone, 274, 279
prednisone, 289
pregnancies, 115, 196, 261,
   368–369, 447
Premarin, 162–163, 166
Preparation H, 440
Prescription Assistance
   Program for Seniors, 57
Prescription Drug Assistance
   Program, 61
prescription drugs
   advertising of, 4–5
   as tax deduction, 86
   effects of on aging, 22–24
   expiration dates, 78

mistakes made in dispensing
    drug interactions and aller-
        gies, 20–21
    drugs with similar-sound-
        ing names, 16–18
    medical shorthand mis-
        read, 18–19
    poor handwriting, 13–16
    protecting yourself from,
        24, 26
    substituting drugs, 19–20
    transcription errors, 18
patents for, 4–5, 40–41, 67, 72
patient assistance programs,
    51–64
pricing of, influences from
    lobbyists on, 3
pricing of. *See* pricing of pre-
    scription drugs
questions to ask before
    accepting from doctors, 11
samples of, 10–11
saving money on
    at Internet pharmacies,
        27–36
    buying generic drugs,
        67–72, 85
    buying in larger quantities,
        72–74
    comparing prices of, 85–88
    comparing to over-the-
        counter drugs, 76–78
    cutting tablets, 78–84
    finding less expensive
        alternatives, 74–76
    in Canada, 37–49
    in Mexico, 49–50
    making the most of insur-
        ance benefits, 84–85
total annual spending by
    consumers for, 3
See also specific drug names
Prescription Drugs I Take
    worksheet, 25
Prescription (Massachusetts

pharmaceutical assistance
    program), 59
prescription membership pro-
    grams, 85
Prescriptions By Mail, 35
Prevacid, 76, 260
priapism, 217
pricing of over-the-counter
    drugs
    antitussives and expecto-
        rants, 333, 470
    bulk purchases, 309, 344
    combination products,
        327–329
    combination vs. single-ingre-
        dient products, 303–305
    cough drops and throat
        lozenges, 335
    diabetes treatments, 422–427
    eye-care products, 385, 387,
        389, 391
    for children
        cough, cold, flu, and
            allergy remedies,
            463–465, 467–473
        diaper rash remedies,
            486–487
        gastrointestinal conditions,
            478–483, 485
        pain relievers, 467–468,
            475–476
    gastrointestinal remedies
        antacids, 360–364
        antidiarrheals, 370–371
        antiemetic products, 368
        for children, 478–480
        gas-reducing products, 381
        H2 blockers, 366
        laxatives, 373–374,
            376–378
    head lice treatments,
        445–446
    hemorrhoid treatments,
        442–443
    motion-sickness (antivertigo)

products, 437–438
    mouth-care products,
        394–395, 397, 399
    name-brand vs. generic, 306
    nasal decongestants, 321–322
    osteoarthritis, 452–454
    pain medications
        acetaminophen, 349–350
        aspirin, 345–346
        for children, 467–468,
            475–476
        menstrual discomfort
            treatments, 429–430
        nonsteroidal anti-inflam-
            matory drugs (NSAIDs),
            352–353
        topical analgesics, 355–356
    skin-care products
        acne treatments, 419–420
        burn care, 407
        moisturizers, 402–405
        sunscreen, 415–416
        topical antifungal, 409–410
        topical first-aid, 411–412
        wart removers, 417
    sleep aids, 433–434
    smoking-cessation products,
        448–449
    stimulants, 435
    urinary irritation relief, 456
    vaginal products, 431–432
pricing of prescription drugs
    antibiotics, 94–102, 107,
        109–111, 113–114
    antihistamines, 205
    asthma, 197, 199, 201–203
    central nervous system con-
        ditions
        Alzheimer's disease,
            233–234
        antianxiety drugs, 211–213
        antidepressants, 218–221,
            252–254
        antipsychotic drugs,
            224–225

antiseizure drugs, 228–229
attention deficit disorder
   (ADD) drugs, 235–237
Parkinson's disease,
   231–232
comparing at different pharmacies, 85–88
eye conditions
   glaucoma, 271–273
   inflammation, allergies,
      congestion, and infec-
      tions, 277–279
gastrointestinal conditions
   intestinal problems,
      266–267
   stomach acid reduction,
      261–262
generic, 68
genitourinary conditions
   male erectile dysfunction,
      190
   urinary alkalinizers and
      acidifiers, 184–185
   urinary tract infections,
      188
   urinary tract relaxers, 186
   urine flow through
      prostate, 191–192
heart conditions
   angina, 128–129
   beta–blockers, 133–136
   blood thinners, 120–121
   calcium channel blockers,
      131–133
   cardiovascular drugs, 123
   high blood pressure,
      138–143, 145–147
   irregular heartbeats,
      125–126, 131–133
   lower blood cholesterol
      and triglycerides,
      152–153
hormones
   androgens, 169
   diabetes treatments,

174–176
   estrogen replacement
      products, 164–166
   gout treatments, 181–182
   hypothyroidism treat-
      ments, 178–180
   oral contraceptives,
      157–160
   osteoporosis treatments,
      170
   progesterone replacement
      products, 167
influences from lobbyists on,
   3
at Internet pharmacies,
   27–28, 33
newly–released, 5
pain medications
   arthritis, 242–245
   migraines, 255
   muscle relaxers, 252–254
   narcotics, 248–250
skin conditions
   acne, 280–283
   bacterial and viral skin
      infections, 285
   dry skin, 293–294
   fungal infections, 287–288
   psoriasis, skin inflamma-
      tion, and rashes,
      291–292
Prilosec, 76, 114, 260
primidone, 226
privacy, invasion of, 7–9
probenecid, 181
procainamide, 124
Procan, 124
pro-time (prothrombin time),
   119
Prodium, 455
"productive" cough, 332
progesterone, 166–167
progestin, 156–157, 166
propellants, 195
Propine, 270

Propionibacterium acnes
   (P.acnes), 418
propoxyphene, 246, 250
ProSom, 210
prostaglandin levels, 428
prostate, 102, 191–192
prostate cancer, 168
proteins, 386
prothrombin time (pro-time),
   119
proton pump inhibitors, 257,
   260
Protonix, 260, 263
Proventil, 76, 195, 197
Provera, 166, 170
Prozac, 216, 221
pseudoephedrine, 318–320,
   325, 439, 464
Pseudogest, 318, 465
Pseudotabs, 318, 465
psoriasis, 288–292
psychotic disorders, 222–226
psyllium seeds, 373
puberty, 167
Pulmicort, 198–199
purines, 181
Pyridium, 455
pyrilamine maleate, 428

Q
QD, 19
QID, 19
QOD, 19
quazepam, 210
Questran, 76, 149
quetiapine, 223

R
rabeprazole, 260
raccoon bites, 102
radiation, UV-A and B, 412
raloxifene, 168–169
ranitidine, 258, 365–367
rashes, 288–292
Realfastdrugstore.com, 44

rebates, 6–7, 425
Red Cross Toothache kit, 396
Relafen, 241
Remeron, 215
Reno, Janet, 229
Requip, 230
resistance to antibiotics, 89–90
Restoril, 210, 213
Retin-A, 280–281
Reye's syndrome, 342, 347, 370, 466
Rezulin, 172
rhabdomyolysis, 150–151
rheumatoid arthritis, 245–246
Rheumatrex, 245
Rhode Island Pharmaceutical Assistance for the Elderly (RIPAE), 61
Rickettsia, 112
rimexolone, 274
RIPAE (Rhode Island Pharmaceutical Assistance for the Elderly), 61
risedronate, 169
Risperdal, 223
risperidone, 223
Ritalin, 234–235, 237
Rite-Aid, 34
rizatriptan, 255
Robaxin, 251, 254
Robitussin, 317, 331–334, 468, 474
Roche Pharmaceuticals, patient assistance program, 53
Rocky Mountain spotted fever, 112
rofecoxib, 241
Rogaine, 298
ropinirole, 230
rosiglitazone, 171–172
Rowasa, 266
RxAssist, 54–55
RXMPSS, 35

S
s-adenosylmethionine (SAMe), 452, 454
SAD (social anxiety disorder), 216
Saffola, 487
sales on over-the-counter drugs, 309–311
sales representatives, 5–6, 10–11
Saleto-200, 316
salicylates
    in antidiarrheals, 369–370
    in aspirin, 342–343
    in skin treatments, 289, 414, 416–418
    in topical analgesics, 354
salmeterol, 195, 197
salt-restricted diets, 375, 377
salt-water gargles, 336
SAMe (s-adenosylmethionine), 452, 454
samples of drugs, 10–11
Sam's Club, 344
Schedule II narcotics, 239, 247
Schering Laboratories, patient assistance program, 53
schizophrenia, 222
Scope, 393
seasonal allergies, 204
second-degree burns, 286, 406
second generation cephalosporins, 108
seizure disorders, 226–229
seizures, 217
selegiline, 230
Senecot, 484–485
Senior Citizen Drug Program, 59
Senior Citizen Subsidy for Drugs, 60
seniors
    effects of drugs on, 22–24
    prescription drug assistance for, 55–56
senna, 377
Senokot, 377, 484
Senokot-S tablets, 372
Septra, 104, 115, 188
Serax, 209
Serevent, 195, 197
Seroquel, 223
serotonin, 217, 248, 254, 256, 265
serotonin reuptake inhibitors (SSRIs), 216–217, 221–222, 256
sertraline, 216
Serzone, 217
sex drive, 167
shampoo, 77, 288
shark liver oil, 440
shingles, 284
shipping charges for drugs, 33
shorthand, medical, 18–19
side effects
    acarbose, 173
    acetaminophen, 347–348
    alendronate, 169
    allopurinol, 181
    Alzheimer's disease treatments, 233
    amplification by caffeine, 201
    androgens, 167
    antacids, 360
    antianxiety drugs, 210, 216–217
    antibiotics, 103–116
    antidepressants, 214–215
    antihistamines, 75, 205
    antipsychotic drugs, 222–223
    aspirin, 342–343
    beta agonists, 196
    cimetidine, 259
    colchicine, 182
    Cytotec, 261
    Detrol, 185
    dimethyl sulfoxide (DMSO), 451
    Ditropan, 185

dopamine, 231
estrogen, 163
eye congestion treatments,
    276
eye drops, 270–271
ipratropium, 200
lodoxamide, 275
metformin, 172
migraine medications,
    255–256
Motrin IB, 299
muscle relaxers, 251
narcotics, 247, 250
nonsteroidal anti-inflamma-
    tory drugs (NSAIDs),
    241–242, 245, 274, 343, 352
oral contraceptives, 156–157
probenecid, 181
rosiglitazone and pioglita-
    zone, 172
Sporanox, 287
steroids, 198–199
stimulants, 234–235, 435
tricyclic antidepressants, 265
Urispas, 185
vasoconstrictors, 441
Viagra, 189
vitamin C, 337
xanthine derivatives, 200–201
sildenafil, 189
silicone oil, 398
Silvadene, 286
silver sulfadiazine, 286
SilveRxCard, 61
simethicone, 380, 479
simvastatin, 150
Sinapils Tablets, 317
Sinarest, 317
Sine-Off Sinus Medicine
    Tablets, 317
Sinemet, 230, 233
Sinequan, 215, 251
single-component products,
    302, 326
Singulair, 201, 203

sinus congestion, treatments
    for, 317–320
sinus problems, 396
sinusitis, 99–100, 102
sitz baths, 441
Skelaxin, 251
skeletal muscle relaxers,
    251–254
skin-care products
    burn treatments, 406–407
    moisturizers, 400–406
    sunscreen, 280, 398, 412–416
    topical antifungal, 407–410
    topical first-aid, 410–412
    wart removers, 416–417
skin conditions
    acne, 280–283
    burns, 286, 406–407
    dry skin, 293–294, 400–406
    infections, 102, 104, 283–288
    irritation, 288–292
    itching, 288–292
    psoriasis, 288–292
    rashes, 288–292
skin moisturizers, 400–406
skunk bites, 102
SL, 19
sleep aids, 432–434
Sleepinal, 432
Slo-bid, 200
small intestines, 343
Smart Buys on Prescription
    Drugs worksheet, 88
smoking-cessation products,
    446–450
SMZ/TMP DS, 102, 115
soap, 401, 418
social anxiety disorder (SAD),
    216
soda (soft drinks), 260, 264,
    331, 368–369, 428
sodium acid phosphate, 184
sodium bicarbonate, 183
sodium citrate, 183
soft drinks, 260, 264, 331,

368–369, 428
Solarcaine, 406–407
Soma, 76, 251
Sominex, 432
Sonata, 210, 213
sorbitol, 264
sore throats, 90–91, 336–337
"SOS Worksheet" for Saving
    Money on Over-the-Counter
    Drugs, 312–314
sour stomach, 360
South Carolina Senior Pre-
    scription Drug Program, 61
Spec-T Sore Throat/Decon-
    gestant Lozenges, 317
SPF (sun protection factor),
    413–414
splitting tablets, 78–84
Sporanox, 286–287
sports drinks, 483–484
Sportscreme, 354
SSRIs. See serotonin reuptake
    inhibitors
St. Joseph's Cold Tablets for
    Children, 317
Stadol nasal spray, 247
staph, 90
staphylococcus, 283
state pharmaceutical assistance
    programs, 56–62
statins, 148–151
stepped approach, 147
steroid drops, 276–277
steroids, 193, 197–200, 203,
    288–290
stimulant laxatives, 377–380,
    484–485
stimulants, 234–235, 434–436
stomach, 258, 343–344,
    367–369, 477–479. See also
    gastrointestinal conditions
stomach acid, reduction of,
    257–263
stool softeners, 372, 375–376,
    379

storage, nitroglycerin, 127
store sales, over-the-counter drugs, 309–310
strep, 90
strep throat, 335–336
stress, 398
Stridex, 280
strokes, 151
stuffy noses, treatments for, 317–320
subsalicylate, 343
substance P, 354
sucralfate, 261
Sudafed, 298, 318, 330, 464
Sulamyd, 97, 102, 276
sulfacetamide, 276
sulfacetamide eye drops, 97, 102
sulfamethoxazole, 115
sulfas, 105, 114–116
sulfasalazine, 265
sulfonylureas, 171–173
sulindac, 240
sumatriptan, 255
Sumycin, 281
sun protection factor (SPF), 413–414
sunscreen, 280, 398, 412–416
supermarkets, pharmacy departments in, 308
supplements, 163, 169, 363
suppositories, 431, 484
Suprax, 104, 108
Surfak, 372, 377
Surmontil, 215
survival mutation, 89
Susphrine, 318
Swim Ear, 393
swimmers, ear infections in, 391–393
Symmetrel, 230
Synthroid, 177, 180
syringes, 392–393, 422–424, 460–461
systemic (whole-body) side effects, 271

T
tablet cutting, 78–84
tacrine, 233
Tagamet, 189, 258–259, 365–366
Tagamet HB, 298
Talwin, 247
tardive dyskinesia, 222
Tasmar, 230
Tavist, 298, 323
Tavist-D Tablets, 317
tax deductions for prescriptions, 86
TCN, 19
tea tree oil, 408–410
Tegretol, 114, 226–227
temazepam, 210
Tenex, 234–235
Tenormin, 136
Tequin, 104–105, 110–111
terazosin, 143–144, 191
terbutaline, 196
Terumo, 424
Tessalon, 206
testicular development, 167
Testoderm, 168
testosterone, 168
tetracyclic antidepressants, 215
tetracyclines, 19, 105, 112–113, 281
tetrahydrozoline, 386
Thecanadiandrugstore.com, 44
Theo-24, 200
Theo-Dur, 200
theophylline, 114, 200
therapeutic index, 69
thiazide diuretics, 144
thiazolidinediones, 171–172
thinning blood, drugs used for, 119–122
thioridazine, 222
thiothixene, 223
third-degree burns, 286, 406
third generation cephalosporins, 108

Thorazine, 22, 222
throat infections, 101–102
throat lozenges, 334–336
throats
    sore, 90–91, 336–337
    tickles in, 331
thymol, 354
thyroid disease, 435
thyroid treatments, 176–181
Thyroid USP, 177
tickles in the throat, 331
Ticlid, 121
ticlopidine, 121
TID, 19
Tigan, 24
timolol, 270
Tinactin, 298, 407, 410
tioconazole, 430
Titralac, 380
TIW, 19
tizanidine, 251
Tobradex, 277
tobramycin, 276–277, 280
Tobrex, 276, 280
tocainide, 124
toenail fungus, 407–409
Tofranil, 215, 251
tolazamide, 171
tolbutamide, 171
tolcapone, 230
Tolinase, 171
tolnaftate, 407
tolterodine, 185
Tonocard, 124
tooth decay, 216
toothaches, 395–398
Topamax, 227
topical analgesics, 354–356, 395
topical antifungal products, 407–410
topical first-aid products, 410–412
topical nasal decongestants, 320–323, 325
topical steroids, 288–290

topiramate, 227
Toradol, 241
toxicity, 123
tramadol, 247–248
transcription errors, 18
transethinyl estradiol, 163
Tranxene, 209–210
tranylcypromine, 214
Travel-Eze, 437–438
traveler's diarrhea, 371
trazodone, 217
Trental, 120–121
Tri-Levlen, 156–157
triamcinolone, 198, 289–290
Triaminic, 317
Triaminicin Tablets, 317
Triaminicol, 317
triazolam, 210, 213
Tricor, 148, 151
tricyclic antidepressants,
    215–216, 250–251, 254, 265
triethanolamine salicylate, 354
triglycerides, 147–154, 172
trihexyphenidyl, 230
Trilafon, 222
Trilisate, 343
trimethoprim, 276
trimethoprim DS, 115
trimipramine, 215
Trimoptic, 270
triphasic oral contraceptives,
    156, 159–160
Triphasil, 160
triple antibiotic ointment, 412
Trivora, 156–157, 160
Trocosal, 343
troglitazone, 172
trolamine salicylate, 354
trovafloxacin, 110
Trovan, 104–105, 110
Trusopt, 270
Tuck's pads, 441
Tums, 360, 362, 365
turpentine, 354
tussin, 331, 333, 468, 474

Ty-Pap, 466, 477
Tylenol, 122, 298, 330
Tylenol Arthritis Strength,
    348–349
Tylenol Cold Plus Cough Sus-
    pension, 473–474
Tylenol for children, 462, 466,
    474–477
Tylenol PM, 433
Tylenol with Codeine, 246
Type 1 herpes simplex virus
    (HSV-1), 398
type 2 (adult onset) diabetes,
    171
typhus, 112
tyramine, 214–215

U
Udder Cream, 400
ulcerative colitis, 265–268
ulcers, 257, 260–263
Ultram, 247–248
unblistered burns, 286
Uniphyl, 71
unique patents, 40–41
Unisom, 298, 432
United Research Laboratories
    (URL), 320
Univasc, 83
University of Maryland School
    of Pharmacy, 450
upset stomachs, 367–369,
    477–479
Urecholine, 187
urgency, 186
uric acid, 181
urinary acidifiers, 184
urinary alkalinizers, 183
urinary antispasmodics, 185
urinary irritation, 455–456
Urinary Relief Tablets, 455
urinary tract infections,
    186–188
urinary tract relaxers, 185–187
urinary tract stimulators, 187

Urispas, 185
Uristat, 455
URL (United Research Labora-
    tories), 320
U.S. Food and Drug Adminis-
    tration (FDA)
    advice on giving aspirin to
        children, 342
    approval of over-the-counter
        drugs by, 298–299, 346
    findings on newly patented
        drug improvements, 4
    generic drug definition, 69
    narrow therapeutic index
        (NTI) definition, 69
    Office of Postmarketing
        Drug Risk Assessment, 17
    products containing phenyl-
        propanolamine (PPA)
        pulled by, 316–317,
        438–439
    regulations enforced by
        illegal drug sales over the
            Internet, 31
        importing drugs into U.S.,
            41–42
    statistics on deaths from
        drug interactions and
        errors in seniors, 24
U.S. Government Accounting
    Office, 55
U.S. Surgeon General's Office,
    342
uterine cancer, 163
UTI Relief 32, 455
UV-A and B radiation, 412

V
vaginal creams, 163
vaginal products, 430–432
Vagistat-1, 430
valacyclovir, 284
Valium, 114, 209, 209–210, 227
valproic acid, 226
Valtrex, 284

Vanceril, 198

Vantin, 104, 108

Vaseline, 417, 440

Vasocon, 276

vasoconstrictors, 441

vasodilators, 126–127, 137

Vasotec, 137, 143

vegetable oil, 401

Velosef, 108

venlafaxine, 217

Ventolin, 76, 195–197

verapamil, 143

Verified Internet Pharmacy Practice Site (VIPPS), 31, 33

Vermont Health Access Program (VHAP), 61

veterans, prescription drug assistance for, 55

Vexol, 274

VHAP (Vermont Health Access Program), 61

Viagra, 189

Vibramycin, 281

Vicks, 327

Vicks Chloraseptic, 336

Vicks Head and Chest Liquid, 317

Vicodin, 247

Vioxx, 241, 244

VIPPS seal, 30–31, 36

VIPPS (Verified Internet Pharmacy Practice Site), 31, 33

viral skin infections, 283–286

virtual pharmacies, 27–36, 43–45

viruses, 90–92, 416

Visine, 276, 386

vitamin B12, 260

vitamin C (ascorbic acid), 184, 337–338

Volmax, 17

Voltaren, 76, 241, 274

vomiting, 367–369, 479

W

Wal-proxen, 351, 353–354

Wal-Zan 75 Acid Reducer, 367

Walgreens, 35

Walgreens Ultra-Strength Rub, 356

Wall Street Journal, 7

warfarin, 114–115, 343

warm drinks, 263

wart removers, 416–417

water, 293, 331–332, 398, 400, 406

Water-Jel Burn Jel, 406–407

water pills. *See* diuretics

wax-removal products, 391–393

Web-based pharmacies, 27–36, 43–45

Weight Watchers, 439

Wellbutrin, 217

West Virginia, pharmaceutical assistance programs in, 61

wheezing, 196

whole-body (systemic) side effects, 271

witch hazel, 441

worksheets

    Prescription Drugs I Take, 25

    Smart Buys on Prescription Drugs, 88

    "SOS Worksheet" for Saving Money on Over-the-Counter Drugs, 312–314

wounds, treatments for, 100–101

wrinkles, 281

wristbands, acupressure-type, 438

Wyoming, pharmaceutical assistance programs in, 61

X

Xalatan, 269–270, 273

Xanax, 114, 209–210, 213

xanthine derivatives, 200–201

xanthine oxidase, 181

Y

Yale University School of Medicine, 316

yeast infections, 104, 407, 430–432

yohimbine, 188–189

"Your Plan" by Merck Medco, 33, 35

Z

Zaditor, 279

zafirlukast, 201

zaleplon, 210

Zanaflex, 251

Zantac, 17, 258, 263, 365, 367

Zantac 75, 298, 367

zinc, 386

Zithromax, 76, 113

Zocor, 114, 149–150

zolmitriptan, 255

Zoloft, 216, 222

zolpidem, 210

Zomig, 255

Zostrix, 354, 356

Zovirax, 284–285

Zyban, 217

Zyprexa, 223, 226

Zyrtec, 17, 76, 204–205